The Consumer's
Medical Desk Reference

The Consumer's Medical Desk Reference

Information Your Doctor Can't Or Won't Tell You—Everything You Need To Know For The Best In Health Care

Charles B. Inlander and the Staff of The People's Medical Society

A Stonesong Press Book

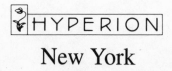

HYPERION

New York

A Stonesong Press Book

Library of Congress Cataloging-in-Publication Data

Inlander, Charles B.
     The consumer's medical desk reference : information your doctor can't or won't tell you—everything you need to know for the best in health care / Charles B. Inlander and the staff of the People's Medical Society.
          p.   cm.
     Includes index.
     ISBN 0-7868-6056-1
     1. Medicine, Popular—Handbooks, manuals, etc.   I. People's Medical Society (U.S.)   II. Title.
RC81.I46 1995
362.1—dc20   94-22256
                                                                      CIP

Text design and typography by Noble Desktop Publishers

First Edition

10 9 8 7 6 5 4 3 2 1

Contents

ACKNOWLEDGEMENTS

As any reader will observe, this book was a massive undertaking. Scores of people were involved in making it a reality, and our gratitude is extended to all. There are, however, individuals who must be acknowledged for their special contribution and dedication to this project.

Karla Morales, Vice President for Communications and Editorial Services at the People's Medical Society, deserves the highest accolades and heartfelt appreciation. She served as the editor on the entire book, overseeing and supervising every aspect of its development. Her dedication to striving for excellence, and commitment to deadlines made this book the definitive work that it is. This is truly her book.

Special thanks to Mike Donio, People's Medical Society's Director of Projects, who was also intimately involved with each stage of the book. From entry ideas to liaison with writers, Mike conducted himself in his usually competent and patient manner.

Other Peoples' Medical Society staff deserving singular recognition are Karen Kemmerer, Ellen Greene, Linda Swank, Gayle Ebert, Jennifer Hay, and Julie Bryfogle.

Major editorial contributors to the book were: Catherine Bachochin, Joyce Mann, Kurt Pfitzer, and Carrie Schaller.

Paul Fargis, of The Stonesong Press, had the vision to create this book. The partnership between Paul and the People's Medical Society in every aspect of this book's development has been without conflict or dispute. Paul deserves additional praise for coordinating the design and production of the project.

Gareth Esersky, with whom we have worked on an earlier book, was indispensable as our insightful consulting editor.

Leslie Wells, our editor at Hyperion, guided us with knowing and gentle hands throughout the process. She never failed to lead us down the right path.

Bob Miller, Hyperion president, immediately saw the need and value of this book and we greatly cherish the trust he had in all of us.

Gail Ross, our literary agent, has been a major reason why the People's Medical Society has become a part of consumer health publishing. We gratefully acknowledge her contribution and wisdom in this project.

Many individuals, from many organizations, provided us materials that have been used or incorporated in this book. Therefore, we especially want to thank: Terri Lowe, National Abortion and Reproductive Rights Action League; Martina Kellner, HCIA, Inc.; Elizabeth C. Hunko, The National Association of Children's Hospitals and Related Institutions, Inc.; Arlene Wheaton, Northwestern National Life Insurance Company; Julia Curry, Choice in Dying, Inc.; Robert Simmons, Jr., Health Care Systems, Inc.; Moira DeWilde, American Academy of Otolaryngology; Susan J. LeClair, *U.S. News and World Report*; Janet Glassman and Lynn Donches, Rodale Press Library; Peter Brigham, Philadelphia Burn Foundation; Dr. Jean Rubel, Anorexia Nervosa and Related Eating Disorders, Inc.; Abbey S. Meyers, National Organization for Rare Disorders; Ed Madara, American Self-Help Clearinghouse; Robin Ungerleider, National Safety Council; Chris Burgston, Group Health Association of America; John A. Bogert, D.D.S., American Academy of Pediatric Dentistry; Diane Solomon, M.D., National Cancer Institute; Cheryl van Tilburg, Blue Cross/Blue Shield Associations; Debbie Weiner, The St. Paul Companies, Inc.; and Becky Hire, American Cancer Society, Inc.

Finally, we thank the more than 80,000 members and supporters of the People's Medical Society without whom none of this would be possible.

Charles B. Inlander
President
People's Medical Society

INTRODUCTION

This is the book where *your* health care begins!

For more than a decade, the People's Medical Society has been the American consumer's authoritative source of health care information. In the many thousands of letters and phone calls we receive each year, we are asked about diseases, operations, insurance policies, and hospitals. Consumers want to know how to file a complaint against a doctor or where they can buy medications at a discount. We are asked to explain medical bills or if a hospital has the right to demand payment before a person is discharged. If there is a health care question, we have had it asked, and we have researched the subject and provided an answer.

Your health care is much more than a visit to a doctor or a stay in the hospital. Your health care may be an insurance policy or an over-the-counter medication. It might be a diagnostic test or an immunization for a child. Health care is your medical record or the phone number of a major medical school where special research is being done on a condition you may have. In other words, health care is a myriad of subjects, people, places, and facts. And all of them have a tremendous impact on you and your family.

In *The Consumer's Medical Desk Reference,* we at the People's Medical Society have put together an important and empowering health care resource book. We believe it is unlike any other book ever published. In it you will find just about everything you need to make informed and educated health care decisions. It answers the majority of questions you are likely to ask about matters relating to your health and those providing health and medical services to you. If you are unable to find the precise answer to your question, *The Consumer's Medical Desk Reference* directs you to resources that have the exact answer. The book has thousands of names, addresses, and phone numbers of organizations, medical institutions, and government entities that can respond to your specific need. We think that you will not be able to find as complete a one-volume resource as this book.

Most consumers wander through the health care system in the dark. We know little about what is being done to us and even less about those who are doing it. We don't understand our health insurance policy. The language on our medical chart is gibberish. We can hardly pronounce the name of the specialty many of our doctors practice. We hear about alternative medicine, but know little about what those different approaches to health care actually do.

Until the People's Medical Society was formed in 1983, consumers had no place to turn to get their questions answered. And they have not had a *book* that provides those answers.

This literally is the book where your health care begins. And we encourage you to use it in the best of health.

Charles B. Inlander
President
People's Medical Society

Described as "one of the most prolific publishers on health matters" by Knight-Ridder News Service, the People's Medical Society has been the consumer's voice in health care since its founding in 1983.

The People's Medical Society is a nonprofit consumer health advocacy organization dedicated to the principles of better, more responsive, and less expensive medical care. The group's mission for more than a decade has been to put previously unavailable medical information into the hands of consumers so that they can make informed decisions about their own health care.

1. The Body and Its Parts

INTRODUCTION

The human body is a complex of systems miraculously interconnected and engineered to make you the unique individual that you are. All human beings have the same basic construction, but individual variation within body parts (even minor ones) often make the difference between health and sickness.

Knowing and understanding your body, from head to toe, from heart to skin, is a useful and important aspect of your own personal health care. Often described as the "ultimate machine," your body and its parts are what make you work. Knowing how they work helps you to take better care of yourself and be more in command of your own health.

In this section, you will learn the most important components of your body, how they work, and how they interact. In addition, a complete glossary of the basic components of the human anatomy will assist you in better understanding the need and function of the elements that make up your body.

Circulatory System

The purpose of the circulatory system is to supply the body's tissues with necessary nutrients and to collect waste from these tissues, via the bloodstream. The blood is pumped by the heart (the center of the circulatory system) and flows through the blood vessels (arteries and veins) of the body.

COMPONENTS OF THE CIRCULATORY SYSTEM

Blood consists of red cells, leukocytes (white blood cells: granulocytes, lymphocytes, and monocytes), platelets, cholesterol, sugar, salts, enzymes, fats, and liquid plasma to float everything in. The blood absorbs almost all of the water that is consumed to ensure liquidity for safe blood volume and pressure. Excess water is removed via urine, sweat, and exhaled air.

Blood vessels (arteries and veins) are the highways that carry blood to all parts of the body. Arteries carry highly oxygenated and nutrient-rich blood away from the heart, while veins are the return paths that carry deoxygenated blood back to the heart. The human body contains some 60,000 miles of blood vessels.

The heart, the strongest muscle in the body, hangs by ligaments in the center of the chest in an area called the mediastinum. It weighs about 12 ounces and is reddish brown in color. It is about 6 inches long and 4 inches wide, its shape resembling that of a cone. A hollow muscle divided into a left and right side, each with two chambers (atrium and ventricle) attached to a complex freeway of arteries and veins (complete with cloverleafs), the heart is the pump at the center of your circulatory system.

The heart is a well-protected piece of machinery. Though fragile in its own right, the heart is like an oyster within a sac, called the pericardium, inside a hard shell made up of the rib cage and lungs around it, the diaphragm under it, and the backbone behind it.

HOW DOES THE CIRCULATORY SYSTEM FUNCTION?

The Heart and Blood Vessels
The heart is composed of two pumps, one to pump blood into the lungs, the other to push it to the rest of the body. The blood begins in the left ventricle. It takes three-tenths of a second for the left ventricle to contract and push blood out into the body, then it rests for half a second.

The blood, tingling with oxygen and ready to travel, is then propelled into the body's primary artery, the aorta. Coursing along the arterial system, countless blood cells (and nutrients) are transported through progressively tinier and tinier arteries and capillaries, the smallest blood vessels linking the arteries to the veins.

Capillaries are so small that red blood cells squeeze themselves through in single file. During passage, oxygen is "unloaded" to neighboring cells of the body, while carbon dioxide is picked up by the red blood cells. Other items are delivered as well, such as minerals, vitamins, hormones, glucose, fat, and amino acids. Skin flushes during exercise because capillaries are operating at full capacity. During sleep, over 90 percent of the capillaries close down. The only place capillaries are visible is in the retinas of the eyes, which is why physicians are able to examine them with an ophthalmoscope.

The blood cells bathe the body's tissues when passing through the capillaries. They deliver oxygen to the eagerly awaiting tissues, which need it to stay alive. And then, after they've collected waste products and carbon dioxide, they turn around, a little blue and winded, and follow the flow through the body's network of veins, arriving finally at the superior and inferior vena cava, and back to the heart.

In the heart, the oxygen-and-nutrient-deficient blood collects in the right atrium. It is then pumped out through the right ventricle into the pulmonary artery and off to the lungs, where the blood gladly gives up the carbon dioxide and waste (which is exhaled) and sucks up its fill of oxygen (which is inhaled). The blood flows from the lungs to the left atrium, where it collects, ready to move into the left ventricle, to be pumped out through the aorta to the rest of the body.

Over and over, again and again, this cyclical process—the blood moving from the upper reservoir atrium chamber to the lower pumping ventricle chambers, and out and back through 60,000 miles of veins, arteries, and capillaries—goes on day in and day out, the heart thumping to the rhythm of an average of 72 beats every minute (an average of 6 quarts of blood every minute), 55 beats during sleep.

Nourishing the Heart

Despite the huge volume of blood flowing through the heart each day (some 8,000 quarts), it does not directly nourish the heart. Like other parts of the body, the heart receives its "diet" via a system of arteries. These are called the coronary arteries—so called because to some anatomists' eyes these arteries seem to form a thorny crown around the heart. There are four such arteries: the right and left main, the circumflex, and the anterior descending. As with the rest of the body's arterial system, the heart's blood supply derives from arteries that come off the aorta and split into capillaries that feed the muscle. Then a system of veins returns the deoxygenated blood to the right atrium. Coronary heart disease, then, is a severe health problem affecting not so much the heart's muscle directly as the flow of the blood through this "crown" surrounding and feeding the heart.

Valves

The valves of the heart are extremely thin, powerful, and efficient "floodgates" made of endocardial tissue (endocardium is also the substance that lines the walls of the atria and ventricles). The valves, when closed, act as barriers to keep blood in areas where it should be (and prevent it from flowing back instead of forward), and then, upon opening, allow the blood to move on.

There are four valves, and the blood, in the course of its journey through the heart, meets these valves somewhat in this order: As the deoxygenated blood accumulates in the reservoir of the right atrium, it is kept there by the tricuspid valve. When the tricuspid opens, the blood flows into the right ventricle and is then pumped through the pulmonary valve into the lungs. The now-oxygenated blood arrives in the left atrium and is kept within that chamber by the closed mitral valve; when the mitral opens, the blood flows into the left ventricle and is pumped through the open aortic valve into the aorta and off to the rest of the body.

The actual rhythm has the mitral and tricuspid valves opening then closing in unison. This causes the "lub" sound of the heartbeat—as one of the two sounds heard through the stethoscope is described. Then the pulmonary and aortic valves, upon the heart's contraction, open in unison to allow the blood to flow to the lungs and into the aorta. This causes the "dub" sound of the heartbeat—in the wording of the popular description.

Heartbeat

What makes the heart contract and beat in the first place? It has to do with the heart's conduction system. If the term "conduction" sounds like something out of electrical engineering, that's just about right. In the wall of the right atrium of your heart, so small that only a powerful microscope can pick it out, is something called the sinus, or sinoatrial (S-A) node. In simple terms, it is your heart's natural pacemaker.

What happens is that an electrical impulse from the S-A node is conducted through the atria, down to the atrioventricular (A-V) node and, via right and left bundle branches, to the ventricles, which, upon receiving the impulses, contract. This whole process takes less than a second. This contraction is what you call your heartbeat.

So the heart, unlike other muscles in the body, doesn't need to be stimulated by electrical nerve impulses outside itself—it can do it all, consistently and rhythmically. A human heart, even after being disconnected from all other nerves in the body, will continue to beat 70 to 80 times a minute. The conduction system even has a self-adjusting feature to alter the force of the contraction if the need should arise.

Heart rate increases during exercise and dreams. Occasionally, you may wake up to find your heart "racing," or beating very rapidly. You need not worry about this situation; you should just relax to bring your heart rate down. The heart rate can also be brought down if the vagus nerves are massaged. The vagus nerves pass through the neck and behind the ears, at the hinge of the jaw.

A word or two about the nature of the beat. There are two components to it: The diastole is that portion of the heartbeat when the heart is at rest—that is, when blood from the atrium is pouring into the ventricle, just before the ventricular contraction; the systole is the contraction. The two numbers in blood pressure readings correspond to these heartbeat phases, the systolic (or higher number) being a measurement of the blood's pressure during the heart's relaxation period. In a normal blood pressure reading of 120/80—or "120 over 80"—the systolic pressure is indicated by the 120, the diastolic by the 80.

Other Functions of the Circulatory System

The blood serves other purposes in the body besides supplying tissues with nourishment. It also patches wounds and fights bacteria, viruses, and other invading organisms.

When the skin is cut or punctured, platelets in the bloodstream rush to the site of the wound or injury to make a temporary patch and prevent blood loss. As the platelets arrive at the site, they become sticky and adhere to injured blood vessel walls.

Enzymes, released by the platelets, then stimulate the production of fibrin filaments that trap red and white blood cells, eventually closing off and sealing the wound. The hard outer covering of this seal is called the scab, which protects the wound until it heals.

Intruders in the blood, such as bacteria, viruses, pollen, and other foreign bodies, are fought off by antibodies. Each antibody fights off one individual enemy. B cells are equipped with "memories," acquired during previous infections, that permit them to recognize and attack viruses such as mumps and chicken pox. Once combatants have perished, white blood cells called phagocytes come along to clean up the mess, and produce replacement antibodies ready to do battle with other invading enemies.

MAJOR PROBLEMS AND COMMON DISORDERS OF THE CIRCULATORY SYSTEM

Blood

Anemia is a condition where the blood is deficient in red blood cells, in hemoglobin, or in total volume.

Agranulocytosis, a drop in white cell count, can be fatal if not treated with antibiotics to prevent infection.

Hemochromatosis is an inherited condition in which too much iron is present in the blood, the opposite of anemia.

Hemophilia is an inherited bleeding disorder caused by the lack of a protein, called factor VIII, that is essential to blood clotting.

Leukemia is a cancer of blood-forming organs characterized by the replacement of bone marrow with immature white blood cells, and the presence of abnormal numbers and forms of immature white cells in circulation.

Blood Vessels

An *aneurysm* is a weak spot in an arterial wall that can be serious or life-threatening if a major artery bursts. Blood rushes out of the artery and causes blood pressure to drop quickly, causing death. Aneurysms may be congenital, present at birth, or they can develop as a result of arteriosclerosis.

Arteriosclerosis, also called hardening of the arteries, results when calcium deposits collect on the arterial walls, reducing the elasticity of the artery. This rigidity may eventually lead to the development of a weak spot on the artery called an aneurysm.

Atherosclerosis is the buildup of fatty deposits on the walls of the arteries which could eventually lead to reduced blood flow to organs and other tissue. As these deposits enlarge, they have a tendency to invade the deeper layers of the arterial wall, causing calcium deposits and scarring. Fatty deposits may also break loose and circulate through the system, eventually clogging other arteries and causing gangrene, heart attack, or stroke.

Cerebrovascular accident, also called a stroke, occurs when the blood flow to the brain is disrupted, by either a blockage or a break in an artery. Risk factors for stroke include high blood pressure, being overweight, hardening of the arteries, diabetes, smoking, using birth control pills, and stress. Treatment includes medications designed to reduce the likelihood of blood clots, measures to control high blood pressure, and learning to deal with stress.

Gangrene is a condition caused by poor circulation to any tissue, especially the extremities such as feet and hands. The normal blood flow is restricted, usually as the result of a blockage, preventing oxygen and nutrients from reaching tissue. As a result, the tissue begins to die.

Hypertension, or high blood pressure, is a condition in which the heart is pumping blood through the circulatory system with a force greater than needed for normal blood flow. Untreated, high blood pressure can have very serious consequences on the entire circulatory system.

Phlebitis is an inflammation of a vein, usually as a result of a varicose vein. Sometimes this condition can lead to the formation of clots, which may become detached and travel to another part of the circulatory system and possibly cause a blockage.

Varicose veins occur when valves in the blood vessels are defective or become damaged, and too much blood stays too long in one place. Veins may become knotted and swollen to four or five times normal size. Most varicose veins develop in the legs, where blood must flow against gravity. Occasionally these fragile veins may burst and bleed. Varicose veins can be inherited, but people are also susceptible to them if they must stand for hours during the day, are pregnant, or are obese. Treatment ranges from wearing elastic hose to surgery.

Heart

Angina pectoris is a medical term for severe, suffocating chest pain caused by an insufficient amount of blood being supplied to the heart muscle. This condition may sometimes be mistaken for a heart attack. Angina is treatable with medications called vasodilators (for example, nitroglycerin tablets), which quickly open the vessels carrying blood to the heart.

Cardiomyopathy is a serious disease that severely affects the functioning of the heart muscle. It may be linked to nutritional deficiencies, or it may occur as a result of changes in the thickness of the heart wall.

Congestive heart failure is the inability of the heart to adequately keep the blood flowing to the rest of the body. More specifically, it has to do with myocardial failure, especially defects of the valves, and affects the right or left ventricle. Water and sodium

are inadequately eliminated, remain in the body, and can cause fluid overload leading in many cases to death by total heart failure.

Constrictive pericarditis is a condition in which the pericardium (the outer membrane, or sac, surrounding the heart) becomes scarred and hard and full of calcium deposits. The heart is no longer free to move about, and its duties are interfered with.

Pericarditis is an inflammation of the pericardium, leading in many cases to chest pain and fever.

Endocarditis is an inflammation of the internal lining of the heart, particularly the valves, caused by an infection.

Myocardial infarction, also called heart attack, is the damage or death of an area of the heart muscle resulting from a reduced blood supply to that area.

Heart Valves

The four heart valves—aortic, mitral, pulmonary, and tricuspid—are responsible for the flow of blood between chambers of the heart and into the circulatory system. These valves are generally susceptible to three types of conditions: stenosis, prolapse, and regurgitation. *Stenosis* is a narrowing of the opening of the valve reducing the flow of blood; *prolapse* occurs when the valve begins to lose its shape and sag, causing an extra clicking sound or murmur; and *regurgitation* occurs when a valve fails to close tight enough and blood flows backward.

Digestive System

The digestive system is basically a tubelike system that converts the three main constituents of food (carbohydrates, proteins, and fats) into energy and other substances that are used to fuel the body.

COMPONENTS OF THE DIGESTIVE SYSTEM

The digestive system consists of the mouth, teeth, tongue, esophagus, stomach, small intestine, large intestine, rectum, and anus. Other glands or organs involved in the process are salivary glands, liver, gallbladder, and pancreas.

First, food is taken into the mouth. It is moved about the mouth by the tongue and ground by the teeth. Food is partially broken down into sugar by saliva, which is produced by salivary glands, located at the sides of the face below each ear.

From the mouth, the food is swallowed and passed into the esophagus (about 10 inches long), which is the tube leading from the mouth to the stomach. The stomach churns with rhythmical contractions and begins digestion of food with the secretions it produces. Alcohol is directly absorbed into the blood through the stomach. Carbohydrates, some proteins, and some fats also pass through the stomach. It takes about 2 hours for food to pass through the stomach and on to the small intestine.

From the stomach, food enters the duodenum (about 10 inches long), the first part of the small intestine. The duodenum secretes enzymes and receives bile from the liver and enzymes from the pancreas to help further digest food. Here, proteins are broken down into their original building blocks, amino acids (which are used by cells to grow, heal, and fight off infection), starch and complex sugars are converted into simple sugars (used for energy), and fats are broken down into fatty acids and glycerin. Nutrients are converted and absorbed into the blood through the approximately 22 feet of small intestine, a process that takes about 4 hours. Once in the blood, nutrients are carried to the rest of the body.

Remaining substances move on to the colon, or large intestine (about 5½ feet long), where more digested material is absorbed. The remainder of undigestible material is stored in the large intestine as waste, the liquid portion of which passes into the blood to the urinary system, and the solid portion of which is later eliminated through the rectum and anus. This process may take 5 to 24 hours.

MAJOR PROBLEMS AND COMMON DISORDERS OF THE DIGESTIVE SYSTEM

Diverticulosis and *diverticulitis* are conditions affecting the large intestine (colon) and are characterized by the formation of small pouches (called diverticula) at weak spots on the intestine wall and inflammation of those pouches. These conditions generally affect people over the age of 60, although they have been diagnosed in people as young as 40.

It is often difficult to know if you have diverticulosis, since there are few symptoms other than some tenderness or muscle spasms in the lower abdomen. Diverticulitis, on the other hand, usually produces abdominal pain, fever, and increased white blood cell count. If not diagnosed and treated, diverticulitis may result in bowel blockages and bowel abscesses.

When diverticulosis produces no symptoms, no treatment is required, although some doctors may recommend a change in diet to include more high-fiber foods. Most cases of diverticulitis can be treated with antibiotics and bed rest; however, serious cases may also require high-protein intravenous fluids.

Gallstones are formed in the gallbladder, the small bladderlike organ that stores bile from the liver, when the liver manufactures too much cholesterol. The excess cholesterol begins to form tiny round or oval lumps of solid matter, usually less than an inch in length. Many people are unaware that they have gallstones until a stone becomes lodged in the bile duct (the tube leading from the gallbladder to the small intestine).

The first symptoms of gallstones are severe and steady pains in the upper abdomen, pain and tenderness on the right side of the abdomen, indigestion, nausea, vomiting, or chills, fever, and jaundice when the bile duct is blocked.

Medications may be prescribed to dissolve the gallstones or they may be broken up with the use of shock waves (a procedure called lithotripsy). When conservative treatment has failed, the gallbladder itself is removed. In recent years, great strides have been made in removing the gallbladder through the abdomen wall in what is called a laparoscopic cholecystectomy.

Inflammatory bowel disease (IBD) is a general term used to describe the chronic conditions of Crohn's disease and ulcerative colitis. Crohn's disease is an inflammation of the walls of the intestines and occasionally may extend to the anus, esophagus, mouth, and stomach. Ulcerative colitis causes ulcers and inflammation of the lining of the large intestine (colon).

The most common symptoms experienced by someone with IBD are abdominal pain and diarrhea. A definitive diagnosis of IBD can be made only after extensive examination using a proctoscope or sigmoidoscope and an X-ray study of the entire digestive tract.

Thus far, no effective treatments have been found for IBD; however, anti-inflammatory medication such as sulfasalazine and cortisone are effective in controlling symptoms. Surgery may be used in severe cases of ulcerative colitis.

Peptic ulcers are raw, open sores that occur in the lining of either the stomach or the duodenum (the first part of the small intestine). Most people associate ulcers with a high-stress lifestyle; however, that is not necessarily the case. A much stronger link is heredity, especially if blood relatives have ulcers.

Ulcers occur when stomach acid and pepsin (an enzyme) break through the protective mucous lining of the stomach. Ordinarily, this lining protects the cells of the stomach; however, when too much stomach acid is produced, it can eat away the protective lining. Symptoms of ulcers may include a gnawing or burning feeling in the stomach, loss of appetite, bloating, nausea, and vomiting. A definitive diagnosis can be made after a barium X-ray study or endoscopic (viewing through a lighted tube) examination of the stomach.

Treatment generally consists of antacid medications to neutralize excess acid or prevent the production of excess acid (cimetidine, ranitidine). Other medications (such as sucralfate) may be used to form protective coatings around the ulcer, shielding it from stomach acid and permitting it to heal. Recent findings from a Canadian study appeared to demonstrate a link between ulcers and the presence of a bacterium known as *Helicobacter pylori*. Eliminating the bacterium promoted faster and longer healing of the ulcer. Changes in diet may also lessen the symptoms of ulcers, as will avoiding such substances as alcohol and tobacco. In severe cases, surgery may be required to treat the ulcer and prevent further complications.

Constipation is the inability to move the bowels and pass stool or the infrequent passage of stool. Generally speaking, constipation is not all that serious and may be treated with home remedies (increased fiber in diet) or commercially available laxatives. A leading cause of constipation is a lack of sufficient fiber in the diet as a result of eating overrefined foods. Some people may think they're constipated just because they don't have a certain number of bowel movements per day or week. But this isn't true, since there is no required number of bowel movements. Regularity, not frequency, is the key to good bowel health.

In addition to dietary changes, constipation may also be treated with glycerin suppositories, laxatives, and purgatives, although their use should be limited and then only under the supervision of a doctor. Persistent constipation should be a sign that further professional medical attention is needed.

Diarrhea is just the opposite of constipation and is characterized by frequent bowel movements. While not a disease, diarrhea could signal some underlying condition that may warrant further professional attention. However, most diarrhea can be self-treated and should resolve in about 2 or 3 days.

The probable cause of diarrhea is food or water that contains an organism (generally bacteria) that upsets the delicate balance of the large intestine. When this occurs, the normal process of passing food through the intestines is disrupted and the food passes too quickly.

Most cases of diarrhea may be treated with over-the-counter medications; however, if symptoms do not resolve within 2 or 3 days, then professional assistance is needed.

Diarrhea in infants is quite serious, and professional medical attention should be sought at the first sign of it.

Heartburn is probably the most frequently experienced digestive disorder in the world. It usually occurs after a meal in which quantities of fried or fatty foods have been consumed. Also contributing to heartburn are citrus fruits and juices, tomato products, chocolates, and coffee.

The one universal symptom experienced by all heartburn sufferers is a burning feeling in the chest. This is often mistaken for a heart attack. The burning sensation is caused by stomach acid that moves up the esophagus from the stomach. When the acid comes into contact with the sensitive lining of the esophagus, burning—often along with excruciating pain—is felt. Most cases of heartburn can be relived by taking an antacid that helps to neutralize the stomach acid (a popular home remedy is baking soda). Products that add a protective coating to the esophagus and stomach may also be used to relieve the pain.

If symptoms of heartburn persist or worsen, then it is time for professional medical attention. Doctors can run a complete series of tests to help determine the exact cause of the heartburn and prescribe appropriate treatment.

Hiatal hernias occur where the esophagus enters the abdomen through an opening in the diaphragm (the sheet of muscle that separates the chest from the abdomen) called the hiatus. An upper portion of the stomach moves into the chest cavity through a weakness in the diaphragm. These hernias occur when pressure in the abdominal cavity increases as a result of physical exertion, coughing, or vomiting.

Generally hiatal hernias do not require treatment unless they are causing other problems such as acid reflux into the esophagus. When this occurs, the strong acid burns the sensitive lining of the esophagus. Constant irritation of this lining could lead to ulcers, or the hernia could become strangulated (twisted, cutting off blood supply), causing more serious problems. Surgery can correct this condition, and is recommended when all other treatments have failed.

Irritable bowel syndrome (IBS) is a condition characterized by alternate bouts of constipation and diarrhea, abdominal pain, gas, and bloating. The exact cause of these symptoms is unknown; however, it has been linked to some disturbance of the wavelike motion of the intestines. Stress is also thought to contribute to this condition. IBS tends to affect middle-aged to older adults and is more common in women than men.

While there is no specific treatment for this condition, the addition of dietary fiber as well as antidiarrheal and antispasmodic drugs has been prescribed for temporary relief of symptoms.

Hemorrhoids are varicose veins located in the anus. Their cause, more often than not, is pressure in the anal area usually as a result of straining during bowel movements. Pregnant women are also likely to develop hemorrhoids because of the tremendous pressure the developing fetus puts on the abdomen, especially in the area of the rectum and anus.

It is not unusual for most people over the age of 50 to have experienced hemorrhoidal problems. Hemorrhoids are usually detected when you notice bright red blood on toilet tissue or you feel a fullness after a bowel movement.

There are two types of hemorrhoids, internal and external. Internal hemorrhoids begin above the internal opening of the anus. If they become so large that they protrude from the anus, they can become squeezed and painful. External hemorrhoids appear outside of the anal opening. Serious problems may develop when blood clots form in external hemorrhoids, causing severe pain. When this occurs, it is necessary to have a physician remove the clot to relieve the condition and pain.

Where no other symptoms are present, hemorrhoids may be treated using a sitz bath (soaking in warm water), applying lubricants (petroleum jelly), or using medicated suppositories. If the hemorrhoids protrude from the anus (called prolapsed hemorrhoids), they must be removed. Fortunately, there are several options for treating hemorrhoids in addition to surgery. Some doctors place rubber bands around the hemorrhoids to cut off circulation. This causes the hemorrhoids to fall off within a few days. Another method involves injecting irritating agents into the veins that cause the hemorrhoids to shrink. Still other methods use electrical currents, lasers, or infrared light to destroy the hemorrhoids.

Immune System

The immune system of the human body protects it against all sorts of invaders, including bacteria, viruses, toxins, and foreign tissues and germs. These invaders, called antigens, can be any chemical substances that stimulate antibody production and are identified, recognized, and eventually attacked by various components of the immune system. Antibodies are produced by white blood cells (lymphocytes) and are specifically designed to destroy different antigens. This process of antibody production in which specific resistance to an antigen is achieved is termed *immunity*.

HOW DOES THE IMMUNE SYSTEM FUNCTION?

The immune system offers two types of immunity: humoral and cell-mediated immunity. Humoral immunity indicates the production of antibodies in order to combat an invading agent. Cell-mediated immunity occurs when the lymphocytes themselves attack and destroy an invading agent. These types of immunity differ from nonspecific types of immunity, such as the natural barrier of protection formed by the skin, because the skin is not specifically programmed to destroy any one microbe.

The functioning of the immune system relies upon central lymphoid organs, which give rise to the antigen-fighting lymphocytes; peripheral lymphoid tissues and organs that provide an environment for the lymphocytes; the lymphocytes themselves; and accessory cells, such as microphages, which aid in the process of antigen destruction.

ROLES OF LYMPHATIC TISSUE AND ORGANS

The central lymphoid organs—the bone marrow and the thymus gland—are responsible for lymphocyte production and maturation. There are two types of lymphocytes produced: T cells and B cells. These cells are derived from lymphatic stem cells in the bone marrow. The T cells first migrate to the thymus gland in order to be processed into mature T cells, and then embed themselves in lymphoid, or peripheral, tissue. The B cells are processed, either in the bone marrow or in other lymphatic tissues, before migrating to lymphoid tissue.

Locations of lymphoid tissue include the lymph nodes, the spleen, the gastrointestinal tract, and other mucosa-associated lymphoid tissue (MALT). Lymphoid tissue is strategically placed in areas that are particularly susceptible to infection, and thus it may readily intercept invading antigens. Both T and B cells remain in separate areas of the lymphoid tissue where they respond to antigens. T cells, which possess cell-mediated immunity, are lymphocytes that directly attack and destroy an antigen. B cells, which have humoral immunity, produce plasma cells, which are responsible for the production of antigen-fighting antibodies. Both T and B cells utilize various accessory cells, macrophages in particular, which phagocytose (ingest) and present antigens to the T and B cells.

T AND B CELLS

T cells are activated (sensitized) when they react with certain antigens for which they been specifically programmed. The T cell is presented the antigen by macrophages, it is sensitized, and it begins to enlarge and eventually divide into a population of cells called a clone. There are four types of T cells within the clone itself: killer T cells, helper T cells, suppressor T cells, and memory T cells.

Killer T cells attach themselves to the antigen and release cytotoxic substances that kill the antigen. Additionally, killer T cells can stimulate macrophages to phagocytose antigens and can make other lymphocytes take on killer-T-cell characteristics and thus make them participate in an immune response. *Helper T cells* aid B cells with antibody production, *suppressor T* cells regulate cell production of the immune system, and *memory T cells* recognize and remember the chemical composition and nature of the antigen. Memory T cells, whose B cell counterpart is called a memory B cell, are important in attacking and fighting the antigen quickly and efficiently in a secondary response, if the antigen should be introduced again into the body.

B cells are likewise activated for specific antigens when microphages present antigens to B cells. B cells

differentiate into memory B cells and clones of plasma cells. Plasma cells secrete antibodies that respond to the antigen: They recognize the foreign microbe, form an antibody-antigen complex, and utilize a complement (plasma proteins) to attack and destroy the antigen. Antibodies are composed of proteins called immunoglobulins (Ig). The five types of immunoglobulins are IgG (neutralizes toxins, contributes to phagocytosis), IgA (participates in mucosal surface protection), IgM (responsible for agglutination and destruction of microbes), IgD (assists in allergic responses), and IgE (plays a role in allergic responses).

The antibody connects with the antigen at locations called antigenic determinant sites and forms an antibody-antigen complex. Finally, the antibody activates plasma proteins so that they may destroy the antigen by cell membrane destruction, phagocytosis, and the release of histamines or other chemotoxic agents.

For more information on the disease-fighting abilities of the body, see the "Lymphatic System" below.

Lymphatic System

The lymphatic system is a system of glands, tissues, and passages involved in producing lymph and lymphocytes and includes the lymph vessels, lymph nodes, thymus, and spleen. The lymphatic system plays a vital role in defending the body against invading pathogens and other dangerous organisms.

COMPONENTS OF THE LYMPHATIC SYSTEM AND HOW IT FUNCTIONS

Lymphocytes are white blood cells important in the production of antibodies to fight off infection. Two main types of lymphocytes are T cells and B cells. The T cells are often referred to as killer cells, and the B cells are called helper cells. These cells are circulated through the body via lymph, a clear, yellowish fluid that contains mainly lymphocytes and fats. Lymph is carried through the bloodstream and released through the thin walls of the capillaries (the body's smallest blood vessels). The lymph then bathes all of the cells in the tissues of the body, supplying them with oxygen and nutrients and picking up wastes and foreign particles.

Once the lymph has bathed the cells and picked up unwanted material, it flows into small channels. These channels empty into larger ones known as lymphatics or lymphatic vessels. The lymph is then filtered through the lymph nodes, spongelike masses of tissue ranging from the size of a pinhead to the size of a penny. One of the largest lymph nodes is called the thymus, a butterfly-shaped gland at the base of the neck, which aids in the production of T cells, the cells of the immune system that fight off bacteria. Swelling of lymph nodes can indicate the presence of an illness, such as an infection or a common cold.

After filtration, clean lymph travels back into the bloodstream. This is how the body rids itself of waste products, such as bacteria and carbon dioxide.

Should a predicament arise whereby the lymph nodes are bombarded with a great deal of bacteria that enter the bloodstream directly, the spleen aids in the process of filtration. The spleen, a fist-sized organ under the lower portion of the rib cage, filters all of the blood in the body. Although its structure is similar to that of lymph nodes, the spleen filters blood rather than lymph.

The spleen and lymph nodes also aid in the production of lymphocytes, the cells responsible for producing antibodies, the chemical agents that fight off infection. Antibodies are produced in the following manner: The lymphocyte acquires a "template" or "blueprint" of the chemical structure of the antigen, or foreign body, present. By doing this, it can then synthesize a neutralizing chemical for the antigen so that it is rendered inactive. The lymphocyte also begins producing large numbers of new lymphocytes that will produce the same neutralizing chemical.

After the battle, the mess is cleaned up by cells called histiocytes, which collect particles of tissue debris, dead bacteria, and dead granulocytes, digest the material, and make it ready for excretion from the body.

If there are too many bacteria to kill initially, the bacteria and lymph are collected into nearby lymph nodes, where the antibody is concentrated. The biggest bacteria battles are fought here, and it is for this reason that the lymph nodes can become swollen during some illnesses.

MAJOR PROBLEMS AND COMMON DISORDERS OF THE LYMPHATIC SYSTEM

Hodgkin's disease is a cancer that develops in the lymphatic system and may spread to other organs. Symptoms of Hodgkin's disease are swelling of the lymph nodes, fever, itching skin, night sweats, tired-

ness, and weight loss. The mere appearance of these symptoms does not automatically mean Hodgkin's disease; however, it does mean that if you are experiencing any of these symptoms, you should see a doctor for a thorough examination.

A definitive diagnosis of Hodgkin's disease is made only after extensive testing that includes blood work, X rays, and a tissue biopsy. Tissue taken from swollen lymph nodes is examined under a microscope for any signs of abnormal cellular growth or structure. If abnormal cells (called Reed-Sternberg cells) are present, doctors examine the entire lymphatic system to determine the degree to which the cancer may have spread to other parts of the body, especially the bones, chest, liver, and spleen.

Chemotherapy and radiation therapy are the preferred treatment methods for Hodgkin's disease. Radiation therapy is usually given in the early stages of the disease; chemotherapy is used for more advanced cases. Sometimes, though, a combination of these treatments is used, depending upon the stage of the disease and the recommendation of the doctor.

Non-Hodgkin's lymphoma is the name of a group of cancers that develop in the lymphatic system. They occur when normal cells suddenly begin to reproduce themselves at an abnormal rate, replacing normal cells and growing into tumors. If not detected and treated early, they may easily spread to other parts of the body.

Symptoms of non-Hodgkin's lymphoma are swelling of the lymph nodes, fever, itching skin, night sweats, tiredness, and weight loss. The mere appearance of these symptoms does not automatically mean cancer; however, it does mean that if you are experiencing any of these symptoms, you should see a doctor for a thorough examination.

A definitive diagnosis of lymphoma is made only after extensive testing that includes blood work, X rays, and a tissue biopsy. Tissue taken from swollen lymph nodes is examined under a microscope for any signs of abnormal cellular growth or structure. If abnormal cells are present, doctors examine the entire lymphatic system to determine the degree to which the cancer may have spread to other parts of the body, especially the bones, chest, liver, and spleen.

Treatments for non-Hodgkin's lymphoma are similar to those for Hodgkin's disease, except for the use of surgery when large tumors must be removed. Chemotherapy uses powerful anticancer drugs to seek out and kill the abnormal cells; unfortunately, it also affects normal cells, resulting in unpleasant side effects. Radiation therapy is also used to damage the cancer cells and interrupt their growth. Sometimes radiation therapy is used in conjunction with chemotherapy, depending upon the stage of the disease and the recommendation of the doctor.

Lymphedema is characterized by an abnormal accumulation of lymph in the tissues, causing swelling of an arm or leg. The lymph is unable to drain normally because the vessels are blocked, damaged, or removed. Vessels may become blocked by cancer cells that collect in the lymph system, or they may be damaged by radiation therapy given for cancer.

Some of the early signs of lymphedema are puffiness of an arm or leg, gradual swelling, and a feeling of heaviness in the limb. It's sometimes difficult to recognize lymphedema because the swelling occurs slowly and often without pain.

While there is no known cure for lymphedema, treatment generally consists of diuretics (drugs that promote the elimination of fluids), massage (to move the excess lymph fluid), elastic pressure bands and compression sleeves (to maintain pressure and promote drainage), and exercise (to keep the limb mobile).

Lymphadenopathy, or swollen glands, occurs as a result of inflammation of the white blood cells in the lymph nodes. Swollen glands are very common and occur whenever the body's immune system is fighting off an invading organism or pathogen. Lymph glands are distributed throughout the body, but the ones most people are familiar with are in the neck, underarms, and groin.

Lymph glands in the neck usually swell when you have a cold and sore throat; however, they also swell if you have an allergy to some substance such as dust, mold, pollen, or an insect bite. Generally speaking, once the cause of the swelling has been eliminated, the glands return to their normal size until they are called upon again to ward off another body invader. When swelling continues without a definite cause, it may indicate a serious underlying condition and calls for professional medical attention.

Lymph glands are one of the body's frontline defenses in fighting disease. For more information, see the preceding discussion of the immune system.

Muscles

Muscles, in conjunction with bones and joints, allow the body to move, to maintain posture, to produce heat, and to maintain the body's homeostasis. Muscle tissue has four general properties: the ability to respond to stimuli, to contract, to extend and stretch, and to return to its original shape. Muscle tissue is either striated or smooth (nonstriated), either voluntary (under conscious control) or involuntary, and is categorized according to its location in the body.

The three types of muscle tissue are skeletal (muscle attached to bones), visceral, or smooth (found in internal structures such as the walls of the stomach, intestines, and blood vessels), and cardiac (found in the walls of the heart).

In addition to the heart muscle, some other well-known muscles are biceps and deltoids (arm), pectoralis major (chest), and gluteus maximus (buttocks). The trapezius is a diamond-shaped muscle that extends from the middle of the back and across the shoulders to the base of the skull. The abdominal muscle is called the rectus abdominis and gives support to the abdominal organs.

COMPONENTS OF THE MUSCULAR SYSTEM

Skeletal Muscle

Skeletal muscles, which number close to 700 in the entire body, permit body movement through the process of contraction and relaxation. Skeletal muscles are striated and move voluntarily, which means they can be made to move by the body.

Skeletal muscles are attached by tendons (cords of connective tissue) to bones at a junction known as the periosteum. Fascia, a band or sheet of fibrous connective tissue, is found surrounding muscles and around organs. Fasciae not only connect and hold muscles together, but several types of fascia also store water and fat, protect and insulate the body, line the walls of the body, separate muscles into groups, and carry nerves and blood vessels. Skeletal muscles are made up of muscle fibers, or cells, which are arranged into bundles called fasciculi or fascicles.

Muscle fibers are cylindrical-shaped cells and are arranged next to one another in a parallel fashion. Skeletal muscle fibers are multinucleate (have several nuclei) and are composed of various components: a plasma membrane (sarcolemma), cytoplasm within the muscle fibers (sarcoplasm), nuclei and mitochondria within the sarcoplasm, and a network membrane called the sarcoplasmic reticulum. Muscle fibers themselves are composed of myofibrils, long, thin, threadlike structures, which are further made up of thin and thick myofilaments. Thick myofilaments are arranged in dark, dense bands called anisotropic bands. Thick myofilaments contain the protein myosin and have structures protruding from them called cross bridges. Thin myofilaments, arranged in light, less dense bands named isotropic bands, are composed of the protein actin and a protein molecule called the tropomyosin-troponin complex.

Cardiac Muscle
Cardiac muscle is the muscle that makes up the walls of the heart. It is striated muscle tissue, its fibers containing one centrally located nucleus. Cardiac muscle tissue is involuntary, and its fibers are stimulated collectively by an impulse. Cardiac muscle tissue is divided into two sections: the muscle tissue comprising the atria, the upper part of the heart; and the muscle tissue comprising the ventricles, the lower part of the heart.

Different from skeletal muscle tissue, cardiac muscle contracts in a rhythmic, rapid, and continuous fashion.

Visceral Muscle
Visceral muscle tissue comprises the walls of the stomach, intestines, uterus, blood vessels, and bladder. Visceral tissue, or smooth muscle tissue, is nonstriated and involuntary. Smooth muscle fibers have single centrally located nuclei and contract more slowly than skeletal muscles.

How Does the Muscular System Function?
Skeletal muscles, working in muscular groups in conjunction with connective tissue, make up the muscular system of the body. Muscles in the muscular system are categorized in numerous ways. A muscle could be named according to its location, size, direction of its fibers, shape, action, and the nature of its origins and insertions. Muscles move by making tendons pull on bones, which form joints.

When a skeletal muscle contracts, one bone moves toward another bone, which remains stationary. The point at which the tendon attaches to the stationary bone is the origin. The other point at which the tendon joins the nonstationary bone is the insertion. Within the muscular group, there are several muscles working to produce a desired movement: The agonist is the muscle that contracts; the antagonist is the muscle that relaxes; and synergists are the muscles that aid the agonist in executing a smooth, clean movement.

Muscle Contraction
In order for muscles to contract, they need to receive nerve impulses, nutrients and oxygen via the bloodstream, and energy from the breakdown of ATP (a compound, adenosine triphosphate, that supplies energy to cells). A muscle contracts by first receiving impulses from motor neurons. Neurons, or nerve cells, receive a stimulus and carry the impulse through its fibers (axons) to the muscle cells. The point at which the muscle receives the impulse is named the motor end plate. The impulse then stimulates the muscle fibers, and thin and thick myofilaments slide past each other, thus producing movement. This process of the myofilaments sliding past each other is termed the sliding-filament theory of contraction.

On a cellular level, the contraction of a muscle begins with nerve impulses at the nerve ending traveling to the motor end plate of the muscle. This occurs as calcium ions cause a chemical, ACh (acetylcholine), to be released. ACh allows the nerve impulses to be carried eventually to the sarcoplasmic reticulum. There, calcium ions are released from storage into the sarcoplasm, which envelops the myofilaments. The calcium ions travel to the cross bridges of the myofilaments and activate the myosin there. Calcium ions also bind to the tropomyosin-troponin complex, which separates the complex from the thin myofilaments. In the presence of calcium ions, myosin catalyzes the breakdown of ATP. Thin myofilaments attach themselves to myosin cross bridges, and the thick and thin myofilaments slide past each other. Energy is released from the ATP breakdown and permits the thick and thin myofilaments to slide back and forth, thereby allowing the contraction of the muscle fibers and of the muscles themselves.

In order for the muscle to return to a relaxed state, ACh is eradicated, thus inhibiting the nerve impulses from moving across to the motor end plate. The nerve impulses cease, calcium ions move back into the sarcoplasmic reticulum, and the myosin stops its enzymatic activity. ATP is resynthesized and binds to the myosin cross bridges. These cross bridges detach from the protein actin, and actin in turn reattaches to the tropomyosin-troponin complex, allowing the thin myofilaments to rejoin with actin. The myofilaments slide back to a relaxed position, and the muscle fibers return to a relaxed state.

Muscle fibers follow the all-or-none principle of contraction: They either contract all the way or do not contract at all. When a muscle contracts, its length measures a little more than half its relaxed length. Some common types of contractions are twitches, abnormal contractions (cramps, spasms, tics, convulsions), isotonic contractions (produces body movement, muscle shortens), and isometric contractions (produces no movement, limited shortening of the muscle). However, muscles may be in a state of partial contraction despite the all-or-none principle.

Partial contraction results in muscle tone, which is essential in maintaining posture. Contractions of muscles can be categorized as either fast or slow. Fast muscle fibers, or white muscle, have few capillaries and contract rapidly for quick movements such as eye movements. Slow muscle fibers, or red muscle, have many capillaries, which contain red blood cells, and contract slowly.

With any contraction, though, energy is released as heat, which helps the body maintain its internal temperature.

Use of Levers in the Muscular System

To create movement, the bones of the body act as levers and the joints act as fulcrums (fixed points). Some kind of resistance (force working against the muscles) and effort (force used to overcome the resistance—a muscle contraction) are also needed to make the lever system of muscles work.

Levers are classified according to the location of their fulcrums, resistance, and effort. There are three types of levers: first-class, second-class, and third-class. Third-class levers are the most common kind of lever found in the muscular system. Its configuration consists of the fulcrum on one end, the resistance on the other, and the effort in the middle. A good example of the third-class lever is the movement of the forearm bending at the elbow. The elbow serves as the fulcrum, the forearm itself is the resistance, and the effort is the contraction of the biceps muscle.

MAJOR PROBLEMS AND COMMON DISORDERS OF THE MUSCLES

Muscular dystrophy (MD) is an inherited, progressive disease that causes a weakness of muscle tissue and eventually death. MD is the name given to a family of muscle diseases, including Duchenne's dystrophy. This condition strikes only males and is usually diagnosed before the age of 5.

Symptoms of MD are muscle weakness, lack of coordination in movement, and difficulty lifting the arms. These symptoms are observed in toddlers who fail to develop normal motor skills such as climbing, balancing, and walking. There is also a marked inability to lift the arms much above the head.

While the exact cause of MD is unknown, it has been discovered that males with MD lack a protein essential to muscle function. As the disease progresses, muscles are gradually replaced by fat tissue, and a general body deformity is noted. Most people with MD also become very susceptible to chest infections, especially pneumonia, which is responsible for many deaths.

There is no known treatment for muscular dystrophy.

Myasthenia gravis is a rare autoimmune disorder that affects the transmission of nerve impulses to the muscles. The first sign that something might be wrong is the appearance of drooping eyelids. Other symptoms include double vision and problems eating, speaking, and swallowing. In some cases, mobility is affected because of a general weakness in the arms and legs.

The exact cause of myasthenia gravis is unknown; however, it does appear as though some factor causes the immune system to turn against muscle tissue. A possible link to the thymus, a component of the immune system, has been discovered.

Only a thorough physical, including X rays and blood work, can diagnose myasthenia gravis. While there's no effective cure, medications can lessen the effect of the condition.

Myofascitis is inflammation of the muscles and the tissues that surround them (the fasciae). It usually occurs as a result of putting strain on the muscles and connective tissue by strenuous exercise. The result is tenderness and pain around the muscle. The best treatment is to rest the affected area and improve overall muscle tone before beginning any exercise program. In rare instances, cortisone is given to reduce inflammation.

Tumors in muscle tissue are rare; however, when they are discovered, they should be examined by a physician. The tumor grows between the muscle and the layers of skin. It is usually visible and appears as a lump on the skin. Most such tumors are benign; however, when one is malignant, it must be treated quickly.

A *muscle pull* occurs when too much of a strain is placed on a muscle and it is overstretched. Many weekend athletes suffer pulled muscles when they fail to adequately warm up prior to physical activity. Most minor muscle pulls may be treated with ice packs and abstention from strenuous activity for a few days.

A more serious muscle pull occurs when the muscle fiber tears and internal bleeding occurs. When this happens, the person needs to apply ice quickly to reduce the swelling, followed by an application of heat and possibly an elastic bandage wrap. If pain is present, an over-the-counter analgesic may provide relief.

Any muscle pull that does not respond to basic treatment after a few days should be examined by a physician to determine if the muscle has been ruptured, the most serious type of muscle pull. In severe cases, surgery is required to repair the muscle.

Sprains occur at joints where muscles, tendons, and bones meet. Because these three are interconnected, any trauma to one affects the others. A sprain is caused by an activity that causes the joint to move outside its normal range, such as when a joint is twisted or stretched. In this instance, the tendons at the end of the muscles are stretched and quickly swell. The entire joint feels sore and is painful to the touch. An application of ice is recommended to reduce the swelling and speed the healing. A support bandage may strengthen a weak joint and prevent or lessen further sprains.

Muscle spasms (also called cramps) are painful, involuntary contractions of muscles that occur for no apparent reason. Some cramps may be traced to over-strenuous exercising or prolonged sitting or standing, but there is no known cause. Cramps may occur at any time and may affect any muscle from the foot to the face. Most cramps will resolve by themselves, although pain relief may be gained by massaging the muscle and gradually moving it.

Nervous System

The nervous system is a collection of nerve cells, called neurons, and their neurochemicals, which are responsible for receiving sensory stimuli, generating and coordinating responses, and, in turn, controlling bodily activities. Our nervous system is divided into the central nervous system (brain and spinal cord) and peripheral nervous system (nerves extending from the brain and spinal cord to other parts of the body). We are wired much like a giant electrical network, with messages being passed along the nerves, through the spinal cord, and finally to the brain.

COMPONENTS OF THE NERVOUS SYSTEM

The major components of the nervous system are the brain, spinal cord, nerve cells, and ganglia (concentrated masses of interconnected nerve cells). The nervous system is protected by the skull and spinal vertebrae in addition to layers of membranes known as meninges. When these layers become infected or inflamed, the condition is called meningitis.

Your brain is the center of the nervous system and is responsible for processing the information received from the rest of your body. It literally is the computer that keeps your body organized and functioning, whether you're breathing, sleeping, or taking a walk.

The brain is an organ that weighs about 3 pounds and is composed of cells called neurons, some 100 billion in all. Its cells are grayish white in appearance, hence the term "gray matter" when referring to the brain. Like all organs, the brain must be nourished and protected from injury. In order to accomplish this, the brain is encased within the skull and is fed via a system of arteries and capillaries that supply it with blood and nourishment.

Your brain is divided into three distinct parts: the brain stem, the cerebellum, and the cerebrum. The brain stem is what joins the brain and the spinal cord; it is also responsible for many of the involuntary functions of your body, such as blood circulation and breathing.

The cerebellum is composed of nerve tissue and is divided into hemispheres known as the right and left hemispheres. It is responsible for many of the conscious activities of living, such as intelligence, memory, speech, and vision. These hemispheres are further subdivided into lobes known as the frontal, parietal, occipital, and temporal, with each having a specific function.

The cerebrum is located beneath the cerebellum and is responsible for maintaining balance, coordination, and other subconscious functions.

The trunk line of the nervous system is the spinal cord, which is encased within the bony protection of the spine. Think of it as a large cable where wires enter from near and distant parts of the body. The nerves entering the cord are named for the sections of the spine where they enter, such as the sacral nerve roots (at the bottom of the spine), lumbar, thoracic, and cervical (neck).

Nerve cells (called neurons) are the basic components and building blocks of the entire nervous system. A neuron consists of a cell body with a nucleus and branching fibers called dendrites. Neurons also have projections called axons, which branch out to form terminals that connect to dendrites of other cells, muscles, or glands. The space between the axons and the receptor, or receiving, cells is called the synapse, and this is where signals are passed by neurotransmitters. (We have more to say later about the functions of nerve cells.)

Ganglia are bundles of nerve cells found outside of the central nervous system and may be located within the brain or spinal cord. They play a role in directing the reflexive actions of the sympathetic nervous system when the body needs to guard against being injured, such as when you pull your hand away when you touch a hot stove.

How Does the Nervous System Function?

Scientists once believed that the nervous system operated much like the electrical system of a house or car, that stimuli such as light, heat, cold, and pain were transmitted from nerve cells to the brain through electrical impulses. However, neurons are not physically connected; rather, the process by which stimuli are transmitted to the brain is primarily chemical.

Cells in the distant parts of the body receive stimuli from the outside world. These cells are called receptor cells or neurons. As we said earlier, neurons are separated by a gap called the synapse. When a stimulus is being transmitted to the brain, the neuron produces specific chemicals called neurotransmitters, which filter across this gap and stimulate neighboring neurons. This stimulation causes a charge within the neighboring neurons, resulting in their production of neurotransmitters to stimulate the next neurons, and so on in a chain, until the charge reaches the spinal cord and finally the brain. The system of receptor cells that first receive stimuli is known as the peripheral nervous system, while the brain and spinal cord make up what is known as the central nervous system.

The brain's neurotransmitters monitor all of our senses from hunger to pleasure to pain. The brain also formulates responses to these stimuli. One type of neurotransmitters, called endorphins, for example, gives the body the ability to suppress pain, such as when a person is running a marathon. This and all other neurotransmitters produced in the body are more effective at reducing pain than chemical painkillers produced in a lab.

When the body is in danger of being injured, such as when a hand is suddenly exposed to something very hot, reflexes take over and cause the hand to snap away quickly and involuntarily. Reflexes are the body's response to danger. They are involuntary in that the stimulus being received is reacted upon before it even reaches the brain. If the message being transmitted is one of emergency, it is received by a mass of nerve cells called a ganglion in the spinal cord. An immediate response is sent back to the motor cells in the area from which the stimulus came, causing the muscles to respond by pulling away from the danger.

Reflexes make up what is known as the sympathetic nervous system. But because these reflexive reactions could get out of hand, the body developed a monitoring system called the parasympathetic nervous system, which controls reflexive reactions. The sympathetic and parasympathetic nervous systems make up what is known as the autonomic nervous system, so called because the reactions to stimuli in this system are automatic and do not require any input from the brain, although the brain may process feelings of pain.

The brain is made up of sections called lobes, which receive stimuli and formulate responses. Visual stimuli is transmitted by nerves in the eyes and received by the occipital lobe. Nerves in the nasal passages send messages to the olfactory lobe. Sensory nerves in the skin, which produce messages of temperature and touch, send messages to the parietal lobe. Other lobes are responsible for hearing and tasting, and other portions of the brain formulate responses to these stimuli, completing the cycle of the nervous system.

Major Problems and Common Disorders of the Nervous System

Alzheimer's disease is a progressive degeneration of brain cells leading to loss of memory, confusion, anxiety, depression, and eventually death. The exact cause of Alzheimer's is not known; however, it is known that certain abnormalities occur within the cells of the brain. Some researchers have investigated a link between the degeneration of the brain cell and the neurotransmitter called acetylcholine (ACh). Unfortunately, there is no effective treatment for Alzheimer's disease, although some medications may lessen the symptoms.

Amyotrophic lateral sclerosis (ALS) also causes progressive degeneration of nerve cells in the brain and spinal cord that control muscle movement. Also known as Lou Gehrig's disease, ALS leads to a wasting away of the muscles once the nerve cells are destroyed. As the muscle tissue is destroyed, paralysis results, ultimately leading to death. Its cause is unknown and there is no effective treatment.

A *brain tumor* is any abnormal growth of tissue that forms in the brain, and may be a primary or secondary tumor. These tumors can be either benign or malignant. A primary tumor is one that develops in the brain tissue; a secondary tumor is one that originates elsewhere and migrates to the brain.

Brain tumors may produce symptoms of double vision, headache, memory loss, impaired thinking, personality changes, weakness, and vomiting. Diagnosis of brain tumors can be made using computed tomographic scanning (CT scanning) or magnetic resonance imaging (MRI). Treatment may include surgery, radiation therapy, and chemotherapy.

Encephalitis is a condition marked by inflammation of the brain and is caused by a virus. Very often the brain is affected secondarily to an existing viral infection in another part of the body. For example, the virus that causes chicken pox, measles, or mumps could spread to your brain and cause encephalitis. Early symptoms are headache and fever; if these symptoms persist and worsen, a physician should be consulted. Diagnosis is made by examining the cerebrospinal fluid obtained through a spinal tap (removing fluid from the spinal column).

Huntington's disease is a fatal, inherited, progressive, degenerative disorder of brain cells with actual shrinkage of tissue. It has been linked to an abnormal gene found on chromosome 4; however, researchers are still searching for the exact gene. The condition produces involuntary movements of the arms, face, trunk, and feet. It also leads to mental deterioration and psychiatric symptoms. If a parent is affected with this disease, each child has a 50 percent chance of developing it as well. Huntington's disease is usually diagnosed around the age of 35; however, even though it is fatal, death may not occur for ten or twenty years following diagnosis.

Meningitis is an inflammation of the membranes covering the brain and spinal cord. The symptoms usually include headache, fever, and a stiff neck. Its cause is attributed to both bacteria and viruses, with bacterial meningitis being the more serious illness. Diagnosis is made by examining the cerebrospinal fluid, obtained by performing a spinal tap. Bacterial meningitis is treated with antibiotics, while viral meningitis has no specific treatment other than bed rest, fluids, and analgesics.

Multiple sclerosis (MS) is a condition that results when the insulating cover that protects nerve fibers, the myelin, is destroyed or damaged. An unknown agent attacks the myelin, damaging it and causing scarring (sclerosis); this in turn affects the way nerve cells conduct signals and coordinate movement. The symptoms of MS are impaired vision, rapid eye movement, numbness (tingling) or weakness in a limb or paralysis in one or more limbs, lack of coordination, and tremor or unsteady gait.

Heredity may play a factor in who gets the disease, which tends to strike slightly more women than men. Although the exact cause of MS has not been determined, it has been linked with a defect in the immune system. MS is a very difficult condition to diagnose and may take repeated electroencephalographic (EEG) studies and other nerve stimulus studies before a definite diagnosis is made. Magnetic resonance imaging (MRI) scans are also often performed.

Medications may be prescribed to control the immune response or muscle movements; however, they cannot cure the condition. Relatively new on the scene is betaferon, approved by the Food and Drug Administration in 1993. In short supply—because it is a biological (any substance made from living organisms or the products of living organisms) and therefore difficult to produce—and suitable for mild to moderate cases of MS, betaferon is administered by self-injection every other day. There are possible side effects, including flulike symptoms, irritation at the site of the injection, and sudden depression.

Physical therapy is often prescribed to help the person adapt to limitations and learn how to overcome them.

Narcolepsy is a neurologic condition characterized by sudden periods of sleepiness during normal daily activities. People affected by narcolepsy very often become sleepy when they are engaged in other activities, such as working or driving. In addition to the sleepiness, many people also experience periods of cataplexy, a condition characterized by sudden muscle weakness which causes them to fall or collapse.

The exact cause of narcolepsy remains a mystery; however, it is thought that REM (rapid eye movement) sleep patterns somehow intrude during waking hours. A diagnosis of narcolepsy can be made using special electroencephalographic (EEG) studies. Medications are prescribed to control the periods of sleepiness and muscle weakness.

Seizure disorders (at one time called epilepsy) occur when the normal electrical patterns of the brain cells become disrupted for some unknown reason. This disorganization of signals causes the body to go into spasms, called seizures. There are two classes of seizures: grand mal and petit mal. The grand mal seizure is the most serious because there are convulsions and loss of consciousness. They may come on suddenly with no warning. Once the seizure begins, the person loses consciousness, followed by violent movement, then a period of sleep. After these phases, the person regains consciousness, although he or she may be confused.

A petit mal seizure, as the name implies, is a small seizure that lasts for only a few seconds or minutes. Loss of consciousness is not accompanied by any violent body movements, and when consciousness is regained, there is no confusion. These types of seizures typically begin in children between the ages of 6 and 12.

Diagnosing seizure disorders involves compiling a complete medical history and may include brain scans and electroencephalographic (EEG) studies. Antiseizure medicines may be prescribed to control both grand mal and petit mal seizures.

Spinal cord trauma is a general term that applies to anything that injures the spinal cord, possibly affecting the way it conducts nerve impulses to the brain. Injury to the spinal cord may result in weakness and loss of sensation from a part of the body to complete paralysis if the cord is severed.

Bleeding within the spinal cord and compression of the cord (caused by swelling) generally produce weakness in the limbs and a loss of sensation. Once the cause of the bleeding is stopped and the swelling is reduced, normal functioning usually returns—although, depending upon the degree of injury, there may be some residual effects.

However, in the case of major trauma to the spinal cord, resulting from a work accident, shooting, stabbing, or sports injury, permanent paralysis may result. The worst possible case is the severing of the cord, thereby cutting off all communication between the brain and the limbs. Depending upon the number of limbs affected, a person would be classified as either a paraplegic (two limbs paralyzed) or a quadriplegic (four limbs paralyzed).

Once the tissue of the spinal cord has been severely damaged, there is very little chance the cells will regenerate and reattach themselves. Physical therapy and mechanical aids can enable people with physical disabilities to lead full and complete lives.

Bell's palsy is a condition that results in the paralysis of facial muscles due to nerve damage. It is typically characterized by sagging muscles and a general weakness on one side of the face. When nerve damage occurs, the electrical signals that usually flow to the muscles are disrupted. There is some research that suggests that an agent, such as a virus, causes the facial nerves to swell, and this is what interrupts the normal electrical patterns. While its exact cause is unknown, the condition is temporary, with full recovery expected within a few months. Some physicians may prescribe cortisone to reduce the swelling and speed the healing, whereas others consider Bell's palsy to be a self-limiting condition that will take care of itself.

Headache is probably the most common complaint among the human race, as there are very few people who have never experienced the pain of headache. While you may think your brain is hurting, the truth is that the brain doesn't really feel pain. It is the pain-sensing structures around the brain that react when something goes wrong. There are nerve cells, blood vessels, and muscles all reacting to stimuli that are perceived as headaches.

Structures in the skull, such as eyes, ears, and teeth, have thousands of nerve cells surrounding them. A painful tooth, for example, can cause pain to radiate throughout the face and head. Disturbances in any one of these cause the nerves to fire, resulting in the sensation of pain we call headache.

There are three recognizable types of headaches: tension, migraine, and cluster. Tension headaches occur when the muscles of the neck contract due to stress or other psychological factors. As these muscles contract, they produce the pain we feel as a headache.

Migraine headaches are caused by the dilation of blood vessels in the face, neck, or scalp, and may produce nausea, vomiting, or visual symptoms such as auras, sparkling lights, or blind spots.

Cluster headaches produce a steady burning pain in and around the eyes or temple. The eyes may appear irritated with redness and constant watering, accompanied by sinus stuffiness. These headaches have a sudden onset with very little warning, tend to follow a pattern of occurrences, and may last for up to 2 hours.

Headaches may be relieved with a variety of over-the-counter analgesics including aspirin, acetaminophen, and ibuprofen; however, prescription medications may be necessary to relieve more serious attacks. Recently, new medications such as sumatriptan are being used to treat migraines once they have developed, and a class of drugs called beta-blockers (propranolol, nadolol) are taken to prevent the migraine from developing. Headaches associated with stress and tension may respond to psychotherapy and tranquilizing drugs, as well as so-called alternative therapies such as biofeedback, relaxation techniques, and meditation.

Reproductive System

Without the human reproductive system, the continuation of the human race would not be possible. In fact, no species would prosper long were it not able to reproduce itself and foster future generations. The entire process of creating new life is dependent upon the joining of two different cells in a biological environment singularly designed for that purpose.

Humans, being mammals (bearing their young live), reproduce sexually through a process called intercourse. Females carry a cell called the ovum or egg, and males carry a cell called sperm. In order to reproduce the species, the egg must be fertilized by sperm in the fallopian tube and then move to the uterus (womb), where the fetus grows and matures until birth.

COMPONENTS OF THE FEMALE REPRODUCTIVE SYSTEM

Except for the external genitalia (vulva), the female reproductive system is internal and consists of the fallopian tubes, ovaries, uterus (womb), and vagina. Mammary glands, although not a part of the reproductive system per se, produce milk that is used to nourish newborn infants.

Fallopian tubes

These two tubelike structures extend from the top of the uterus to the ovaries. The purpose of the fallopian tube is to catch the egg that is released by the ovary at the time of ovulation, and also provide a place for the sperm to fertilize the egg. Small, hairlike structures called cilia propel the egg on its journey from the ovary to possible implantation in the womb if the egg has been fertilized.

Ovaries

The two almond-shaped whitish ovaries hang by ligaments on either side of the pelvis. They are about 1¼ inches long and, together, weigh about ¼ ounce. They produce the ovum, or egg, the largest cell in the body.

Ovaries play a very important role in preparing females for childbearing by bringing about bodily changes when a girl enters puberty, usually around the age of 12. At this time, the pituitary gland signals the ovaries to release hormones that cause the pelvis to widen, hips to develop fat pads, and breasts and pubic hair to develop.

The ovaries regulate the menstrual cycle throughout the childbearing years until the woman is between 45 and 50 to 55, on average. They also supply the egg, or ovum, with nutrients it needs for survival. Women are born with about 500,000 egg cells; however, only about 400 mature eggs are produced that are capable of being fertilized during childbearing years.

During the first few days of the menstrual cycle, the pituitary gland secretes FSH (follicle-stimulating hormone), a hormone that awakens several of the dormant egg cells in the ovary. One egg is pushed to the surface, and in about 2 weeks, it appears as a blister the size of a marble protruding from the surface of the ovary. The pituitary gland then secretes another hormone (LH, or luteinizing hormone) that causes the follicle around the egg to burst and the ripe egg to drop into the fallopian tube for transport to the womb, and for possible fertilization in route.

The ovaries also produce testosterone and convert it into estrogen, the female hormone, which helps the body to develop female sexual characteristics. The ovaries then produce progesterone, which causes rhythmic contractions of the womb and causes its walls to thicken and blood vessels to form. This makes the womb ready to nourish the egg, should it become fertilized.

When a woman reaches the age of 45 to 50 or 55, menopause begins, and the ovaries begin to shrink and hormone production decreases. Skin may dry, muscles may stiffen, and she may become prone to osteoporosis, a disease that causes bones to become brittle.

Uterus

The uterus, or womb, is a pinkish, hollow, regularly contracting muscular organ suspended by ligaments in the lower abdomen. Its interior space could hold about a teaspoonful of liquid. Roughly the shape of a small pear, it weighs about 2 ounces. Its reproductive function is to house and nurse a fertilized egg as it grows into a human being.

Each month, the womb prepares for pregnancy and undergoes the construction of an intricate network of new blood vessels, glands, and tissues. When the womb receives a signal from the hormone estrogen (released from the ovaries), its blood-red, velvet-smooth lining (the endometrium) thickens and the glands enlarge. This will allow the womb to provide nourishment for a new life, should the need arise.

At midcycle, the ovaries begin producing the hormone progesterone. This hormone relaxes the muscles of the womb, prepares its lining for implantation, and prods its glands to secrete nourishing substances for a fertilized egg.

Each month, a single egg is delivered into the womb from one of the two ovaries via the fallopian tubes, which feed into the top of the womb. A third opening through the cervix, or neck of the womb, provides an entrance for sperm and an exit for a baby. When an ovary releases an egg, the mucous glands in the cervix provide a stream through which the male sperm can swim toward the egg to fertilize it.

In order for a sperm cell to fertilize an egg, it must first reach the egg and then break through its barrier. The womb is now prepared to receive the fertilized egg. However, if the egg does not become fertilized in a given month, the lining of the uterus must be shed, a process known as menstruation, or having a period. Menstruation takes place during the final week of the menstrual cycle. On average, a period lasts from 3 to 5 days. After menstruation, the menstrual cycle begins again, and the shed lining is replaced by a new one.

If the egg does become fertilized, it begins dividing right away. As the egg travels down the fallopian tube, it is nourished by its yolk. When it reaches the womb, it attaches to the lining of the womb, and it is from here that the egg will receive food for the duration of the pregnancy.

Another organ called the placenta performs the functions of the baby's lungs, liver, kidneys, and digestive tract until the baby is born. The placenta develops from the chorion, the outermost layer of the fertilized egg, and attaches itself to the wall of the uterus. By the end of pregnancy, the placenta weighs about 2 pounds and is 7 inches in diameter and about 1 inch thick.

The umbilical cord serves as the baby's lifeline. It ranges in length from 5 inches to 4 feet. The cord carries wastes from the baby to the placenta, where they are removed by the mother's bloodstream. The cord also carries vitamins, oxygen, minerals, carbohydrates, and amino acids to the baby via an artery that runs through it.

During pregnancy, the capacity of the uterus becomes 500 times its original size and becomes much stronger, with muscles increasing in size and weight so that it can sustain the labors of birth.

Until the seventh month, the baby changes position frequently, but then gravity causes the baby to assume a head-down position. As the baby grows, the mother's organs, such as the bladder, stomach, and intestines, are pushed to the side. This causes the need for frequent urination and also causes digestive upsets.

A *hysterectomy* is the surgical removal of the uterus, and ends menstruation and childbearing. Sometimes the ovaries and fallopian tubes are also removed. This operation is often performed to attempt to save a woman's life if she is being threatened by cancer or if the uterus has been damaged during childbirth, miscarriage, endometriosis, or infection.

Vagina

The vagina, a tube 4 to 6 inches long, connects the uterus with the external world. It serves as a receptacle for the male penis and sperm and as an exit for the baby. The vagina is made of muscle and fibroelastic tissue, which can expand to more than 4 inches in diameter.

The vagina is located behind the urethra and bladder and in front of the rectum. The Bartholin's glands, two small oval-shaped glands on either side of the vagina, secrete a fluid that lubricates the vulval area. Each month during ovulation, the secretions become thin and watery to help sperm move it to the uterus.

Vulva

The vulva, or mons pubis, is the rounded pad of fatty tissue that covers pubic bone. Extending downward from this are the labia majora, two folds of fatty tissue that protect the genitals. The labia minora lie just underneath and enclose the urethra and the vagina. The upper end of the labia minora forms the prepuce, which encloses the clitoris, a highly sensitive organ with specialized nerve endings that becomes filled with blood during sexual arousal.

Breasts

The function of the breasts is to change blood into milk. The left breast is larger than the right in most women. The breast is nothing more than a modified, and infinitely complex, sweat gland. Around the age of 12, hormones cause fat deposits to develop in the breasts, and they begin to swell. The nipples grow, and the areola, the halo around the nipple, takes on a heavier pigmentation.

Each breast contains about seventeen independent milk-producing units filled with microscopic alveoli, which produce invisible droplets of milk. The milk filters into branching ducts and finally into the main stem, which ends at the nipple.

During pregnancy, the breasts receive estrogen from the placenta, and the weight of the breasts doubles. When the baby is born, milk production begins. For the first few days, the milk is yellowish and watery. This fluid, called colostrum, contains lymphocytes (disease-fighting white blood cells) and immunoglobulins (antibodies) that protect the baby from diseases the mother might have. By the fifth day, the milk begins to provide nourishment for the baby.

The breasts take glucose from the mother's blood, which is changed into lactose with the help of enzymes. Also brought to the baby through the breasts are minerals, especially calcium, which helps develop bone, and vitamins essential for health. Nursing provides the baby with exactly what he or she needs.

During menopause, the things that happened in puberty are reversed. The breasts lose some but not all of their fat deposits. The glandular structure withers, and nearly disappears, and the breasts shrink.

Androgens

Androgens, male sex hormones also produced in small quantities by women, are the powerful stimulators of sexual desire. These hormones can be triggered by emotions or thoughts about love or sex, and by foreplay. During sexual arousal, nerve impulses cause blood supply to sexual organs to increase, the clitoris to become erect, and the vagina to become lubricated.

The female climax, or orgasm, is similar to that of the male except that there is no ejaculation. When sexual excitement reaches its peak, muscle tension also increases, and at orgasm, the muscles in the uterus and vagina contract rhythmically. At this point, blood begins to leave the pelvic area.

MAJOR PROBLEMS AND COMMON DISORDERS OF THE FEMALE REPRODUCTIVE SYSTEM

Cancer

The female reproductive system is prone to cancer of the breast, cervix, ovaries, and uterus.

Cancer is a malignant growth that can affect any of the female reproductive organs. Cancer invades the normal cells and begins growing at a faster rate than normal cells, crowding them out and depriving them of nourishment.

Breast cancer strikes more than 180,000 people (primarily women) each year, and claims over 40,000 lives annually. The answer to surviving breast cancer involves early detection and treatment. Improved breast cancer awareness, with the emphasis upon self-detection and monitoring, plus advances in diagnostic imaging (mammography) have all combined to improve survival rates. Experts agree that a woman is more likely to get a safe, accurate mammogram if the mammography center is accredited by the American College of Radiology and has equipment designed and used only for breast X rays and adjusted each year for correct radiation doses.

Women can perform self-examination of the breasts to detect small lumps. (Menstruating women should perform breast self-examination in the first half of the menstrual cycle when the breasts are easiest to examine. Postmenopausal women should pick a specific, easily remembered time of the month.) Further, any woman should watch for any depression in either breast; cancer tissue, because of its effect on other structures of the breast, can cause a slight hollowing. Any twisting of the nipple from normal position is also a signal to watch for. And any abnormal discharge from the nipple should be considered something to be checked.

Cancer of the cervix, the neck of the womb, usually has very well defined precancerous stages, which may be detected by a Pap smear. In addition to malignant tumors, the cervix is also at risk from infections, such as sexually transmitted diseases.

Cancer of the ovaries can occur at any age, but is most likely to occur after the age of 50. Unfortunately, this type of cancer does not produce well-defined symptoms, although there is usually some abdominal pain and possibly swelling. Exploratory diagnostic procedures, either a laparoscopy or laparotomy, are the only methods of making a positive diagnosis. If cancer is discovered, the procedure is to remove the malignant tissue as well as other affected organs.

Cancer of the uterus, or endometrium (the lining of the uterus), is the third most common form of cancer among women. Symptoms usually include ..excessive bleeding during menstruation or after sexual intercourse. Diagnosis is made by taking a sample of the endometrium tissue and having it analyzed for abnormal growth. If a positive diagnosis is made, the uterus and ovaries are removed in a procedure called a hysterectomy. Chemotherapy may be recommended if there's any chance the cancer has spread to other parts of the body.

Fibroids
Fibroids are benign growths found in the smooth muscle on the uterus. They are usually firm, round, and gray-white in appearance. Because they develop in the uterine wall, they may distort the wall or protrude into the uterine cavity. Unfortunately, they do not usually produce symptoms except when one becomes twisted and produces abdominal pain. They are usually discovered during routine gynecological examinations. Surgery is recommended only when the fibroids cause serious symptoms or complications.

Infertility
Infertility in females usually occurs as a result of an ovulation problem; however, the cause may also lie in the fallopian tubes or lining of the uterus (the endometrium). If the fallopian tubes are blocked or damaged, the sperm may not be able to reach the egg. Or the cervical mucus may be such that it destroys or damages the sperm, thereby preventing conception. Only a complete physical workup by a specialist in fertility may discover the exact cause of the problem. Where possible, medical treatment (with fertility drugs) or surgery may correct the problem. When more serious problems exist, it may be necessary to consider alternate methods of conception.

Premenstrual Syndrome
Many women suffer from symptoms during their menstrual cycle that may cause such discomforts as emotional unpredictability, slight depression, weight gain from fluid retention, and/or tenderness of the breasts. Some women also experience uncontrolled bouts of anger, spells of crying, food cravings, migraines, and severe depression. This condition is known as premenstrual syndrome and is suffered by many women at some time or another during their childbearing years. These symptoms are caused by chemical changes that take place in the woman's body before menstruation.

COMPONENTS OF THE MALE REPRODUCTIVE SYSTEM
The male reproductive system, unlike the female system, is primarily outside the body. Major components of the system are the penis, testicles, prostate gland, seminal vesicle, and the vas deferens. Sperm, or spermatozoa, is the male sex cell responsible for fertilizing the female ovum, or egg. It carries twenty-three chromosomes, which join the twenty-three in the female egg at fertilization. Sperm also carries the X and Y chromosomes, which determine the sex of the baby.

Penis
The penis, the external male sex organ, is cylindrical in shape and contains erectile tissue which fills with blood during sexual excitation. This causes the penis to enlarge and become hard so that it may penetrate the female vagina more easily and deposit sperm near the cervix. The urethra is a tube that lies inside the penis and is used to pass both urine and semen, but not at the same time. The head of the penis is called the glans, and it is covered by a foreskin unless the male has been circumcised. Circumcision is the surgical removal of the foreskin, the

flap of tissue that covers the head of the penis. This operation is performed, usually on newborns, to reduce the risk of infection by preventing the accumulation of secretions (called smegma) under the foreskin, where bacteria can breed. Many doctors believe that circumcision may also help to prevent cancer of the penis, but the American Academy of Pediatrics holds that circumcision is ultimately unnecessary.

During intercourse, the heart rate increases, blood pressure rises, and the testes begin to contract rhythmically, causing semen to move into the urethra. Once the sperm mixes with fluids (semen) from the seminal vesicles and the prostate gland, contractions of muscles at the base of the penis cause ejaculation, or a release of the semen. Following the climax of sexual excitation, or orgasm, the penis returns to a flaccid state.

Testes (Testicles) and Sperm

The testes, also called testicles, are glistening, pink-white oval-shaped glands that weigh ½ ounce each and are about 1½ inches long. They produce sperm cells and testosterone, the male hormone that helps to create muscle, bone, and other tissues.

At birth, the testes are in the abdomen, but shortly thereafter they descend through the inguinal canal into a pouch called the scrotum. The testes are housed outside the body because they need to be about 3 degrees cooler than the rest of the body, in order to produce fertile sperm. To achieve this, the scrotum contains sweat glands that allow evaporation to cool the testes.

The testes are supported in the scrotum by the spermatic cord, which also contains the vas deferens and the arteries and veins that supply the testes. This cord may lengthen to allow the testes to drop away from the body if they become too warm. If they become too cool, the cord shortens and pulls the testes closer to the body.

Sperm is produced in the seminiferous tubules (a series of canals within the testicles), which empty into the epididymis, where sperm is stored until it is mature. On average, the testes produce about 50 million sperm cells a day. The testes also contain millions of Leydig cells, which produce testosterone.

Sperm cells are the smallest cells in the body, and resemble tiny tadpoles. They contain twenty-three chromosomes, including both the boy-producing Y chromosomes and the girl-producing X chromo-

somes; the woman produces only X chromosomes. Therefore, sperm determines the sex of the baby. Sperm cells can swim 7 inches per hour, a necessary task if it is to reach the female's egg and penetrate it with the help of its enzymes. A man can release up to 600 million sperm cells in a single emission.

When a boy reaches puberty, the pituitary gland releases hormones that cause the tubules to begin to produce sperm and the Leydig cells to release another hormone called testosterone. Testosterone causes muscle to develop, the voice to deepen, a beard to grow. Further, it is normal for males to experience erections during sleep if they are (or are not) dreaming about something sexual.

Most testosterone is produced when the man is between the ages of 25 and 35. After 60, the levels drop as energy and drive decrease; however, there is still enough in the system to retain male characteristics.

A *vasectomy* is the tying off or surgical cutting of the vas deferens so that sperm may no longer be transported out of the testicles. After a vasectomy is performed, semen no longer contains sperm, but sperm production is not inhibited. There is also no effect on the man's ability to obtain an erection or to achieve orgasm. The purpose of a vasectomy is to cause sterilization in the man for the purpose of contraception, or pregnancy prevention. The surgery can be reversed, but only at about a 70 percent rate of success.

Semen

Male fertility, or the ability to impregnate a female, requires not only sperm but also semen, the secretions that suspend the sperm. The seminal vesicles, which lie behind the bladder, produce most of the semen, which contains fructose, vitamins, and amino acids to nourish the sperm, mucus for lubrication, and prostaglandins.

Prostate Gland

The chestnut-sized prostate gland, which lies just under the bladder, secretes a fluid that counteracts acidity in the vas deferens and the vagina.

Under the prostate are two tiny yellow glands called Cowper's glands, which secrete a cleansing fluid into the urethra just before ejaculation to prevent damage to the sperm. Urine and semen are kept from simultaneously exiting the urethra by nervous reflexes. This is to protect the sperm from the urine's acidic contents.

MAJOR PROBLEMS AND COMMON DISORDERS OF THE MALE REPRODUCTIVE SYSTEM

Cancer

Cancer of the prostate is the second most common cancer in men. Early detection and treatment are the keys to a full recovery. Symptoms usually include difficulty in starting urination, weak stream, and increased frequency of urination. A digital examination of the prostate in conjunction with ultrasound and possibly a biopsy can confirm a diagnosis of prostate cancer. Additionally, a blood test, called the prostate-specific antigen test, can help diagnose cancer. If the cancer is confined to the prostate gland, it may be removed or treated with radiation. Since prostate cancer may be linked to the level of testosterone in the system, hormone treatment may be used to reduce the levels.

Cancer of the testicles affects about 2 men in 100,000 per year. Tumors in the testicles can be discovered early by means of periodic self-examination. Fortunately, this form of cancer responds well to chemotherapy when detected early. Any change in the size or consistency of either testicle should be checked by a doctor.

Infertility

Infertility is the inability of the male to produce or deliver enough healthy sperm to bring about conception. A low sperm count, called oligospermia, occurs when the man does not produce enough sperm cells. Or the man may produce defective sperm cells that aren't able to survive very long after ejaculation and never reach the egg. Only a complete physical workup, including an examination of sperm, can locate the cause of male infertility.

Impotence

Impotence, or an inability to attain an erection adequate to complete sexual intercourse, is common and occurs in many men at one time or another. The cause is usually fatigue, illness, or stress and anxiety. Other causes may be the use of drugs, neurological diseases, diabetes, arteriosclerosis, cancer, radical prostate surgery, infections, and genitourinary injuries. Treatment varies, depending on the exact cause.

SEXUALLY TRANSMITTED DISEASES

Sexually transmitted diseases (STDs), once known as venereal diseases, are common in both men and women. See "AIDS" and "Sexually Transmitted Diseases and Sexual Problems" in section 2, "Medical Conditions."

Skeletal System

WHAT IS THE SKELETAL SYSTEM?

The skeletal system is the framework that gives the body its shape. It is made up of about 206 separate bones and weighs about 20 pounds. Without the skeleton, we would be little more than an amorphous collection of tissue without shape and definition.

The skeleton serves several important purposes. It protects the internal organs as well as allows for standing and walking. In addition, bone marrow, the fluid found inside the bones, produces red blood cells that carry nutrients to the tissues of the body, and produces white cells that help protect the body from potentially harmful diseases.

Each bone is covered with a thin layer of skin called the periosteum. The periosteum contains nerves and blood vessels that supply the bones with nutrients. Beneath the periosteum lies the dense, rigid compact bone, which contains thousands of tiny holes and passageways. Through these run more nerves and blood vessels that carry nutrients into the bone. Inside the layer of compact bone lies spongy bone which encases a gelatinlike substance, the bone marrow.

Bone marrow produces white blood cells (which fight infection), red blood cells (which carry oxygen), and platelets (which help stop bleeding).

COMPONENTS OF THE SKELETAL SYSTEM

The skull, vertebrae (constituting the spine), and rib cage form the axial skeleton. The skull and vertebrae protect your brain and spinal cord. In between the twenty-eight vertebrae are spongy cushions called disks. The vertebrae and disks are held together by a network of muscles and ligaments. The last bone in the line of vertebrae is known as the coccyx, or tailbone.

The rest of the skeletal bones are known as the appendicular skeleton and include the shoulder, arms, hands, hips, legs, and feet. The skull has twenty-eight bones, eight of which are fused to cover the brain. At the base of the skull lies a large hole that surrounds the top of the spinal cord. The shoulder group includes the shovel-shaped scapula and the key-shaped clavicle. The upper arm bone is known as the humerus, which connects with the lower arm bones, a pair known as the radius and ulna. From here extend the wrist bones (carpals), palm bones (metacarpals), and fingers (phalanges).

Along with the thick breastbone, the twenty-four ribs anchored to the spine protect the heart and lungs.

The lower half of the skeletal system begins with the pelvis and continues with the thighbone (femur), kneecap (patella), shinbone (tibia) and fibula, the ankle (talus), the heel (calcaneus), the foot bones (metatarsals), and toes (phalanges).

Bones are connected by joints. There are three types of joints: fixed joints, which hold the bones firmly together, as in the plates of the skull; partly movable joints, which allow some mobility, as in the spine; and freely movable joints, which allow for plenty of mobility, as in major joints such as the knees and elbows.

The male and female skeletons differ slightly in that male bones are somewhat larger and heavier, and the hipbones of the female are spaced farther apart to allow room for the carrying of a baby.

MAJOR PROBLEMS AND COMMON DISORDERS OF THE SKELETAL SYSTEM

The bones, just like other body systems, are subject to diseases and injury. Bones are subject to tumors (cancer), degenerative diseases (arthritis, osteoporosis, scoliosis, spondylolisthesis), and fractures (broken bones).

Bone cancer is a relatively uncommon disease. Back pain and swelling in the joints are the most common symptoms. Bone cancer has often spread to distant organs, such as the lungs, by the time it is diagnosed. Treatment includes radiation and

Fractures

A fracture is a break, rupture, or discontinuity of a bone, which occurs as a result of a physical force being exerted on a bone—a force that is greater than the bone can withstand.

Symptoms of a fracture are local pain, swelling or bruising over a bone, tenderness, and deformity where the injury occurred. Medical attention should be sought. A doctor may be able to tell whether a bone is fractured just by looking at it. In some instances, however, an X ray of the bone may be necessary. Inspection of vessel and nerve damage may also be necessary.

A *simple fracture* is a simple break in which the bone does not pierce the skin.

A *compound fracture* is one in which the broken bone is exposed though a wound in the skin.

A *greenstick fracture* occurs mostly in immature long bones of children, in which one side of the bone is broken and the other side is unbroken but may bend.

A *comminuted fracture* is one in which a part of the damaged bone is broken into fragments or shattered.

A *pathological fracture* is one that occurs in bone already weakened by an existing pathological process such as osteomalacia, metastatic cancer, or tuberculosis.

A *transverse fracture* occurs at right angles to the long part of the involved bone; an *oblique fracture* is one that breaks at a slanting, or oblique, angle.

Treatment of a fracture depends on where the injury occurred; however, the general rule is to immobilize the bone with a bandage dressing, a sling, a splint, a cast, or a combination of these. If the bone has been displaced from its usual position, it must be set in its proper position in order to heal properly. "Reduction" is the medical term for setting the bone. Sometimes surgery is required in order to reset bone, and sometimes not.

Understanding the Medical Terminology

An understanding of the various uses of the medical term "open" is necessary in order to communicate effectively with your practitioner in the treatment and repair of a fracture.

Almost invariably the result of trauma, an *open fracture* is one in which there is an open wound that reaches all the way down to the site of the fracture, with at least part of the bone exposed. A *closed fracture* is one that does not have such a wound associated with it.

Now to treatment: An *open reduction* is a surgical procedure that involves opening of the skin and other soft tissue to gain access to the site of the fracture to align the broken ends properly or to insert a fixation device. Open reductions can be done on both closed and open fractures. Finally, to add to the confusion, some open reductions can be done through a small incision and the use of an arthroscope—an instrument that consists of a tube, an optical system of magnifying lenses, and a fibroscopic light source. Arthroscopy, as the procedure is called, is minimally invasive, does not require a large incision, and is usually cited as an alternative to the open procedure.

chemotherapy, which has dramatically improved the ability to treat the spread of bone cancer. Other treatment includes the surgical removal of the cancerous bone and then the administration of anticancer drugs to treat the cancer that may spread to the lungs and other organs.

Arthritis is simply characterized as pain in the joints. It has many causes, including inflammation of the joint membrane, cartilage breakdown, infection, and metabolic and other disorders. Treatment for arthritis should be sought if the pain interferes with daily activity or with sleep. Treatment ranges from rest and exercise to surgery, in extreme cases.

Osteoporosis is a disease in which the bones become thin and brittle as a result of a deficiency of calcium, an important nutrient for strength and hardness of the bones. If the daily intake of calcium is deficient, the body is forced to pull calcium from the bones. As the calcium is depleted, the bones become porous and very weak, making them more susceptible to fractures. The disease affects mainly the spinal column, causing backaches and rounded shoulders. Osteoporosis is more common in postmenopausal women and is one reason older people tend to shrink in size as they age. Treatment includes a higher intake of calcium, estrogen therapy, and exercise.

Scoliosis is a progressive, degenerative condition that affects the spine, causing it to rotate and become misshapen, often appearing S-shaped. This condition may be diagnosed during infancy or adolescence. Although the exact cause of scoliosis has yet to be determined, it is believed to be a genetic defect.

As the condition progresses, the space between the vertebrae increases, causing them to become thicker on one side. Eventually, the person develops severe deformity such as rounded shoulders, swayback, and sunken chest. Spinal braces may be used to halt the deformity; however, if the condition has progressed to a stage where braces are ineffective, then surgery is the only alternative.

Steel rods, called Harrington rods, are implanted along the spine after it has been straightened surgically. In addition, bone fragments are placed around the rods. As healing takes place, tissue, bone fragments, and rods fuse into a single unit able to support the straightened spine.

Spondylolisthesis is a condition that occurs when one of the vertebra slips over the one below it, especially in the lower back or lumbar region. When the normally bony arch of the vertebrae becomes soft, they tend to slip forward, putting pressure on spinal nerves and causing pain. This condition may also result when osteoarthritis has caused the joints between the vertebrae to become worn and unstable.

Treatment may consist of traction or the application of a plaster cast to immobilize the area. Physical therapy may be helpful in eliminating discomfort and increasing mobility. In those cases where the condition does not respond to conservative treatment, surgery to fuse the vertebrae may be necessary.

Bones are strong—very strong, in fact—but if enough pressure is applied, they will break. When this happens, we call it a fracture. There are five types of fractures: simple, compound, greenstick, pathological, and comminuted (See pg. 23).

After the bone has been set, immobilization is usually necessary to minimize pain and facilitate healing. Casts, splints, and traction are the usual devices or methods used to immobilize bones.

Skin

The skin is the largest and most visible organ in the body. It protects our bodies from the sun, bacteria, and infection. The skin regulates body temperature, stores fat and water, senses the environment, excretes sweat, and aids in the body's synthesis of vitamin D.

COMPONENTS OF THE SKIN

The skin is composed of the epidermis, dermis, and subcutaneous tissue. The epidermis, the outermost layer of the skin, is composed of flat squamous cells, round basal cells, and a stratum corneum (a nonliving keratinous layer). Also found in the epidermis are keratinocytes (producers of keratin), melanocytes (producers of melanin), and Langerhans' cells (linked with immune system surveillance). The epidermis not only regulates water loss (through openings called pores), produces melanin and keratin, and serves as the barrier between the environment and the internal organs, but also is the site of new skin cell production.

The dermis, made up of an upper section called the papillary dermis and a lower section called the reticular dermis, contains reticuloendothelial cells, fibrous connective tissue, follicles, blood and lymph vessels, sweat and sebaceous glands, sensory nerves, and muscle. And the subcutaneous tissue is mainly composed of fat, which protects against injury, insulates the body, and is a reserve for calories.

MAJOR PROBLEMS AND COMMON DISORDERS OF THE SKIN

The occurrence of major problems of the skin has been attributed to cell and follicle dysfunction, parasites, various allergens and irritants, infection, heredity, and excessive sunlight exposure. Common skin disorders and afflictions include acne, rosacea, psoriasis, dermatitis, bacterial infections, and skin cancer.

Acne, a skin disorder resulting in an eruption of pimples on the skin, commonly affects teenagers because changing levels of hormone activity cause the sebaceous glands to produce an excess of oil (sebum). Sebum, skin cells, and bacteria collect and build up in the follicles of the skin and cause pimples to form. The sebum ruptures the follicle walls, allowing whiteheads (a closed pore), blackheads (an open pore), and pimples to appear on the skin's surface. Sebaceous cysts appear when the sebum does not rupture the skin and, instead, forms a lump under the skin.

The treatment of acne usually involves the application of some kind of topical antibacterial product, such as benzoyl peroxide or tretinoin (Retin-A). Or antibiotics may be utilized, in both topical and oral form, to combat the infection. These include oral and topical tetracycline, erythromycin, and topical clindamycin. Other treatment methods are the use of Accutane (oral isotretinoin), cortisone injections, estrogen therapy, and ultraviolet light therapy. In the case of cystic acne, minor surgery and dermabrasion may be implemented to remove sebaceous cysts.

Rosacea is a skin condition that results in redness and inflammation of the skin, primarily affecting the face. As rosacea progresses, the skin flushes and exhibits tiny pimples (papules and pustules) and dilated blood vessels (telangiectasia). Rosacea may escalate into a condition known as rhinophyma. Rhinophyma is characterized by a bulbous nose and red lines and bumps on the skin's surface. The treatment of rosacea involves the use of topical steroid applications and both topical and oral antibacterial products. Rhinophyma may be treated with laser or scalpel surgery and dermabrasion.

Psoriasis is characterized by a scaling of the skin caused by the overproduction of skin cells. The scales may have a silverish appearance and can be removed by softening and scrubbing them. The thickening, pitting, or crumbling of fingernails may also be a result of psoriasis. Common treatments of psoriasis include the use of topical steroid preparations or coal tar preparations, ultraviolet light therapy, drugs such as anthralin and methotrexate, and PUVA therapy (the use of psoralen and ultraviolet light).

Dermatitis, or *eczema*, is a general term used to describe any inflammation of the skin. One type of dermatitis, atopic eczema, results from an allergic reaction to various allergens ranging from wool to detergent. The itching, blistering, and crusting rash that results from atopic dermatitis can be treated with oral antibiotics, ultraviolet light therapy, and topical corticosteroids.

Avoiding the allergen, stress, and extreme temperatures also aid in treating atopic dermatitis. Allergic contact dermatitis results from exposure to any allergen to which the body is sensitive. Allergens include the sun, dyes, cosmetics, plants (poison ivy, oak, sumac), clothing, metal compounds, and ingredients in certain medications.

Contact dermatitis results in inflamed, red, itchy skin and blisters. Treatment consists of the identification and the removal of the offending allergen, and the use of topical corticosteroid cream may be helpful to the patient before the blistering phase of allergic contact dermatitis appears.

Seborrheic dermatitis is a condition where the skin is red and inflamed and causes yellowish, greasy scales to appear on the scalp (dandruff), face, and other areas of the body. The itching and general discomfort of seborrheic dermatitis can be treated with hydrocortisone creams (for facial seborrheic dermatitis) and, for the scalp, shampoos containing zinc pyrithione, selenium sulfide, sulfur and salicylic acid, or tar. Other types of dermatitis include nummular dermatitis, stasis dermatitis, and exfoliative dermatitis.

Common disorders of the skin can also be caused by various types of *fungal* and *bacterial infections*. Fungal infections, which are dermophyte infections (infections where fungi infect dead skin, hair, or nails), include tinea corporis (ringworm), tinea cruris (jock itch), and tinea pedis (athlete's foot). Bacterial infections include impetigo, ecthyma, folliculitis (of hair follicles), carbunculosis, furunculosis, and paronychial infections (of nails). Skin disorders can also stem from viral infections (herpes, warts, cold sores, chicken pox), parasitic infections (scabies, pediculosis), yeast infections (candidiasis), or can be related to problems associated with pigmentation (vitiligo, albinism).

Skin cancer, a steadily growing affliction whose cases increase each year, is primarily caused by skin and skin cell exposure to ultraviolet light (UVL). Prolonged UVL exposure has not only been linked to skin cancer but has also been known to cause premature aging and wrinkling of the skin and damage to the eyes.

Nature of UVL

UVL refers to the light found from 200 to 400 nm on the broad spectrum of solar radiation which reaches the earth's surface. (Light wavelengths are measured in nanometers [nm].) All wavelengths of solar radiation can affect the skin, but UVL is the most damaging. There are three types of UVL: UVA (320 to 400 nm), UVB (290 to 320 nm), and UVC (200 to 290 nm). Two of these three—UVA and UVB—pass through the earth's ozone layer and can damage the skin.

As to which UVL is more harmful, or is the culprit in causing skin cancer, scientists and researchers find themselves in considerable debate. It is thought, though, that UVB is the ultraviolet light that produces sunburns, tans, and cancer. UVA can produce a tan but penetrates the skin more deeply and thoroughly than UVB and contributes to skin damage when coupled with UVB exposure.

When skin is exposed to UVL, skin cells, or more specifically, the cell's DNA, is rearranged and damaged. UVL also damages the body's immune system and its ability to combat tumor cells. In particular, UVB inhibits the Langerhans' cell's function of immune system surveillance. Immediate overexposure to the sun results in a sunburn—a damaging burn of the skin where the blood vessels close to the skin's surface increase their blood flow, producing redness.

Melanin, a dark pigment produced by skin cells, is manufactured as a defensive measure against the sun's rays. Melanin blocks, absorbs, and scatters UVL wavelengths. As a result, the skin tans over a period of time to increase its defense against sun exposure. The skin also has at its disposal keratin and urocanic acid, which both aid in absorbing UVL. However, long-term exposure, in conjunction with other factors, contributes to skin cancer.

There are three types of skin cancer: basal cell carcinoma, squamous cell carcinoma, and malignant melanoma.

Basal Cell and Squamous Cell Carcinomas

Of the three types of skin cancer, basal cell carcinoma and squamous cell carcinoma are nonmelanoma (nonmalignant) cancers and are the most common types of skin cancer. Skin cell carcinomas are cancers that start in the covering or outer layer of the skin. Both round basal cells and flat squamous cells are found in the epidermis, the skin's outer layer, and have the potential to grow into a mass of tissue (tumor) when damaged by the sun. The tumors appear on the skin's surface as bumps or nodules on the face, neck, head, hands, or trunk. Basal and squamous cell tumors manifest themselves in numerous ways on the skin's surface: smooth or bleeding and crusting lumps or scaly, red, and flat patches.

The tumors normally do not metastasize (grow and spread to other areas of the body). However, if neglected or left untreated, the tumors have the capacity to spread. Treatment of nonmelanoma skin cancers is successful 95 percent of the time. There are several treatment procedures, their use contingent on the location, size, type, and progression of growth of the tumors. These procedures are surgery; curettage (in which a small spoon-shaped device scrapes away the tumor); and such specialized types of surgery as cryosurgery (use of subfreezing temperatures to destroy tissue), chemosurgery (application of chemicals to destroy tissue), electrosurgery (surgery done with an electric instrument), and radiation therapy.

Malignant Melanoma

Malignant melanoma may arise from pigmented moles and lesions due to exposure to sunlight or because of hereditary factors. Malignant (cancerous) melanomas develop in the pigment-producing cells of the skin, the melanocytes. The cells grow abnormally and develop into tumors. Malignant melanomas often metastasize through the bloodstream and can affect and invade other organs of the body. Treatment of malignant melanomas largely depends upon the progression of the cancer, the tumor size and the extent of its growth, and how deeply the tumors are embedded into the skin. Treatment procedures include surgery (for tumors that have not metastasized), chemotherapy, and biological therapy.

Risk Factors for Skin Cancer

Many factors contribute to the development of skin cancer. Family history of skin cancer and skin disorders, habitual exposure to UVL, an outdoor occupation, and severe childhood sunburns can all contribute to developing skin cancer. Individuals who are fair-complected, have light-colored eyes and hair, and tan poorly or burn easily are also at risk, as are individuals who have nonhereditary skin disorders such as albinism (marked by partial or total lack of pigment in the body), xeroderma pigmentosum (marked by extreme sensitivity to ultraviolet light), freckles on the upper portion of the back, actinic keratoses (red or brown rough patches on skin due to the sun), or moles.

Cancer Detection in Moles

Since 70 percent of melanoma tumors arise from preexisting moles, it is important to detect any abnormalities in moles. In order to check to see if a preexisting mole is cancerous, there are certain indications one can look for in a self-examination. One should look for any asymmetricality in a mole, one that is not uniform or circular in shape; border irregularities such as rough edges; color differences such as blue, black, or pink, which vary from the normal brown color of moles; diameter changes greater than 6 mm. This monitoring process can be easily remembered as *ABCD*.

Other warning signs for melanoma in moles include itchy, oozing, or bleeding moles, mole pigment spreading, sensations of pain in moles, and abnormalities in the surrounding skin. Moles are usually found on the back and lower extremities; however, men commonly develop them on the neck, head, and trunk, and women usually find them on the arms and lower leg area.

How to Limit Sun Exposure

The best preventive measure to take against skin cancer is to avoid the sun and UVL. Keeping in mind that there is no "safe" way to tan, it is wise to avoid even artificial tans acquired by sunlamps and tanning beds. One can use a self-tanning lotion to achieve a tan color, but this coloration does not protect the skin in any way against UVL. One can limit sun exposure by staying out of the sun during its peak hours (10:00 A.M. to 2:00 P.M.); by wearing polarized sunglasses, broad-rimmed hats, and long-sleeve, tightly weaved, light-colored clothing; and by applying sunscreens and sunblocks.

Sunscreens and Sunblocks

Sunscreens and sunblocks are lotions, oils, sprays, gels, and creams that help screen or block out the UV rays. Sunblocks scatter and deflect UVL, and sunscreens absorb UVL. Sunscreens that absorb

UVB are given an SPF (Sun Protection Factor) number which indicates how long a person can stay in the sun until he or she burns. To calculate how long you can stay in the sun with sunscreen before burning, multiply the SPF number by how long it takes you to burn without sunscreen. If your skin takes 10 minutes of sun exposure in order to burn, with the application of a sunscreen with SPF 15, you may spend 2½ hours in the sun before burning. SPF numbers range from 2 to 50 and contain such ingredients as PABA (para–aminobenzoic acid), cinnamates (octylmethoxy cinnamate and cinoxate), and salicylates for UVB protection; benzophenones (oxybenzone and sulisobenzone), dibenzoylmethane derivatives, and 3 percent avobenzone (Parsol 1789) for UVA protection.

Most skin experts suggest an SPF number of 15 or higher to achieve adequate protection from the sun. Before choosing a sunscreen, however, it is important to consider for which area of the body you are using the sunscreen—for example, the lips and face are more sensitive—which skin type you are (fair, medium, dark), whether you are allergic to sunscreen ingredients (some people are allergic to PABA), whether the sunscreen is waterproof, and what kind of activity you are going to engage in. Two general rules to bear in mind about sunscreen application are: Apply liberally on all exposed areas of the skin 30 minutes to 1 hour before sun exposure and reapply every 2 hours or after sweating or swimming. You should keep in mind that UVL is present all year round, is found in increasingly higher levels due to ozone depletion, is at a stronger intensity at the equator and at high altitudes, and can produce photosensitivity reactions in people taking certain medications (tetracycline, furosemide, and hydrochlorothiazide). Remember, too, that 80 percent of UVL is not affected by cloud cover, and UVL can be reflected and intensified by sand and water.

Further, since severe, blistering sunburns in early childhood have been linked to the development of skin cancer in later life, it is wise to keep small infants out of the sun and to protect the skin of young children.

Research into sunblocks made from ingredients such as titanium dioxide or zinc oxide and which block out most or all of UVA and UVB rays has been hopeful. Efforts to try to decrease the whitish film that appears on the skin and to increase the cosmetic value of such products have also been encouraging.

At this time, however, no sunscreen or sunblock guarantees total UVL protection.

Frankly, the best way to avoid UVL is to avoid the sun—which most people find difficult to accept or even to acknowledge. Deeply entrenched attitudes toward sun exposure and the "healthy" tan may have to change before proper and sensible skin care can develop.

Urinary System

The urinary system, composed of the kidneys, ureters, bladder, and urethra, is responsible for eliminating liquid waste products from the body. It also assists in maintaining a balance of salts and other dissolved minerals in the blood.

During metabolism, a process that releases energy from food and nourishes the cells of the body, waste products are created as the cells use the nutrients delivered by the bloodstream. It is then the responsibility of the urinary system to filter the blood and remove these waste products.

COMPONENTS OF THE URINARY SYSTEM

The kidneys are a pair of bean-shaped, reddish-brown organs, about the size of a fist, located in the back of the abdomen on each side of the spine. Each kidney weighs about 5 to 6 ounces. The kidneys filter urea, uric acid, and creatinine (liquid waste), which have been collected and carried to the kidneys by the blood.

Indeed, blood passes through the kidneys continuously, and the kidneys clean and filter it, ridding it of waste that may be deadly. This is achieved by the kidney's 1 million tiny filtering units, called nephrons. The kidneys prevent red blood cells and protein from passing through the nephrons and return these materials to the bloodstream.

Other functions of the kidneys include the production of red blood cells and the regulation of levels of potassium, sodium chloride, and other substances. Each hour, the kidneys filter twice the amount of blood that is in the body, restoring it and its essential vitamins, amino acids, glucose, hormones, and so on. Kidneys slow their activity to about one-third during nighttime hours.

About 2 quarts of the filtered product, called urine, are produced daily. Tiny droplets of urine pass from the tubules in each kidney and collect in a reservoir at the kidney's center, which is connected to the bladder. Urine is passed to the bladder via wavelike muscular contractions of the ureters every 10 to 30 seconds.

The ureters are two narrow (about the size of pencil lead) 12-inch-long tubes. The ureters empty urine into the bladder, where it is stored over several hours until urination occurs. Special valves between the bladder and ureters prevent urine from flowing back toward the kidneys.

The bladder is a punching-bag-shaped flexible, muscular reservoir, with a urine capacity of 6 to 24 ounces. As urine collects in the bladder, the bladder gradually expands until it becomes full. Reflexes in the bladder help hold the urine until enough has been collected for urination, the process by which urine is excreted from the body. Worry, anxiety, or fear can increase blood pressure and increase the speed at which urine is produced. Although the bladder may not be full, these stresses may tighten the bladder wall and cause the person to feel the need to urinate.

Urination begins when the muscles of the bladder contract, allowing urine to flow out of the bladder through the urethra. The amount of fluid that passes through the urethra varies each day, from 1 pint to 2 gallons, depending on food and liquid intake and fluid losses from sweat glands and lungs. Cold weather can increase frequency of urination, and warm weather can decrease it. Urine production drops by one-fourth during sleep hours.

The components of urine can reveal a great deal about what is happening in the body. This analysis is done through a test called a urinalysis, defined as any physical, chemical, or microscopic examination of urine. If it is cloudy, malodorous or discolored, a person should consult a physician. Cloudiness may indicate the presence of a bladder or kidney infection, or it could just be an effect of strenuous exercise. Normally, urine has a slightly aromatic, distinctive odor; however, this may change if a person is taking certain medications, eating certain foods, or has an unusual or abnormal metabolic condition, such as diabetes.

A number of other medical conditions, such as heart disease, psoriasis, and endocrine disorders, can be diagnosed with the help of a urinalysis. Virtually all organs empty waste products into the bloodstream, which are then filtered through the kidneys and show up in urine. An examination of these waste products can help determine how well a particular organ or gland is functioning. During pregnancy the body secretes the hormone HCG, which can be detected by testing the woman's urine with a home pregnancy test kit.

MAJOR PROBLEMS AND COMMON DISORDERS OF THE URINARY SYSTEM

Bladder tumors, either benign or cancerous, develop inside the lining of the bladder, and occur more often in men than in women. These tumors grow from the walls and tend to resemble small mushrooms.

Most bladder tumors produce no noticeable symptoms. The first sign that there might be a problem is blood in the urine. The doctor performs a digital rectal or vaginal examination to feel for any lumps in the bladder. Urine samples are taken and analyzed for the presence of cells that might be cancerous. A cystoscopic examination permits the doctor to directly view the bladder and obtain tissue specimens for biopsy.

Bladder cancers may be treated by surgery, radiation therapy, chemotherapy, or any combination of these methods. In the most serious cases, the bladder must be removed and an artificial bladder is created outside the body.

Cancer of the kidneys generally falls into three categories: nephroblastoma (also called Wilms' tumor), renal cell carcinoma, and transitional cell carcinoma. Nephroblastoma affects children under the age of 4, and accounts for about 20 percent of all cancers in children. Renal cell carcinoma usually occurs after the age of 40 and accounts for about 75 percent of all kidney cancer. Transitional cell carcinoma affects the cells lining the renal pelvis and usually develops in smokers or those who have taken large quantities of painkillers.

These conditions may be diagnosed by ultrasound, CT scanning, intravenous pyelography (IVP), or renal biopsy. Treatment may involve removing the kidney and the ureters if necessary and, where appropriate, follow-up chemotherapy and radiation therapy.

Glomerulonephritis is the name given to a serious kidney condition that affects the filtering part of the kidney. It may occur as either an acute (short-term) or chronic (long-term) infection. When it enters the chronic stage, it eventually leads to kidney failure, at which point the person must rely on dialysis to artificially filter the blood.

Diagnosing glomerulonephritis requires laboratory examination of the blood and urine to determine the level of functioning of the kidneys. Finding certain antibodies in the blood may indicate the presence of infection, and examination of the urine may reveal certain proteins and other elements ordinarily not present.

Treatment is difficult and may include steroids or immunosuppressant drugs. Another process, called plasmapheresis, may be used to filter the blood of those people with glomerulonephritis. Changes in diet and nutrition—such as restricting potassium, protein, and salt—may reduce the strain put on the kidney by this condition.

Polycystic kidney disease is a hereditary condition that causes large quantities of cysts to grow within the kidney. As these cysts increase in size, they destroy normal kidney tissue, thereby causing the kidney to fail. As kidney function is reduced, it is necessary to artificially cleanse these people's blood through a process called dialysis. The only effective treatment for polycystic kidneys is a kidney transplant.

Cysts are fluid-filled sacs that grow within the kidney. It is not unusual for people over the age of 50 to have some growth of cysts in their kidneys, but in most cases these cause no problems.

Discolored urine usually indicates that the urine is very concentrated, which may be the result of decreased fluid intake, the recent completion of strenuous exercise, certain drugs or medications being taken, or a number of other factors. Light-colored urine indicates an increase in the amount of fluids consumed and the kidneys' ability to eliminate excess water.

Hematuria, the presence of blood in the urine, is very serious, as this could indicate injury to the kidney and subsequent bleeding or the presence of an infection, or it could be the result of strenuous exercise, such as jogging or bicycle riding. In any event, a physician should be consulted immediately whenever blood is noticed.

Kidney stones may indicate a high level of uric acid in the kidneys, ureters, or bladder. Stones are formed when the mineral content of urine becomes too concentrated due to a lack of fluid intake, chronic infections, misuse of medication, blockages, or certain metabolic disorders. Lack of exercise and loss of water through perspiration during warm weather can increase the risk of stones. These stones may vary from the size of tiny bits of gravel to extreme cases of 14 pounds.

Urinary tract infection (UTI) is a term that may be used to describe *urethritis* (inflammation of the urethra), *cystitis* (inflammation of the bladder), or *pyelonephritis* (inflammation of the kidney). These infections are most often caused by bacteria that have spread from the rectum to the urethra and bladder.

Symptoms associated with urethritis and cystitis are generally a need to pass urine and pain upon urination. The urine may or may not have a distinctive odor and there may or may not be blood present. The symptoms associated with pyelonephritis are chills, fever, and lower-back pain.

Women tend to experience a higher incidence of UTI than men because of the shortness of their urethras (the tube through which urine is expelled from the body) and diaphragm use. UTIs such as nonspecific urethritis are most likely contracted as a result of sexual activity.

A diagnosis is made by examining a urine sample, taken midstream to avoid further contamination, under a microscope and looking for pus cells. Another method involves adding a few drops of urine to a culture dish and attempting to grow the particular bacterium responsible for the infection.

UTIs respond well to antibiotics, and in many cases physicians will begin a regimen of antibiotics before all lab results are completed.

Glossary of Basic Components of the Human Anatomy

Adenoids—masses of glandlike lymphatic tissue located behind the nose and on the back wall of the upper throat. In children, adenoids help, with the tonsils, to protect the body against inhaled germs. Around age 9 or 10, they begin to shrink. By adolescence, the adenoids have usually disappeared.

Adrenal glands—two tiny glands lying atop the kidneys that are divided into outer cortex and inner medulla and have two separate functions. The cortex produces hormones called steroids, which are important in sexual development, in maintaining body strength, and in metabolizing fats, carbohydrates, proteins, sodium, and potassium. The medulla, which is part of the sympathetic nervous system, releases the chemical adrenaline to prepare muscles, heart, and blood vessels for instant action.

Aorta—the largest artery in the body, leading from the left ventricle of the heart, over and down through the chest, through the diaphragm and into the abdomen, ending near the fourth lumbar vertebrae. Branches of the aorta supply blood to all parts of the body.

Appendix—a 3-to-6-inch-long appendage or sac jutting out from the cecum of the colon near the junction of the colon and the small intestine. Roughly the size and shape of an earthworm, it can become inflamed, causing appendicitis. The appendix's function is unknown.

Auditory nerve—the nerve that connects the inner ear to the brain and transmits impulses to the brain.

Bladder—an elastic organ, located below the kidneys in the pelvis, whose function is to store urine until it is released through the urethra. It is composed of a strong network of muscle fibers that stretch as urine collects. Long tubes called ureters carry urine from the kidneys to the bladder.

Blood—the body's life fluid, approximately 10½ pints of which flow through the average body, performing three vital functions. Blood transports oxygen, nutrients, fats, and waste products. It controls body functions and temperature by carrying hormones to all parts of the body, and it combats infection with seven main types of white blood cells. Blood is 40 percent red and white blood cells and platelets and 60 percent plasma. Plasma is a watery solution of proteins and salts in which blood cells are suspended.

Bone—the substance of which the skeleton is composed, bone is a mixture of calcium carbonate, calcium phosphate, and fibrous tissue. The body's 200-plus bones are all made up of compact and cancellous bone. Compact bone is a hard tube surrounded by membrane and enclosing the bone marrow. Cancellous bone has a fine lacework structure and forms the body's short bones and the ends of its long bones. The marrow of cancellous bone produces new red blood cells.

Brain—the central organ of the nervous system and, after the liver, the second largest of the body's internal organs, weighing about 3 pounds. Fitting inside the skull, the brain is made up of soft, pinkish-gray tissue and is buffered from the skull by tough membranes called meninges. The brain is divided into the cerebrum, the cerebral cortex, the brain stem, and the cerebellum. The brain, which has billions of cells, interprets all sense impressions, controls more than 600 voluntary muscles, regulates the nervous system, and stores information in the memory. The brain also functions as a gland, manufacturing chemicals that act like painkillers.

Breast—in women, one of two milk-secreting glands, consisting of fifteen to twenty lobes divided by fibrous tissue and extending from the nipple to armpit. The breast's lobes produce milk after the birth of a baby. Pressure by the infant's mouth on the areola (circle of dark skin surrounding the nipple) causes milk to be released from tiny surfaces on the nipple. Breasts have no muscle and take their shape from a large pad of fat cells.

Cartilage—tough, whitish, elastic tissue joined with the bone to form the skeleton. The types of cartilage include hyaline cartilage, fibrocartilage, and elastic cartilage. Hyaline cartilage, strong and slippery, makes up the ends of bones at joints and acts as a shock absorber. The nose is made of hyaline cartilage. Fibrocartilage, densely packed fibers, is the material that forms the disks between spinal vertebrae. Elastic cartilage, of which the outer ear and larynx are made, is the most flexible type of cartilage. Deteriorating cartilage can accompany osteoarthritis.

Colon—the tubelike digestive organ, about 5½ feet long, situated in a rectangular shape around the perimeter of the abdomen, connected by the ileum to the small intestine and by the rectum to the anus. The colon receives about 1 quart of material daily from the small intestine and processes it (by squeezing out liquid) into about 4 ounces of stool, which is excreted from the body through the anus.

Cornea—transparent tissue forming the outer layer of each eyeball, covering the iris and the lens. The curvature of the cornea enables it to serve as a convex lens, bending light rays inward and beginning the focusing process.

Diaphragm—a large muscle lying across the middle of the body and separating the thoracic and abdominal cavities. The diaphragm receives a signal from the brain to flatten and tense, causing the thoracic cavity to expand and enabling the lungs to breathe. Involuntary spasms of the diaphragm cause hiccups.

Ear—one of two organs of hearing and equilibrium located on either side of the head and consisting of three parts: the outer ear, the middle ear, and the inner ear.

Eardrum—a thin layer of tissue located in the auditory canal just before the ossicles of the middle ear. The eardrum vibrates when sound waves are transmitted through the auditory canal to the middle ear and the inner ear.

Esophagus—a 10-inch-long muscular tube responsible for moving food from the mouth to the stomach. The esophageal sphincter is a ring of muscles that opens to allow food to descend into the stomach and closes to prevent food from flowing back from the stomach to the esophagus.

Eustachian tube—the canal connecting the middle ear with the back of the pharynx. It equalizes pressure on either side of the eardrum and can provide a path for infection to travel from the nose to the ear. Swallowing forces air into the eustachian tube to correct the stuffy feeling in the ears caused by a change in air pressure.

Eye—one of two organs of vision located in bony sockets of the skull. Eyes consist of a pupil, through which light enters; a retina (end of the optic nerve); an iris, which gives the eye its color and narrows or widens to expand or contract the pupil; the cornea, a membrane covering the iris and pupil and refracting light; and the vitreous humor, a transparent jelly forming the main part of the eyeball. Lacrimal ducts constantly supply the eye with tears to clean and lubricate them and to protect them from infection. A set of six external ocular muscles controls and coordinates eye movement.

Fallopian tubes—two tubes, about 4 inches long, extending from the ovaries to the uterus, through which an egg passes during each menstrual period from the ovaries to the uterus, and where fertilization of an egg by a sperm occurs.

Gallbladder—a membranous sac, about 3 inches long, located below the liver. It drains bile from the liver, stores it, and sends it on to the duodenum, where it neutralizes the acidity of digested food and breaks down fatty compounds. When the gallbladder is removed, in extreme cases of infection or blockage, bile goes directly from the liver to the intestine with no ill effect on digestion.

Gums—pink, firm, fibrous tissue covering the areas of the upper and lower jaw, inside the mouth, where the teeth are located, and forming a collar around the neck of each tooth. The mucous membrane covering the gums helps carry blood and lymph from the jaws to the face.

Hair—a specialized body growth covering most of the body and consisting of dead skin cells filled with the protein keratin. The main function of hair is to help the body retain heat by standing erect to diminish the loss of body warmth. The average head can contain more than 100,000 hairs. Each hair root on the body is encased in a follicle beneath the skin. Hair color and texture, along with baldness and graying, are determined largely by heredity.

Heart—a large hollow mass of muscles that pumps blood (and with it oxygen) to every cell in the body. The heart is composed of four chambers: the right atrium and ventricle, and the left atrium and ventricle. The first two collect blood returning from the body and pump it to the lungs, where it is oxygenated. The second two pump the oxygenated blood to the body. The heart relaxes and contracts during the two phases of its beat. Its activity is controlled by electrical impulses.

Hemoglobin—a complex protein in the red blood cells containing iron and red pigment and carrying oxygen to the tissues and removing carbon dioxide from the tissues. Normal blood contains 14 to 15 mg of homoglobin per 100 ml of blood.

Hypothalamus—a gland located at the base of the brain responsible for coordinating the activities of nine glands of the endocrine system. Hormones secreted by the endocrine glands regulate growth, sexual development, activities of other glands, metabolism, and emotions. The hypothalamus secretes at least ten substances that control the activities of the pituitary gland just below it. Some scientists think the hypothalamus detects levels of hormones circulating in the blood and acts through the pituitary to achieve the required hormonal balance.

Inner ear—innermost of the three portions of the ear, which contains the cochlea and the vestibule. Sound waves cause the eardrum to vibrate, set in motion the fluid within the cochlea, and trigger a delicate membrane to stimulate thousands of sensory hair cells, which trigger the auditory nerve to send messages to the brain. The vestibule houses the utriculus and the sacculus, the two saclike organs of balance, whose sensory hair cells also stimulate nerve impulses.

Kidney—one of a pair of maroon-colored, bean-shaped organs, located at the base of the rib cage, beneath the liver and spleen, and weighing about 8 ounces each. The kidneys are connected to the circulatory system by the renal artery and renal vein. They filter waste material from the blood, forming, one drop at a time, about 1½ quarts of urine daily. About 400 gallons of blood flow daily through the kidneys.

Larynx (voice box)—a cartilaginous structure containing the vocal cords. Located in front of the throat, the larynx is held together by ligaments and moved by muscles. Besides producing sound for speech, the larynx is part of the respiratory system. In men, the largest ring of cartilage forms the Adam's apple. The epiglottis at the base of the tongue is the lid that closes the larynx during swallowing, preventing food and liquid from entering the larynx.

Ligaments—bands of tough, fibrous tissue that connect and stabilize bones at the joints. When stretched or partially torn, a sprain results. The four ligaments on the knee are especially susceptible to injury, particularly during sports.

Liver—the largest internal organ in the body, the liver is a dark red, wedge-shaped organ, weighing 3 to 4 pounds, located beneath the lower right rib cage. It has several vital functions: to produce bile to digest fat; to produce and store glycogen for conversion to glucose; to synthesize protein and form urea; to store vitamins A, D, E, and K; and to produce blood-clotting agents.

Lung—one of two spongelike organs located on either side of the chest where respiration (exchange of gases) takes place. The right lung has three lobes, the left has two. The lungs are connected to the trachea (windpipe) by the bronchial tree. As the tree extends into the lung, it separates into smaller and smaller branches called bronchioles. Oxygen is exchanged for carbon dioxide at the alveoli, or air sacs, at the end of the bronchioles. Breathing occurs when the brain signals the diaphragm to thrust down, allowing the lungs to fill with air.

Lymph nodes—glandlike organs located throughout the body that manufacture lymphocyte cells to fight disease. The nodes also filter foreign agents and bacteria from the lymph, which is the fluid that carries lymphocytes to the circulatory system. The nodes are located behind ears, between the jaw and neck, in the armpits and groin, and in other places. Tonsils, spleen, and thymus gland are also lymphatic tissue that produces white cells to counteract infection.

Middle ear—a group of three bones, or ossicles, called the hammer, anvil, and stirrup because of their shapes, located in the auditory canal just beyond the eardrum. The ossicles concentrate incoming sound waves as they are transmitted along the auditory canal to the inner ear. The middle ear is connected to the throat by the eustachian tube.

Nerve cell (neuron)—one of billions of specialized cells in the body, half of them contained in the brain, that make up the body's central and peripheral nervous systems. Nerve cells receive chemical signals through branchlike extensions called dendrites and transmit electrical impulses, or messages, to other nerve cells along long, rodlike structures called axons. The junction between the terminal fibers of a transmitting axon and the dendrites of a recipient neuron is called a synapse. Dendrites and axons are called nerve fibers. A nerve is a bundle of nerve fibers.

Nose—a facial structure above the mouth responsible for the sense of smell and for inhaling and filtering air. The nose is made of cartilage and bone. Its internal nasal passage has two chambers, lined with mucous membranes, where inhaled air is moistened and warmed, and where the air is filtered by nostril hairs. Small receptors at the top of the nasal cavities detect odors by dissolving stimuli in mucous secretions.

Optic nerve—a nerve stretching from the eyeball to the middle of the brain. The nerve begins at the retina, which contains 126 million receptors, or nerve cells, which are sensitive to light and color. The receptors are divided into rods and cones. They supply information to occipital lobes of the brain.

Outer ear—the visible portion of the ear, consisting of a skin-covered flap of cartilage and the auditory canal, which leads to the eardrum. The auricle collects sound waves and sends them through the auditory canal to the eardrum.

Ovary—in women, one of a pair of reproductive organs that produces eggs and the female sex hormones estrogen and progesterone. The ovaries are located to the left and right of the uterus, in the lower abdomen.

Pancreas—a 6-inch-long gland, below and in back of the stomach and liver, with two functions. The pancreas secretes enzymes into the digestive tract to help break down fats, carbohydrates, and proteins in the small intestine. It also secretes insulin, which stabilizes the body's metabolism of sugars and starches.

Patella—the kneecap, which forms a covering for the lower end of the femur (thighbone) and makes up the knee joint. The patella is susceptible to injury, especially among young people.

Pelvis—the basinlike framework of bones supporting the lower abdomen, surrounding the reproductive organs and the organs that eliminate waste. The bones of the pelvis are the ilium, the pubis, the coccyx, the ischium, the pubic arch, and the sacrum. The pelvic bones connect to the spinal column and also to the femurs. A woman's pelvis is broader and flatter than a man's, with a larger central cavity that accommodates the birth canal.

Penis—the shaftlike external male sex organ. When aroused, it fills with blood and becomes erect to enable sexual intercourse. Located just below the bladder and pubic bone, the penis contains a tip, or glans, and also the urethra, a tube through which semen and urine leave the body.

Pharynx (throat)—the tube of muscles and membranes forming the cavity extending from the back of the mouth to the esophagus. Composed of three chambers, the pharynx aids in breathing, ventilates the middle ears via the eustachian tube, and also assists in swallowing. The lowest part of the pharynx contains the larynx (voice box).

Pituitary gland—pea-sized gland, located at the base of the brain just above the back of the nose. Controlled by the hypothalamus and by hormones from the brain, the pituitary itself secretes eight hormones that guide the main body functions, including growth, metabolism, reproduction, and reaction to stress. Pituitary hormones also stimulate hormonal secretions by other glands.

Placenta (afterbirth)—the organ attached to the wall of the uterus during pregnancy. Via the placenta, the developing fetus obtains nourishment from the mother, because it serves as an exchange of vascular systems between mother and fetus.

Prostate gland—in men, the gland partly composed of muscle surrounding the neck of the bladder and the beginning of the urethra. The prostate manufactures prostatic fluid, which mixes with sperm to produce semen.

Scrotum—the bag of skin that holds the testicles.

Seminal vesicle—either of the paired, saclike glands behind the bladder in the male reproductive system. The seminal vesicles release a fluid that forms part of the semen.

Sigmoid colon—the S-shaped part of the colon between the descending colon and the rectum, forming a right angle with the rectum. The sigmoid colon and the descending colon are the two parts of the colon where colon cancer is most likely to occur. The sigmoid is also susceptible to ulcerative colitis.

Sinuses—cavities within bones or other tissues, including the paranasal sinuses, which are eight hollow spaces within the skull and which open to the nose. The functions of the paranasal sinuses include resonation of the voice, filtering of dust and foreign objects from inhaled air, and lightening of the weight of the skull on the vertebrae of the neck. The paranasal sinuses are lined with mucous membranes.

Skin—the body's outer surface and largest organ, weighing about 6 pounds and covering about 25 square feet. Composed of three layers—epidermis, dermis, and inner fatty tissue—the skin provides a barrier against infections and injury, regulates the body's temperature, helps rid the body of wastes, transforms the sun's rays to vitamin D, guards the body against ultraviolet rays, and transmits sensory messages of pain, pleasure, pressure, and temperature.

Small intestine—the longest part of the digestive tract, a tubelike organ measuring 22 feet in length and ½ inch in diameter, extending from the top opening of the stomach to the ileum. It is divided into the duodenum (the shortest, widest portion that joins the stomach and pyloric valve), jejunum (the middle portion, which is slightly larger in diameter and with a thicker wall than the ileum), and ileum (the portion that opens into the large intestine). Inside the small intestine, bile from the liver and juices from the pancreas begin to break down proteins, starches, and sugars, and to metabolize fats. Nutrients are absorbed into the blood through the lining of the small intestine. Waste is passed along to the colon.

Spinal column (backbone)—twenty-six bones, or vertebrae, that encase the spinal cord and provide a strong, flexible support for all of the body's upright movement. Seven cervical vertebrae support the neck and head, twelve thoracic vertebrae support the rib cage, and five lumbar vertebrae support the lower back. The sacrum, near the base of the spine, is composed of five vertebrae fused into one bone. The coccyx at the base of the spine contains four bones fused into one. Disks of cartilage separate the vertebrae and absorb shocks to the body and protect nerves. Displacement of a disk can cause extreme pain to an impacted nerve.

Spinal cord—a portion of the central nervous system extending 18 inches from the base of the brain down through the spinal column. The spinal cord is ½ inch in diameter and weighs only about 2 ounces, but it is connected to all but twelve of the body's nerves (the cranial nerves are the exception). It relays messages from the brain to the muscles, organs, glands, and blood vessels. Messages returning from these parts of the body are relayed by the spinal cord to the brain or responded to with spinal reflexes. The spinal cord forms, with the brain, the central nervous system.

Spleen—an organ roughly the shape and size of a cupped hand located underneath the lower left ribs, behind the stomach, and weighing about 6 ounces. The spleen stores red blood cells and releases them to the bloodstream in an emergency, to boost the body's oxygen supply. The spleen also removes parasites, foreign substances, and damaged red blood cells, and manufactures white blood cells called lymphocytes to help fight infection.

Stomach—a pouchlike digestive organ, located below the diaphragm in the upper left abdomen, that receives food from the esophagus. Its three layers of muscle fibers expand to accommodate food and contract to release digestive juices on food and churn it into a semiliquid consistency. The stomach also contains glands in its mucous membrane lining that secrete hydrochloric acid and digestive enzymes. The full stomach holds approximately 2½ quarts.

Teeth—peg-shaped bonelike structures, consisting of a visible crown and a root, that fit into bony sockets of the jawbone, inside the mouth, and protrude through the gums. Adults have thirty-two teeth. The primary function of teeth is to tear and grind food to prepare it for digestion. Teeth also assist in speech.

Tendon—the tough, spindled ends of muscle fibers attached to bones to give stability and motion to the joints. Inflammation of the tendons, called tendinitis, is usually caused by injury, by excessive repetitive activity (such as typing), or by misuse or overuse of a joint. Symptoms include pain and swelling of the joint.

Testicle (testis)—in men, one of a pair of the principal organs of reproduction located within the scrotum. The testicles produce sperm cells along with the hormone testosterone, which causes the deep voice, body hair, body build, and sex drive in the developing male. The testicles are connected by the vas deferens to the urethra.

Thyroid—a tiny gland, the size and shape of a walnut, that is located in front of the neck, weighs 1 ounce, and takes iodine from the blood and converts it into two hormones, which are secreted on a signal from the pituitary gland. These hormones maintain body metabolism by enhancing the consumption of oxygen, helping the brain develop, speeding chemical reactions, and determining when the body needs food or rest.

Tongue—an organ of the mouth, stretching from the front teeth to the pharynx, whose muscles are vital for speaking and for chewing and swallowing food, and whose taste buds determine taste.

Ureter—one of a pair of tubes that carries urine from the kidney into the bladder.

Urethra—a small, tubular structure that drains urine from the bladder.

Uterus—in women, the hollow, pear-shaped organ of reproduction that holds the embryo/fetus from the time of fertilization until birth. Located within the pelvis, between the bladder and rectum, the uterus is about 3½ inches long, 2 inches wide, and 1 inch thick. The uterus is connected by the fallopian tubes to the ovaries and by the cervix to the vagina. Its muscles can increase in weight from 1 ounce to 36 ounces (2¼ pounds) during pregnancy.

Vagina (birth canal)—in women, the tubelike, muscular sex organ stretching from the vulva upward and back to the uterus. The vaginal walls expand and contract during intercourse, and stretch greatly during childbirth. The walls also secrete fluid to lubricate the vagina, keep it clean, and maintain acidity.

Vas deferens—in men, a tube passing from the testicles through the scrotum and joining the seminal vesicle.

Vulva—in women, the outer genitals.

2. Medical Conditions

INTRODUCTION

Despite the complexity and intricacies of our body systems, most of us live the majority of our lives illness- and disorder-free. But when maladies or ailments strike, our lives are altered, sometimes forever.

Understanding the conditions that can beset us is an essential aspect of curing or coping with them. Individuals informed about their own maladies are in a better position to care for themselves and to interact with medical professionals. Knowing about the diseases, ailments, and conditions that afflict us allows us to make better, more educated decisions about available treatments.

In this section, you will learn about the most common medical and health conditions affecting us. You will better understand what the condition is and what is done to correct it. By having more knowledge about what is happening to you, the better able you will be to participate in your own health care.

AIDS (Acquired Immune Deficiency Syndrome)

Acquired immune deficiency syndrome (AIDS) is a progressive disease characterized by the breakdown and eventual failure of the immune system. AIDS, once considered primarily an affliction of homosexual men, has now grown into a pandemic that affects many individuals. By the year 2000, the World Health Organization predicts that 40 million people will be infected with the virus that causes AIDS.

This virus, called the human immunodeficiency virus (HIV), attacks the cells of the immune system, disables and destroys them, thereby allowing the body to be subjected to various "opportunistic" infections. AIDS may be transmitted through sexual contact, infected blood and blood products, or a perinatal relationship (mother to fetus).

In 1981 epidemiologists (people who study and track diseases) began noticing cases of a very rare type of pneumonia known as *Pneumocystis carinii* affecting homosexual men. It is usually found in people whose immune system has been suppressed as a result of medical treatment. However, none of the patients identified was taking any immune-system-suppressing medications; their only link was their homosexuality. Not long after that, a rare type of cancer,

called Kaposi's sarcoma (a kind of cancer on skin and in the gastrointestinal tract and respiratory system), was also diagnosed in male homosexuals.

Because these individuals shared a similar life style, it was suspected that transmission of this disease occurred though sexual contact. At first doctors thought this acquired immune disease affected only male homosexuals; however, it was later diagnosed in intravenous drug users, Haitians, and hemophiliacs who used blood products. At this point, scientists began looking for a common causative agent, most likely a new, and as yet undiscovered, virus.

The virus, HIV, discovered in 1983 by French and American scientists, has probably been the most extensively researched virus in laboratories and the bane of the scientific community. Despite the best efforts of biomedical researchers, many questions remain as to the origins of HIV, how it mutates within the body, and how effective preventive measures such as vaccines can be developed.

Once HIV invades the body, AIDS may not develop for years as the virus lies dormant before becoming active again. During this time, infected individuals may not exhibit any signs or symptoms of AIDS; however, they are asymptomatic HIV carriers and can pass along the infection. Or they may exhibit general symptoms, such as fever, loss of weight, night sweats, or tiredness, that could mimic other diseases. Because of these varied immune responses and because of the mutable and unstable nature of the AIDS virus itself, there is yet no cure or vaccine.

The Immune System and HIV

The AIDS virus attacks and cripples the body's immune system, specifically affecting the cells that are integral to the correct functioning of the immune system. The immune system protects the body against all sorts of invaders, including bacteria, viruses, toxins, and foreign tissues and germs. These invaders, called antigens, can be any chemical substance that stimulates antibody production and that is identified, recognized, and eventually attacked by various components of the immune system. Antibodies are produced by white blood cells (lymphocytes) and are specifically designed to destroy different antigens. This process of antibody production in which specific resistance to an antigen is achieved is termed immunity.

Deaths Attributable to HIV Infection/AIDS

During the 1980s, human immunodeficiency virus (HIV) infection emerged as a leading cause of death in the United States. The latest reports from the Centers for Disease Control and Prevention and the National Center for Health Statistics indicate that HIV infection/AIDS continues to cause an increasing proportion of all deaths.

According to a 1993 *Monthly Vital Statistics Report,* in 1991 there were 29,555 deaths due to HIV infection, 17.3 percent more than the 25,188 deaths recorded in 1990. Of these deaths, 62 percent (18,366 deaths) were for white males; 25 percent (7,440 deaths) for black males; 7 percent (1,997 deaths) for black females; and 5 percent (1,484 deaths) for white females. The largest numbers for males and females were for the age groups 25–34 and 35–44 years. Although the numbers of deaths were greatest for white males, the age-adjusted death rates and almost all age-specific death rates were highest for black males, followed by white males, black females, and white females.

Overall, HIV infection was ranked as the ninth leading cause of death in 1991. For the black population it ranked sixth and for the white population it ranked tenth among the leading causes of death.

However, the AIDS virus is difficult to combat, since it attacks the immune system cells that play a central role in fighting antigenic activity in the body. Of the two kinds of lymphocytes produced (B cells and T cells), the AIDS virus attacks and destroys the T cells. Ordinarily, it is the responsibility of the T cells to attack and destroy an antigen, while B cells produce plasma cells which give rise to antigen-fighting antibodies. T and B cells both utilize various accessory cells, principally macrophages (also affected by HIV), which phagocytose (ingest) and present antigens to the T and B cells.

There are four types of T cells: Killer T cells destroy antigens; helper T cells stimulate antibody production; suppressor T cells regulate the actions of killer and helper cells; and memory T cells remain in the bloodstream and recognize invading antigens. HIV attacks the CD4 lymphocytes (helper T cells) in such a way that the immune system cannot function and, as a result of CD4 lymphocyte depletion, the body is subject to a variety of infections and diseases. It is not known how HIV attacks CD4 lymphocyte cells. A major theory postulates that HIV directly attacks CD4 lymphocytes, causing them to implode (called cell lysis) or clump together (called syncytia). It has also been suggested that

the HIV can program CD4 cells to self-destruct (called apoptosis). Furthermore, some scientists believe that HIV, through unknown indirect mechanisms, causes CD4 cells to destroy other CD4 cells.

Once in the CD4 cell, HIV hides undetected by the immune system in the cell's genes. HIV, being a retrovirus with only RNA, has a protein called reverse transcriptase that allows the viral RNA to change into a mirror image of itself—viral DNA. As viral DNA, HIV can replicate itself by instructing the infected cell to produce new HIV cells. With more HIV cells in the body's system, HIV is capable of destroying even more CD4 cells.

Researchers believe that by developing antiviral drugs that can either halt the HIV life cycle at some point or inhibit the action of the protein (glycoprotein 160) that regulates HIV replication, the viral replication can be controlled and the progress of the disease slowed down. However, even these antiviral drugs, such as zidovudine (AZT), have a limited effectiveness on a virus that can readily develop a tolerance to the drug or can mutate in such a way that the drug cannot work. Multidrug therapy (using a combination of drugs so that HIV cannot become accustomed to any one drug) has been met with considerable skepticism because HIV could conceivably develop multiple resistances.

As far as the prospect of developing an effective vaccine for AIDS, scientists are still puzzled about what part of the immune response to concentrate on. The AIDS virus has the ability to make itself unrecognizable to memory antibodies that were formed during an earlier invasion. It does this by changing its recognizable outer covering that would ordinarily be attacked by the memory cells, therefore escaping destruction. Scientists concede that while the development of a preventive vaccine may be a possibility in the foreseeable future, the vaccine should not be a replacement for other prevention methods (sexual behavioral changes, for example) devised to control the spread of AIDS.

STAGES OF HIV INFECTION

Despite the fact that HIV affects and progresses in an individual in various ways and at different rates, there are general stages of HIV infection. The initial infection of HIV is accompanied by transient flulike symptoms, though the period of time between the infection and the onset of chronic symptoms varies from one to seven years. Usually at this stage, antibodies for HIV have developed and can be detected by two blood tests: ELISA (enzyme-linked immunosorbent assay) and the Western blot test.

Through the early stage of HIV infection (seroconversion), symptoms include fatigue, malaise, swollen lymph glands, rash, loss of appetite, weight loss, headaches, fever, night sweats, and diarrhea. As HIV infection progresses and the immune system has sustained considerable damage, symptoms of AIDS-related complex (ARC) can appear: fever, loss of weight, severe diarrhea, swollen lymph glands, and night sweats. Also at this stage, characteristic disorders of ARC are recognized. These disorders include severe dermatitis, arthritis, intellectual impairment, pneumonias, nephritis, personality changes, yeast infections of the mouth, and neurological disorders.

Finally, full-blown AIDS occurs as the immune system is severely impaired and as indicator diseases and infections plague the body. The most common indicator diseases are *Pneumocystis carinii* pneumonia, HIV wasting syndrome (acute HIV infection), yeast infection of the mouth and esophagus, Kaposi's sarcoma, and tuberculosis and other respiratory infections. Other indicator diseases include various cancers, viruses, and parasitic, fungal, and protozoan infections: toxoplasmosis of the brain, heart, and lungs; cryptococcosis infection; chronic herpes simplex virus infections of the mouth, esophagus, and lung; various forms of lymphoma (cancer); disseminated strongyloidiasis (causes pneumonia); cytomegalovirus infection of the retina; yeast infection of the respiratory system; and cryptosporidiosis infection of the intestine (causes diarrhea).

TREATMENT OF AIDS

The treatment of AIDS focuses on three areas: arresting the progression of HIV replication through the use of antiviral drugs; treating the opportunistic infections and diseases through antimicrobial drug therapy; and attempting to restore the health of the immune system through such methods as bone marrow transplants and immunoglobulin therapy. Antiviral drugs include zidovudine (AZT, Retrovir), the only FDA-approved drug; didanosine (DDI, Videx); and the investigational drug zalcitabine (dideoxycytidine, DDC, Hivid). Other experimental or new antiviral drugs are Soluble CD4, interferon, Inosine pranobex (isoprinosine), and IMREG-1. One, two, or multiple antiviral drugs can be administered; however, as with any kind of drug therapy, these drugs are not without side effects.

If AIDS patients desire to try out experimental AIDS drugs, they may participate in clinical drug trials. A clinical drug trial, run by a pharmaceutical company, independent investigators, and the FDA, uses human subjects to test the particular drug's efficacy and safety. While on one hand the patient may receive free, excellent medical care by participating in the clinical trial, on the other hand the patient is inconvenienced by frequent testing and visits, may have to pay a portion of the total cost, and may have his or her health put at risk.

There are, of course, alternative methods of treatment to drug therapy. Although physicians are skeptical concerning their overall value of effectiveness, these methods offer the patient little or no side effects and may be a more comforting mode of treatment than drug therapy. Alternative methods of treatment include acupuncture, use of herbal medicine, dietary modification, chiropractic therapy, homeopathic medicine, and body and mind relaxation exercises.

PREVENTION METHODS

Since no cure or vaccine for AIDS has been developed, the best defense against contracting AIDS is prevention. AIDS is transmitted only through sexual contact, contact with infected blood or blood products (for example, transfusion, IV needle sharing, accidental needle punctures), transplantation of infected tissue and organs, artificial insemination, and from mother to fetus. AIDS cannot be transmitted through casual contact, touching, sharing cutlery or crockery, hugging, nonsexual contact, or closed-mouth kissing.

Preventive methods include avoiding IV drug use and modifying one's sexual behavior by practicing "safe sex": wearing latex condoms, using spermicidal jellies, reducing the number of sexual partners, knowing the sexual history of the partner, avoiding unprotected anal, oral, and vaginal intercourse and "wet" kissing with saliva exchange (HIV has been isolated in saliva).

AIDS RESOURCES

The following sources may be contacted to learn more about the prevention, detection, and treatment of AIDS.

AIDS Hotlines

American Social Health Association
P.O. Box 13827
Research Triangle Park, NC 27709
800-342-2437
800-344-7432 Spanish
800-243-7889 Hearing-impaired

Clinical Trials Information Service
P.O. Box 6421
Rockville, MD 20849-6421
800-874-2572
800-243-7012 Hearing-impaired

National AIDS Clearinghouse
P.O. Box 6003
Rockville, MD 20849-6003
800-458-5231

National Association of People with AIDS
2025 I Street N.W., Suite 1118
Washington, DC 20006
800-673-8538

Project Inform
220 Market Street
San Francisco, CA 94103
800-822-7422
800-334-7422 in California

AIDS Agencies, Foundations, Associations, and Services

Governmental Agencies

Centers for Disease Control and Prevention
Department of Health and Human Services
5600 Fishers Lane
Rockville, MD 20857
301-443-2610
Headquarters in Atlanta:
1600 Clifton Road N.E.
Atlanta, GA 30333
Research, public awareness, education, monthly reports.

Food and Drug Administration
Department of Health and Human Services
Center for Biologics Evaluation and Research
8800 Rockville Pike
Bethesda, MD 20892
301-496-3556
Testing standards, focus of AIDS activities in FDA, regulates biological therapeutics.

Health Resources and Services Administration
Department of Health and Human Services
AIDS Program
5600 Fishers Lane
Rockville, MD 20857
301-443-4588
Administers grants, provides reimbursements to patients, ambulatory care, education and training activities.

National Commission on Acquired Immune Deficiency Syndrome
1730 K Street N.W.
Washington, DC 20006
202-254-5125
Studies national AIDS policy, recommends to Congress and the President.

National Institute of Allergy and Infectious Diseases
National Institutes of Health
Department of Health and Human Services
AIDS
6003 Executive Boulevard
Bethesda, MD 20892
301-496-8000
Information 301-496-5717
Hotline 800-342-2437
Institute at NIH for AIDS, conducts research of AIDS drugs and vaccines, conducts clinical trials.

Public Health Service
Department of Health and Human Services
Minority Health
5515 Security Lane, #1102
Rockville, MD 20852
301-443-5084
Information 301-443-9870
Provides grants for minority AIDS education and prevention projects.

Public Health Service
Department of Health and Human Services
National AIDS Program
200 Independence Avenue S.W.
Washington, DC 20201
Information 202-245-6867
Develops policies, recommends funding, provides
government and private organizations with information.

Nongovernmental Agencies

ACT UP (AIDS) (AIDS Coalition to Unleash Power)
135 W. 29th Street, 10th Floor
New York, NY 10001
212-564-2437
Promotes public awareness of AIDS and government
involvement, organizes rallies and demonstrations.

AIDS Action Council
2033 M Street N.W., Suite 802
Washington, DC 20036
202-293-2886
Promotes and monitors legislation on AIDS research
and education, lobbies in Congress for funding of
AIDS research.

AIDS Hotline
c/o American Social Health Association
P.O. Box 13827
Research Triangle Park, NC 27709
919-361-8400
800-342-2437
800-344-7432 Spanish
800-243-7889 TTY
National STD hotline 800-227-8922
Public policy office hotline 202-543-9129
Provides information on AIDS and HIV transmission and
prevention, referrals for testing and counseling.

AIDS Prevention League
c/o Saiom Shriver
136 Westwood Avenue
Akron, OH 44302
216-376-4384
Promotes nondairy vegetarianism for AIDS prevention,
education.

AIDS Resource Foundation for Children
St. Clare's Home for Children
182 Roseville Avenue
Newark, NJ 07107
201-483-4250
Operates homes for children with AIDS, HIV, and ARC,
foster parent recruitment and support programs, provides
support services to families, workshops, and outreach
programs, referrals.

AIDS Services and Prevention Coalition
23416 Highway 99, Suite A
P.O. Box C-2016
Edmonds, WA 98020
206-778-6162
Health care organizations, associations, and advocacy
groups that promote public AIDS policy and prevention,
education, offers patient services.

AIDS Task Force for the
American College Health Association
c/o Dr. Richard Keeling
University of Virginia
Department of Student Health
Box 378
Charlottesville, VA 22908
804-924-2670
Provides information to college students about AIDS.

American Association of Physicians for
Human Rights (Gay/Lesbian)
2940 16th Street, Suite 105
San Francisco, CA 94103
415-255-4547
Promotes education about the health needs of homosexuals
concerning AIDS, offers referral and support program for
HIV- infected physicians.

American Civil Liberties Union
(Civil Rights and Liberties)
132 W. 43rd Street
New York, NY 10036
212-944-9800
Maintains and operates AIDS and Civil Liberties Project.

American Foundation for AIDS Research
5900 Wilshire Boulevard, 2nd Floor
E. Satellite
Los Angeles, CA 90036
213-857-5900
Organizes fund-raising for AIDS research, develops
educational programs.

American Red Cross
17th and D Streets N.W.
Washington, DC 20006
202-737-8300
Research and public education campaigns.

Americans for a Sound AIDS Policy
P.O. Box 17433
Washington, DC 20041
703-471-7350
24-hr. AIDS information service 900-INF-AIDS
Promotes the formulation of effective AIDS public policy,
testifies before Congress, supports treatment and health
care of AIDS patients.

Artists Confronting AIDS
684½ Echo Park Avenue
Los Angeles, CA 90026
213-250-4487
Promotes AIDS awareness in the creative and
performing arts.

Association of Nurses in AIDS Care
704 Stony Hill Road, Suite 106
Yardley, PA 19067
215-321-2371
Nurses and health care professionals who provide
leadership and educational services for members, promotes
public awareness of AIDS.

**CAVDA (Citizens Alliance for VD Awareness)—
Citizens AIDS Project**
P.O. Box 1073
Chicago, IL 60648
312-236-6339
Project of CAVDA, provides information, educational
programs to professionals and the public, conducts
research and surveys.

Clinical Trials Information Service
P.O. Box 6421
Rockville, MD 20849-6421
800-874-2572
800-243-7012 TTY
Provides information on drug trials for AIDS and HIV.

Education, Training and Research Associates
P.O. Box 1830
Santa Cruz, CA 95061-1830
408-438-4060
Provides AIDS Education Training program, sponsors
California AIDS Clearinghouse, education, surveys,
and research.

**Foundation of Pharmacists and Corporate America for
AIDS Education**
700 5th Street N.W., Suite 303
Washington, DC 20001
202-371-1830
Pharmacists and members of the pharmacy industry who
provide information and AIDS prevention services for the
public, sponsors workshops and seminars.

Gay Men's Health Crisis (AIDS)
129 W. 20th Street
New York, NY 10011
212-807-6664
212-645-7470 TDD
AIDS hotline 212-807-6655
Provides support and therapy groups for AIDS patients and
families, also provides legal, financial, and health care
services, sponsors lectures and prevention programs.

Haitian AIDS Hotline
8037 N.E. 2nd Ave.
Miami, FL 33138
800-772-7432
Provides information to Haitians concerning AIDS
and HIV.

Haitian Coalition on AIDS
50 Court Street, Suite 605
Brooklyn, NY 11201
718-855-0972
Promotes education and public awareness of AIDS,
especially within the Haitian community, provides
counseling and other social services.

Health Education Resource Organization (AIDS)
101 W. Read Street, Suite 825
Baltimore, MD 21201
301-685-1180
Provides education and patient services to Maryland
residents, promotes information on AIDS nationally,
provides counseling, funding, referrals.

HIV/AIDS Program
c/o U.S. Conference of Mayors
1620 I Street N.W.
Washington, DC 20006
202-293-7330
United States Conference of Mayors which promotes
AIDS awareness, lobbies for legislation concerning AIDS.

Human Rights Campaign Fund
1012 14th Street N.W., 6th Floor
Washington, DC 20005
202-628-4160
Promotes legislation for AIDS research.

International AIDS Prospective Epidemiology Network
c/o David G. Ostrow
155 N. Harbor Drive, #5103
Chicago, IL 60601
312-565-2109
Public health workers and organizations who provide
support services and medical care for AIDS patients.

Mattachine Society of Washington
5020 Cathedral Avenue N.W.
Washington, DC 20016
202-363-3881
Referrals and education on AIDS.

Mothers of AIDS Patients
1811 Field Drive N.E.
Albuquerque, NM 87112-2833
619-544-0430
Provides education presentations on AIDS and support for
families of AIDS patients.

Multicultural Training Resource Center
1540 Market Street, Suite 330
San Francisco, CA 94102
800-545-6642 in California
Provides AIDS and HIV information to diverse cultural
groups.

Names Project
2362 Market Street
P.O. Box 14573
San Francisco, CA 94114
415-863-5511
800-872-6263 in California
Provides information on the AIDS quilt names list.

National AIDS Clearinghouse
P.O. Box 6003
Rockville, MD 20849-6003
301-217-0023
800-458-5231
800-243-7012 TDD/TTY
Provides information on educational materials, clinical
drug trials, publications.

National Association of People with AIDS
1413 K Street N.W., 10th Floor
Washington, DC 20005
Mail to: P.O. Box 34056
Washington, DC 20043
202-898-0414
800-866-2992 Voice/TDD
Provides membership to those with AIDS or HIV, health
care and services, contributes to educational campaigns.

National Gay Rights Advocates
540 Castro Street
San Francisco, CA 94114
A public interest law firm that provides advice to lawyers
involved with AIDS and gay/lesbian cases, operates AIDS
Civil Rights Project.

National Leadership Coalition on AIDS
1730 M Street N.W., #905
Washington, DC 20036
202-429-0930
Creates AIDS health policies and education programs with
businesses, provides information and a business support
network.

National Minority AIDS Council
300 I Street N.E., Suite 400
Washington, DC 20002
202-544-1076
Provides AIDS educational and research programs,
monitors legislation and regulations, distributes
information on AIDS concerning minority communities.

National Mobilization Against AIDS
1540 Market Street, Suite 160
San Francisco, CA 94102
415-863-4676
Promotes governmental support, research, and funding of
AIDS organizations, public action supporting AIDS
patients, organizes Memorial Day marches and vigils.

National Native Americans AIDS Prevention Center
3515 Grand Avenue, Suite 100
Oakland, CA 94610
800-283-2437
Provides referrals to counseling and testing centers,
information.

National Resource Center on Women and AIDS
Center for Women Policy Studies
2000 P Street N.W., Suite 508
Washington, DC 20036
202-872-1770
Provides assistance and information on women and AIDS
to various groups, develops AIDS policy through the
National Collaboration for AIDS Policy for Women.

Pediatric AIDS Coalition
1331 Pennsylvania Avenue N.W., Suite 721-N
Washington, DC 20004
202-662-7460
800-336-5475
Promotes pediatric AIDS prevention, education,
research and treatment programs, monitors legislation
and regulations.

Pediatric AIDS Foundation
2407 Wilshire Boulevard, Suite 613
Santa Monica, CA 90403
213-395-9051
800-552-0444
Funds pediatric AIDS research, provides assistance to
AIDS health care, promotes public awareness of pediatric
AIDS issues.

People with AIDS Coalition
31 W. 26th Street
New York, NY 10010
212-532-0290
800-828-3280
NY hotline 212-532-0568
Provides local support networks for AIDS patients, offers
social services.

Project Inform
1965 Market Street, Suite 220
San Francisco, CA 94103
415-558-8669
800-822-7422
800-334-7422 in California
Provides information on AIDS and HIV treatment,
organizations that provide treatment, outreach and
advocacy program.

Ryan White National Fund (AIDS)
c/o Athletes and Entertainers for Kids
Nissan Motor Corporation
P.O. Box 191, Building B
Gardena, CA 90248-0191
213-768-8493
800-933-KIDS
Provides social services to children and their families,
referral and counseling services, operates an AIDS clinic,
promotes AIDS awareness and education through various
programs.

San Francisco AIDS Foundation
P.O. Box 6182
San Francisco, CA 94101-6182
415-864-5855
415-864-6606 TDD
N. CA hotline 800-FOR-AIDS
San Francisco hotline 415-863-AIDS
Promotes education on the prevention of AIDS, provides social services, workshops and seminars, referral services, educational materials.

Stamp Out AIDS
240 W. 44th Street
New York, NY 10036
212-354-8899
Assists organizations in AIDS fund-raising.

Teens Teaching AIDS Prevention
3030 Walnut Street
Kansas City, MO 64108
816-561-8784
800-234-8336
Provides information on AIDS and HIV for teens, referrals to AIDS organizations.

Women's Action Alliance
c/o Shazia Z. Rafi
370 Lexington Avenue, Suite 603
New York, NY 10017
212-532-8330
Maintains the Women's Center Program which operates the AIDS Project.

World Hemophilia AIDS Center
10 Congress Street, Suite 340
Pasadena, CA 91105
818-577-4366
Serves as an information clearinghouse for AIDS, conducts surveys.

Alcoholism

Many people enjoy responsibly consuming alcoholic beverages from time to time. But the overconsumption of alcohol can lead to numerous problems, including a disease called alcoholism.

DEFINITION OF ALCOHOLISM

Alcoholism is a disease that is characterized by a person's periodic or continuous inability to control drinking, a preoccupation with alcohol, the use of alcohol despite its consequences, and distortions in thinking, most notably denial, according to the National Council on Alcoholism and Drug Dependence (NCADD). The symptoms of alcoholism, a long-lasting illness, develop in stages and create problems in major life areas such as work, family and social life, health, and economic functioning.

The myth that alcoholics are simply weak-willed people is harmful because it often prevents the victim from admitting to his or her problem, which is the first step in treating the disease. Knowing that alcoholism is a disease makes it easier for the alcoholic to seek treatment and for the family to admit the problem and seek help.

CAUSES OF ALCOHOLISM

There is no single cause for alcoholism, although research is being done to help better understand this complex disease. One theory is that alcohol is a habit-forming drug. Another theory is that a person may become addicted to the drug by first using it to relieve stress and then becoming dependent on it.

Quite a few studies show a familial connection. They show that a person whose parents or other relatives were alcoholics is more likely to become alcoholic than a person with abstinent parents or relatives. The cause of this is not known—it may be genetic, environmental, or both. The problem could be genetic if a person is hereditarily unable to properly metabolize alcohol. If this occurs, the drinker could build a tolerance and even an addiction to alcohol. The addiction results from a feeling of painful physical withdrawal when alcohol is no longer in the system. The manifestations of withdrawal can be fatal.

Other studies have shown antisocial behavior and other personality traits may be linked with alcoholism.

SIGNS OF PROBLEM DRINKING

If a person misuses alcohol—for example, uses it to forget a problem, to get through the day, to "escape," or simply to become intoxicated—he or she may have an alcohol problem. While only 10 percent of people who drink become alcoholics, a person should be warned that consuming more than four drinks in succession, 3 days a week, every week, can be considered pre-alcoholic. A habit of six drinks per day for most men (three for most women) can do considerable damage to bodily organs. An estimated 4 million people in the United States are problem drinkers today (excluding the estimated 6 million alcoholics).

The following questions developed by the National Institute on Alcohol Abuse and Alcoholism may be used to help determine if a person has a drinking problem or is possibly an alcoholic:

Do you think and talk about drinking often?

Do you drink more now than you used to?

Do you sometimes gulp drinks?

Do you often take a drink to help you relax?

Do you drink when you are alone?

Do you sometimes forget what happened when you were drinking?

Do you keep a bottle hidden somewhere at home or at work for a quick "pick-me-up"?

Do you need a drink to have fun?

Do you ever start drinking without really thinking about it?

Do you ever drink in the morning to relieve a hangover?

Do you ever feel that you need a drink?

Do you become irritable when drinking?

Do you drink to get drunk?

Has your drinking harmed your family or friends in any way?

Does drinking change your personality, creating an entirely new you?

Are you more impulsive when you are drinking?

People should keep in mind that not everyone who enjoys drinking is an alcoholic and that not everyone who drinks every day is an alcoholic. Alcohol can be safe when consumed in moderation. On the other hand, there are alcoholics who do not drink every day.

PHASES OF ALCOHOLISM

Alcoholism generally develops in phases over the course of five to seven years. Although these phases are not always experienced by alcoholics, they are characteristic of what most developing alcoholics go through.

The first stage, the warning stage, is characterized by the drinker's use of alcohol frequently or daily to relieve tension and to feel good. The person might also search for more occasions or reasons to drink. On these occasions, he or she begins to increase the amount of alcohol being consumed and begins to build a tolerance to that alcohol.

During the second stage of alcoholism, the danger stage, the drinker consumes larger amounts of alcohol to obtain the same relief. The drinker might also begin sneaking drinks, drinking alone, and gulping drinks, experience the inability to remember something that occurred during or after drinking, feel guilty about drinking habits, and occasionally shun responsibilities, such as working.

In the third stage, the drinker shows signs of having lost control of his or her drinking by drinking more than intended and by making excuses for drinking. He or she may behave aggressively toward others and withdraw from social interaction. He or she may also protect the liquor supply by hiding it. At this point, the drinker may have fallen victim to an illness related to his or her consumption.

During the final stage of alcoholism, the drinker may well be intoxicated most of the time, due to a complete loss of control. The drinker will lay his or her hands on anything that will intoxicate. He or she may experience shaking, which prevents the body from performing everyday tasks and renders him or her unable to function with any degree of normality.

GETTING HELP

There are many places to turn for an alcoholic who wishes to recover. By the time an alcoholic searches for help, he or she may have already become addicted to the substance and may require it in order to func-

Alcohol-Induced Deaths

According to the National Center for Health Statistics, in 1991 a total of 19,233 persons died of alcohol-induced causes in the United States. The category "alcohol-induced causes" includes not only deaths from dependent and nondependent use of alcohol but also accidental poisoning by alcohol. It excludes accidents, homicides, and other causes indirectly related to alcohol use.

tion. For this reason, he or she may need physical and emotional assistance to stop drinking.

An alcoholic can turn to many people for help. Doctors, members of the clergy, or community health or social workers can help an alcoholic seek treatment. Most hospitals have inpatient or outpatient clinics to aid alcoholics. There are also public and private hospitals exclusively designed for the treatment of alcoholism.

Alcoholics Anonymous (AA) is a group that emphasizes mutual support, a commitment to abstinence, and anonymity in a twelve-step program toward recovery from alcoholism. AA has helped thousands of people suffering from alcoholism to overcome their disease.

Families of alcoholics can seek help from Al-Anon, a group for alcoholics' spouses, and Alateen, a group for teenage children of alcoholics. These groups can help families of alcoholics understand and deal with their problems.

TREATMENT

The first step in recovering from alcoholism is to get the alcohol out of the body. This step may require that the person be placed in a medical facility, because of the severe reactions he or she may experience during withdrawal from alcohol. After detoxification, the person may undergo both medical and psychiatric aid for a healthy, full recovery.

Psychiatric counseling and consultation are often used. "Halfway houses" are treatment facilities that can help a recovering alcoholic return from the disease to his or her normal life in a healthy environment. An outpatient clinic, which is available at many hospitals, is another option where a recovering alcoholic can receive treatment without being hospitalized.

Alcoholics Anonymous Worldwide Services Office
68 Park Avenue S.
New York, NY 10016

PREVENTION

Alcoholism can be prevented if a person understands the effects of alcohol on the body and if he or she is aware that alcohol is a drug. These factors can be a basis for personal prevention. Avoiding overconsumption of alcohol, being aware of one's family history with alcohol as well as one's own history with alcohol, and knowing places to turn for help can reduce the chances of becoming an alcoholic.

STATISTICS ABOUT ALCOHOL

Blood Alcohol Concentration

The effects of alcohol on a person depends on the person's body weight and on how much alcohol is consumed. Blood alcohol concentration (BAC) is often expressed as a percentage, such as .05 percent for 50 mg of alcohol per deciliter of blood. One "drink," such as 12 ounces of beer, 4 ounces of wine, or a 1½-ounce shot of whiskey, gin, or vodka, contains approximately the same amount of ethyl alcohol, 8 grams, or 8,000 mg. It is recommended that drinkers keep their blood alcohol concentration below .4 percent.

It takes the average adult nearly 1 hour to break down 8 grams of alcohol, depending on factors such as body weight and the amount of water contained in the body. Alcohol is absorbed through the mouth, esophagus, stomach, and intestines.

Women and Alcohol

Because the average woman's volume of total body water is lower than that of men, the same drink given to men and women will have a greater effect on women. Concentrations of alcohol are usually higher during the first 2 weeks of the menstrual cycle for women who are taking oral contraceptives. In addition, damages to the fetus are found in women who have consumed moderate amounts of alcohol during pregnancy. Miscarriages can occur when a pregnant woman drinks four to seven drinks a week, although damage to the fetus may occur at a lower level of consumption.

Effects of Alcohol on the Body

Brain—Alcohol directly affects brain cells. This may result in dizziness, unclear thinking, staggering, slurred speech. It makes some people feel they can do things they really can't do. Large amounts may result in unconsciousness or death.

Eyes—Because of alcohol's effects on the nervous system, it is difficult for the eye muscles to function, resulting in blurred vision.

Mouth/throat—Alcohol is not digested like other beverages. Absorption into the body begins through the mouth and throat. It is an irritant to the lining of the mouth and throat and can cause sores and ulcers.

Alcohol Impairment Chart

Approximate Blood Alcohol Percentage

Drinks	Body Weight in Pounds								
	100	120	140	160	180	200	220	240	
0	.00	.00	.00	.00	.00	.00	.00	.00	ONLY SAFE DRIVING LIMIT
1	.04	.03	.03	.02	.02	.02	.02	.02	
2	.08	.06	.05	.05	.04	.04	.03	.03	
3	.11	.09	.08	.07	.06	.06	.05	.05	
4	.15	.12	.11	.09	.08	.08	.07	.06	
5	.19	.16	.13	.12	.11	.09	.09	.08	
6	.23	.19	.16	.14	.13	.11	.10	.09	
7	.26	.22	.19	.16	.15	.13	.12	.11	
8	.30	.25	.21	.19	.17	.15	.14	.13	
9	.34	.28	.24	.21	.19	.17	.15	.14	
10	.38	.31	.27	.23	.21	.19	.17	.16	

Subtract .01% for each 40 minutes or drinking
One drink is 1¼ oz. of 80 proof liquor, 12 oz. of beer, or 4 oz. of table wine.

Heart—Alcohol can increase the workload of the heart. Irregular heartbeat and high blood pressure can result.

Liver—Alcohol can poison the liver. Most of the alcohol a person drinks is processed by the liver, which is why alcohol can seriously damage the liver. The damage can result in liver failure.

Stomach—Alcohol irritates the digestive system. Vomiting and sores called ulcers may result.

Kidneys—Alcohol can stop the kidneys from maintaining a proper balance of body fluids and minerals.

Veins/arteries—Alcohol widens blood vessels, causing headaches and loss of body heat.

Blood—Alcohol reduces your body's ability to produce blood cells, resulting in anemia and/or infection.

Muscles—Alcohol can cause muscle weakness. This may result in staggering and falling.

Effects of Increased Blood Alcohol Level by Percentage

.02 (one drink)—Some drinkers may feel warmth and relaxation.

.04—Most people feel relaxed, talkative, and happy. Skin may flush.

.05—The first sizable changes begin to occur. Lightheartedness, giddiness, lowered inhibitions, and less control of thoughts may be experienced. Both restraint and judgment are lowered; coordination may be slightly altered.

.06—Judgment somewhat impaired; normal ability to make a rational decision about personal capabilities is affected, such as one's driving ability.

.08—Definite impairment of muscle coordination and a slower reaction time; driving ability suspect. Sensory feelings of numbness of the cheeks and lips. Hands, arms, and legs may tingle and then feel numb. Legally impaired in Canada and in some states.

.10—Clumsy; speech may become fuzzy. Clear deterioration of reaction time and muscle control. Legally drunk in most states, and in California, it is illegal to operate a motor vehicle with this or greater BAC.

.15—Definite impairment of balance and movement. The equivalent of a ½ pint of whisky is in the bloodstream.

.20—Motor and emotional control centers measurably affected; slurred speech, staggering, loss of balance, and double vision can all be present.

.30—Lack of understanding of what is seen or heard; individual is confused or stuporous. Consciousness may be lost at this level ("passes out").

.40—Usually unconscious; skin clammy.

.45—Respiration slows and can stop altogether.

.50—Death can result.

Source: U.S. Department of Health and Human Services, Public Health Service, National Institute on Alcohol Abuse and Alcoholism, Rockville, Maryland.

How Long to Wait Before Driving

According to NCADD, almost half of all traffic fatalities are alcohol-related. Although alcohol-related accidents are declining, almost 10 percent of the licensed driving population was arrested in 1991 for driving under the influence of alcohol. People between the ages of 21 and 24 cause the highest number of fatal crashes due to driving under the influence.

Drinking and driving *do not* mix, and, frankly, liquor affects everybody differently. So the best rule is never drive after drinking. The following table is a general guideline for how long to wait after imbibing before attempting to drive. (One drink equals 1 mixed drink or 12 ounces of beer or 4 ounces of wine or champagne.)

Body Weight (lbs.)	1 drink	2 drinks	3 drinks
100–119	0 hrs	3 hrs	6 hrs
120–139	0 hrs	2 hrs	5 hrs
140–159	0 hrs	2 hrs	4 hrs
160–179	0 hrs	1 hr	3 hrs
180–199	0 hrs	0 hrs	2 hrs
200–219	0 hrs	0 hrs	2 hrs
Over 200	0 hrs	0 hrs	1 hr

Body Weight (lbs.)	4 drinks	5 drinks	6 drinks
100–119	10 hrs	13 hrs	16 hrs
120–139	8 hrs	10 hrs	12 hrs
140–159	6 hrs	8 hrs	10 hrs
160–179	5 hrs	7 hrs	9 hrs
180–199	4 hrs	6 hrs	7 hrs
200–219	3 hrs	5 hrs	6 hrs
Over 200	3 hrs	4 hrs	6 hrs

Source: U.S. Department of Health and Human Services, Public Health Service, National Institute on Alcohol Abuse and Alcoholism, Rockville, Maryland.

State Alcohol Abuse Treatment Offices

These agencies provide programs for the prevention, detection, treatment, and rehabilitation of alcohol abusers. They also coordinate the implementation of alcohol abuse prevention programs in the community, school, and workplace.

Alabama

Alabama Department of Mental Health and Mental Retardation
Substance Abuse Division
200 Interstate Park Drive
P.O. Box 3710
Montgomery, AL 36193-5001
205-271-9253

Alaska

Alaska Department of Health and Social Services
Office of Alcoholism and Drug Abuse
114 2nd Street
Pouch H
Juneau, AK 99811-0607
907-586-6201

Arizona

Arizona Department of Health Services
Office of Community Behavioral Health Services
411 N. 24th Street
Phoenix, AZ 85007
602-220-6478

Arkansas

Arkansas Department of Human Services
Office of Alcohol and Drug Abuse Prevention
400 Donaghey Plaza N.
P.O. Box 1437
Little Rock, AR 72203
501-682-6656

California

California Health and Welfare Agency
Department of Alcohol and Drug Programs
111 Capitol Mall, #450
Sacramento, CA 95814
916-445-1943

Colorado

Colorado Department of Health
Office of Health Care Services
Division of Alcohol and Drug Abuse
4210 E. 11th Avenue
Denver, CO 80220
303-331-8201

Connecticut

Connecticut Alcohol and Drug Abuse Commission
999 Asylum Avenue
Hartford, CT 06105
203-566-4145

Delaware

Delaware Department of Health and Social Services
Division of Alcoholism, Drug Abuse, and Mental Health
Bureau of Alcoholism and Drug Abuse
Delaware State Hospital
1901 N. DuPont Highway
New Castle, DE 19720
302-421-6101

District of Columbia

District of Columbia Department of Human Services
Commission of Public Health
Alcohol and Drug Abuse Services Administration
801 N. Capitol Street N.E.
Washington, DC 20002
202-727-0740

Florida

Florida Department of Health and Rehabilitative Services
Alcohol, Drug Abuse and Mental Health Program Office
Alcohol and Drug Abuse Program
1317 Winewood Boulevard
Tallahassee, FL 32399-0700
904-488-8304

Georgia

Georgia Department of Human Resources
Division of Mental Health, Mental Retardation and Substance Abuse
Alcohol and Drug Abuse Services
47 Trinity Avenue S.W.
Atlanta, GA 30334-1202
904-894-4785

Hawaii

Hawaii Department of Health
Mental Health Division
Alcohol and Drug Abuse Branch
1270 Queen Emma Street, Room 706
Honolulu, HI 96813
808-548-4280

Idaho

Idaho Department of Health and Welfare
Governors Commission on Alcohol and Drug Abuse
450 W. State Street, 3rd Floor
Boise, ID 83720
208-334-5740

Illinois

Illinois Department of Alcoholism and Substance Abuse
100 W. Randolph Street, Suite 5-600
Chicago, IL 60601
312-814-3840

Indiana

Indiana Department of Mental Health
Division of Addiction Services
117 E. Washington Street
Indianapolis, IN 46204
317-232-7837

Iowa

Iowa Department of Public Health
Division of Substance Abuse and Health Promotion
Lucas State Office Building, 4th Floor
Des Moines, IA 50319
515-281-3641

Kansas

Kansas Department of Social and Rehabilitation Services
Alcohol and Drug Abuse Services
2700 W. 6th Street
Topeka, KS 66606
913-296-3925

Kentucky

Kentucky Human Resources Cabinet
Department of Mental Health and Mental Retardation Services
Substance Abuse Division
275 E. Main Street
Frankfort, KY 40621
502-564-2880

Louisiana

Louisiana Department of Health and Hospitals
Division of Alcohol and Drug Abuse Prevention
P.O. Box 4049
Baton Rouge, LA 70821
504-342-6717

Maine

Maine Department of Human Services
Office of Alcoholism and Drug Abuse Prevention
35 Anthony Avenue
Statehouse Station 11
Augusta, ME 04330
207-626-5404

Maryland

Maryland Department of Health and Mental Hygiene
Addiction Services Administration
201 W. Preston Street
Baltimore, MD 21201
410-225-6925

Massachusetts

Massachusetts Executive Office of Human Services
Department of Public Health
Community Health Services Bureau
Division of Substance Abuse Services
150 Tremont Street, 6th Floor
Boston, MA 02111
617-727-1960

Michigan

Michigan Department of Public Health
Office of Substance Abuse Services
3500 N. Logan Street
P.O. Box 30206
Lansing, MI 48909
517-335-8809

Minnesota

Minnesota Department of Human Services
Chemical Dependency Division
444 Lafayette Road
St. Paul, MN 55155
612-296-4610

Mississippi

Mississippi Department of Mental Health
Division of Alcohol and Drug Abuse
1101 Robert E. Lee Building
Jackson, MS 39201
601-359-1288

Missouri

Missouri Department of Mental Health
Division of Alcohol and Drug Abuse
1706 E. Elm Street
P.O. Box 687
Jefferson City, MO 65102
314-751-4942

Montana

Montana Department of Institutions
Division of Alcohol and Drug Abuse
1539 11th Avenue
Helena, MT 59620
406-444-4927

Nebraska

Nebraska Department of Public Institutions
Division of Alcoholism and Drug Abuse
P.O. Box 94728
Lincoln, NE 68509-4728
402-471-2851

Nevada

Nevada Department of Human Resources
Rehabilitation Division
Bureau of Alcohol and Drug Abuse
Kinkead Building
505 E. King Street
Carson City, NV 89710
702-687-4790

New Hampshire

New Hampshire Department of Health and Human Services
Office of Alcohol and Drug Abuse Prevention
105 Pleasant Street
Concord, NH 03301
603-271-6100

New Jersey

New Jersey Department of Health
Alcohol, Narcotic and Drug Abuse Division
129 E. Hanover Street, CN-362
Trenton, NJ 08625
609-292-5760

New Mexico

New Mexico Department of Health and Environment
Division of Behavioral Health Services
Substance Abuse Bureau
1190 St. Francis Drive
Santa Fe, NM 87501
505-827-2589

New York

New York State Division of Alcoholism and Alcohol Abuse
194 Washington Avenue
Albany, NY 12210
518-474-5417

North Carolina

North Carolina Department of Human Resources
Division of Mental Health, Developmental Disabilities and Substance Abuse Services
Albemarle Building
325 N. Salisbury Street
Raleigh, NC 27603-5906
919-733-4670

North Dakota

North Dakota Department of Human Services
Division of Alcoholism and Drug Abuse
State Capitol, Judicial Wing
Bismarck, ND 58505
701-224-2769

Ohio

Ohio Department of Health
Bureau on Alcohol Abuse and Alcoholism Recovery
246 N. High Street
P.O. Box 118
Columbus, OH 43266-0588
614-466-3445

Oklahoma

**Oklahoma Department of Mental Health and
Substance Abuse Services**
1200 N.E. 13th Street
P.O. Box 53277
Oklahoma City, OK 73152
405-271-8777

Oregon

Oregon Department of Human Resources
Office of Alcohol and Drug Abuse Programs
1178 Chemeketa Street N.E.
Salem, OR 97310
503-378-2163

Pennsylvania

Pennsylvania Department of Health
Office of Drug and Alcohol Programs
809 Health and Welfare Building
Box 90
Harrisburg, PA 17108
717-787-9857

Puerto Rico

Puerto Rico Department of Addiction Control Services
2114 Río Piedras Station
Río Piedras, PR 00928-1414
809-763-7575

Rhode Island

**Rhode Island Department of Mental Health,
Retardation and Hospitals**
Division of Substance Abuse
600 New London Avenue
Cranston, RI 02920
401-464-2091

South Carolina

**South Carolina Commission on Alcohol and
Drug Abuse**
3700 Forest Drive, Suite 300
Columbia, SC 29204
803-734-9520

South Dakota

South Dakota Department of Human Services
Division of Alcohol and Drug Abuse
Kneip Building
700 Governor's Drive
Pierre, SD 57501-2291
605-773-3123

Tennessee

**Tennessee Department of Mental Health and Mental
Retardation**
Division of Alcohol and Drug Abuse Services
706 Church Street
Nashville, TN 37243-0675
615-741-1921

Texas

Texas Commission on Alcohol and Drug Abuse
1705 Guadalupe Street
Austin, TX 78701
512-463-5510

Utah

Utah Department of Human Services
Division of Substance Abuse
120 North 200 West
P.O. Box 45500
Salt Lake City, UT 84145-0500
801-538-3938

Vermont

Vermont Agency of Human Services
Office of Alcohol and Drug Abuse Programs
State Complex
103 S. Main Street
Waterbury, VT 05676
802-241-2175

Virginia

**Virginia Department of Mental Health, Mental
Retardation and Substance Abuse Services**
Office of Substance Abuse Services
109 Governor Street
Richmond, VA 23219
804-786-3906

Washington

Washington Department of Social and Health Services
Division of Alcohol and Substance Abuse
Mail Stop OB-44
Olympia, WA 98504
206-753-5866

West Virginia

**West Virginia Department of Health and Human
Resources**
Public Health Bureau
Office of Mental Health and Community Rehabilitation
Services
Division of Alcoholism and Drug Abuse
State Capitol Complex
Building 3, Room 519
Charleston, WV 25305
304-558-2276

Wisconsin
Wisconsin Department of Health
Division of Community Services
Office of Alcohol and Other Drug Abuse
One W. Wilson Street
P.O. Box 7850
Madison, WI 53707
608-266-3442

Wyoming
Wyoming Department of Health
Division of Community Programs
Substance Abuse Program
Hathaway Building
Cheyenne, WY 82002
307-777-6494

Allergies and Allergens

An allergy is a hypersensitive reaction of the body to certain agents it perceives as harmful. These agents, called allergens, are normally harmless and common substances. However, in some people, these substances can cause mild to very severe reactions, discomfort, and coldlike symptoms. Allergens can be taken into the body by inhalation, through contact with the skin, or by ingestion of foods or medications.

As allergens enter the body, the body's immune system perceives them as harmful and produces antibodies to combat the invaders. White blood cells, or lymphocytes in the form of B cells and T cells, produce antibodies or attack the allergen directly. The reaction between allergen and antibody releases chemicals, most notably histamine, that cause the body to experience a variety of uncomfortable symptoms. Symptoms can range from a runny nose, a skin rash, and congestion in the lungs to anaphylaxis (a life-threatening reaction), severe respiratory distress, and shock. General treatment of allergies consists of recognizing and identifying the allergen, avoiding the offending agent, and taking medications (usually antihistamines) to ease symptoms or to cope with the allergy. Common reactions to allergies include hay fever, asthma, hives and angioedema (swelling of the face and extremities), contact and atopic dermatitis, and food, drug, and insect sting allergies.

Hay fever, or allergic rhinitis, results as the body inhales various substances such as pollens, mold spores, dust and dust mites, and animal dander (the scales of skin shed by animals with feathers or hair). A host of symptoms occurs as a result of a person's sensitivity to these substances: nasal and bronchial congestion, sneezing, itchy eyes, nose, and throat, coughing, runny nose, headache, and sinus pain. Treatment of allergic rhinitis may include taking antihistamines such as terfenadine, using immunotherapy (allergy shots), and applying topical steroids such as beclomethasone, flunisolide, and triamcinolone.

Asthma is a lung disorder characterized by wheezing, difficulty in breathing (due to swollen bronchial tubes), a constricted feeling in the chest, and coughing. A common chronic disorder in children, asthma and its symptoms may be brought on or aggravated by allergens, temperature changes, exercise, emotional stress, hormonal changes, or bronchial or sinus infections.

The treatment for asthma involves avoiding those allergens that bring on attacks, taking inhaled medications such as steroid drugs Azmacort, AeroBid, Beclovent, and Vanceril, or other drugs such as theophylline, cromolyn sodium, and albuterol.

Hives, or urticaria, appear on the skin as red, raised, swollen, and itchy patches almost immediately after exposure to the allergen. Hives may be brought on by the ingestion of drugs (penicillin, sulfa), the consumption of certain foods (fish, nuts, eggs, berries, milk, shellfish), or the exposure to various other common allergens (pollens, animal dander, insect bites) and reactions to temperatures, light, stress, and illness. The condition of *angioedema* results in large, subcutaneous welts which have the potential to threaten life if they occur in the throat and block the airway.

Treatment of hives and angioedema involves avoiding the allergen and taking antihistamines such as terfenadine or diphenhydramine, histamine blockers such as cimetidine or ranitidine, or oral corticosteroids.

Allergic contact dermatitis results in a skin eruption, rash, or skin irritation due to any allergen to which the body is sensitive. Allergens include the sun, dyes, cosmetics, plants (poison ivy, oak, sumac), clothing, metal compounds, and ingredients in certain medications. Contact dermatitis reactions appear as inflamed, red, itchy patches or blisters on the skin. Treatment consists of the avoidance of the allergen and the application of topical corticosteroid creams.

Atopic eczema, a type of dermatitis, results from an allergic reaction to various allergens ranging from wool to detergent. The blistering and crusting rash that appears on the skin can be treated by avoiding the allergen or by using oral antibiotics or oral histamines, ultraviolet light therapy, and topical corticosteroids.

Food, drug, and insect sting allergies result from the consumption of various foods or food components (milk, berries, nuts, shellfish, wheat, corn, vegetables, food dyes, preservatives), the ingestion or injection of certain types of drugs (most common is penicillin), or the sting venom of certain insects (yellow jacket, hornet, fire ant, wasp, bee). Skin tests, RAST (radioallergosorbent) testing, and double-blind food allergy tests are helpful in detecting food allergies and other allergens as well. Often, those persons experiencing reactions to certain foods do not have allergies, but instead have an intolerance to the food. Symptoms of food allergies include dermatitis, hives, abdominal pain, vomiting and nausea, swelling, diarrhea, and nasal congestion. Drug allergies cause a person to experience difficulty in breathing, wheezing, hives, itching, and skin rashes. The most common drugs to provoke allergic responses are penicillin, barbiturates, sulfas, insulin, anesthetics, and anticonvulsant drugs. Allergic responses to insect stings can produce symptoms such as hives, itching, and constricted sensations in the throat and chest.

With all of these three types of allergies, symptoms can escalate to a potentially life-threatening reaction called anaphylaxis. Anaphylaxis, a severe systemic reaction, can immediately occur from exposure to any allergen. Symptoms of anaphylaxis include airway constriction, swollen throat, difficulty in breathing, nausea, vomiting, hives and angioedema, dizziness, shock, low blood pressure, rapid pulse, mental confusion, and anxiety. Anaphylaxis must be treated immediately with injectable adrenaline (epinephrine, EpiPen, Ana-Kit), which opens the constricted airway and blood vessels. Treatment of food, drug, and insect sting allergies includes avoiding the allergen, using immunotherapy (for food and insect sting allergies), and taking antihistamines and corticosteroids.

15 Common Birth Defects

Note: For additional genetic diseases and for information on the roles of dominant and recessive genes and X-linked inheritance, see "Genetic and Familial Diseases" later in this section.

Down syndrome. The #21 chromosome pair does not divide normally at conception. Increase in maternal age can lead to more babies with this defect.

Woman between 20 and 25: 1 in 2,000 risk. Woman at 45: 1 in 32 risk. Children have short stature; slanting eyelids; broad, flat nose; small ears; short, stubby fingers; moderate to severe mental retardation; congenital heart defects common; tendency toward middle-ear infections.

Huntington's disease. Dominant gene results in lethal disease not apparent at birth. Early symptoms, clumsiness or tics, appear between ages 35 and 45. Symptoms worsen to include twisted facial expressions, uncontrollable writhing of the body, and severe emotional problems that resemble manic-depression or schizophrenia. Deterioration can go on ten to twenty years until death.

Cystic fibrosis. Most common fatal genetic disease among Caucasians. Caused by recessive, defective gene. Some cases not diagnosed until age 4. Children prone to bacterial lung disease throughout life eventually die of respiratory failure by age 21.

Sickle-cell anemia. Crescent-shaped, rather than round, hemoglobin (pigment) in red blood cells. Abnormal cells more likely to get caught in spleen and die, leaving person with shortage of red blood cells, thus shortage of oxygen. Symptoms may not appear until 6 months of age. Usually found in people of African descent. Sickle cells stuck in arteries can result in injury to brain, lungs, and kidneys. Can lead to death.

Tay-Sachs disease. Recessive, defective gene results in body's inability to produce enzyme that normally breaks down fatty deposits in the brain and nerve cells. Gene carried by 1 in 25 American Jews. Symptoms may not appear until 6 months of age. No treatment available.

Hemophilia. Most well known of X-linked disorders. Defective gene is located on the X, or female, chromosome and is recessive. Blood does not clot normally, and even minor scrapes can lead to uncontrolled, even fatal bleeding. Disorder most associated with males, but a female has a 50 percent chance of inheriting disorder if she is the daughter of an affected father and carrier mother.

Duchenne-type muscular dystrophy. X-linked disorder. Fatal muscle disorder appears in boys between ages 6 and 9. Muscles weaken over time, forcing child into a wheelchair by the teen years. Affects all muscles, including heart and those used in breathing.

Spina bifida and anencephaly. Together these neural tube defects are among the most common birth defects in the United States. Anencephaly (missing brain) is always fatal. Spina bifida, which results in a gap in the bone that surrounds the spinal cord, can be slight or severe. Severe cases include paralysis, lack of bladder and bowel control, and hydrocephalus (water on the brain). Caused by combination of hereditary and environmental factors.

Rh disease. Problems can arise for unborn baby of mother who lacks the Rh factor in her blood (Rh negative) and father who does not (Rh positive). If fetus is Rh positive and is a second or later pregnancy, mother's antibodies will attempt to destroy baby's blood cells. Vaccine now available to prevent antibodies from forming in mother's blood.

Phenylketonuria (PKU). Enzyme deficiency that prevents proper breakdown of the amino acid phenylalanine. Can lead to severe mental retardation and physical problems. However, special diet low in this amino acid can avert these problems. Routinely screened for at birth.

Cerebral palsy. Refers to movement and posture problems resulting from brain injury. Considered a birth defect if injury occurs before or during birth. Does not get worse over time.

Cleft lips and palate. Incomplete fusion in lip or palate (roof of mouth) caused by hereditary and/or environmental factors. Problems in infant's ability to suck are common, as are speech disorders. Heredity responsible in 25 percent of cases. Environmental factors include maternal diabetes, alcohol abuse, anticancer drugs, and seizure medications. Can be corrected with plastic surgery.

Clubfoot. Second most common birth defect in the United States. Scientists not sure why boys are twice as likely as girls to develop clubfoot. Entire foot twisted inward and downward in worst cases. Most cases probably caused by hereditary and unidentified environmental factors.

Rubella. Severe birth defects can result if mother exposed to rubella (German measles) in early pregnancy. Defects include blindness, deafness, microcephaly (small head), mental retardation, cerebral palsy, and congenital heart defects. Mother is immune to rubella if she already has had the disease, or if she is vaccinated prior to becoming pregnant.

Fetal alcohol syndrome (FAS) and *drug-addicted infants.* Severe birth defects can be brought on by mother's inability or refusal to stop ingesting alcohol and drugs during pregnancy. Intoxicants pass through the placenta to developing baby. FAS infants are undersized at birth, have small heads, mild to moderate retardation, short attention spans, and behavioral problems. May have joint abnormalities and congenital heart disease. Narrow eyes and short, upturned nose characteristic of FAS children. Infants born to heroin addicts are often born addicted themselves and may suffer withdrawal symptons severe enough to cause brain damage or death. Cocaine and marijuana users give birth to infants smaller than usual.

Cancer

Cancer is the uncontrolled growth and spread of abnormal cells. When cells divide over and over, a tumor results. Tumors can be either benign or malignant. Benign tumors are not cancer, but malignant ones are.

Healthy, noncancerous cells of the body grow, divide, and replace themselves in an orderly process, which keeps the body in a healthy state and good repair. When cells become cancerous, they lose their ability to do their particular job; they invade nearby tissues and take over the blood supply intended for normal cells. Cancer can strike any body organ or tissue. Cancerous cells can spread to other parts of the body, carried through the lymphatic or circulatory systems. Cancer's ability to spread to different parts of the body is called metastasis. Most cancers form solid tumors.

Carcinoma is the name given to cancers whose cells were originally part of linings, such as skin or the lining of the digestive tract. Carcinomas are the most common types of cancer and include lung, skin, and colon cancer. *Sarcomas* are cancers whose cells come from tissues that hold the body together. Bone and muscle cancers are two examples. No solid tumors are formed when cells in the blood or other body fluids become cancerous. Examples of this type of cancer are leukemia and lymphoma.

CAUSES OF CANCER

Cancer is caused by mutations, or changes, in genes; these mutations are brought about by internal and external environmental factors, including exposure to chemicals and radiation. When these factors enter cells, they can harm the cell's DNA, by either breaking or tangling the DNA molecules. Other factors can change the chemical composition of the DNA molecule. If a mutation causes the cell to become cancerous, the factor involved is known as a carcinogen.

Family history appears to play an important role in certain forms of cancer. This may help explain why some heavy smokers develop lung cancer while others do not. More than 100 distinct forms of cancer exist, and the cause of each may be different. However, research shows that the role of heredity is irrefutable in 5 to 7 percent of all cancer patients.

TWENTY TYPES OF CANCERS AND THEIR TREATMENTS

1. Bone and Connective Tissue

The two major types of bone sarcoma are osteosarcoma and Ewing's sarcoma. Osteosarcoma mostly affects the fast-growing bones in children. It starts in cells that form bone and often affects the leg bones, beginning on or near the knee. Common symptoms are pain and swelling. Tumors in the hip and spine can cause pain in the leg and thigh.

Treatment includes surgical removal of the tumor and chemotherapy to destroy the metastases in the lung that are common with this type of cancer.

Ewing's sarcoma is a cancer that develops in the bone marrow. Ewing's sarcoma, like osteosarcoma, is most common in young people, in this case, those 10 to 20 years old. It often occurs in the shafts of long bones, and symptoms include pain and swelling as well as fatigue, weight loss, and fever. Metastasis to

the lungs is common. Radiation treatment is the most common treatment.

2. Brain Tumors

Most brain cancers are the result of metastases of other cancers, usually from the lung and breast. Cancers that originate in the brain account for only a small portion of brain tumors; in incidence of these, heredity plays a major role, especially in children.

Gliomas form the largest group of primary brain cancers, about 45 percent. A glioma is a tumor made of glial cells, a type of nerve tissue. Symptoms include headache, vomiting, and pressure on nerve tracts. Most primary brain cancers are not curable, but surgery can help relieve the symptoms and prolong life. Radiation therapy can be effective in some cases of primary brain cancer as well as with cancers originating in the lungs or breast.

3. Cancer of the Esophagus

Tobacco and alcohol seem to be the main instigators where this cancer is concerned, at least within the United States. Geography also plays a role. Cases are increasing in the southeastern United States, and in the Hunan province of northern China, such cancer is quite common.

It is one of the more difficult cancers to treat; fortunately, it is somewhat rare compared to other can-

Annual Deaths Attributed to 10 Cancers

Lung	143,758
Colon	56,243
Breast	43,849
Prostate	33,564
Pancreatic	25,536
Stomach	14,225
Ovarian	13,028
Brain/Nervous System	11,952
Kidney	10,774
Bladder	10,406

Source: Monthly Vital Statistics Report, vol. 42, no. 2 (Supplement) (August 31, 1993). Centers for Disease Control and Prevention, U.S. Department of Health and Human Services, Public Health Service.

cers of the digestive tract. The two methods to treat these tumors are surgery and radiation therapy.

4. Cancer of the Eye

Eye cancer can be divided into three categories: the eyeball itself; the socket and its surrounding soft tissues; and the eyelids and conjunctiva. Eye cancers usually produce noticeable symptoms that lead, fortunately, to early diagnosis and treatment. These symptoms include double vision, protrusion of the eyeball or other obvious changes.

Malignant melanomas and retinoblastoma are the two most common cancers of the eyeball itself. Malignant melanoma usually occurs in adults; retinoblastoma occurs in infants and young children.

If detected at an early stage, eye cancers can often be treated without loss of vision.

5. Liver Cancer

Liver cancers can be either primary or secondary, depending on the site of origin. Primary cancers, or cancers that originate in the liver itself, are rare in the United States but common in Africa and Asia. Secondary liver cancers are the results of cancers that originated elsewhere in the body, often the breast, lung, or colon. Cirrhosis predisposes a person to liver cancer.

In its early stages, liver cancer usually does not produce obvious symptoms. Later symptoms include weight loss, malaise, loss of appetite, abdominal swelling, and pain. Treatment is either surgery or chemotherapy or a combination of the two.

6. Lymphomas and Hodgkin's Disease

Hodgkin's disease most often strikes young people between the ages of 15 and 35. A second peak in the disease occurs in those 50 to 60. The first symptom is often an enlarged lymph node in the neck, armpit, or groin. Other symptoms include fever, night sweats, weight loss, and uncontrollable itching.

A classification system for Hodgkin's and other lymphomas has been devised based on the extent of the cancer. The levels are:

Stage One: cancer that involves a single node or region of nodes

Stage Two: cancers involving two regions of nodes, restricted either above or below the diaphragm

Stage Three: cancers present both above and below the diaphragm

Stage Four: cancers that have spread beyond the lymph nodes to other organs

Radiation therapy and chemotherapy, either alone or in combination, are the treatment of choice.

Symptoms of non-Hodgkin's lymphomas are enlarged lymph nodes, fever, weight loss, intestinal disturbances, bleeding, infection, and the buildup of fluids in the membranes that line the chest or abdominal cavities.

7. Mouth, Pharynx and Larynx Cancers

Most of these cancers occur in men over 45 who have a history of using cigarettes, pipes, cigars, chewing tobacco, or snuff. Excessive alcohol consumption can also play a role. These cancers usually form in the mucous membranes lining the upper respiratory and digestive tracts.

If detected in the early stages, these cancers have a high cure rate. In some cases reconstructive surgery is necessary in addition to radiation treatments.

8. Breast Cancer

Breast cancer is the second leading cancer killer among women. Its suspected causes include family history, early menarche (onset of periods), late menopause, late first pregnancy or no pregnancy, diet, alcohol, smoking, and local radiation.

Signs include nipple discharge, scaling, or bleeding; change in nipple direction; change in breast contour; skin dimpling; and persistent lumps. Monthly self-examination and regular exams by a doctor are recommended. Mammography aids in detection. Treatment is surgical removal of a lump, a part of the breast or the entire breast, or the entire breast and supporting muscle tissue. Surgery is often followed by chemotherapy or radiation therapy in the event the cancer has spread to surrounding lymph nodes.

9. Colon Cancer

Cancer of the colon is the second biggest cancer killer in the United States, after lung cancer. Twenty percent of cases are thought to be traceable to genetic predisposition. Other suspected causes include a diet high in fat and red meat and low in fiber. Symptoms include benign and malignant polyps (small, mushroomlike abnormalities of the intestine); generally, the larger the polyp, the greater the chance that it will be malignant. People who have long-term ulcerative colitis, diverticulosis, and polyps of the colon have a greater chance of developing this type of cancer. Rectal examinations and tests that screen for excessive blood in the stool are effective screening tests. Treatment includes surgery (to remove the tumor) and chemotherapy.

10. Lung Cancer

This cancer has surpassed breast cancer as the leading cancer killer of women, and now kills more than twenty-five times as many men as it did in 1930. Cigarette smoking is the primary cause of lung cancer—only 10 percent of patients are nonsmokers—but other risks include exposure to industrial substances such as asbestos, nickel, chromium, arsenic, radon, and halogenated ethers. Lung cancer often invades neighboring lymph nodes and spreads to other parts of the body.

Symptoms include weight loss, general fatigue, chest pain, coughing of blood, and a tumor that can be discovered by X rays. Treatment includes surgical removal of the tumor, a lobe of the lung, or the whole lung, depending on the extent to which the disease has spread. Drug therapy and radiotherapy (administration of X rays) are also prescribed for patients whose tumors have spread.

11. Prostate Cancer

This cancer is the second most common cancer among American men; it is a slow-developing cancer of the prostate gland, the accessory male sex gland below the bladder. Detection is through a rectal examination and the prostate-specific antigen (blood) test. Men over 50 are advised to undergo annual exams. Like other cancers, prostate cancer can metastasize, or spread, to other parts of the body. In many cases, however, prostatic cancer is a very slow-growing malignancy. Autopsy studies have shown that about one-third of men over the age of 50 have microscopic evidence of prostate cancer, yet the vast majority of these cancers grow so slowly they never become a threat to life. Hence the common statement that "most men die *with* prostate cancer, not *of* it."

12. Cervical Cancer and Cancer of the Uterus

Cervical cancer is one of the most common female cancers. Symptoms include polyps, bleeding, and lesions. Treatments include radiation and radical hysterectomy (removal of the uterus, adjoining tissue and lymph nodes, and ovaries). Early detection, which is accomplished by having regular Pap smears done, is crucial.

Cancer of the uterus usually begins in the lining of the uterus (the endometrium). This cancer has increased considerably in the past fifty years. Heredity plays a role, and this disease is more common among the affluent. Obesity is also a factor.

Abnormal bleeding is usually the first sign. When precancerous conditions exist, a dilation and curettage (D&C) and hormone treatment are often sufficient therapy. More advanced cases require a hysterectomy.

13. Leukemia

This group of diseases is characterized by a proliferation of white blood cells in the bone marrow that impedes the manufacture of red blood cells. The exact causes are unknown, although there appears to be increased risk associated with exposure to radiation, chemicals, and drugs. Symptoms are unexplained weight loss, low energy, fever, subcutaneous hemorrhaging, anemia, and lowered resistance to infection. Once fatal, leukemia can now be treated successfully in some cases with radiation and chemotherapy, anticancer drugs, antibiotics, steroids, and transfusions.

14. Skin Cancer

Of all the cancers, skin cancer is the most common and the easiest to diagnose. Basal cell carcinoma and squamous cell carcinoma are the two most prevalent types of skin cancer and are easily cured in most cases. Treatment includes surgery or topical medication.

Malignant melanoma is the most serious form of skin cancer as well as the most rare. An estimated 5,500 Americans die of this disease yearly.

All skin cancers are easily detected. Symptoms include growths or nodules on the skin that break and bleed. Melanoma usually begins as a brown spot on the skin; the lesion gradually forms an irregular border, variations in color, and an irregular surface. Radiation and chemotherapy offer little help in combating malignant melanoma.

Prolonged exposure to the sun increases the chances of contracting skin cancer. People who sunburn easily are especially susceptible. We cover this in detail in the discussion of the skin in section 1, "The Body and Its Parts."

The Great Debate:
Alternative Versus Conventional Treatments

In the hunt for the optimal cancer therapy, cancer patients inevitably witness the great debate about alternative methods of cancer treatments. While consumers watch, practitioners from both the alternative and mainstream cancer treatment camps proffer success stories and decry the other camp. Many in the medical world label alternative practitioners "quacks"; practitioners on the other side of the fence criticize the establishment for their "cut, burn, and poison" therapies.

The great debate between alternative and conventional cancer practitioners has been going on for decades—and it shows no signs of abating. Although unconventional methods of treatment are loudly and repeatedly denounced by mainstream medical associations, alternative (or complementary) cancer treatments continue to have an audience.

Why are consumers and physicians turning to unconventional techniques despite the recommendations of the medical giants?

The reason may well be twofold: First, patients and doctors have become frustrated with the limited effectiveness of mainstream medicine against major common cancers. Alternative therapies are attractive because they are frequently nontoxic, noninvasive, and do not endanger normal tissue. This, combined with the emphasis on quality of life, makes the alternative approach immensely appealing—especially since conventional therapies fail. It is no wonder, then, that they turn elsewhere for assistance and hope.

Second, alternative practitioners spend more time with each patient, emphasizing the patient's uniqueness and giving fuller explanations of treatment, according to an article some years back in the *Canadian Medical Association Journal.*

Interestingly enough, alternative practitioners don't fit the quack stereotype projected by the conventional medical world. According to one study, the majority of practitioners are physicians and some are verifiably board-certified. Nor are people who use alternative treatments ignorant and gullible, as the conventional medical world once claimed. The study, by Barrie R. Cassileth, Ph.D., of the University of Pennsylvania Cancer Center, found that patients who used alternative treatments exclusively or in conjunction with conventional therapy tended to be better educated than patients who used chemotherapy, radiation, and surgery only.

But how effective are alternative therapies? Unfortunately, unconventional therapies have not undergone the kind of scientific support and testing that the mainstream-endorsed therapies have received, or their results have not been published by "accepted" medical journals. Much of the evidence of their effectiveness is anecdotal, and the medical mainstream says this lack of proof makes these treatments unacceptable. That situation may change, as the U.S. Office of Technology Assessment is preparing guidelines for scientifically evaluating alternative therapies.

Despite the handful of articles that evaluate alternative therapies, consumers who are attracted to alternative approaches find it difficult to get an objective view of how these compare with standard, conventional methods. Many mainstream physicians have so little knowledge of alternative therapies that they cannot offer accurate guidance—assuming that they are willing to discuss the subject at all, which many are not.

Given the difficulty in getting straightforward information, how can the consumer decide between alternative and conventional therapies? Patrick McGrady, Jr., of CANHELP, Inc. (in the Seattle, Washington, area), has spent years helping cancer patients make treatment decisions. He offers these guidelines for making a decision:

• **Begin by evaluating conventional treatments.** As a cancer patient, McGrady says, you must scrupulously ask to see published studies of proposed therapies. Examine the mean survival time of each therapy.

"You are much better off with a treatment with a track record of success," McGrady says. "But if the published studies on conventional treatment do not offer the kind of long-term survival results you want, then consider alternative treatments. You must inform yourself of the availability of options. If you don't do that, you are selling yourself short."

• **Approach *all* therapies with suspicion.** "One has to be as suspicious of alternative therapies as of conventional treatments," says McGrady. "Just because they are less toxic doesn't mean they'll be more efficacious."

It's important to pin down what the doctor—any doctor—means by "response." Is that short-term survival, long-term survival, reduced pain, enhanced well-being, or what? Regard all cure and remission rates with caution; statistics can promise more than might apply to your situation, and some practitioners are fond of fabricating their own statistics.

In the absence of published studies to help you evaluate a treatment, you'd be smart to talk with patients of the doctors whose services you are considering using. "This is a burden for the doctor, but it is only fair for the doctor to give you names of patients who have successfully undergone treatment. Talk to the patients," McGrady says.

By and large, McGrady recommends dealing with M.D.'s. "You need to be monitored not just as a cancer patient but as a person susceptible to infections and illness. The practitioner needs a solid grounding in allopathic medicine."

On the other hand, the letters M.D. don't automatically mean that the practitioner will deliver the best treatment. McGrady advises that you approach all doctors with a healthy dose of skepticism. "I deal with the best doctors in the world, and I love them dearly, but I know they are all unreliable," he says. "Even the best of doctors does not have the time to do the best job. Nurses too are not perfect. The patient must bring all the support he or she can muster—families, friends, and support groups. You need a watchdog, someone who is really alert, who can also ask questions—such as `Why a green pill today when yesterday she took a white pill?'"

• **Ask questions and more questions.** "Learn to insist that physicians talk to you; learn to walk away from any doctor who doesn't meet your needs," McGrady advises.

"It's also very important to examine all the doctor's pieties. What is the doctor's biological theory? nutritional theory? Do these pieties conceal useless treatment? They often do," McGrady states. There are indeed quacks out there—"doctors who absolutely waste valuable time with useless treatment."

• **Act quickly.** "People do delay getting down to brass tacks," McGrady observes. "Yes, you want to get a third, fourth, even tenth opinion. But once the evidence is in, make up your mind and go for it right away.

"If the therapy works, stay with it," he says. "If the tumor is not shrinking, change treatment immediately." One advantage of doing all this homework, time-consuming though it may be, is that you'll have a Plan B waiting in the wings.

15. Multiple Myeloma
This cancer affects the skeleton and blood and is characterized by an imbalanced proliferation of plasma cells. Skeletal pain is usually the first symptom. As the disease progresses, skeletal deformities can result, particularly to the ribs, sternum, and spine. Anemia usually accompanies this cancer. Aspirin with or without codeine helps the skeletal pain. Other treatments include radiation and chemotherapy. Maintaining adequate body fluids is important in managing myeloma.

16. Gastrointestinal Cancers
These cancers include those of the pancreas, gallbladder, and bile ducts. In gallbladder cancer, it is estimated that 80 to 90 percent of patients also have gallstones; however, most people with gallstones never develop this cancer. If the cancer is discovered early, simple removal of the gallbladder is often sufficient. In more advanced cases, the outlook isn't as bright; chemotherapy seems to have limited success.

The pancreas has the highest incidence of cancer of sites within the gastrointestinal tract. Pancreatic cancer is the fifth most common cause of death from cancer in the United States, after lung, colorectal, breast, and prostate gland cancers. The usual warning sign in pancreatic cancer is jaundice.

In cancer of the bile duct, location plays a role in the outcome; cancers near the intestine seem to have a better long-term outlook.

17. Cancer of the Ovary
Ovarian cancer is rare among women under 35 but is more easily cured in younger women. This cancer can range from low- to high-grade. In low-grade cancers, the disease is limited to one or both ovaries and treatment is the removal of the ovaries, tubes, and uterus. In the most severe form, the cancer can spread to distant organs such as the lungs or bones. In these cases, radiation and chemotherapy are indicated.

18. Cancer of the Stomach and Small Intestine
Stomach cancer was once one of the most common cancers in the United States; now it is quite rare. It occurs most often in people from low social and economic classes, leading researchers to believe that diet plays a role. It is a common cancer in Japan, however.

The first symptoms of stomach cancer are abdominal pain and discomfort. Complaints of gas, indigestion, and a full feeling are common. Surgery to re-move all or part of the stomach offers the best chance of a cure.

Cancer of the small intestine is rare; the number-one predisposing factor is chronic inflammatory bowel disease. This cancer can be treated with surgery and chemotherapy.

19. Cancer of the Thyroid Gland
This cancer is suspect when a noticeable bulge appears on the throat near the Adam's apple. Most tumors turn out to be benign and are common among women of childbearing age. If malignant, surgery is recommended.

20. Urinary Tract Cancers
Blood in the urine is the number-one warning sign of these cancers. Environmental agents—such as dyes, leather, paints—seem to play a role in bladder cancer. Treatment can include the introduction of chemotherapeutic agents into the bladder or removal of the bladder.

CANCER TREATMENTS
It's frightening when the diagnosis is cancer. Amid the fear and anger, the question comes up: What is the best treatment for me?

Cancer treatments consist of both conventional and alternative therapies.

Conventional Cancer Therapies
Surgery involves the physical removal of tumors as a way of stopping their growth.

Radiation therapy uses X rays to kill cancer cells by producing biochemical changes that interfere with the cancer cell's ability to reproduce. Radiation is also used to relieve symptoms of cancer.

Chemotherapy is the use of cytotoxic (cell-destroying) drugs that circulate through the body to destroy cancerous cells. (Unfortunately, chemotherapy is also toxic to normal, healthy cells, and unpleasant side effects are common.) "Chemo" is frequently used as "adjuvant therapy"—in conjunction with surgery or radiation treatment. The idea is to destroy any cancer cells that escaped previous treatment so that they will not cause a recurrence.

Hormone therapy makes use of chemicals to halt the growth of cancer cells, but it doesn't kill cells directly. It stymies a tumor's growth by changing the hormonal environment.

Stamp of Approval

Thousands of hospitals treat cancer patients; some have received special designations or stamps of approval. The implication is that these organizations stand on the cutting edge with their research, clinical trials, and cancer treatments.

The National Cancer Institute has created several categories of cancer care groups and facilities that it funds:

- Comprehensive cancer centers, a select group of institutions (about twenty-three of them), investigate new methods of diagnosis and treatment and offer patients state-of-the-art treatment according to each center's specialty.
- Clinical and laboratory cancer centers. On a smaller scale, these centers also explore new methods of cancer treatment or do cancer research.
- Clinical cooperative groups bring together cancer research physicians from around the country into groups that each specialize in one kind of cancer.
- Community clinical oncology programs introduce new clinical research findings to community doctors and community hospitals and clinics.

Additionally, about 800 hospitals have cancer programs approved by the American College of Surgeons, which means they have multidisciplinary cancer conferences, a cancer registry, and requirements for the continuing education of health care professionals.

But here's a key point to remember: Approval of a cancer program only assures that certain program elements are in place and are functioning satisfactorily. Approval doesn't necessarily mean that you will receive the right care for your condition. Also, many cancer hospitals or clinics that feature alternative treatments—therapies that are not endorsed by mainstream medicine—will be excluded from these lists by the very nature of their programs.

Immunotherapy (also called biotherapy) seeks to control cancer by enhancing the body's disease-fighting systems. There are many branches of biotherapy in the investigative phase. One branch uses natural substances, such as interferon and interleukin-2, which are proteins found in the body that interfere with a virus's ability to replicate itself.

Bone marrow transplants replace a cancer patient's damaged bone marrow with healthy marrow—often in the form of an autologous transplant, in which some of the cancer patient's own marrow is removed, frozen, and stored, and then reintroduced *after* the patient has undergone radiation and chemotherapy. The bone marrow may also be taken from a compatible sibling or even an unrelated donor. Although these are complicated and hazardous procedures, in some cases they bring about a remission.

Research is being done in new areas of cancer control. Some of the hot projects today include research on monoclonal antibodies (using antibodies as guided missiles to deliver anticancer drugs directly to tumor cells, sparing healthy tissue); hyperthermia (using heat to stimulate white blood cells to attack cancer cells or to make cancer cells more vulnerable to radiation or chemotherapy); and laser treatment (projecting a laser beam onto a tumor to destroy cancer cells).

Because many of today's conventional treatments have limited effectiveness against cancer when used alone, combination therapy is becoming common. Radiation and chemo may be given to a patient before surgery, and combinations of radiation therapy and chemo may be administered to patients whose cancers are inoperable. The idea is to use one therapy to enhance the effect of another or to supply a strength when another treatment is weak.

Cancer Research Trials— Are They for You?

Modern medicine has yet to devise the perfect cancer cure. But coming up with a new generation of refined and sophisticated cancer combatants is one of the goals of clinical research trials. In the United States, clinical trials are a stepping-stone along the road to Food and Drug Administration approval of new cancer therapies. To work, they need participants—people with cancer who are willing to try an investigative therapy that may or may not meet with success.

Usually, each clinical trial is designed to answer one specific question about cancer. The idea behind these research ventures is that until people are given a new therapy in a controlled situation, there is no way physicians can scientifically measure its effectiveness. And so a carefully controlled trial is constructed to plumb the merits of the new approach.

Naturally, the question the study hopes to answer determines who can participate. Some investigations evaluate a therapy's effectiveness in the early stages of disease and are open to almost anyone. Others are designed for patients for whom there is no present effective treatment. Certain experiments will not accept people who have already undergone another form of cancer treatment.

One thing all clinical research trials share is uncertainty. There are no guarantees that a new treatment will succeed. In that regard, an investigative therapy may not offer you any advantage over existing treatment methods.

Out of the close to 1 million people diagnosed with cancer each year, about 25,000 participate in research trials. National Cancer Institute officials would like to double that figure, and so have announced plans for a major recruitment campaign.

As with any other medical encounter, the consumer needs to question the purpose of a study and to carefully balance its goals with his or her own cancer care needs.

Trial and Error: Questions to Ask

If you wish to participate in a cancer experiment, you can learn about openings in research trials by calling the National Cancer Institute's cancer information hotline, 1-800-4-CANCER. Your physician can also give you details on upcoming trials by tapping into NCI's Physician Data Query system, a computerized data bank of cancer information for doctors.

If you qualify to participate, you'll be given an informed-consent document that states the purpose of the investigation and discusses potential benefits and risks. But before you sign on the dotted line, be a smart consumer and ask these questions:

• How does this option compare with your other options? This entails looking at the possible treatments for your disease, their side effects, and their probability of success and then comparing that data with the goal of the clinical trial. Or, to put it another way: "The greatest need of the patient in making the decision to participate is thorough information about his or her condition," writes Emil J. Freireich, M.D., in *The American Cancer Society Cancer Book*. "The best source of information is the physician . . . [and] a major source of additional information is a second opinion."

• **What are the benefits of participation?** Many clinical trials have control groups—participants who are treated with a placebo or a conventional therapy instead of the new treatment. The control group is compared with the experimental group to measure the new therapy's success. Which group will you be placed in? If you aren't selected to try the experimental therapy, what therapy will you be given? How effective is that therapy? It should offer you a real benefit.

• **What are the predicted side effects?** Researchers pick promising drugs to explore in a clinical study. Although one goal of medicine is to develop anticancer drugs with few side effects, clinical trials are after all experimental and risks are not always foreseen. Some side effects can be serious, permanent, even life-threatening.

• **What checks and balances have been set up to monitor patient safety?** What rights do you have if you are dissatisfied with the quality of care or if you are harmed by research (either through unforeseen side effects or through human error)? Find out what treatment you would be entitled to and who would pay for it. In the same vein, query about the follow-up care you'll be entitled to after the study and how long it will continue.

• **What is the cost of participation?** More insurance companies these days are refusing payment for treatments that they term experimental. Check your insurance plan for details. Clinical trial participants can sometimes get financial assistance from foundations or social agencies. But quite often participation will mean payments for medical bills and incidental expenses—money out of your own pocket.

• **Can you withdraw from the trial?** Find out what will happen if you and the research project part paths. Will you be given another form of treatment? Will the research trial treatment interfere with getting another form of treatment later on? The National Cancer Institute claims that participants may leave any of its research studies at any time and that participants may refuse to take part in any aspect of the research.

Deciding to participate in a clinical trial is like any other consumer decision: You do it with eyes open to both the possible advantages and the possible disadvantages of the investigative therapy. Your doctor can help you weigh this option (as can family, friends, and clergy). But no one should pressure you by saying you "owe" medical science your illness to be researched, and you certainly shouldn't be afraid to say no. Ultimately, electing to participate or not participate is your decision.

Drawbacks of conventional techniques—especially the three standard therapies: surgery, radiation, and chemotherapy—are their mutilating and destructive properties. Some of the current research efforts strive to find the therapy that will extend survival while making treatment less painful. And while conventional medicine has not found the cure for most cancers, real progress has been made in treating some specific forms of the disease.

Alternative Cancer Therapies

Alternative cancer treatments (also called unconventional, complementary, or unproven treatments) can resemble investigative therapies, yet they exist for the most part outside the world of mainstream medicine. Rather than treating the symptom—the tumor—many of these therapies attempt to treat the cause, be it faulty physical health or spiritual well-being.

Michael Lerner's "A Report on Complementary Cancer Therapies" (*Advances,* winter 1985) offers an insightful description of the range of alternative therapies available to consumers, and although it was written some years back, its contents are still applicable. Lerner investigated complementary cancer therapies for three years and developed this classification of popular therapies:

Psychological approaches, including psychotherapy and imagery. Of all the alternative therapies, these approaches have the greatest credibility in conventional medicine, Lerner says. "In major cancer centers, imagery, relaxation, and patient-support groups are increasingly accepted, but their effects are believed to be limited to enhancing the quality of life, promoting acceptance of treatment, or relieving discomfort and pain. These are by no means trivial accomplishments."

Diet and nutritional-metabolic approaches include dietary regimens and nutritional supplement programs. Interestingly enough, says Lerner, in many cases "current research findings coincide with the nutritional recommendations of complementary cancer therapists."

Health-promoting lifestyles. This approach suggests that a healthful way of life can heal damaged cells. It can include yoga, aerobic exercise, deep relaxation exercises, and an emphasis on harmony with nature.

Spiritual approaches emphasize internal or transcendent methods of healing. These therapies "suggest that healing can take place for the patient at different levels—that a patient may die physically yet heal spiritually."

Alternative immune therapies, including herbal or so-called high-technology programs to bolster the immune system.

Alternative medical therapies are high-tech approaches such as the unconventional use of high-dose chemotherapy, radiation, and hyperthermia.

Other approaches include folk medicine systems.

In his concluding points, Lerner refers to the movement toward ethical complementary cancer therapies as part of a larger movement toward the rehumanization of medicine. "Gradually," he predicts, "the emphasis on good nutrition, psychological support, and more humane staff-patient relationships will become therapeutic ingredients of quality-care institutions."

Which of these techniques are most commonly used? According to Barrie R. Cassileth, Ph.D., and Helene Brown in *Ca—A Cancer Journal for Clinicians,* the most popular therapies are, in descending order of frequency of use, metabolic therapy (the detoxification, cleansing, and restoration of cells so that "impurities" will no longer interfere with the body's metabolism and healing abilities), diet treatments, megavitamins, mental imagery applied for antitumor effect, spiritual or faith healing, and immune therapy.

When looking for the right doctor and the right hospital, consider these criteria:

- Experience. The number of cancer patients treated is a better barometer than the size of the institution.
- Environment. Finding a hospital that treats you in a positive and pleasant manner influences the speed of your recovery and your frame of mind.
- Tumor registry and tumor committee. This information network helps review cancer patients and treatment plans.
- Complete staffing. Twenty-four-hour-a-day physician staffing and a full range of skilled nursing practitioners are recommended.

SOURCES OF CANCER TREATMENT INFORMATION

Information on Standard Cancer Treatments and Clinical Trials

American Cancer Society
1599 Clifton Road N.E.
Atlanta, GA 30329-4251
800-ACS-2345
404-320-3333

Leukemia Society of America
733 3rd Avenue
New York, NY 10017
212-573-8484

National Cancer Institute
Office of Cancer Communications
9000 Rockville Pike
Building 31, Room 10 A 31
Bethesda, MD 20892
800-4-CANCER
800-638-6070 in Alaska
800-524-1234 in Hawaii
301-496-5583

Information on Alternative Cancer Treatments

Cancer Control Society
2043 N. Berendo Street
Los Angeles, CA 90027
213-663-7801

Committee for Freedom of Choice in Cancer Therapy
1180 Walnut Avenue
Chula Vista, CA 92011
619-429-8200

International Association of Cancer Victors and Friends
7740 W. Manchester, Suite 110
Playa del Rey, CA 90291
213-822-5032

People Against Cancer
P.O. Box 10
Otho, IA 50569-0010
515-972-4444

Cancer Researchers

The following are researchers who, for a fee, will conduct a detailed literature search of your disease, often including conventional and alternative treatments.

Cancer Consulting Group
990 Grove
Evanston, IL 60201
312-866-7711

CANHELP, Inc.
Patrick McGrady, Jr.
3111 Paradise Bay Road
Port Ludlow, WA 98365-9771
206-437-2291

The Health Resource
Janice R. Guthrie
209 Katherine Drive
Conway, AR 72032
501-329-5272

Planetree Health Resource Center
2040 Webster Street
San Francisco, CA 94115
415-923-3680

Hospitals

The following hospitals are associated with a National Institutes of Health cancer research center.

Alabama

University of Alabama Hospitals
2451 Fillingim Street
Birmingham, AL 36617
205-471-7110

Arizona

University Medical Center
1501 N. Campbell Avenue
Tucson, AZ 85724
602-626-4660

California

City of Hope National Medical Center
1500 Duarte Road
Duarte, CA 91010-3012
818-359-8111

University of California at Los Angeles Medical Center
10833 Le Conte Avenue
Los Angeles, CA 90024-6972
213-825-9111

University of California at San Diego Medical Center
225 Dickinson Street
San Diego, CA 92103-6999
619-453-7500

University of Southern California
The Kenneth Norris Jr. Cancer Hospital
1441 Eastlake Avenue
P.O. Box 33804
Los Angeles, CA 90033-1085
213-224-6600

Colorado
University of Colorado Health Sciences Center
University Hospital
4200 E. 9th Avenue
Denver, CO 80262
303-399-1211

Connecticut
Yale–New Haven Hospital
20 York Street
New Haven, CT 06504
203-785-4242

District of Columbia
Georgetown University Hospital
3800 Reservoir Road N.W.
Washington, DC 20007
202-784-2000

Illinois
Northwestern Memorial Hospital
Superior Street and Fairbanks Court
Chicago, IL 60611
312-908-2000

Rush–Presbyterian–St. Luke's Medical Center
1653 W. Congress Parkway
Chicago, IL 60612-3833
312-942-5000

University of Chicago Hospitals
5841 S. Maryland Avenue
Chicago, IL 60603-1470
312-947-1000

University of Illinois
1740 W. Taylor Street
Chicago, IL 60611-4494
312-996-3900

Maryland
Johns Hopkins Hospital
600 N. Wolf Street
Baltimore, MD 21205-2182
410-955-5000

Massachusetts
Dana-Farber Cancer Institute
44 Binney Street
Boston, MA 02115-6084
617-732-3000

Michigan
Harper Hospital
3990 John R Street
Detroit, MI 48201-2097
313-745-8040

University of Michigan Hospitals
1500 E. Medical Center Drive
Ann Arbor, MI 48105-2300
313-769-7100

Minnesota
Mayo Clinic and Foundation
200 First Street S.W.
Rochester, MN 55902
507-284-2511

New Hampshire
Dartmouth-Hitchcock Medical Center
2 Maynard Street
Hanover, NH 03756
603-646-5000

New York
Memorial Sloan-Kettering Cancer Center
1275 York Avenue
New York, NY 10021-6094
212-639-2000

Montefiore Medical Center
Jack D. Weiler Hospital
Albert Einstein College of Medicine
1825 Eastchester Road
Bronx, NY 10461-2396
212-904-2000

New York University Medical Center
550 First Avenue
New York, NY 10016-6451
212-263-5111

Presbyterian Hospital in New York
Columbia-Presbyterian Medical Center
622 W. 168th Street
New York, NY 10032-3796
212-305-2500

Rochester General Hospital
1425 Portland Avenue
Rochester, NY 14621-3086
716-338-4000

Roswell Park Cancer Institute
666 Elm Street
Buffalo, NY 14203-1155
716-845-2300

Strong Memorial Hospital
University of Rochester
601 Elmwood Avenue
Rochester, NY 14642
716-275-2644

North Carolina
Duke University Medical Center
3000 Erwin Road
Durham, NC 27705
919-684-8111

North Carolina Baptist Hospital
Medical Center Boulevard
Winston-Salem, NC 27103
919-748-2011

University of North Carolina Hospital
Manning Drive
Chapel Hill, NC 27514-4216
919-966-4131

Ohio
Ohio State University Hospitals
410 W. 10th Avenue
Columbus, OH 43210-1236
614-293-8000

University Hospitals of Cleveland
2074 Abington Road
Cleveland, OH 44106-5001
216-844-1000

Pennsylvania
American Oncologic Hospital
Fox Chase Cancer Center
7701 Burholme Avenue
Philadelphia, PA 19111-2497
215-728-6900

Hospital of the University of Pennsylvania
3400 Spruce Street
Philadelphia, PA 19104-4228
215-662-4000

Montefiore University Hospital
3459 5th Avenue
Pittsburgh, PA 15213
412-648-6000

Presbyterian University Hospital
DeSoto at O'Hara Street
Pittsburgh, PA 15213-2593
412-624-2100

Rhode Island
Roger Williams Hospital
825 Chalkstone Avenue
Providence, RI 02908-4735
401-456-2000

Texas
Cancer Therapy and Research Center
4450 Medical Drive
San Antonio, TX 78229
512-690-1111

University of Texas
M.D. Anderson Cancer Center
1515 Holcombe Boulevard
Houston, TX 77030-4095
713-792-2121

Utah
University of Utah Hospital and Clinics
50 N. Medical Drive
Salt Lake City, UT 84132
801-581-2121

Vermont
Medical Center Hospital of Vermont
Colchester Avenue
Burlington, VT 05401-1726
802-656-2345

Virginia
Virginia Commonwealth University
Medical College of Virginia Hospitals
401 N. 12th Street
Richmond, VA 23219
804-786-9000

Washington
Fred Hutchinson Cancer Research Center
1124 Columbia Street
Seattle, WA 98104
206-467-5000

Wisconsin
University of Wisconsin Hospital and Clinics
600 Highland Avenue
Madison, WI 53792
608-263-6400

Cholesterol and Its Health Hazards

WHAT IS IT?

Cholesterol is a soft, fatlike substance found in all the body's cells. It is used to form cell membranes, certain hormones, and other necessary substances. Besides being present in human tissues, cholesterol is also found in the bloodstream—and is called serum cholesterol. The blood transports it to and from various parts of the body. Hypercholesterolemia is the term for high levels of cholesterol in the blood.

But the cholesterol most people know about is dietary cholesterol, which we talk about below.

HOW IS IT PRODUCED?

The liver provides the body with cholesterol in varying amounts, usually about 1,000 mg a day. An additional 400 to 500 mg or more can come directly from foods, most of which the liver processes. (Typically, the body makes all the cholesterol it needs, so it's not something people need to consume to maintain their health.)

Foods from animals—especially egg yolks, meat, fish, poultry, whole-milk products (such as cheeses, yogurt, sour cream, ice cream, and butter), and organ meats—contain it; foods from plants don't.

TYPES OF CHOLESTEROL

Cholesterol doesn't dissolve in water, the main component in blood, so the liver processes it into protein carriers called lipoproteins.

High-density lipoproteins (HDL), manufactured in the small intestine and the liver and released into the bloodstream, carry cholesterol back to the liver to be processed and disposed. HDL escorts excess cholesterol from the body and helps excrete it and is therefore sometimes referred to as the "good" cholesterol.

Low-density lipoproteins (LDL) carry cholesterol to cells in the body where it is used to form cell membranes. Excess LDL cholesterol is returned to the liver, broken down, and disposed of. Extra LDL cholesterol attracts and hangs onto fatty cholesterol and helps deposit it in arteries and cell walls, and is therefore sometimes referred to as the "bad" cholesterol. Very low-density lipoproteins (VLDL) carry the largest amount of triglycerides, lipids (body fats), that

are important in fat metabolism and the manufacture of cholesterol. High levels of VLDLs have also been linked to an increased risk of coronary artery disease.

CHOLESTEROL AND HEART DISEASE

In many medical studies over the past few decades, high levels of serum cholesterol—that is, the level of cholesterol in the blood—have been implicated in the formation of atherosclerosis (in which layers of artery walls become thick and irregular due to deposits of fat, cholesterol, and other substances) and coronary artery disease.

How cholesterol is involved in forming atherosclerotic plaque isn't perfectly clear. Much of the recent research into cholesterol and lipids has focused not so much on total serum cholesterol levels, but rather on the proportion of HDL to the total cholesterol picture. The way some medical researchers put it is that the problem is not how much cholesterol there is, but how it circulates and what company it keeps—HDL or LDL.

HOW MUCH CHOLESTEROL SHOULD I HAVE?

Doctors disagree on what is a good cholesterol level. Some are on the lenient side and choose numbers that cause their more cautious colleagues to question their recommendations. The more conservative doctors then promote numbers that others feel strongly are far too low.

Conservatively and safely, under 200 mg/dl (milligrams per deciliter of blood)—preferably in the 160–180 range—is considered a good level for minimum heart disease risk. Various doctors have different levels for alarm, but, conservatively, a reading higher than about 200 mg/dl is considered problematic by most experts. On the other hand, cholesterol that drops to noteworthy lows sometimes indicates a disease present in the body: perhaps pernicious anemia or hyperthyroidism.

A high HDL level means less chance of atherosclerosis and heart disease, and a low HDL or high LDL reading indicates trouble ahead. Exercise and moderate alcohol consumption have been shown to increase HDL levels. The higher the HDL level and the lower the total serum cholesterol level, presumably the more protected you are. Some studies have indicated even a regression in plaque when total cholesterol and LDL are lowered and HDL increased.

A recent examination of data from the Framingham Heart Study has confirmed that high cholesterol levels mean increased risk among people recovering from heart attacks. Compared to subjects who had a cholesterol level under 200 mg/dl (within a year after their heart attack), subjects with a cholesterol level over 275 mg/dl had a 3.8 times greater risk of a second heart attack. As reported in the *Annals of Internal Medicine* in late 1991, risk of death from coronary heart disease was found to be 2.6 times greater among the higher-cholesterol subjects. The message from this is loud and clear: If you're recovering from a heart attack, it's critical that you manage your cholesterol level.

Triglycerides are another form of fat in the body, and having a high serum triglyceride reading is as risky as having a high serum cholesterol level. According to the American Heart Association, triglyceride levels normally range from about 50 to 250 mg/dl, depending on age and sex. As people get older (or fatter or both), their triglyceride and cholesterol levels tend to rise. Women also tend to have higher triglyceride levels.

Several clinical studies have shown that an unusually large number of people with coronary heart disease also have high levels of triglycerides in the blood (called hypertriglyceridemia). However, some people with this problem seem remarkably free from atherosclerosis. Thus, elevated triglycerides, which are often measured along with HDL and LDL, may not directly cause atherosclerosis but may accompany other abnormalities that speed its development.

CAN CHOLESTEROL LEVELS BE CONTROLLED?

Scientists still disagree on methods aimed at lowering total serum cholesterol levels and whether or not a low-cholesterol diet is effective to any large degree. They do agree, however, that people who already have heart disease ought to be on low-cholesterol diets, but that's about all they agree on. It's probably wise and generally healthier to eat a low-fat, low-cholesterol diet, just in case.

Even though the jury's still out on the effectiveness of dietary cholesterol reduction in lowering total serum cholesterol—and the role of diet in heart disease altogether—here are some things that might work:

- Eat fewer calories, because losing weight helps. It isn't as important as other risk factors, but it shouldn't be ignored.
- Eat foods rich in fiber. (A word of caution here: Although there is research to support the popular—and commercially successful—notion that daily servings of oat bran can help reduce cholesterol, such findings also indicate that the amounts needed to do so are somewhere around 6 cups a day. Furthermore, oat bran and other fibers may combine with calcium in the gut to form a substance that your body cannot absorb.)
- Eat more fruits and vegetables, and replace animal fats—especially those that are solid at room temperature—with vegetable oils like corn, safflower, soybean, and sesame. A vegetarian diet may be protective.
- Get yourself a chart of foods and their dietary cholesterol content and place a ceiling of 300 mg a day on your meals.
- Cut down on coffee. One study linked high cholesterol to men who drank three cups a day or more. Besides, caffeine can elevate heart rate and cause arrhythmias that are not of benefit to anybody with heart disease.

There are drugs that lower serum cholesterol levels, although as with nearly everything else associated with the study of and research into cholesterol, atherosclerosis, and heart disease, results have been mixed. One of the more recent, more successful experiments saw a drug called cholestyamine reduce serum levels, but under very rigid clinical conditions.

Other drugs used to reduce serum cholesterol levels include colestipol hydrochloride, lovastatin, nicotinic acid, gemfibrozil, and sodium dextrothyroxine.

The consensus among experts is that only if dietary therapy and weight loss regimen have failed over the course of a year or so should drugs be used. Except in dire emergencies, they should not be the first treatment turned to.

Chronic Pain and Pain Management

Pain is not necessarily a bad thing. It's your body's warning system that all is not well. Caused by the signals from sense nerve endings, pain is a basic symptom of inflammation. But more than that, it's

Taking Control of Pain

When suffering from chronic pain, either you or the pain is in charge. To take control of the pain in your life, you should consider the following.

1. **Free yourself from strong pain medications.** Medications that were helpful following any surgery can be habit-forming. Ask your doctor to help you wean yourself from these drugs so that your body can start producing endorphins.

2. **Get moving physically.** Ask your doctor and therapist to help you develop an exercise program that is right for you. By building up endurance, you'll soon be feeling better.

3. **Eat properly for your whole body's sake.**

4. **If you smoke, try to quit.** This may be one of the best ways you can help yourself.

5. **Be of good cheer.** The more you laugh, the sooner it will stop hurting.

Adapted from the Comprehensive Pain Management Program, Good Shepherd Rehabilitation Hospital, Allentown, Pennsylvania.

important to the diagnosis of the cause of many disorders. And imagine the damage that would occur if you did not feel pain when touching a hot stove. This pain, by the way, is called acute pain: It is a normal sensation triggered in the nervous system to warn you of possible injury and the need to take care of yourself.

Chronic pain, however, is a different matter. It is persistent and often difficult to treat. Living with it can cause great emotional stress on the individual as well as loved ones.

Many people with chronic pain are otherwise healthy; for some of these people a change in lifestyle combined with a holistic, or comprehensive, approach to pain management may be helpful. Exercise and psychological support can allow the body to correct itself.

For others, chronic pain is a result of severe illness, such as arthritis or cancer, or is a side effect of a treatment, such as chemotherapy. Perhaps there was an initial injury, such as a broken leg or sprained back, from which the person has long since recovered, yet pain remains.

Older adults are often the victims of chronic pain, for many chronic pain conditions—cancer, arthritis, and angina (cramping chest pain caused by lack of oxygen to the heart muscle) associated with coronary heart disease—commonly afflict them.

THE SCIENCE OF PAIN

Pain relief occurs, either naturally or through the help of man-made painkillers, because of a "lock and key" system that involves special sites on cells called receptors. Painkilling chemicals are the keys that fit the receptors' lock.

When the brain receives a pain signal, it stimulates the release of the body's natural opiates (endorphins) from the nerve cells. Mu receptors (the most important of three known opiate receptors on nerve cells) are keyed to respond to the endorphins, or a drug that is similar, such as morphine. The endorphins then plug into the mu receptors, taking the edge off the pain.

TYPES OF PAIN CLINICS AND PAIN SPECIALISTS

Your doctor should be able to direct you to individual clinicians (doctors, dentists, therapists, and so on) who specialize in treating chronic pain or direct you to a nearby pain clinic or pain center. The three types of pain clinics are:

1. Comprehensive or multidisciplinary pain clinic or pain center. Usually based at a university medical center or major hospital; specializes in treating all kinds of chronic and acute pain, including cancer pain.

2. Syndrome-oriented clinic. Treats only one kind of pain problem—for example, a headache clinic or a low-back-pain clinic.
3. Treatment-oriented clinic. Specializes in using only one type of treatment for a pain problem— for example, acupuncture, biofeedback, nerve blocks.

To obtain a list of accredited pain treatment centers, write: The Commission on Accreditation of Rehabilitation Facilities, 2500 Pantzano Road, Tucson, AZ 85715.

MEDICATIONS IN CHRONIC PAIN RELIEF

Aspirin. Studies in patients with chronic pain show that two aspirin tablets are as potent as 30 to 60 mg of codeine in relieving pain. Many experts believe that related drugs like ibuprofen (a nonsteroidal anti-inflammatory agent) may be as potent as a morphine injection in relieving pain after surgery. Aspirinlike drugs are also effective in chronic pain conditions where inflammation is a factor, such as in arthritis. The advantage of aspirinlike drugs is that they have relatively few side effects; nonetheless, they do have them. Among the most serious are stomach and intestinal problems, blood clotting defects, and liver and kidney damage (associated with large doses over a long time).

Nerve blocks (or conduction anesthesia). Also known as a local anesthetic, a nerve block causes a loss of feeling in a part of the body through injection of a local anesthetic into a nerve, thus stopping the nerve signals from moving up and down the nerve. This type of pain relief has only limited effectiveness in dealing with chronic pain because nerve blocks wear off within a few hours. Nerve blocks affect an area larger than necessary to relieve pain; they also affect fibers needed for movement and other body sensations. Doctors can perform permanent nerve blocks that kill the pain; this is done in some cases of advanced cancer.

Opiate medications. Most cancers, surgery, burns, and kidney stones can be treated with these analgesics, which are narcotic drugs that contain opium, drugs made from opium, or any of several artificial or partly artificial drugs that behave like opium. The opiates include morphine, methadone, codeine, hydromorphone (Dilaudid), and meperidine (Demerol). Opiates eliminate pain, suppress cough, relieve shortness of breath, and stop diarrhea. However, for many people, they are not without unwanted side effects, such as nausea, vomiting, dizziness, and constipation.

Antidepressants. In some cases even antidepressant drugs have been known to benefit chronic pain sufferers, in part—experts believe—because such drugs increase the supply of a naturally occurring neurotransmitter, serotonin. According to the *Johns Hopkins Medical Handbook* (New York: Medletter Associates, 1992), "Scientists now have evidence that cells using serotonin are also an integral part of a pain-controlling pathway that starts with endorphin-rich nerve cells high up in the brain and ends with inhibition of pain-conducting nerve cells lower in the brain or spinal cord."

Pain

New clinical practice guidelines have been issued by the Agency for Health Care Policy and Research, a branch of the Department of Health and Human Services, in an effort to correct the problem of inadequate treatment of pain in patients with cancer.

The guidelines recommend the following clinical approach:

1. Ask about pain regularly

   Assess pain systematically

2. Believe the patient and family in their reports of pain and what relieves it

3. Choose pain control options appropriate for the patient, family, and setting

4. Deliver interventions in a timely, logical, coordinated fashion

5. Empower patients and their families

   Enable patients to control their course to the greatest extent possible

Undertreatment of Pain

Relief of pain and suffering should be the fundamental goal of every physician, yet new research indicates that physicians chronically underprescribe medications, thereby causing patients needless suffering. According to a survey undertaken at Rush–Presbyterian–St. Luke's Medical Center in Chicago and published in the journal *Pain,* 65 percent of hospitalized patients reported experiencing unbearable pain at some point.

Why are doctors reluctant to give adequate doses of painkilling drugs? After all, isn't the ancient medical dictum "to cure sometimes, to comfort always"? Doctors underprescribe largely because they fear that heavy doses of drugs will create addicts. They hold back even when their patients have only weeks or months to live. Russell Portnoy, M.D., director of analgesic studies at Memorial Sloan-Kettering Hospital, calls this a practice based on "a medical myth." Unfortunately, this misconception persists despite an important study published a decade ago in the *New England Journal of Medicine.* Out of 11,882 hospital patients treated with painkilling drugs, only 4 were found to have become addicted.

Still, the myth thrives, and not only among prescribing physicians but caregiving nurses as well. The Rush–Presbyterian–St. Luke's survey found that, on the average, nurses gave patients only one-fourth of the doses of painkillers allowed by the physicians. From this and other studies, it's clear that misinformation concerning effective doses, duration of effects, and dangers of addiction is rampant and, according to Portnoy, persists in part because of gaps in medical education. Currently, the typical 4-year medical curriculum devotes 4 hours or less to pain, and most experts agree that is not enough.

This state of affairs is echoed in a 1987 report by the Hastings Center, an eminent think tank specializing in medical ethics. "Guidelines on the Termination of Life-Sustaining Treatment and the Care of the Dying" concluded that "many health care professionals have inadequate knowledge about the pharmacology of pain relief and the appropriate use of narcotics and similar agents for dying patients."

So much for the problem. Now, what can you do? If you find yourself in such a situation, realize that you (or your surrogate) must play a major role.

- Specify in your living will that you wish medication to keep you as pain-free as possible. (See "Death and Dying Issues" in section 10, "Consumer Protection: Your Legal and Medical Rights," for more information.)
- Discuss with your doctor your fear of or concern about pain and your desire for adequate medication for control of pain. Pain is a complex symptom, and not all of it is physical in origin; much derives from anxiety, a sense of hopelessness, family stress, fear, spiritual concerns, and more—and all can lower your threshold for pain, thereby creating the perception of more and more pain.
- But also ask what the adverse side effects of the painkilling drugs are. A June 1988 article in *Postgraduate Medicine* points out that pain control measures often fail because the patient cannot anticipate the adverse side effects.

- **Communicate as honestly as you can the extent of your pain.** Some experts recommend that doctors ask two key questions: Does the medicine ever take the pain away completely? Does the pain return before it's time for the next dose of medicine? According to Robert G. Twycross and Sylvia A. Lack in *Symptom Control in Far Advanced Cancer: Pain Relief,* if no is the first answer, then the dose should be increased. If the second answer is yes, then the dose should be increased. But don't wait for your doctor to ask the questions. Give him or her the answers right away.
- **Discuss with your physician the alternative therapies for pain relief**—for example, biofeedback, hypnosis, relaxation techniques, and acupuncture. While they may not work in your case, they have in many others.

OTHER TREATMENTS OR METHODS FOR CHRONIC PAIN RELIEF

Acupuncture. Although practiced in China for thousands of years, acupuncture remains a controversial therapy for pain in Western medicine. In it, fine, wire-thin needles are inserted under the skin at selected sites. The needles are twirled, given a slight electric charge, or warmed. Opinion is divided as to acupuncture's efficacy, with its proponents arguing that the local needling of the skin activates endorphin systems of pain control. Its detractors maintain that chronic pain patients show no long-term benefit from the treatment.

Transcutaneous electrical nerve stimulation (TENS). This method of pain control applies brief pulses of electricity to nerve endings. Electrodes are placed on the skin, preferably near where the pain is felt, and joined by wires to a machine. Experts describe this method as fairly safe and with no known side effects (although it is important to note that TENS is not done on people with pacemakers).

Brain stimulation. Like TENS, this is an electrical method for controlling chronic pain. It utilizes surgically implanted electrodes in the brain in sites known to be rich in receptors and endorphin-containing cells. The person actually determines when and how much stimulation is needed to control pain, doing so by operating the external transmitter that beams electronic signals to a receiver under the skin that is connected to the electrodes. Clearly, a disadvantage is that this technique requires brain surgery and the risks and costs associated with it.

Relaxation techniques. Broadly speaking, these are therapies in which patients are taught to do breathing and relaxation exercises to relax stiff or tense muscles, reduce anxiety, and alter their mental states. *Biofeedback,* for example, teaches the person to monitor certain functions of the body, such as muscle tension, and to alter the functions through relaxation. The belief behind any relaxation technique is that tension, if it is not actually at the root of the chronic pain, can make any pain worse. *Meditation,* in a manner of speaking another relaxation technique, aims to produce a state of relaxed but alert awareness—a state, it is hoped, in which a person tries to stop awareness of his or her surroundings so that the mind can focus on a single thing, such as a key word or image.

Hypnosis. This technique induces a passive, trancelike state resembling normal sleep and resulting in increased responsiveness to suggestion. Hypnosis is used to help reduce pain, aid relaxation, and reduce anxiety sometimes associated with chronic pain; however, not every person is a good subject for this technique, and hypnosis is not without its critics.

CHRONIC PAIN RESOURCES

American Chronic Pain Association
P.O. Box 850
Rocklin, CA 95677
916-632-0922

International Pain Foundation
909 N.E. 43rd Street, Suite 306
Seattle, WA 98105-6020
206-547-2157

National Chronic Pain Outreach Association
7979 Old Georgetown Road, Suite 100
Bethesda, MD 20814
Send SASE.
301-652-4948

Common Infectious Diseases

Infectious diseases are diseases caused by germs, or microbes. These tiny, living cells can be divided into three types: bacteria, protozoa, and viruses.

When these tiny microbes either invade tissue or release poisons, they cause disease. Some viruses multiply within a cell then destroy it; this is the case with polio, for example. Some bacteria, like the ones that cause tetanus or diphtheria, release strong poisons (toxins) that spread throughout the body. Some common bacteria interfere with body functions; this, for example, is what happens when bacteria enter the intestines and cause diarrhea.

The symptoms of the onset of infectious disease often include: headache, body ache, weakness, fatigue, listlessness, fever, and poor appetite.

GASTROINTESTINAL INFECTIONS

These infections generally affect the stomach or the intestines.

Gastroenteritis. The most common causes of this infection of both the stomach and intestines are bacteria and viruses. Food contaminated with the toxin staphylococci causes a form of food poisoning: Suspect foods are those that are made from dairy products, such as salad dressings and cream-filled desserts. Dehydration can occur if vomiting becomes severe.

Many viruses also cause gastroenteritis. This "intestinal flu" is marked by nausea, vomiting, and diarrhea and usually goes away within a few days. The best treatment is to drink plenty of liquids to prevent dehydration.

Diarrhea. Diarrhea is a bowel movement that is looser and more frequent than is usual for the individual. A doctor needs to be seen if the illness lasts more than 1 or 2 days; if the patient is an infant, young child, or elderly person; if the patient is already dehydrated from some other illness; if the diarrhea is accompanied by high fever, cramps, rashes, jaundice, or blood, pus, or mucus in the stools.

Hepatitis. Type A hepatitis is a viral disease caused by the ingesting of contaminated food. The infection is spread by direct contact or through fecal-contaminated food or water, and the symptoms—nausea, vomiting, loss of appetite, fatigue, muscle and joint aches—usually develop within 2 to 5 weeks of exposure. Other symptoms can include dark urine,

clay-colored stools, jaundice, and fever. Injections of human gamma globulin provides protection against the spread of Type A hepatitis. This illness tends to clear up within 1 or 2 weeks. In rare cases it can cause cirrhosis, the scarring of the liver; in rarer cases, it can lead to death.

Type B hepatitis is more severe than Type A and is a virus commonly spread from the blood of an infected individual to others. Hemophiliacs, those who receive transfusions or other blood products, homosexual men, and drug users who exchange needles are at a high risk. Type B hepatitis is more likely to scar the liver and is slower to heal. Prolonged bed rest is the only treatment. A vaccine is available for those at risk.

Researchers are still gathering information about this disease, but it appears that non-A, non-B hepatitis is spread through sexual activity and contact with infected blood. The symptoms are similar to those of hepatitis A and hepatitis B, but they are often milder.

RESPIRATORY INFECTIONS

The common cold. A variety of viruses causes the common cold, a contagious disease readily spread by close contacts with others. Certain over-the-counter drugs, such as aspirin and nasal decongestants, can relieve symptoms but do not actually offer a cure. The best treatment is bed rest and liquids. The most serious complications of the common cold are secondary infections, such as bronchitis, sinusitis, and tonsillitis.

Influenza. The flu is caused by a specific group of viruses. It differs from the common cold in that the illness comes on suddenly. Symptoms include fever, chills, muscle aches, fatigue, and weakness. The cough is dry and the eyes may become red. The flu can be dangerous to the elderly, and vaccines are recommended for them as well as for pregnant women and infants. Treatment includes bed rest, aspirin, and liquids. A dangerous complication is pneumonia.

Sinusitis. When bacteria or viruses enter the air-filled spaces within the facial bones, infection occurs. If the ducts connecting the sinus cavities become inflamed, the sinuses become unable to drain mucus, and they swell and become painful. Antibiotics can help, and drainage can be restored by drugs that shrink the swollen tissues.

Sore throat. Most sore throats are caused by viruses, but the common bacterium hemolytic streptococcus causes a sore throat that, if not treated with antibiotics, can lead to complications such as rheumatic fever. To test for strep throat, cells are scraped from the back of the throat and later studied.

Tonsil infection. Sometimes strep bacteria invade the tonsils. High fever, severe sore throat, and difficulty swallowing are the usual symptoms. Infected tonsils are treated with antibiotics.

Laryngitis. Laryngitis is the inflammation of the larynx and vocal cords. If bacterial in nature, it is treated with antibiotics. For viral laryngitis, bed rest and liquids are recommended. Croup is a form of laryngitis that occurs in young children. Its first symptom is a barking cough and hoarse voice. Because airways can become constricted, croup is a serious illness. Treatment with steam usually suffices.

Pneumonia. Pneumonia is the infection of the air spaces of the lung and can be either viral or bacterial in nature. The most common viral pneumonia is caused by the influenza virus. Symptoms include those commonly associated with the flu as well as chest pain, shortness of breath, cough, and high fever. Treatment consists of bed rest, fluids, and aspirin. Of the bacteria causing pneumonia, the most common one is the *Streptococcus pneumoniae*. Most bacterial pneumonias respond to antibiotics, usually within 3 weeks.

OTHER INFECTIOUS DISEASES

Urinary infections. Urinary infections are more common in women than in men and are particularly bothersome to elderly women. Most of these infections are caused by common bacteria found in the intestinal tract: In women, these bacteria travel through the short, female urethra, find their way into the bladder, and multiply in the urine. In elderly men, urinary infections can be brought on by enlargement of the prostate gland.

Drinking lots of water helps prevent these infections. Treatment is antimicrobial drugs that relieve symptoms within 1 to 2 days.

Meningitis. This is a serious bacterial infection that results in the inflammation of the membranes that cover the brain and spinal cord. When caused by viruses, it usually is not as serious.

Symptoms of bacterial meningitis are fever, difficulty in waking up, confusion, irritability, and stiffness and pain in the neck. Bacterial meningitis caused by the *Hemophilus influenzae* is most common in children 18 months old to 4 years old. Treatment is with antibiotics.

The symptoms of viral meningitis are less severe. They include headache, pain in neck muscles, fever, and sometimes a rash.

Tetanus (Lockjaw). The symptoms of this disease caused by bacterial-producing spores are restlessness, irritability, stiffness of muscles, and sometimes difficulty in swallowing.

The spores enter the body through cuts and other wounds. If tissue closes over the wound, the lack of oxygen can cause these spores to grow and resulting toxins then travel along the nerves and affect the central nervous system. This disease is easily prevented by keeping up to date on tetanus shots. Treatment includes oxygen if respiratory nerves have been affected. Antibiotics can help.

Herpes simplex. This viral infection is caused by a herpes simplex virus, which attacks the skin and nervous system and usually produces small, short-lived, fluid-filled blisters on the skin and mucous membranes. Herpes simplex I (called oral herpes) infections tend to occur on the face, most commonly where the lips meet the skin or around the nose. (These blisters are often called cold sores or fever blisters.) This recurring infection is often brought on by stress; heat compresses can help skin rashes.

Herpes simplex II (called genital herpes) infections are usually limited to the genital area and usually passed along by sexual contact. Painful sores appear on the skin and moist lining of the sex organs of men and women. Antibiotics are the usual treatment. The blisters can be cleaned with soap and water to help prevent secondary infections.

Depression

Major depressive disorder (depression) is a common illness that affects 1 in 20 Americans each year and twice as many women as men. Important to note is that a depressive illness is a "whole body" illness, involving body, mood, thoughts, and behavior. It is not a passing blue mood, nor is it a sign of personal weakness or a condition that can be willed or wished away. Without treatment, symptoms can last for weeks, months, or years. Appropriate treatment, however, can help over 80 percent of those who suffer from depression, according to the National Institute of Mental Health.

As to the causes of depression, research conducted by the National Institute of Mental Health indicates there is a risk for developing depression when there is a family history; in other words, a biological vulnerability can be inherited. The risk may be somewhat higher for those diagnosed with bipolar depression or manic-depressive illness. However, not everybody with a genetic vulnerability develops the illness. Additional factors, possibly a stressful environment and other psychosocial factors, are involved in the onset of depression.

Though major depression seems to occur generation after generation in some families, it can also occur in people who have no family history of depression. So, whether the disease is inherited or not, it is evident that people with major depressive illness often have too little or too much of certain neurochemicals.

Obviously, too, psychological makeup plays a role in vulnerability to depression. People who have low self-esteem, who consistently view themselves and the world with pessimism, or who are readily overwhelmed by stress are prone to depression. A serious, chronic illness, difficult relationship, financial problem, or any unwelcome change in life patterns can also trigger a depressive episode.

The major treatments for depression are antidepressant medication, psychotherapy, and a combination of the two.

Depression is generally divided into three types: psychological, biological, and a mixture of psychological and biological. The main symptom of all depressions is a persistent unhappy, sad, anxious, or "empty" mood.

Psychological depression. Triggered by psychological or emotional events, such as the breakup of a marriage or loss of a job. Symptoms are exclusively psychological and emotional. Biological functioning is most likely unaffected.

Biological depression. Triggered by physiological event within the body, rather than painful life experience. Often accompanied by a variety of physical symptoms caused by chemical imbalances in the nervous and hormonal systems.

Psychological depression with biological symptoms (mixed). Triggered by psychological or emotional events, but symptoms are both emotional and physical.

List 1
Psychological Symptoms of Depression
Sadness and despair
Low self-esteem
Apathy; no motivation
Interpersonal problems
Guilt feelings
Negative thinking (cognitive distortions)
Suicidal thoughts

List 2
Physical Symptoms of Depression
Sleep disturbances
Appetite disturbances
Loss of sex drive
Fatigue and decreased energy
Inability to experience pleasure (anhedonia)
Family history of depression, suicide, eating
    disorders, or alcoholism
Panic attacks

List 3
Symptoms That May Be Seen in Both Psychological and Biological Depressions
Poor concentration and poor recent memory
Hypochondria—excessive concerns with one's health
Drug/alcohol abuse
Excessive emotional sensitivity (including anger and
    irritability)
Pronounced mood swings
Any or all of the symptoms in Lists 1 and 2

List 4
Diseases and Disorders That Can Cause Depression

Addison's disease	Malignancies (cancer)
AIDS	Malnutrition
Anemia	Menopause
Asthma	Multiple sclerosis
Chronic infection	Porphyria
(mononucleosis, TB)	Postpartum mood
Congestive heart	changes
failure	Premenstrual syndrome
Cushing disease	Rheumatoid arthritis
Diabetes	Syphilis
Hyperthyroidism	Systemic lupus
Hypothyroidism	erythematosus
Infectious hepatitis	Ulcerative colitis
Influenza	Uremia

BIOLOGICAL FACTORS IN DEPRESSION

Endogenous (produced from within) depressions are the most common of the biologically caused depressions. They occur in susceptible people for unknown reasons but tend to run in families.

Manic-depression (bipolar depression) is one such disorder. Not nearly as prevalent as other forms of depressive illness, manic-depressive illness involves cycles of depression and elation or mania. Sometimes the mood switches are dramatic and rapid, but most often they are gradual.

A second endogenous depression is seasonal affective disorder (SAD). The gray skies and reduced daylight of winter can trigger a chemical imbalance in susceptible individuals, resulting in a severe biological depression. "Light therapy" is helpful for individuals with this disorder. Patients sit 3 feet away from full-spectrum fluorescent lights for 2 to 3 hours a day during the winter.

Medication side effects can trigger biological depression. These drugs include antihypertensives (medications for high blood pressure), cortisone acetate, estrogen, progesterone, anti-Parkinson drugs, antianxiety drugs, and birth control pills.

Other triggers in biological depression include chronic drug and/or alcohol abuse, physical illness, and hormonal changes.

ANTIDEPRESSANT MEDICATIONS

Three groups of antidepressant medications have been used to treat depressive illnesses: tricyclics (Tofranil, Elavil), monoamine oxidase inhibitors (MAOIs—Marplan, Nardil, Paranate), and lithium. Lithium is the treatment of choice for manic-depressive illness and some forms of recurring, major depression.

There are now newer antidepressants available that are neither tricyclics nor MAOIs and that generally lack the side effects associated with these two

Helping Yourself

Depressive illnesses make you feel exhausted, worthless, helpless, and hopeless. Such negative thoughts and feelings make some people feel like giving up. It is important to realize that these negative views are part of depression and typically do not accurately reflect your situation. Negative thinking fades as treatment begins to take effect. In the meantime:

- Do not set yourself difficult goals or take on a great deal of responsibility.
- Break large tasks into small ones, set some priorities, and do what you can as you can.
- Do not expect too much from yourself. This will only increase feelings of failure.
- Try to be with other people; it is usually better than being alone.
- Participate in activities that may make you feel better. You might try mild exercise, going to a movie or a ball game, or participating in religious or social activities. Don't overdo it or get upset if your mood is not greatly improved right away. Feeling better takes time.
- Do not make major life decisions, such as changing jobs or getting married or divorced, without consulting others who know you well and who have a more objective view of your situation. In any case, it is advisable to postpone important decisions until your depression has lifted.
- Do not expect to "snap out" of your depression. People rarely do. Help yourself as much as you can, and do not blame yourself for not being up to par.
- *Remember,* do not accept your negative thinking. It is part of depression and will disappear as your depression responds to treatment.

Source: "Depression: What You Need to Know," a pamphlet published by the National Institute of Mental Health.

traditional classes of drugs. One type, SSRIs (serotonin-specific reuptake inhibitors—Desyrel, Prozac, Zoloft), selectively blocks the reuptake of one of the major neurotransmitters, serotonin.

Antidepressants may cause mild and usually temporary side effects in some people. The most common ones usually associated with tricyclic depressants are dry mouth, constipation, bladder problems, sexual problems, blurred vision, dizziness, and drowsiness. According to the National Institute of Mental Health, the newer antidepressants have different types of side effects, including headache, nausea, nervousness and insomnia, and agitation.

Antidepressant drugs are not habit-forming, says the National Institute of Mental Health. However, as is the case with any type of medication prescribed for more than a few days, antidepressants have to be carefully monitored to see that a person is getting the correct dosage.

If someone is taking MAO inhibitors, he or she will have to avoid certain foods, such as cheese, wine, and pickles. Other forms of antidepressants require no food restrictions.

Another important rule is that a person should never mix medications of any kind—prescribed or over-the-counter—without consulting his or her doctor.

PSYCHOTHERAPIES

There are many forms of psychotherapy used to help depressed individuals, including some short-term therapies (usually defined as 10 to 20 weeks). "Talking" therapies help people gain insight into and resolve their problems through verbal "give-and-take" with the therapist. So-called behavioral therapists help people learn how to obtain more satisfaction and rewards through their own actions and how to unlearn the behavioral patterns that contribute to their depression.

Two of the short-term psychotherapies that research has shown helpful for some forms of depression are interpersonal and cognitive/behavioral therapies. Interpersonal therapists focus on the patient's disturbed personal relationships that both cause and aggravate the depression. Cognitive/behavioral therapists help people change the negative styles of thinking and behaving often associated with depression.

Psychodynamic therapies, sometimes used to treat depression, focus on resolving the patient's internal psychological conflicts that are typically thought to be rooted in childhood.

Drug Abuse

Drug abuse is any deliberate misuse of a drug for nonmedical purposes or for reasons other than its intended purpose. Found at all social levels and backgrounds, the drug abuser is dependent upon drugs to alter his mood or perception of reality and to gratify his physical desires or enhance his abilities to such a degree that harm to his health and others results.

Drug abuse is normally characterized by certain drug-dependent states (addictions) in which the abuser finds himself: psychologically dependent, physically dependent, and functionally dependent. *Psychological dependence,* or habituation, is a type of compulsive neurotic behavior in which there is an emotional need and craving for and reliance upon drugs to maintain a sense of well-being. *Physical dependence,* or true addiction, is a state in which the body physically needs the drug in such a way that, if the drug dosage were drastically reduced or stopped, withdrawal symptoms appear. Another manifestation of physical dependence is the tolerance the drug user gains in continued, repeated use of a drug. The user is tolerant of a drug when increasingly higher doses of the drug are needed to maintain the same drug effect. *Functional dependence* describes the dependence of the body's functions on a certain drug to maintain a sense of well-being (a person may become functionally dependent even on laxatives or nasal sprays). One or all of these drug dependencies are characteristically present in patterns of excessive and/or regular drug abuse.

All drugs, chemical entities that create a specific response in a biological system, are dangerous and have the potential of being misused. Any drug, be it an illicit street drug or a prescription medication, can be misused and/or abused. The ways in which a drug may be abused depends upon the drug itself, its dosage and effects, its route of administration in the body, the availability of the drug itself, and its addictive quality.

Addiction, a chronic, uncontrollable, and compulsive behavior which is the hallmark of the drug abuser, results after continued exposure to certain drugs. Some drugs are more addicting than others—narcotics and cocaine, for example, have highly addictive properties.

In general, abusers take drugs at regular, short intervals and exercise little or no self-control over their drug usage. Drugs may offer the users a euphoric sense or "high"; relieve feelings of inadequacy, depression, and pain; improve performance or abilities (such as with anabolic steroids); or give the user a way to escape from reality, stressful problems, or an unpleasant environment. In any case, no matter which reason prompts them to take drugs, abusers continue using drugs to experience a certain state of euphoria and well-being and eventually to maintain and cope with everyday life. This type of drug dependence can lead to many health complications, including disease (hepatitis, lung and heart disease, for example), mental problems, and even AIDS.

Drugs, specifically psychoactive drugs (those drugs that influence the mind), can be inhaled, ingested, or injected. These different routes of administration allow drugs to be carried through the bloodstream, eventually to the central nervous system. Those drugs that are intravenously injected or inhaled affect the drug user at a faster rate than ingested ones.

Drugs are classified into general categories:

Depressants. Drugs that slow down and relax signals passing through the central nervous system and are able to produce a physical dependency: alcohol, barbiturates, sedatives, and tranquilizers.

Narcotics or narcotic analgesics. Painkillers that are addicting and produce an intense high: opium, codeine, heroin, and morphine.

Stimulants. Addicting drugs that speed up signals to the central nervous system and produce alert, energetic behavior: cocaine, amphetamines, caffeine, nicotine.

Hallucinogens. "Psychedelic" drugs that produce hallucinations or changes in sensory perceptions: LSD, ecstasy, mescaline, PCP, psilocybin, and cannabis (marijuana, hashish).

Drug users can take any of these various drugs and experience different effects; however, drug users can eventually develop addictions and become physically and psychologically dependent on the drug.

The signs and symptoms of drug abuse vary from person to person, but general signs of addiction and abuse can be recognized:

1. Changes in personality or behavior, such as violent mood swings of euphoria, apathy, and depression, changing friendships, secretiveness, lying, denial of problems, and demanding or stealing money.
2. Decline in job performance or academic performance; poor work effort or poor grades, inattentiveness or distraction at job or at school.
3. Changes in physical habits or appearance, including weight loss, loss of appetite, change in sleeping habits, appearance of unusual skin lesions, puncture wounds, appearance of symptoms indicating the onset of severe health problems or diseases, persistent cough, nasal congestion, red, bloodshot eyes, physical exhaustion, different clothes, or indifference to personal grooming.
4. Withdrawal from parents, family, friends; solitary drug use, little or no communication with those around the user.
5. Discovery of drugs or drug paraphernalia: hypodermic needles, tubes, plastic bags, or other suspicious articles found on or around the user.
6. Frequent intoxication of user. User is consistently intoxicated or high and exhibits abnormal or hazardous behavior.

Drug addiction may also be suspected if a reduced dosage or complete cessation of the drug produces pronounced withdrawal symptoms.

General withdrawal symptoms include aches and pains, anxiety, chills, cramps, convulsions, dehydration, diarrhea, dizziness, fever, hot flashes, insomnia, nausea, perspiration, psychotic behavior, tremors, vomiting, and weakness. These symptoms occur because the body becomes dependent on the continuous presence of the drug in the body's system. When the drug is eliminated or reduced, the body experiences mental and physical symptoms. Some of the drugs that can produce marked withdrawal symptoms are alcohol, narcotics, nicotine and caffeine, tranquilizers, amphetamines, marijuana, and cocaine.

The treatment of drug dependence and abuse consists of various treatment programs, most of them employing gradual detoxification and continued psychotherapy. Treatment can be drug-free or maintenance, residential (halfway houses, therapeutic communities, etc.) or ambulatory (outpatient treatment facility), voluntary or involuntary (complete hospitalization), or a combination of several of these methods. Drug-free programs are aimed at abstinence, total withdrawal from the drug—for example, Alcoholics Anonymous (AA). Maintenance treatment involves detoxification by the administration of other drugs that relieve and prevent unpleasant withdrawal symptoms—for example, Antabuse (an antagonist drug for alcohol); methadone or naltrexone (antagonist of heroin).

Drug-Induced Deaths

According to the August 31, 1993, *Monthly Vital Statistics Report* from the Centers for Disease Control and Prevention and the National Center for Health Statistics, in 1991 a total of 10,388 persons died of drug-induced causes in the United States. The category "drug-induced causes" includes not only deaths from dependent and nondependent use of drugs (legal and illegal use) but also poisoning from medically prescribed and other drugs.

The age-adjusted death rate for drug-induced causes increased by 35 percent from 1983 to 1988, then declined 14 percent between 1988 and 1990, and increased again in 1991 by 6 percent. The age-adjusted death rate for drug-induced causes for males was 1.9 times the rate for females, and the rate for the black population was 1.8 times that for the white population.

With any drug abuse treatment program, psychological and emotional support for the user is essential for the recovery of his or her mental stability. Local or community support groups (for example, AA and Narcotics Anonymous) and family members can provide invaluable support and encouragement for the rehabilitation of the drug user. Other support groups exist to help family members cope with another member's addiction (Alateen and Al-Anon, for example, for alcoholism). Further, local agencies, abuse centers, clinics, and abuse hotlines can give information about drugs and drug abuse.

DRUG ABUSE RESOURCES

Listed below are telephone numbers and addresses of various governmental and nongovernmental agencies that provide information and advice on drug abuse.

Al-Anon Family Groups Headquarters
P.O. Box 862, Midtown Station
New York, NY 10018
800-356-9996
800-245-4656 in New York
800-443-4525 in Canada

American Council for Drug Education
204 Monroe Street, Suite 110
Rockville, MD 20850
301-294-0600
800-488-3784

Drug Abuse Information and Treatment Referral Line
11426 Rockville Pike, Suite 410
Rockville, MD 20852
800-662-4357
800-662-9832 Spanish
800-228-0427 Hearing-impaired

National Clearinghouse for Alcohol and Drug Information
Substance Abuse Prevention
P.O. Box 2345
Rockville, MD 20852
301-468-6433
800-729-6686

National Council on Alcoholism and Drug Dependence
12 W. 21st Street
New York, NY 10010
212-206-6770
800-622-2255

State Drug Abuse Treatment Offices

These agencies provide programs for the prevention, detection, treatment, and rehabilitation of drug abusers. They also coordinate the implementation of drug abuse prevention programs in the community, school, and workplace.

Alabama
Drug Abuse Office
Mental Illness and Substance Abuse
Department of Mental Health
200 Interstate Park Drive
P.O. Box 3710
Montgomery, AL 36193
205-270-4648

Alaska
Drug Abuse Office
Alcoholism and Drug Abuse Division
Health and Social Services Department
P.O. Box 110607
Juneau, AK 99811
907-586-6201

Arizona
Drug Abuse Office
Community Behavioral Health Services
411 N. 24th Street
Birch Hall
Phoenix, AZ 85008
602-220-6488

Arkansas
Drug Abuse Office
Alcohol and Drug Abuse Prevention
Department of Human Services
P.O. Box 1437
Little Rock, AR 72203
501-682-6656

California
Drug Abuse Office
Alcohol and Drug Programs Department
1700 K Street
Sacramento, CA 95814
916-445-1943

Colorado
Drug Abuse Office
Alcohol and Drug Abuse Division
4210 E. 11th Avenue
Denver, CO 80220
303-331-8201

Connecticut
Drug Abuse Office
Alcohol and Drug Abuse Commission
999 Asylum Avenue
Hartford, CT 06105
203-566-4145

Delaware
Drug Abuse Office
Alcoholism and Drug Abuse Bureau
Health and Social Services Department
1901 N. DuPont Highway
New Castle, DE 19720
302-421-6101

District of Columbia
Drug Abuse Office
Department of Human Services
1300 First Street N.E.
Washington, DC 20002
202-727-0740

Florida
Drug Abuse Office
Alcohol, Drug Abuse and Mental Health
1317 Winewood
Building 6, Room 183
Tallahassee, FL 32399
904-488-8304

Georgia
Drug Abuse Office
Substance Abuse Section
Division of Mental Health, Mental Retardation and
Substance Abuse
Department of Human Resources
878 Peachtree Street N.E.
Atlanta, GA 30309
404-894-4200

Hawaii
Drug Abuse Office
Alcohol and Drug Abuse Division
Department of Health
1250 Punchbowl Street
Honolulu, HI 96813
808-586-4007

Idaho
Drug Abuse Office
Division of Family and Children
Department of Health and Welfare
450 W. State Street, 3rd Floor
Boise, ID 83720
208-334-5934

Illinois
Drug Abuse
Department of Alcoholism and Substance Abuse
100 W. Randolph, Suite 5-600
Chicago, IL 60601
312-793-9500

Indiana
Drug Abuse Office
Division of Addiction Services
402 W. Washington
Indianapolis, IN 46204
317-232-7816

Iowa
Drug Abuse Office
Substance Abuse and Health Division
Department of Public Health
Lucas State Office Building
Des Moines, IA 50319
515-281-3641

Kansas
Drug Abuse Office
Alcohol and Drug Abuse Services
Department of Social and Rehabilitation Services
300 S.W. Oakley
Biddle Building
Topeka, KS 66606
913-296-3925

Kentucky
Drug Abuse Office
Division of Substance Abuse
Department of Health Services
275 E. Main Street
Frankfort, KY 40601
502-564-2880

Louisiana
Drug Abuse Office
Office of Prevention and Recovery
2744 B Wooddale Boulevard
Baton Rouge, LA 70808
504-922-0730

Maine
Drug Abuse Office
Office of Substance Abuse
Executive Department
Statehouse Station 159
Augusta, ME 04333
207-289-2595

Maryland
Drug Abuse Office
Drug Abuse Administration
Health and Mental Hygiene Department
201 W. Preston Street, 4th Floor
Baltimore, MD 21201
410-225-6925

Massachusetts
Drug Abuse Office
Department of Public Health
150 Tremont Street
Boston, MA 02111
617-727-0201

Michigan
Drug Abuse Office
Office of Drug Control Policy
P.O. Box 30026
Lansing, MI 48909
517-373-4700

Minnesota
Drug Abuse Office
Chemical Dependency Program Division
Department of Human Services
444 Lafayette Road
St. Paul, MN 55101
612-296-3991

Mississippi
Drug Abuse Office
Division of Alcohol and Drug Abuse
Department of Mental Health
1101 Robert E. Lee Building
239 N. Lamar Street
Jackson, MS 39201
601-359-1288

Missouri
Drug Abuse Office
Alcohol and Drug Abuse Division
Department of Mental Health
P.O. Box 687
Jefferson City, MO 65102
314-751-3090

Montana
Drug Abuse Office
Alcohol and Drug Abuse Division
Department of Institutions
1539 11th Avenue
Helena, MT 59620
406-444-4927

Nebraska
Drug Abuse Office
Alcoholism and Drug Abuse Division
Department of Public Institutions
226 Coliseum—UNL
Lincoln, NE 68588
402-472-6046

Nevada
Drug Abuse Office
Bureau of Alcohol and Drug Abuse
Department of Human Resources
505 E. King Street
Carson City, NV 89710
702-687-4790

New Hampshire
Drug Abuse Office
Office of Alcohol and Drug Abuse
Department of Health and Welfare
Hazen Drive
Concord, NH 03301
609-271-4627

New Jersey
Drug Abuse Office
Division of Alcohol and Drug Abuse
Department of Health
129 E. Hanover Street, CN-362
Trenton, NJ 08625
609-292-5760

New Mexico
Drug Abuse Office
Behavioral Health Services Division
Department of Health
P.O. Box 26110
Santa Fe, NM 87502
505-827-2601

New York
Drug Abuse Office
Division of Substance Abuse
Stuyvesant Plaza
Executive Park
Albany, NY 12203
518-457-2061

North Carolina
Drug Abuse Office
Alcohol and Drug Abuse Services
Department of Human Resources
325 N. Salisbury Street
Raleigh, NC 27603
919-733-4670

North Dakota
Drug Abuse Office
Alcoholism and Drug Abuse
Department of Human Services
State Capitol, Judicial Wing
600 E. Boulevard
Bismarck, ND 58505
701-224-2769

Ohio
Drug Abuse Office
Alcohol and Drug Addiction Service
2 Nationwide Plaza, 12th Floor
Columbus, OH 43215
614-466-3445

Oklahoma
Drug Abuse Office
Alcohol and Drug Abuse Division
Department of Mental Health
P.O. Box 53277, Capitol Station
Oklahoma City, OK 73152
405-521-0044

Oregon
Drug Abuse
Alcohol and Drug Problems
Department of Human Resources
301 Public Service Building
Salem, OR 97310
503-378-2163

Pennsylvania
Drug Abuse Office
Drug and Alcohol Programs
Department of Health
809 Health and Welfare Building
Harrisburg, PA 17120
717-787-9857

Puerto Rico
Drug Abuse Office
Addiction Control Service
2114 Río Piedras Station
P.O. Box 21414
Río Piedras, PR 00928
809-764-3795

Rhode Island
Drug Abuse Office
Governor's Justice Commission
222 Quaker Lane, Suite 100
West Warwick, RI 02893
401-277-2620

South Carolina
Drug Abuse Office
Commission on Alcohol and Drug Abuse
3700 Forest Drive, Suite 300
Columbia, SC 29204
803-734-9520

South Dakota
Drug Abuse Office
Division of Alcohol and Drug Abuse
Kneip Building
700 Governor's Drive
Pierre, SD 57501
605-773-3123

Tennessee
Drug Abuse Office
Bureau of Alcohol and Drug Abuse
Department of Health
Cordell Hull Building
Nashville, TN 37247
615-741-1921

Texas
Drug Abuse Office
Commission on Alcohol and Drug Abuse
720 Brazos Street, Suite 403
Austin, TX 78701
512-867-8700

Utah
Drug Abuse Office
Division of Alcoholism and Drugs
Department of Social Services
120 North 200 West, 4th Floor
Salt Lake City, UT 84103
801-538-3941

Vermont
Drug Abuse Office
Alcohol—Drug Programs
Agency of Human Services
103 S. Main Street
Waterbury, VT 05671
802-241-2170

Virgin Islands
Drug Abuse Office
Assistant Commissioner
Department of Health
St. Croix Hospital
St. Croix, VI 00820
809-778-6311

Virginia
Drug Abuse Office
Special Assistant for Drug Policy
Office of the Governor
State Capitol Building, 3rd Floor
Richmond, VA 23219
804-786-2211

Washington
Drug Abuse Office
Alcohol and Substance Abuse Bureau
Social and Health Services Department
Office Building 2
Mail Stop OB-21W
Olympia, WA 98504
206-753-5866

West Virginia
Drug Abuse Office
Division of Alcohol and Drug Abuse
State Capitol Complex
Building 3, Room 402
Charleston, WV 25305
304-348-2276

Wisconsin
Drug Abuse Office
Alcohol and Other Drug Abuse
Health and Social Services Department
125 S. Webster, Room 120
Madison, WI 53703
608-266-9923

Wyoming
Drug Abuse Office
Division of Community Programs
Health and Social Services
Hathaway Building, Room 350
Cheyenne, WY 82002
307-777-6945

Eating Disorders

Millions of people suffer from eating disorders, such as anorexia nervosa, bulimia, and compulsive overeating. These syndromes are the result of many biological, psychological, and sociological factors. Typically, people who suffer from food addiction are females, but these syndromes occur in males as well. Most people with eating disorders are obsessed with their weight and try to balance eating with exercise or fasting. The addiction is usually used to overcome feelings of discomfort or anxiety.

According to Anorexia Nervosa and Related Eating Disorders, Inc., about .5 percent of women between ages 10 and 30 have anorexia nervosa. About 5 percent of college-aged women have bulimia. One in 10 people with anorexia or bulimia is male.

ANOREXIA NERVOSA

Anorexia nervosa is an eating disorder characterized by the relentless pursuit of thinness, a refusal to eat (which can lead to extreme loss of weight, hormonal disturbances, and even death), a fear of becoming fat, a distorted body image, and excessive dieting leading to emaciation. Anorexia nervosa is commonly coupled with a high amount of physical activity and ritualistic eating habits. These rituals center on how food is prepared, arranged, and eaten, its type, and its amount.

Primarily an illness that affects adolescent girls, anorexia nervosa is treated as an illness in and of itself, although it is also a symptom of other psychological problems associated with family background.

If the condition is not treated, muscle weakness, including the heart muscle, may be experienced, along with menstrual irregularity and numerous problems in the digestive tract, such as cramps, flatulence, and bloating. These symptoms may persist for years after prolonged low weight and in some cases become life-threatening.

Treatment for this condition includes medical assistance (with hospitalization often recommended even in the disease's early stages), psychotherapy, and family therapy. Self-help groups are also successful in helping patients overcome this condition.

Physical Consequences of Prolonged Dieting

- Hunger, cravings, preoccupation with food, and, in many cases, binge eating
- Dry, scaly skin. Skin may be yellow or gray.
- Dull, brittle, thin hair
- Loss of muscle as well as fat. Person may look like a skeleton covered only with skin.
- Loss of menstrual periods and, sometimes, fertility in women
- Loss of sexual desire
- Icy hands and feet. Person is cold when others are warm.
- Downy fuzz on face, limbs, and body
- Shrunken, weakened heart
- Anemia. Liver and kidney damage in some cases.
- Loss of bone minerals. A young person may have the soft, brittle bones of an 80-year-old.
- Constipation, digestive discomfort, abdominal bloating
- Dehydration, muscle cramps, tremors
- Dental problems
- Death. Up to 20 percent of the people who have anorexia die.

BULIMIA

Bulimia is a habitual disturbance in eating behavior characterized by bouts of excessive eating followed by self-induced vomiting, purging with laxatives, strenuous exercise, or fasting. Bulimics are preoccupied with their weight and will do almost anything to control it. Bulimics maintain their usually normal weight by using these methods to ease fears of obesity or to relieve bloated feelings. Tooth erosion, caused by stomach acid coming into contact with the teeth, may occur if excessive vomiting is induced.

Some characteristics of bulimia are bingeing, eating secretly, repeated attempts to lose weight, depression, and fear of becoming fat. Psychotherapeutic techniques are used to treat this condition.

Physical Consequences of Binge Eating and Purging

- Weight fluctuations because of alternating diets and binges
- Swollen glands in neck and jaw
- Loss of tooth enamel
- Broken blood vessels in face; bags under eyes
- Upset of the body's fluid/mineral balance leading to rapid or irregular heartbeat and possible heart attack
- Dehydration, fainting spells, tremors, blurred vision
- Laxative dependency, damage to bowels
- Indigestion, cramps, abdominal discomfort, bloating, gas, constipation
- Liver and kidney damage in some cases
- Internal bleeding; infection
- Death. Heart attack and suicidal depression are the major risks.

COMPULSIVE OVEREATING

Compulsive overeating, leading to obesity, is a condition usually caused by a pattern of overeating and/or a lack of exercise that begins in childhood. However, there are other contributing factors, such as genetic makeup, cultural background, physical and psychological characteristics, and socioeconomic status.

Treatment usually follows a plan that combines dieting with exercise and is geared toward maintaining body tone as weight is gradually reduced. Foods containing excess calories are eliminated while the balance of protein, carbohydrates, and fat required for growth are maintained. Exercise is encouraged because even a moderate increase in physical activity can lead to weight loss and appetite control. Self-help groups play an important role by providing moral support to help people overcome their disorder.

Some compulsive overeaters tend to binge, while others eat continuously. Bingeing is characterized by the intake of large amounts of food in a short period of time, eating high-calorie food, or sometimes eating secretly. Bingeing may be coupled with repeated attempts to lose weight through fasts or diets, resulting in weight fluctuation. Depression can also occur. Food intake can be used as a way to deal with stress or to relieve anxiety. Other compulsive overeaters use their fat to hide or protect themselves from others, almost like a shell.

Bingers often have the lack of fulfillment of one of three basic human needs: identity (Who am I?); relationship (Am I lovable?); or power (Am I in charge of my life?). The binge cycle usually begins with a trigger, something to cause the person to want to eat. The person then decides to eat. However, after eating, the person usually experiences feelings of failure for having given in to the desire to eat. This feeling then acts as a trigger for the person to eat again. Common feelings that lead to binges are anger, loneliness, rejection, resentment, helplessness, self-depreciation, depression, boredom, and even extreme happiness.

According to Dr. Frank M. Webbe of the Florida Institute of Technology, food addiction occurs in both men and women. Most are depressed over their uncontrolled eating. Most eat until the food is gone. Most have immediate family members who have alcohol or food addictions. Nearly 40 percent of people who call the Food Addiction Hotline (800-872-0088) say they gave up hope of overcoming their addictions, and almost 18 percent say they have attempted suicide at least once.

Physical Consequences of Compulsive Overeating

- Weight gain, sometimes obesity
- Increased risk of high blood pressure, clogged blood vessels, heart attack, and stroke
- Increased risk of some cancers
- Increased risk of bone and joint problems
- Increased risk of diabetes

Lists reprinted with permission from *Eating and Exercise Disorders,* Anorexia Nervosa and Related Eating Disorders, Inc., P.O. Box 5102, Eugene, OR 97405.

Eye Conditions and Disorders

NORMAL VISION

When someone with normal vision looks at an object, light rays travel from the object to the eyes. The light rays enter the eye through the cornea (the transparent front part of the eye), pass through the lens of the eye, and converge when they reach the retina. The retina transmits images to the brain via the optic nerve.

The same cannot be said about eyes afflicted by any of the four most common eye problems: nearsightedness, farsightedness, astigmatism, and presbyopia. These, too, are the most common reasons for the need for glasses or contact lenses. These four conditions are not diseases; they are considered simply "optical errors." Although nothing, including exercises, surgery, and corrective lenses, will cure the eye conditions, these errors can be corrected and normal vision achieved.

NEARSIGHTEDNESS

Nearsightedness, or myopia, is a condition of the eye in which a person has difficulty seeing objects that are far away. Very nearsighted people have difficulty seeing objects, whether close or far away. Nearsightedness results when the growing eyeball becomes elongated, or too long, thereby causing the light rays of distant objects to focus in front of, and not upon, the retina, and creating blurred vision.

The shape of the eyeball cannot be physically changed to eliminate nearsightedness; however, corrective lenses, in the form of glasses or contact lenses, are prescribed to help the eye perform its task more effectively. An experimental form of surgery, called radial keratotomy, involves making a series of spokelike cuts in the cornea to flatten its curvature. While this procedure changes the focal length of the eye, it does nothing to alter the original shape of the eyeball. Some ophthalmologists are currently investigating the use of lasers to reshape the cornea, but these procedures have not been perfected, are infrequently done, and remain controversial.

Nearsightedness usually stabilizes by adulthood (when the eyeballs stop growing); the degree of nearsightedness generally does not become progressively worse thereafter.

FARSIGHTEDNESS

Farsightedness, or hyperopia, is a condition of the eye in which the light rays of an object do not come into focus on the retina but instead converge behind it. This results when the eyeball is too short from front to back. Initially, people who are farsighted have difficulty seeing objects that are in their near vision; however, as they age, distant objects also become blurred. Some people mistakenly believe that farsightedness is the opposite of nearsightedness, but this isn't the case. A farsighted person, just like a nearsighted person, sees all objects out of focus. The ability to see distant objects clearly results when the farsighted person squints, thereby changing the shape of the lens and bringing about a slight improvement in vision. Therefore, while the farsighted person may be seeing clearly, he or she is putting strain on the eyes, possibly resulting in headaches.

Many farsighted people may not know they have this condition until they reach their 50s, because at this time the lens-bending muscles of the eye will begin to lose their ability due to strain. The result is blurred vision, sometimes both close and far away. It is important to receive yearly eye examinations, because an optometrist or an ophthalmologist will be able to catch the problem and prescribe corrective lenses that will take strain off of the eyes.

PRESBYOPIA

Everyone is certain to develop presbyopia at some point, as it is part of the aging process. It is the loss of our ability to use near-focusing muscles. Around their mid-40s, people find the need to buy reading glasses because their eyes are no longer able to focus on close objects. By the mid-50s to 65 years of age, all of a person's ability to use these muscles is lost, and the condition cannot get any worse.

ASTIGMATISM

In an astigmatic eye, the rays of light entering the eye do not come together at the same point, due to an error in the shape of the cornea. The image does not focus on the retina properly and, whether near or far away, is blurred. This condition is inherited and may be present at birth. Astigmatism stabilizes when a person reaches adulthood and changes very little throughout life. Corrective lenses are the solution for overcoming astigmatism.

OTHER EYE DISORDERS

Cataracts

A cataract is any imperfection in the clarity of the lens resulting in a loss of transparency and diminished vision. Aging is the number-one cause of cataracts; eventually, nearly everyone develops them. Changes in the chemistry of the body often cause the lens to become cloudy and less transparent.

The solution to cataracts is surgical removal of the clouded lens and insertion of an artificial lens. Although this is not always necessary for clearer vision—sometimes cataracts are small and in places that do not block the vision a great deal—cataract surgery is one of "the safest and most effective of all surgical procedures," according to Dr. John Eden of St. Luke's–Roosevelt Medical Center in New York City.

Either general or local anesthesia can be used on the patient undergoing cataract surgery. The eyelid and eye muscles are paralyzed to prevent eye movement. The virtually painless operation lasts about an hour. Another surgical technique involves a frozen probe (called a cryoprobe), which sticks to the lens so that it may be drawn out. Yet another technique uses sound waves to break up the lens, which is then removed with a vacuum needle.

In most cases, an artificial lens (called an intraocular lens) is placed in the lens capsule inside the eye. The use of the implantable artificial lens eliminates the need for the patient to wear thick glasses or contact lenses, although there are other possible solutions if a lens implant cannot be performed.

While most cataract surgery is done on an outpatient basis, some doctors may wish their patients to remain in the hospital for an overnight stay. In rare instances, when there are additional complicating factors present, a patient may be hospitalized 4 to 7 days. Only an ophthalmologist can recommend and perform cataract surgery. An optometrist is not certified to do so but may detect cataracts and refer the patient to an ophthalmologist.

Glaucoma

While glaucoma is one of the leading causes of blindness, it is also the easiest to prevent. Glaucoma is a disease of the eye in which there is an increased amount of pressure inside the eyeball, generally after the age of 40. This increased pressure is caused by a decrease in drainage of fluid in the eye. The resulting pressure kills cells in the optic nerve and causes a decrease in vision and sometimes blindness.

Glaucoma can be diagnosed and treated early on; however, in its early stages it has no noticeable symptoms. So a person may not know he or she has the disease unless an eye care professional diagnoses it during a regular examination. Obviously, then, the key to detecting and treating glaucoma is regular visits to an optometrist or ophthalmologist, especially after the age of 40.

The most common type of glaucoma, called chronic simple or open-angle glaucoma, is characterized by a small and gradual increase of pressure to and damage to the eye.

The most common treatment for glaucoma is daily eyedrops. Oral medication and, in some cases, surgery are also used. These treatments do not cure glaucoma; they simply reduce the pressure in the eye and bring it down to a normal level.

Sty

A sty is an infection of one of the glands of the eye along the eyelid. It is characterized by a painful red lump on the edge of the eyelid. The treatment is a hot compress, such as a warm, damp washcloth, applied to the area. Sometimes a doctor may prescribe antibiotic eyedrops or ointment to control the infection.

Conjunctivitis (Pinkeye)

Conjunctivitis, or pinkeye, is any inflammation of the transparent membrane that covers the front surface of the eyeball and laps over onto the inner eyelids.

Infectious conjunctivitis is caused by bacteria or a virus and is characterized by redness, inflammation, excessive tearing, scratchy eyes, and a sticky feeling in the eyes in the morning due to excessive discharge not blinked away during sleep. Bacterial conjunctivitis is treated with antibiotic eyedrops, while viral conjunctivitis is treated by the body's own defense system. Since infectious pinkeye is contagious, a person who

has it should wash his or her hands before and after applying medication, keep his or her hands away from the eyes, and never share washcloths or towels with others.

Allergic conjunctivitis is caused by anything that causes an allergic reaction and is characterized by redness, itching and burning in the eyes. This type of pinkeye is not contagious and can be treated by removing the cause of the allergy, such as animal fur, flowers, or soap. Eyedrops with a mild local anesthetic are sometimes used as well.

Chemical or *toxic conjunctivitis* is caused by irritants in the environment, such as a contact lens solution, air pollution, or chlorine in swimming pools, and can be relieved by removing the irritant and/or with lubricating eyedrops.

Corneal Infections

The cornea, the clear tissue layer that lies in front of the iris, can become infected by injury, a lodged foreign object, a scratch, a tear, or an abrasion. These infections can also be caused by diseases, such as pinkeye, herpes, or chlamydia. Normally, tears prevent corneal infection, but should a person be suffering such symptoms as pain, tears, redness, sensitivity to light, or a scratchy feeling during blinking, medical attention should be sought at once.

Antibiotic eyedrops and sometimes an eye patch are the usual treatment for corneal infection. Infection

Eye Examinations

Everyone should have regular eye exams, as our visual needs change with age and certain diseases and disorders may develop that can go unnoticed without regular checkups.

During an eye examination, the doctor asks about the medical history of the patient so that the cause of any disorders can be pinpointed.

The actual examination consists of a series of tests, including the reading of an eye chart (called a Snellen chart), a physical exam of the eye, and eye muscle tests. The doctor then uses a biomicroscope to examine the eye in great detail, checking for the presence of any diseases or disorders. Next, the doctor asks the patient to look through a masklike device called a phoroscope. This device enables the doctor to randomly change lenses in order to determine if the patient's eyes perform better using corrective lenses or if any change is required in a patient's current corrective lenses.

A person should have routine eye examinations every year before the age of 40 and every 6 months thereafter in order to keep vision at its sharpest. Early detection and treatment of diseases and disorders of the eye is the key to good vision.

can be prevented through protection, such as using protective goggles in situations that could be potentially hazardous to the eyes, avoiding ultraviolet light from the sun and sunlamps, washing hands before contact with the eyes, and avoiding rubbing the eyes.

Scleritis

Scleritis is an inflammation of the white of the eye. Symptoms of scleritis are redness and inflammation caused by an infection or irritation, often an allergy. Eyedrops with cortisone are the usual treatment.

Blepharitis

Blepharitis is an infection of the glands of the eyelid. Symptoms, if any, include reddened and encrusted eyelids. The treatment for this condition is eyedrops containing an antibiotic and cortisone.

Bearing similarities to dandruff, blepharitis can also affect the eyebrows and lashes, so some doctors advise patients to use dandruff shampoo and to clean their eyebrows and eyelids with a tearless baby shampoo. Though not contagious and usually mild, the condition should not go untreated, as a loss of lashes may result.

Subconjunctival Hemorrhage

Subconjunctival hemorrhage simply refers to a broken blood vessel in the eye. Although the condition may seem serious and frightening, it is no more serious than a bruise on any other part of the body. The hemorrhage appears as a bright spot of blood in the eye. It can be caused by a knock or blow to the eye, but usually occurs spontaneously. There is no treatment for it, but the blood will be reabsorbed within two weeks.

Eyelid Tics

Another common concern among patients is a twitching of the eyelid. This is caused by stress or anxiety. Although it feels obvious and visible, it is barely noticeable. It is not a disease or disorder, and ignoring it is the best treatment. The problem often goes away once the patient realizes that the cause is tension.

Ptosis

Ptosis is a drooping of an eyelid due to defect or injury to the nerve that supplies the eyelid. It can be present at birth, having developed during fetal formation. If vision is impaired as a result, plastic surgery can lift the eyelid.

Color Blindness

Color blindness is still somewhat of a mystery to doctors. It is an untreatable condition in which a person, usually a male, is less perceptive of one or more colors (usually reds and greens), and instead sees grays or browns in place of these colors. A hereditary condition that can be genetically transmitted through the mother, color blindness is present at birth, never worsens or improves later in life, and, in most cases, is easily adjusted to.

Retinal Disorders

The retina is the thin, delicate tissue that transmits images to the brain via the optic nerve. Any problem with the retina, such as scarring or tearing, may result in a slight visual impairment or even blindness.

Retinal detachment, or the inability of the retina to remain attached to the back of the eyeball, can result from a blow to the eye, a cyst, tumor, scar tissue, or hemorrhage, infection, or other disease of the eye.

Symptoms of a detached retina include spots before the eyes, visual loss, and light flashes, but pain is not a symptom. Not everyone who experiences these symptoms has a detached retina; for instance, tiny specks before the eyes in most cases can be dismissed as "floaters," cells that float around in the fluid that covers the eyeball. These groups of cells will probably disappear eventually. However, if a person notices other such problems with his or her eyes, they should be checked immediately by an eye doctor.

Treatment of retinal detachment is always surgical, involving the reattachment of the retina to the back of the eyeball.

Retinal hemorrhage, or a break in a blood vessel of the retina, will cause blood to interfere with the ability of the retina to transmit images to the brain. Although in severe cases the retina can become detached through a hemorrhage, this is a rare occurrence. In most cases, this condition heals by itself. However, any loss or impairment of vision should be checked by an eye doctor so that a proper diagnosis can be made.

Macular degeneration is another serious retina problem that encompasses a broad spectrum of diseases, all of which result in the same symptoms—loss of the central vision we use for reading, watching TV, driving, etc. The macula is a specialized part of the retina that is needed for seeing straight ahead and seeing fine detail, as opposed to the part of the retina that involves peripheral vision. Although macular degeneration primarily affects people over the age of 50, it is known to strike even children. It is estimated that 6 million people in the United States are victims of macular degeneration.

The problem begins when the insulating layer that separates the retina from the blood vessels behind it breaks down. As a result, new blood vessels grow into the retina, destroying vital nerve tissues. Because the condition is painless, a person is unaware of early macular changes. The first signs or symptoms may be a blurring of reading matter, a distortion of letters, or even a loss of part of the letter. However, as the condition progresses, central vision is impaired to the point where circular blind spots begin to appear in the field of vision.

While the condition cannot be cured, a form of treatment using a laser (called photocoagulation) is available to slow down, and in some cases even stop, the loss of vision if applied early in the course of the illness. Unfortunately, most cases of macular degeneration cannot be treated.

OTHER VISUALLY IMPAIRING DISEASES

Arteriosclerosis is a condition of the arteries in which they become clogged with fatty deposits, making them less elastic and making it difficult for blood to pass through them. This condition affects the retina of the eye, slowing circulation to this part of the eye and killing the cells there. When retinal cells die, the brain receives less information about the image the eyes are looking at. How much vision is impaired depends on which area of the retina is being affected. Arteriosclerosis should be treated by a family doctor, although an eye doctor can diagnose the condition.

Hypertension, also called high blood pressure, is another condition that can have adverse effects on the retina. Hypertension can cause hemorrhages in the retina and cause vision to become impaired. Scar tissue left after hemorrhages can pull the retina, and, in severe cases, detachment may result.

Diabetes, a condition whereby the body does not produce enough insulin to process its own sugar, can affect the eyes only in severe or untreated cases. Severe cases of diabetes may result in hemorrhaging of the retina and cause scarring and impaired vision, similar to the effects of hypertension on the retina. To avoid this hemorrhaging, also known as diabetic retinopathy, a person must control his or her diabetes

through the use of insulin injections and diet, which can be prescribed by a family doctor.

Foot Care

The feet are two of the most important parts of the body. After all, they are counted on to support all of the body's weight and to carry a person to the places he or she wants to go. Aching feet can slow a person down considerably and make easy tasks seem extremely difficult, so it is important to take good care of the feet. Regular exercise, frequent massages, and comfortable shoes are the keys to happy feet. Without proper attention, the feet can develop a number of diseases and disorders. Here are a few of these disorders and some tips on how to avoid them.

ATHLETE'S FOOT

Athlete's foot is a contagious disease of the feet, caused by a fungus that thrives on moist surfaces. It is characterized by its peeling, cracking, and itching.

People are most likely to develop athlete's foot if their shoes do not allow the feet to breathe, causing warmth and moisture on the soles and between the toes where the fungus can attack.

In a majority of cases, athlete's foot will not disappear by itself. In fact, the fungus, if left alone, can soon cause the skin to crack, allowing bacteria to enter and cause infection.

An over-the-counter preparation (such as Tinactin, Halotex, or Desenex) can be used to relieve the itching, cracking, and burning. After showering or bathing, the feet should be dried thoroughly, especially between the toes, and cornstarch or powder should be applied to keep them dry. The feet should be exposed to light and air whenever possible. A person should not walk barefooted, especially in locker rooms or around swimming pool areas. Socks should be changed often, and white socks should be worn if possible, since colored socks will add to heat buildup inside the shoes.

For a severe case of athlete's foot, a doctor may prescribe clotrimazole (Lotrimin cream or lotion) or an oral antibiotic such as griseofulvin. However, both of these drugs may cause a rash or blistering, and griseofulvin is associated with such side effects as headaches, nausea, and numbness in the extremities, so they should be used with care.

CALLUSES

A callus is an area of dead, thickened yellowish-red skin which the body has built up to cushion the foot from excess pressure and friction. As long as a callus isn't troublesome, it can be forgotten.

However, the body may build calluses on the areas bearing the most weight, causing a great deal of pain. A painful callus can also be caused by a malaligned bone or crooked toe.

The simplest solution to a painful callus is to switch shoes. Women should switch back and forth between high- and low-heeled shoes. All shoes should be comfortable with each step, and the weight of the body should be distributed evenly across the soles of the feet.

More serious calluses are caused by a dropped metatarsal (when one of the sesamoid, or small and round, bones behind the toes is much lower than the ones on either side of it), bunions, hammertoes, and other biomechanical problems. In these cases, a thick, deep callus will build up to help even it all out, but in the process, such a callus can become excruciatingly painful.

Calluses caused by a dropped metatarsal are sometimes treated through the use of collagen injections, which act as a cushion between the underside of the metatarsal and the outer skin. Since the benefits of the injections are not permanent, the collagen material needs to be reinjected annually for maximum results.

A simpler solution is to redistribute body weight by using a callus pad or a moleskin, which is simply a soft cloth with one velvety side and one sticky side to hold it in place over the callus. A callus can also be softened at home by daily soaking the feet and using an abrasive brush on the callus, followed by a cream to soften the callus. More painful calluses can be excised or cut away by a podiatrist.

Here, too, is a solution recommended by podiatrist Suzanne M. Levine of the New York College of Podiatric Medicine: Crush 5 or 6 aspirin tablets into a powder and mix with 1 tablespoon of lemon juice. Apply the paste to the callus. Put the entire foot into a plastic bag and cover with a warm towel for at least 10 minutes. Unwrap the foot and, using a pumice stone (a rough-edged stone that can be purchased in a drugstore), scrub the callus. The dead skin of the callus should come loose and flake away easily.

CORNS

A corn is a hard, thickened, and sometimes painful area of skin found on or between the toes. Like a corn kernel, it's round and yellow. If it is reddish, it has become inflamed. Corns develop as a result of friction and pressure on the feet.

If corn is constantly rubbed against the side of a shoe, it will grow larger and cause pain. The pain of a corn may also be coming from a bursa, a fluid-filled sac that overlies and protects all joints in the body. With friction between the corn and the bone where the bursa lies, the bursa will become swollen and painful.

The only permanent solution to a corn problem is to buy shoes that fit comfortably, even if it means buying a larger size or a different style.

Contrary to what some television commercials may have people believing, over-the-counter corn removal remedies do not work. Most of them contain salicylic acid, a caustic substance that can cause blisters and infection, which will only add to the problem.

But there are solutions. To treat a corn at home, the foot can be soaked in a solution of Epsom salts (which can be found in any drugstore) and warm water. Then moisturizing cream should be applied and the corn covered. The area can be wrapped in plastic for at least 15 minutes. After removal of the plastic, a pumice stone can be rubbed on the corn in a side-to-side motion to remove the hard corn skin. However, the only way to permanently get rid of corns is to change shoes if they cramp the feet.

When corns are due to an imbalance in the feet, a podiatrist might recommend orthotic inserts and order a plaster cast to be made of the feet to make the orthotic fit perfectly. Or a podiatrist can perform minimal incision surgery in the office and cut away the bony prominence of the corn.

HAMMERTOE

A hammertoe is a deformity of one of the middle toes, usually the second or third, in which the joint has become bent and twisted. It looks like the small hammer inside the workings of a piano.

Most hammertoes are the result of heredity. If a person has a high arch or if the second toe is especially long, he or she may be forcing it to bend, especially if there is not a great deal of space for the toes in the person's shoes. Hammertoes may also be due to injury or other congenital foot shapes, such as an arch that sags.

A painful hammertoe is caused by an aggravated bursal sac (a sac of fluid that protects the joints). To relieve the pain, the hammertoe can be covered with any kind of shield or padding, such as a corn pad, lamb's wool, or a bandage. A person might also want to cut open an old pair of shoes to relieve the pain temporarily. Minor surgery may be necessary if surrounding tissue has become inflamed.

BUNIONS

A bunion is a bony bump on the edge of the big toe, causing the joint to become inflamed. It is a form of arthritis, indicating that the bone beneath is degenerating.

Some bunions cause a swinging-in of the big toe, while others simply appear on the side or top of the toe. Bunions often appear on both feet.

A painful bunion is a result of friction and inflammation of the bursal sac (which protects the joint) of the toe. If a person pushes down on the bump and a whitish area appears, and if the area turns red when released, he or she may have bursitis.

While tight-fitting shoes may contribute to bunions, it is more likely that they are there because the person's mother or father had them as well. Women are more susceptible to bunions than are men, possibly due to their different foot shape and possibly because of different hormone levels in women.

Ice is the best treatment for bunions. Three or four 15-minute applications of an ice pack per day will help reduce heat and inflammation. Another treatment is a soak in warm water and vinegar (about 1 cup for every gallon of water), which can help to reduce inflammation. Other treatments include ultrasound, electrogalvanic stimulation, paraffin baths, and whirlpool massages.

Wide sandals or shoes with a hole cut out should be worn to relieve pressure on the bunion. An orthotic shoe insert, special insoles, or arch supports can sometimes also relieve the pressure.

Only surgery can completely eliminate a bunion. There are several types of surgical procedures a doctor may suggest, most of which can be done in the office the same day.

CRACKED HEELS

Heels need moisture. When calluses build up on the backs of the feet, the heels can become cracked. Other causes of cracked heels are fungal infections, dry skin, and being overweight.

The first step to healing the heel is to have a doctor break down the hard, callused skin using salicylic acid. Next, a cream like Whitfield's ointment or cortisone and some plastic wrap can be used for an occlusive dressing, which will keep moisture from evaporating and increase penetration of the creams. Skin creams such as Hydrisinol, Carnol HC, Aquacare/HP, Lubriderm, and Eucerin should be applied two to three times each day.

Cracked heels can also be aided by eliminating open-backed shoes and by using heel inserts or heel cups made of plastic.

INGROWN TOENAILS

Ingrown toenails cut into the skin around the nail, causing them to become sore, especially when shoes are being worn.

The toenails can cut into the skin if they are cut on a curve or if they are kept too short. Nails should always be cut straight across. Tight shoes may also be to blame.

An ingrown nail can be healed by keeping the pressure off of it. Sandals or shoes with a hole cut in them should be worn. If there is an infection present, the feet can be soaked in an iodine solution to reduce the inflammation. The nails should then be cut or trimmed, the nail grooves cleaned, and an antibiotic cream applied. If pain persists, a person should see his or her doctor.

ACHING ARCHES

When walking, the arches of the feet should only dip a little when the feet roll from the heel toward the toes. The foot should spring back from each step without letting the arch touch the ground. If it does, that person is probably experiencing pain.

Ligaments, arthritis, or flat-footedness are all causes of aching arches, as are change of routine, plantar fasciitis (an overstretched band of tissue running from the heel to the ball of the foot), and tendinitis (inflammation of the small tendons that attach the muscles in the feet to their bones).

The best way to treat the pain is to rest first, then follow up with applications of ice. Later, heat may be applied. An elastic bandage wrapped around the arch may help support it. Shoes with extra arch supports should be purchased, along with insoles to help better support the arches. If the person is still experiencing pain, he or she should visit a doctor, who may be able to help analyze the step and help eliminate the pain.

BLISTERS

Blisters are the result of friction between a shoe and the skin. A blister is actually a protective device that defends the foot against this friction. Most blisters start with redness and swelling, and a burning sensation.

Once a blister has formed, it is best left alone. However, the skin may be cleaned with alcohol or an iodine solution, then, using a sterile, sharp instrument, the blister may be punctured and the top part left in place to avoid infection. An antibiotic cream should then be applied, and the blister covered with a bandage or a sterile piece of gauze or tape.

Shoes that are too short or too narrow are most often the problem. A person should be sure to wear shoes that fit well in order to avoid blisters.

WARTS

A wart is a hard circular benign tumor, usually white. Warts can appear alone or in clusters, and can disappear suddenly or survive for years.

Although warts can be contagious, some people never get them, while others seem to be particularly susceptible to them. A lesion can be identified as a wart if it is very painful when squeezed at its sides. Pressure on corns and calluses is not as painful.

Sometimes a wart will disappear on its own—signs of this are redness, swelling, or a black hardened look—or it may simply shrink up. When one wart fades away, others nearby will sometimes follow. However, for the more stubborn wart, there are remedies. One is to cut and attach a 40 to 60 percent salicylic acid pad (which can be purchased at any drugstore) to fit the wart. It should be covered with a bandage to keep it dry and in place. This procedure should be repeated until the wart disappears. Before a new pad is applied, any dead tissue should be removed with a pumice stone.

Other remedies to try are Compound W and Duofilm. The foot should be kept dry if these treatments are being used. Salicylic acid ointment, vitamin A injections, phenol, and nitric acid, sulfuric acid, and silver nitrate can all be used or applied by a doctor as well. Other treatments by doctors include ultrasound, surgery, and laser surgery.

Genetic and Familial Diseases

Birth defects occur in 1 of every 14 births. Some of these defects can be inherited, passed from parent to child in the genes—the information packets that determine human development. Some common hereditary birth defects are described in "15 Common Birth Defects" earlier in this section. These include Huntington's disease, sickle-cell anemia, Tay-Sachs disease, cystic fibrosis, hemophilia, Duchenne's muscular dystrophy, and Rh disease.

Hereditary diseases can be passed from parent to child in three different ways:

Autosomal dominant disorders. If a parent has a dominant gene disorder, there is a 50 percent chance the child will inherit this disorder. Examples include familial high cholesterol and some forms of glaucoma that cause blindness if not treated.

Autosomal recessive disorders. If both parents are carriers of recessive genes—genes that can cause an illness—there is a 25 percent chance that each child will inherit the condition; a 50 percent chance that each child will be a carrier who does not have the disorder; and a 25 percent chance that each child will be unaffected. These diseases are often severe and can lead to early death. Examples of major recessive disorders are sickle-cell anemia and Tay-Sachs disease.

X-linked inheritance. The X and Y chromosomes determine if a child is male or female. If the mother is a carrier of an X-linked recessive disorder, there is a 50 percent chance each male child will receive the abnormal X chromosome and be affected, and a 50 percent chance each daughter will be a carrier. Examples include hemophilia (the inability of blood to clot) and red-green color blindness.

10 HEREDITARY AND FAMILIAL DISEASES

Thalassemia. Blood disease triggered by recessive gene commonly found among those of Italian or Greek descent, but disorder can affect those of Middle Eastern, southern Asian, or African descents.

Thalassemia refers to various types of anemia. The most harmful is Cooley's syndrome. Children appear normal at birth but become pale and weak within the first year or two of life. Without treatment, major organs become enlarged, with heart failure and infection the leading causes of death.

Marfan syndrome. Disease of connective tissue caused by a dominant gene. Symptoms may be mild or severe, may be present at birth or not until adulthood. Affected individuals are often tall, slender, and loose-jointed. A pattern of abnormalities can affect the heart, blood vessels, lungs, eyes, bones, and ligaments. Can sometimes cause sudden death in adults unaware they had disorder, as was the case of U.S. Olympic volleyball player Flo Hyman in 1986.

Achondroplasia. Form of dwarfism caused by dominant gene. Child has relatively normal torso and short arms and legs. Problems can arise due to the common symptoms of this disorder, which include swayback, crowded teeth, spinal cord compression, bowlegs, and ear infections. Psychological problems may also arise.

Neurofibromatoses. These are inherited disorders of the nervous system caused by abnormal genes and gene mutations. Severity of symptoms can vary greatly. A common sign can be six or more large tan spots on the skin, often present at birth. Benign tumors may appear under the skin, often during adolescence. Tumors can also develop on the auditory (hearing) nerves, the brain, and the spinal cord. Most cases are mild, but some children can have learning disabilities, speech problems, and seizures and be hyperactive.

Wilson disease. A liver and mental disorder that does not appear until between the ages of 8 and 20.

Gaucher disease. A disorder affecting the liver, spleen, and bone marrow that appears anytime from childhood on through adulthood. Seen most commonly in Ashkenazi Jews.

Hypertension. High blood pressure triggered by an autosomal dominant gene, but exact genetic functioning unknown. Some researchers claim problem lies in how sodium is carried across cell membranes. Others argue that inherited problems in eliminating sodium from the body are the culprit. Others cite excessive sensitivity to stress.

Familial high cholesterol. This is an autosomal dominant trait. There is a flaw in the gene that controls production of LDL (so-called bad cholesterol) receptors. One person in 500 affected. If left untreat-

ed, person receiving gene from one parent may have first heart attack in 30s or 40s.

Glaucoma. Higher than normal pressure inside the eye which, if untreated, can lead to blindness. Hereditary in 10 to 15 percent of cases. Genetic trigger not well understood, but people of African ancestry suffer from it more than those of European background. Greater pigmentation in very dark eyes may be a factor.

Diabetes mellitus. A disorder of insulin production by the pancreas or interference with the effect of insulin on cells. Up to 25 percent of the U.S. population may carry a predisposition toward diabetes. Screening tests—fasting blood sugar or postprandial blood sugar (sugar levels after eating)—can determine elevated blood sugar levels. But elevated blood sugar may not be a factor. Sometimes a family history of obesity, lipid disturbance, premature cardiovascular disease, or diseases of the eye or kidney can point to underlying diabetes. See "Screenings and Tests for Common Familial Conditions" in section 5, "Procedures," for more information.

Hearing Loss and Hearing Disorders

Hearing loss, or hearing impairment, is any kind of loss in sensitivity of hearing and occurs because of obstructions in the ear, disease and infection, hereditary factors, natural processes of aging, abnormalities of ear structures and functions, or acoustic trauma.

But first, a quick discussion of the anatomy of the ear is necessary for a complete understanding of the disorders.

THE EAR

The ear, made up of the outer ear, middle ear, and inner ear, is responsible for hearing: It collects and receives sound waves and translates these waves into nerve impulses, which are then sent to the brain.

The outer ear, which consists of the ear canal and tympanic membrane (eardrum), collects sound waves and focuses them into the middle ear. The middle ear, whose function it is to further transmit sound vibrations to the inner ear, is comprised of three tiny bones called the ossicles (malleus, incus, stapes) and the oval and round opening (two small openings to the inner ear). The middle ear houses the eustachian tube, which brings air into the ear and helps in equalizing air pressure in the ear.

The inner ear, also called the labyrinth, is made up of several bony canals and chambers and contains the organ of hearing, the cochlea. The cochlea contains hair cells (sensory cells) with tiny projections which, when stimulated by sound waves, initiate sound impulses.

HEARING LOSS DISORDERS

There are two types of hearing loss: conductive hearing loss and sensorineural hearing loss. Hearing loss is described as conductive when there is a failure in the mechanisms in the middle ear, making them physically unable to conduct sound. This type of hearing loss can often be arrested, improved, or prevented. Conductive hearing disorders include otitis media, cholesteatoma, and otosclerosis (see below).

Sensorineural hearing loss indicates a partial or complete loss of hearing due to malfunctions and problems of the sensory organ of the ear (the cochlea) and of the auditory nerves. Sensorineural hearing loss can be treated medically, but usually the kind of damage produced is irreversible and hearing cannot be improved. Sensorineural hearing disorders include tinnitus, Ménière's disease, purulent labyrinthitis, congenital sensorineural hearing loss, acoustic trauma, and presbycusis (see below).

In general, treatment of hearing disorders can involve medications, surgery, and the use of hearing aids.

CONDUCTIVE HEARING DISORDERS

Otitis media is an acute middle ear infection that occurs most commonly in children. In otitis media, the middle ear cavity and eustachian tube become inflamed and infected with bacteria (the most common is *Streptococcus pneumoniae*), due to a cold, allergic reaction, or sinus or throat infection. The infection causes earache, an accumulation of fluid, and a buildup of pus and mucus.

The symptoms of otitis media include earache, feelings of pressure or blockage in the ear, fever, and muffled hearing. Otitis media is not a life-threatening condition, and the hearing loss that accompanies it is temporary. The condition can be treated by alleviating the pressure and pain in the ear, primarily accomplished by draining the excess fluid. However, if otitis media is left untreated, the condition can become chronic or cause further complications such as chron-

ic or permanent hearing loss, a perforated eardrum, mastoiditis, and labyrinthitis. Treatment includes the use of antibiotics (amoxicillin, ampicillin, cefaclor, co-trimoxazole), decongestants (for colds), antihistamines (for allergies), analgesics (for pain), or, in severe cases, a surgical process known as myringotomy (in which an incision is made in the eardrum in order to drain the fluid).

A *cholesteatoma* is a buildup of skin cells in the ear that grows into a benign cyst or tumor behind the eardrum. Caused by repeated infections and poor eustachian tube function, a cholesteatoma has the capacity to grow and enlarge so much that it could damage the bones of the middle ear.

The symptoms of a cholesteatoma include hearing loss, discharge from the ear, earache and headache, feelings of pressure, facial muscle weakness, and dizziness. Treatment of a cholesteatoma consists of careful cleansing of the ear, the use of antibiotics, and in some cases, surgical removal of the growth or a mastoidectomy (removal of the mastoid process). If left untreated, infection could take hold and spread to other parts of the ear and body, causing such complications as brain abscess, permanent hearing loss, and meningitis. *Otosclerosis,* a bone disease, affects the inner ear and occurs when a growth of spongy bone begins to form on the bony capsule that serves as the entrance to the inner ear. The growth can then affect and impede the movement of the stapes, so that vibrations are not carried to the inner ear. Gradual hearing loss results, as well as tinnitus, and may be first detected in people when they are young adults (15 to 25 years old). The hearing loss that accompanies otosclerosis is conductive and can be corrected. However, if left untreated, otosclerosis can produce sensorineural damage to the ear. Treatment of otosclerosis includes a stapedectomy (replacing of the stapes), medications such as sodium fluoride, vitamin D, and calcium, and hearing aids (to cope with hearing loss).

SENSORINEURAL DISORDERS

Tinnitus is an ear disorder in which a constant or intermittent ringing, roaring, or noise is heard in the ear. Tinnitus can be caused by wax buildup or by an ear infection. However, tinnitus can be a symptom of many serious ear disorders. Or the disorder can be caused by blood pressure levels, allergies, diabetes, head and neck injuries, or by exposure to a variety of medications such as aspirin, antibiotics, sedatives,

Is Your Baby's Hearing Normal?

More than 3 million American children have hearing loss. An estimated 1.3 million of these are under 3 years of age. You, the parents and grandparents, are usually the first to discover hearing loss in your babies, because you spend the most time with them. If at any time you suspect your baby has a hearing loss, discuss it with your doctor.

Your baby's hearing can be professionally tested at any age. Computerized hearing tests make it possible to screen newborns. Some babies are in a higher risk category for having hearing loss than others. If you circle any item (a) through (f) on this test, your child should have a hearing test as soon as possible, no later than at 3 months of age.

All children should have their hearing tested before they start school. This could reveal mild hearing losses that the parent or child cannot detect. Loss of hearing in one ear may also be determined in this way. Such a loss, although not obvious, may affect speech and language.

Hearing loss can even result from earwax or fluid in the ear. Many children with this type of hearing loss can have normal hearing restored through medical treatment or minor surgery.

In contrast to temporary hearing loss, some children have nerve deafness, which is permanent. Few, however, are totally deaf.

Most hearing-impaired children have some usable hearing. Early diagnosis, early fitting of hearing aids, and an early start on special educational programs can help maximize the child's existing hearing.

Use this simple test to answer the question "Is your baby's hearing normal?"

Preschoolers Hearing Loss Risk Factors and Test

To determine risk factor score, circle each item that applies:

(a) Family history of hearing loss, including brothers and sisters.

(b) History of illness in the mother during pregnancy, use of drugs during pregnancy, prolonged labor, or premature birth.

(c) Presence of birth defects.

(d) Low birth weight or other physical problems at birth (such as jaundice).

(e) Child has had meningitis or scarlet fever.

(f) Child has chronic middle ear infections and/or chronic upper respiratory allergies.

Give each circled item 3 points, add, and enter risk factor score: _____

Infants (birth through 12 months)

Give 0 points for every time you check the "Almost Always" column, 1 for every "Half the Time," 2 for every "Infrequently," and 3 for every "Never."

	Almost Always (0)	Half the Time (1)	Infrequently (2)	Never (3)
1. Nearby loud noise startles my baby and makes him/her move or even cry.				
2. Unexpected loud noise awakens my baby.				
3. My voice alone comforts or soothes my baby even when I do *not* pick him/her up.				
4. When my baby cannot see me, he/she turns eyes and head in the direction of my voice.				
5. My baby imitates noises.				

Total for Infants: _____

Babies (12 months through 3 years)

Same scoring as Infants.

	Almost Always (0)	Half the Time (1)	Infrequently (2)	Never (3)
1. My baby can point at familiar people or objects when asked.				
2. My *first* call gets a response.				
3. My child can imitate words. (If over 18 months, he/she can use a few words.)				
4. My child's speech and voice sound like other children's his/her age.				
5. My child listens to TV at a normal volume.				

Total for Babies: _____

Total Score: Infants *or* Babies score plus risk factor = _____

Recommendations

The American Academy of Otolaryngology—Head and Neck Surgery recommends the following:

0 to 5: Low risk of hearing loss. No immediate action is required.

6 to 12: Discuss the baby's hearing with your pediatrician, family physician, or a physician who specializes in hearing problems.

13 and above: Strongly recommend that the child's hearing be evaluated by an ear, nose, and throat (ENT) specialist.

© American Academy of Otolaryngology—Head and Neck Surgery, Inc., Alexandria, Virginia.

Hearing screening tests are available over the phone in certain cities and major metropolitan areas. Call the Dial-a-Screening Hotline at 800-222-EARS. Operators will give you a local or nearby number to call for a quick hearing test over the phone.

and inflammatory drugs. Since most instances of tinnitus arise from damage done to sensory nerves in the inner ear, it is possible to experience some hearing loss as well as tinnitus itself from exposure to loud music and other intense noises.

Treatment of tinnitus includes treating the underlying disease or problem, using biofeedback treatments, "masking" the tinnitus with other more pleasant noises, avoiding caffeine, nicotine, salt, and exposure to loud noises.

Ménière's disease, a type of disorder of the labyrinth, causes an individual to experience tinnitus, vertigo attacks with nausea and vomiting, and hearing loss. The cause of the disease is not known, but it is thought that the overproduction and malabsorption of fluid (endolymph) in the cochlea is involved. The excess fluid in the labyrinth creates pressure against the membranes of the labyrinth, causing problems of balance and hearing loss.

Treatment of Ménière's disease includes reducing the amount of fluid in the inner ear, taking medications to relieve vertigo and gastrointestinal symptoms such as meclizine and diazepam, and performing surgery on the central part of the inner ear and a labyrinthectomy (in severe cases). The patient may also be asked to follow a low-salt diet or to take diuretics.

Purulent labyrinthitis may result from a number of ear disorders that worsen and involves malfunctions of the inner ear. An individual suffering with labyrinthitis may experience hearing loss, tinnitus, vertigo, and nystagmus (involuntary rapid eyeball movement). Acute otitis media, brain trauma and hemorrhaging, congenital malformations, allergies, aging, and abnormalities in the blood, the cardiovascular system, and endolymph production all have the potential to cause labyrinthitis. Treatment for labyrinthitis may include surgical procedures such as a radial mastoidectomy or a labyrinthectomy, ultrasound treatments, or antibiotic therapy.

Congenital sensorineural hearing loss is a condition where hearing loss is acquired at birth. Infants may experience hearing loss as a result of different complications incurred in the womb or during delivery. Complications include rubella virus developing in the inner ear, anoxia (lack of oxygen) during birth, exposure to ototoxic drugs (drugs passed from mother to infant), trauma to the skull during delivery, or preexisting hereditary conditions (family history of deafness, malformations of the ear, etc.). Early detection of hearing loss in infants is essential for the simple reason that children need to hear language in order to learn it and communicate.

Parents, through careful observation of their infant, can suspect hearing loss if the child does not respond to the parent's voice or to environmental noises (loud noises) and does not imitate sounds around him or her. Further, if the infant has any one of several risk factors for hearing loss, he or she should be examined by a physician and be given a hearing test (see below). Risk factors include family history of deafness, low birth weight, the infant had meningitis or jaundice as a newborn, sustained a serious head injury, received antibiotic medication intravenously at birth, or the mother had rubella (German measles) or a viral infection or drank alcohol while pregnant. Hearing can be tested at any age, and if any of the risk factors have been identified by the parents, the child should be tested by 3 months of age.

Acoustic trauma describes any hearing loss engendered due to excessive exposure to loud, damaging sounds (any sound that measures above 85 decibels) or severe injury of the ear. Individuals with acoustic trauma experience tinnitus and hearing loss. Acoustic trauma may occur as a result of an individual's occupation (rock musician, construction worker, airline ground crew member) or lifestyle (listening to loud music, using earphones and headphones, etc.). Since acoustic trauma affects and damages the sensory cells in the inner ear, the hearing loss is sensorineural. Lost hearing cannot be restored, but individuals can wear hearing aids to amplify sounds around them. Individuals may also prevent further nerve damage by wearing protective earplugs to shield the ears from intense vibrations and sounds.

Presbycusis, or age-related hearing loss, occurs progressively as an individual ages. Symptoms of presbycusis are gradual hearing loss and tinnitus. The normal process of aging produces changes in the cochlea and the cochlear nerves, damage in the inner ear, and results in permanent sensorineural hearing loss. The only treatment method for presbycusis is the wearing of hearing aids. Hearing aids vary in style and cost. They can be worn in the ear (made from a mold of the ear canal) or behind the ear. Hearing aids must be individually fitted to ensure performance and comfort and should have a guarantee or trial period so that an individual can get accustomed to the hearing aid. Other visual communicative techniques such as lipreading or watching expressions are also helpful in coping with hearing loss.

Heart Attack

A heart attack occurs when the blood supply to the heart is reduced or stopped. Blood carrying oxygen to the heart is cut off and the heart muscle tissue begins to die. The severity of the attack depends on how much of the heart's blood supply has been cut off and for how long.

Symptoms

A person having a heart attack may experience such symptoms as uncomfortable pressure, fullness, squeezing, or crushing pain in the center of the chest that lasts 2 minutes or longer. The pain may seem to extend to the left arm, back, shoulder, throat, neck, or arms. The person may feel dizzy, faint, or experience shortness of breath. The face may become pale and sweaty. Possible vomiting may cause the person to mistake the heart attack for bad indigestion. Many people pass out in panic; some who suffer too much damage to the heart muscle never regain consciousness. Medical attention should be sought immediately for any person who feels he or she may be suffering from a heart attack.

Once the tissue around the heart begins to die, it cannot regrow. However, if the blood flow to that area of the heart can be restored soon enough, the tissue can be saved. It should be noted here that recent studies have added to a growing body of evidence that patients who do not respond to advanced cardiac life support before being rushed to a hospital have little

chance of survival. According to studies published in the September 22, 1993, issue of the *Journal of the American Medical Association*, only about .5 percent of patients who were not revived with a pulse at the scene of their heart attack ultimately survived. And of those few who did survive, virtually all suffered permanent cerebral disability.

Arteriosclerosis (marked by thickening, loss of elasticity, and hardening of the walls of the arteries) is often the cause of heart attacks, because fatty deposits that gather on the walls of the arteries can cause blood to clot, restricting blood flow to the heart. Another cause of heart attack is a contraction or spasm in a coronary artery. The cause of these spasms is unknown, but they can occur in normal arteries or in those that are partially blocked.

Angina

An angina attack, similar to a heart attack, occurs when coronary arteries are partially blocked, and the person experiences a painful, crushing sensation and difficulty breathing. Angina attacks are caused by arteriosclerosis, whereby globs of fatty tissue gather on the walls of the arteries, causing the heart to receive less oxygen. Since angina attacks feel quite similar to heart attacks, a person who is suffering from an actual heart attack may dismiss it as a painful angina attack.

"Silent" Heart Attacks

"Silent" heart attacks are just that—silent, undetected. About one-quarter of all heart attacks are not recognized when they occur. Many people have such "silent attacks" and never know it, although they may vaguely remember an incident where they felt inexplicably ill and full of foreboding or had a bout with unusual "indigestion."

The so-called silent heart attack causes damage to the heart muscle but no noticeable symptoms—and sometimes no lasting problems. On the other hand, most cardiologists say these people have heart disease just as serious and potentially deadly as someone who cannot walk a flight of stairs without chest pain or someone who was hospitalized for weeks with an unmistakable heart attack. Each year approximately 350,000 Americans who had no symptoms die suddenly and are found at autopsy to have had extensive coronary disease.

PREVENTION

There is no sure way to prevent a heart attack. However, there are precautions that can be taken to stack the odds against it. A change of lifestyle habits—eating, smoking, drinking, and fitness habits, for example—often does the trick.

Smoking

According to the American Heart Association, smokers are more than twice as likely to suffer from a heart attack as nonsmokers. A smoker is also more likely to die, and more likely to die suddenly (within an hour), from a heart attack than a nonsmoker. Studies also show that filtered cigarettes are not safer than nonfiltered ones in terms of preventing a heart attack.

High Blood Pressure

High blood pressure indicates that the heart is working overtime to pump needed blood and oxygen to other organs of the body. If high blood pressure isn't treated, the heart may become enlarged and have to work progressively harder to do its job. High blood pressure also speeds the process of arteriosclerosis, causing arteries and arterioles (small branches of arteries that link arteries to capillaries) to scar, harden, and become less elastic. For these reasons, high blood pressure, if not treated, can contribute to heart attack.

Stress

Stress is a natural part of life. It's what keeps us bright and alert, and ready for action, and in the misty past kept us one step ahead of the predators who saw early humanoids as odd-looking cold cuts with legs. But it's today's type of unnatural, work-related stress that does damage to the heart. In some studies, so-called Type A personalities—aggressive, ambitious, competitive, workaholic, explosive—have been identified as prime candidates for heart attack. Interestingly, the Type A traits are said to be not the causes of heart disease, but rather symptoms, which, if detected early enough and modified successfully, can put a stop to the coronary risk factor.

Stress may be a major factor in many heart attacks because it places stress on the heart, it raises blood pressure, it may contribute to arteriosclerosis, and it releases hormones, some of which are not very good for the health of the heart. Stress that follows emotional shock or personal crisis may be the origin of sudden cardiac death.

Stress can be reduced or controlled in countless ways, such as taking vacations, meditation, biofeedback, taking a deep breath and counting to 10 backward, exercising, even changing jobs or getting married. There are community service programs that offer stress-reducing programs as well.

Exercise

The benefits of exercise, especially aerobic exercise, are widely believed, yet are still the subject of some controversy as to effectiveness. What exercise seems to be able to do is create a good psychological and emotional atmosphere, release tension and stress, and help in weight loss. Exercise can lower the heart rate, blood pressure, and cholesterol levels, and can open new pathways for blood to reach the heart.

But exercise can be dangerous, too, for the heart. Overdoing exercise can be fatal. Hard exercising may lead to arrhythmias, although some doctors feel that such heartbeat irregularities in otherwise fit people are not serious.

And isometric exercises for people with heart disease should probably be ruled out. These static, push-and-pull exercises (including weight lifting) tend to raise blood pressure and increase the heart's demand for oxygen, which may bring about a coronary event.

Clearly, a person should consult a doctor before beginning any exercise program, and should exercise in moderation until his or her heart and body can endure a more intermediate program.

Alcohol

Light to moderate drinking seems to reduce the risk of coronary heart disease. What scientists think happens is that alcohol raises high-density lipoprotein (HDL) cholesterol, the so-called good cholesterol, in a way that somewhat resembles the aftereffects of exercise. Beyond moderation, however, alcohol has a destructive effect.

Alcohol in not overly large portions can cause what doctors call holiday heart syndrome: a complex array of arrhythmia disorders. Chronic alcohol consumption can cause cardiomyopathy—a serious disease involving inflammation and decreased function in heart muscle—and conduction disorders. A few drinks downed within an hour negatively affect the muscle fibers of the all-important left ventricle and perhaps cause permanent damage over the long run. And more than modest alcohol use is especially bad for you if you have a preexistent heart condition. Further, excessive alcohol intake (more than 2 ounces daily) raises blood pressure in some people.

DIET AND NUTRITION

Cholesterol

Cholesterol is a soft, fatlike substance found in all the body's cells that is used to form cell membranes, certain hormones, and other necessary substances. Besides being present in human tissues, cholesterol is also found in the bloodstream. The blood transports it to and from various parts of the body. Hypercholesterolemia is the term for high levels of cholesterol in the blood.

Foods such as egg yolks, meat, fish, poultry, and whole-milk products contain cholesterol. Excessively high cholesterol levels cause the formation of plaque in the arteries, reducing blood flow and restricting oxygen flow to the heart. A reading higher than 200 mg of cholesterol per deciliter of blood is considered moderately dangerous, but exercise and moderate alcohol consumption have been shown to help rid the body of excess cholesterol.

To reduce cholesterol levels, a person should eat fewer calories; eat foods rich in fiber; eat more fruits and vegetables and replace animal fats—especially those that are solid at room temperature—with vegetable oils like corn, safflower, soybean, and sesame; and cut down on coffee.

Vitamins and Minerals

Some specific vitamins and minerals, too, are good for heart disease. Here's an overview of the most important of them, according to various studies.

Magnesium. It's been shown to aid in keeping blood pressure from becoming high blood pressure. In clinical studies magnesium administered during acute myocardial infarction seemed to reduce the size of the infarct and reduce ventricular abnormalities, too. Magnesium deficiency has been linked to sudden death in patients with ischemic heart diseases, the deficiency causing coronary artery spasm. It's also been implicated in ventricular tachycardia, a heartbeat irregularity, and in chronic heart failure.

A lack of magnesium in the diet and impaired absorption of it, as well as depletion of it due to digitalis toxicity and the use of some diuretics, are all factors in dangerous magnesium deficiency. People who drink "soft" water—stripped of its natural minerals, including magnesium—may be more at risk of heart disease than those who drink "hard" water.

Foods high in magnesium include tofu, soy flour, black-eyed peas, wheat germ, nuts (cashews, almonds, Brazil nuts, and pecans), peanuts, and kidney and lima beans. Magnesium supplements may be useful. The U.S. recommended daily allowance, or RDA, is 350 mg for men, 300 mg for women.

Potassium. Same story here, and it works in concert with magnesium in a balance with calcium and sodium. Potassium depletion leads to arrhythmias; the presence of potassium in healthy amounts is necessary for certain antiarrhythmia drugs to work properly. There is often a marked potassium deficiency in people who have heart attacks. Potassium deficiency can be caused by the taking of diuretics.

Foods high in potassium include brussels sprouts, cauliflower, avocado, potato, tomato, banana, cantaloupe, peaches, oranges, flounder, salmon, and chicken.

Niacin, once known by the nondescript name of vitamin B_3, is found in a wide variety of foods, such as meat (especially liver), chicken, fish (especially tuna and salmon), whole grains, wheat germ, dairy products, eggs, nuts, dried beans, and peas. It is usually sold as nicotinic acid or, even more commonly, nicotinamide. Niacin's ability to reduce cholesterol levels in the blood has long been recognized, but since it's a vitamin and cannot be patented, no pharmaceutical company has bothered to test and promote it in the fight against heart disease. However, in 1990 researchers from the University of Pennsylvania reported that niacin was the least costly medication available for reducing cholesterol levels. According to their calculations, it can achieve a 1 percent reduction for one-third to one-half the cost of other cholesterol-lowering drugs.

Further, in a collaborative study financed by the National Heart, Lung and Blood Institute, middle-aged men who had already suffered one heart attack and who took large doses of niacin for five years were found to be less likely to have died of a second heart attack. This benefit was seen despite a potentially serious side effect associated with niacin therapy: an increased incidence of abnormal heart rhythms.

Very important to note is the fact that niacin is not without side effects, many of them potentially serious: ranging from flushing, rashes, itching, hives, nausea, diarrhea, and abdominal discomfort to liver malfunction, jaundice, elevated uric acid levels and gout, abnormally high blood sugar levels, peptic ulcers, and the aforementioned abnormal heart rhythms. The soundest advice for anyone is not to self-administer niacin in any form or switch the type already being used without consulting a physician. Further, many experts recommend that people using megadoses of any kind of niacin get liver function tests every few months, as well as periodic checks of blood sugar and uric acid levels.

Selenium and *zinc* are also mentioned frequently as substances that should be found in adequate amounts in the diet (or taken in supplements) to aid in heart health. *Chromium,* too.

New research suggests that *vitamin E* supplements can substantially reduce the risk of heart disease. Researchers at Boston's Brigham and Women's Hospital and the Harvard School of Public Health found that people who took supplemental vitamin E every day had a 40 percent drop in heart attack risk compared to those who did not take vitamin E supplements. The greatest protection was found at levels of about 100 I.U. of vitamin E a day for more than two years.

Vitamin E's most important role may be helping to prevent the oxidation of artery-clogging LDL (low-density lipoprotein) cholesterol. It also helps prevent what's called platelet aggregation. Platelets are disk-shaped blood components that are involved in blood clotting. They can also clot up in blood vessels when they shouldn't. Getting adequate amounts of vitamin E allows this nutrient to be incorporated into the membrane of platelets and prevents the platelets from clumping together and from sticking to blood vessel walls.

Further, according to recent research, having optimal levels of vitamin E in your blood can help prevent the damage to tissues that can occur when blood is first cut off, then resupplied, as might happen in the case of a blood vessel spasm or even during surgery, when a blood vessel might be briefly clamped.

Vitamin A—specifically a type of vitamin A called beta-carotene—has been shown to promote heart health, too. A recent, long-term study found that among men who already had evidence of cardiovascular disease, those taking beta-carotene supplements over six years had half as many strokes, heart attacks, sudden cardiac deaths, or surgeries to open or bypass clogged coronary arteries as those taking placebos. In the study, the doctors took 50 mg of beta-carotene every other day (equivalent to 83,720 I.U.).

A large study of women, by the same researchers, found a 22 percent reduction in the risk of heart attack and a 40 percent reduction in stroke risk for women with high intakes of fruits and vegetables rich in beta-carotene, compared with women whose intakes were low. The low-beta-carotene group was getting fewer than 6 mg of carotene a day, the amount found in less than half a carrot. The high-intake group was getting more than 15 to 20 mg a day—one to two on the carrot scale. So the difference between the two groups was only about 10 to 15 mg, about the amount found in a single serving of a beta-carotene-rich fruit or vegetable.

The research team cautioned, however, that the reportedly protective effect of vitamins does not outweigh other heart disease risk factors such as smoking, fatty diets, and high cholesterol levels.

Fish

Eating fish even one or two times a week may significantly reduce the risk of heart attack. It's the fish oils—eicosapentanoic acid, or omega-3 fatty acid—that do the job, but only the oils of saltwater fish like salmon, tuna, flounder, and cod. The oils in fish are thought to prevent blood clots from forming in the arteries and reduce the risk of heart attack.

Mental Health and Mental Health Disorders

Mental health might best be described as the ability to get along, to function in society. A mentally healthy person is able to sustain relationships with others, family and friends, and to carry on with the responsibilities of home and work.

A mentally healthy person is also able to perceive the motivations of others more or less correctly and has normal thought processes that are reasoned and logical, rather than bizarre.

PERSONALITY DISORDERS

Certain individuals are mentally unhealthy because of personality disorders. Below are the most common types of these disorders.

Antisocial personality disorder. This disorder is marked by a pattern of irresponsible and antisocial behavior that has its roots in childhood. Adults diagnosed as such usually have a history of conduct disorder and attention-deficit hyperactivity disorder (ADHD).

Childhood signs include ongoing truancy; physical cruelty to animals and other people; involvement in or starting of physical fights; setting of fires; lying, stealing, and vandalism. As adults, these people often fail to honor financial obligations. They destroy property, harass others, and may be engaged in illegal occupations.

Avoidant personality disorder. Extreme sensitivity to rejection is the hallmark of this disorder. The person is shy, leads a socially withdrawn life, and shows a pattern of social discomfort and fear of negative evaluation from others. The disorder usually appears in early adulthood. Some of its signs include no, or only one, close friend or confidant, other than a first-degree relative; unwillingness to get involved with people unless certain of being liked; exaggeration of potential difficulties or risks involved in doing something ordinary but outside the person's routine.

Borderline personality disorder. This is a form of severely dysfunctional personality organization. Borderline types suffer from instability of mood, interpersonal relationships, and self-image. Symptoms include extremes of overidealization and devaluation in interpersonal relationships; impulsiveness in the areas of spending, sex, substance abuse, shoplifting; inappropriate, intense anger; recurring suicidal threats; chronic feelings of emptiness and boredom; difficulty tolerating being alone. Studies show that so-called borderline types have a large number of depressed relatives.

Dependent personality disorder. This person subordinates his or her own needs to those of others and gets others to assume responsibility for major areas in his or her life. The onset usually occurs in early adulthood. Signs include inability to make everyday decisions without excessive amount of advice and reassurance; allows others to make important decisions; because of a fear of rejection, agrees with people even when he or she believes they're wrong; volunteers to do demeaning and unpleasant things in hopes of being liked. Traits of dependency appear in almost all psychological diagnoses.

Histrionic personality disorder. This disorder generally develops in early adulthood. These people are known for their excessive emotionality and attention-seeking. They seek reassurance and approval and are uncomfortable when not the center of attention. Often they are inappropriately sexually seductive and overly concerned with physical attractiveness. Their style of speech can be expressionistic, lacking in detail.

Narcissistic personality disorder. Patterns of grandiosity, in fantasy or behavior, and a hypersensitivity to others' evaluations are the hallmarks of this disorder. A lack of empathy is also apparent. Often they have a grandiose sense of self-importance and exaggerate accomplishments and talents. They can be preoccupied with fantasies of unlimited success and power and chronic feelings of envy for those they perceive as more successful. Often their self-esteem is fragile. They also believe their problems are unique and can only be understood by other special people. They fish for compliments and have a sense of entitlement, such as the feeling that they do not have to wait in line when others do.

Obsessive-compulsive personality disorder. This is the personality disorder least often confused with misbehavior. Emotional constriction, orderliness, perseverance, stubbornness, and a restricted ability to show warm and tender feelings mark this disorder. Symptoms include perfectionism that interferes with ability to get the task done; preoccupation with details, rules, and lists; insistence that others follow their way of doing things; excessive devotion to work and productivity; lack of generosity. Adolescents with these traits sometimes grow up to be caring adults; in other young people, these traits can foretell schizophrenia.

Paranoid personality disorder. Persons diagnosed as having this personality disorder have a pervasive and unwarranted tendency to interpret the actions of others as deliberately demeaning or threatening. They feel exploited or harmed by others and often bear grudges for long periods of time. Hypervigilant, they take precautions against perceived threats and feel themselves to be persecuted. Some paranoid personality types may also develop feelings of superiority, owing to their perceived position and power.

Passive-aggressive personality disorder. People with this disorder tend to procrastinate and are sulky and irritable when asked to do something they don't want to. They often avoid obligations by saying "I've forgotten," and they unreasonably scorn those in authority. Moreover, they are not direct about their own needs. Passive-aggressive individuals fight two conflicting desires: the wish to be passive and dependent coupled with a sense of entitlement.

Schizoid personality disorder. These people have a pattern of indifference to social relationships; they neither desire nor enjoy close relationships, including being part of a family. They prefer to be "loners" and have no or only one confidant other than first-degree relatives. They choose solitary activities and are vague about goals, are absentminded, and rarely experience strong emotions such as anger and fear.

Schizotypal personality disorder. Schizotypal people show peculiarities of thinking not severe enough to be schizophrenia. Onset is usually in early adulthood. Criteria include paranoid ideas, suspiciousness, odd beliefs, magical thinking, and bizarre fantasies or preoccupations.

Treating Personality Disorders
Personality disorders represent a lifetime pattern of being and behaving. Because of these long-standing habits, patients often don't recognize how their disorders have contributed to their general unhappiness in life and their interpersonal relationships.

Treatments generally are of three types: psychoanalytically oriented psychotherapy; psychopharmacology (medication); cognitive and behavioral therapy (counseling).

Psychotherapy. The goal is for the person to become aware of the negative impact of his or her personality on others and on his or her own sense of accomplishments and feelings of satisfaction. He or she learns to accept responsibility for negative traits and to understand their origins and develop adaptive behaviors.

Medications. The goal is to provide the person with a medication that reduces the breaks with reality and relieves the agitation, anxiety, panic, and depression of his or her illness, as well as stabilizes impulsiveness and mood swings. Types of drugs include antipsychotics (Haldol, Thorazine), antidepressants (Prozac), antianxiety drugs (Librium, Valium), mood-stabilizing drugs, and anticonvulsants (Dilantin).

Cognitive-behavioral therapy. The goal is to alter the person's set of basic assumptions that has led to the maladaptive behavior by challenging and testing the logic of these assumptions. Many times therapists use talk therapy to help the person overcome negative feelings that are the root cause of the emotional problems.

In conjunction with these therapies, certain disorders respond well to specific treatments. These include:

Avoidant personality disorder. Assertiveness training may be helpful following a solidified relationship with the therapist.

Dependent personality disorder. Behavioral therapies can be very successful, especially assertiveness training.

Obsessive-compulsive personality disorder. Patients often seek treatment on their own; group and behavioral therapy is also helpful.

Passive-aggressive personality disorder. Some promise is seen with cognitive-behavioral treatments. Therapy is needed that helps channel the patient's anger away from resistance into more productive measures.

ANXIETY DISORDERS AND PHOBIAS

Some mentally unhealthy people do not have a disorder of personality, but rather they experience fear in a manner that keeps them from leading fully productive lives. Below are some common anxiety disorders and phobias.

Generalized anxiety disorder. This disorder is marked by unrealistic and excessive anxiety and worry (apprehensive expectations) about two or more life circumstances that go on for 6 months or more. In children and teens, the anxiety often concerns academic, athletic, and social performance. However, onset is often in the 20s and 30s. Symptoms can include trembling, shortness of breath, heart palpitations, and trouble falling or staying asleep. Caffeine intoxication can show identical symptoms.

Obsessive-compulsive disorder (not to be confused with obsessive-compulsive personality disorder). Obsessive, intrusive thoughts plague the person. Thoughts can be persistent with images that are intrusive and senseless. Common are repetitive thoughts of violence, such as killing one's child, or contamination, such as becoming infected by shaking hands. The compulsive aspect of this disorder includes repetitive physical actions such as handwashing, counting, checking, and touching. Depression and anxiety are common with this disorder, which can arise during childhood, adolescence, and early adulthood.

Panic disorder. Commonly known as panic attacks, this disorder is marked by discrete periods of intense fear or discomfort that can last minutes or even hours. The "unexpected" aspect of panic attacks is the main feature of this disorder. The person feels intense apprehension, fear, terror, and impending doom upon entering the trigger situation, which might be driving a car or being in a crowded place. This is not to be confused with a simple phobia. Physical symptoms can include shortness of breath, dizziness, unsteady feelings, faintness, choking, heart palpitations, trembling and shaking, nausea, depersonalization or derealization, numbness or tingling, hot flashes, and chest pain. The average age of onset is late 20s.

Post-traumatic stress syndrome. Symptoms of this disorder arise following a psychologically distressing event outside the range of usual human experience, such as seeing someone being killed or knowing somone who was recently killed as the result of accident or violence; the sudden destruction of one's home or community; or a serious threat to one's life or physical integrity. The person experiences intense fear, terror, and helplessness. Symptoms include re-experiencing the traumatic event; avoidance of stimuli associated with the event; numbing of general responsiveness; increased arousal; exaggerated startle response.

Intense psychological distress occurs when the person is exposed to events that remind him or her of the experience, such as anniversaries. Victims can experience an inability to feel emotions or may suffer recurrent nightmares in which the event is relived. They might suffer from hallucinations or flashbacks, as if the event is recurring. A sense of a foreshortened future—the sense that they cannot expect a long life—can trouble some people.

Social phobia. This is the persistent fear of one or more social situations in which a person is exposed to the scrutiny of others and fears he or she will act in an embarrassing way. Panic disorder and simple phobia often coexist with social phobia. Onset is usually in late childhood and early adolescence.

Simple phobia. This phobia is marked by the persistent fear of a specific stimulus that brings about an intense anxiety response. Stimuli can include dogs, snakes, insects, mice, enclosed spaces (claustrophobia), heights (acrophobia), and air travel.

Treatments of Anxiety Disorders and Phobias
Antianxiety drugs (tranquilizers) are especially helpful in defined circumstances, such as dealing with stress or handling a recent emotional upheaval.

The benzodiazepines (Librium, Valium, Xanax) take the edge off these disorders by enhancing the actions of neurotransmitters in the brain that reduce nerve-impulse transmissions and slow down certain brain activity. However, side effects can include sleepiness, reduced coordination, and addiction.

Often medication combined with other therapies can help. For example, panic attacks are commonly treated with Xanax along with relaxation and deep breathing techniques. Desensitization, in which the person is gradually exposed to the object of his or her phobia, can often alleviate the anxiety.

Relaxation Techniques

Some people use relaxation techniques to deal with situations that contribute to their anxiety. In fact, whether you call it relaxation or meditation, many people find it an effective alternative to medications. And there are instances in which these techniques may be used in conjunction with medications. Here are some general suggestions on relaxation techniques.

- Locate yourself in a quiet environment devoid of radio, TV, or music, assume a comfortable seated position, and close your eyes.
- Slowly relax all of your muscles, beginning with the feet.
- Breathe naturally and easily through your nose, silently repeating a monosyllabic word such as "one" each time you exhale.
- Concentrate on the rhythm of your breathing. If thoughts or images intrude, let them pass and return to your repetitions.
- Try to maintain this state for 10 to 20 minutes daily.

The relaxed state is characterized by decreased heartbeat and respiratory rate, and lowered metabolic rate and blood pressure, just the opposite of what happens during an anxiety attack.

PROBLEMS ASSOCIATED WITH CHILDREN AND TEENS

Attention-deficit hyperactivity disorder (ADHD). This is a common behavioral disorder in children. Children move excessively—even in sleep—have short attention spans and different listening skills, are unable to finish things, and are easily distracted. It is ten times more common in boys than girls. Medications provide promising treatment and include Ritalin, Dexedrine, and Cylert. Ritalin is a stimulant, but in ADHD children it has the paradoxical effect of slowing down the hyperactivity.

Autism. This is a serious disorder involving the lack of development of cognitive and language skills. These children have significant problems in social environments. They are detached and unable to get involved emotionally. They do not respond to cuddling or eye contact. Autism is considered a neurological disorder that often exists in conjunction with some degree of mental retardation. There is no known treatment; these children need supervision and care throughout life.

Learning disabilities. Fifteen percent more boys than girls suffer from the inability to associate sounds with symbols. Most learning disabilities in the recent past were labeled dyslexia, the inability to see the difference between "was" and "saw," for example. Now researchers feel that some of these children may suffer from memory deficiencies. Phonetic approaches geared to the individual child can help.

Nocturnal enuresis (bed-wetting). This is the inability to hold urine while sleeping. Help should be sought if the problem persists beyond age 7. There seems to be some genetic connection; often the families of bed wetters have members who sleepwalk or who suffer night terrors. Treatment includes praising dry nights and the use of alarms that go off when detecting moisture. Two-thirds of children using the alarms soon learn to wake up and go to the bathroom. The treatment usually takes more than a month.

PROBLEMS ASSOCIATED WITH THE ELDERLY

Delirium. Ten to 40 percent of the hospitalized elderly develop delirium, the clouding of conscience with perceptual disturbances, incoherent speech, and disorientation. Overmedication is the biggest contributor to delirium in the elderly.

Dementia syndrome. Five percent of people aged 65 and older suffer from deterioration of the intellect, cognition, behavior, and emotions. In addition, 10 to 30 percent of these suffer from a second illness that impairs their cognitive skills.

Mood disorders. Physical illnesses that cause delirium or dementia in the elderly can bring about a secondary depression marked by mood swings. Mood disorders can also be brought on by drugs (such as antihypertensives), endocrine disorders, and structural brain lesions.

Paranoid personality disorder. Stress in the elderly can overwhelm their defenses and lead to paranoia. The stressors can include physical illness, isolation, and the deaths of family members and lifelong friends.

Sleep disorders. Depression following a heart attack often leads to sleep difficulties in the elderly. Other factors interfering with sleep are anxiety and pain. Insomnia and early-morning waking are common.

MENTAL HEALTH RESOURCES

American Board of Professional Psychology
2100 E. Broadway, Suite 313
Columbia, MO 65201
314-875-1267

American Board of Psychiatry and Neurology
500 Lake Cook Road, Suite 335
Deerfield, IL 60015
708-945-7900

American Mental Health Counselors Association
5999 Stevenson Avenue
Alexandria, VA 22304
800-326-2642
703-823-9800

American Mental Health Foundation
2 E. 86th Street
New York, NY 10028
212-737-9027

American Psychiatric Association
1400 K Street N.W.
Washington, DC 20005
202-682-6000

American Psychological Association
1200 17th Street N.W.
Washington, DC 20036
202-336-5500

Autism Society of America
8601 Georgia Avenue, Suite 503
Silver Spring, MD 20910
301-565-0433

Council on Anxiety Disorders
P.O. Box 17011
Winston-Salem, NC 27116
919-722-7760

Learning Disabilities of America
4156 Library Road
Pittsburgh, PA 15234
412-341-1515

National Alliance for the Mentally Ill
2101 Wilson Boulevard, Suite 302
Arlington, VA 22201
800-950-6264
703-524-7600

National Council on Aging
409 3rd Street S.W.
Washington, DC 20024
202-479-1200

National Institute of Mental Health
Public Inquiries Section, Room I5 C-05
5600 Fishers Lane
Rockville, MD 20857
301-443-4513

Society for Autistic Citizens
1234 Massachusetts Avenue N.W., Suite 1017
Washington, DC 20005
202-561-8527

MAJOR PSYCHIATRIC DISORDERS

Based on the National Institute of Mental Health Epidemiologic Catchment Area Survey—a comprehensive, community-based survey of mental disorders and use of services by adults, aged 18 and older—it is estimated that 1 of every 5 persons in the United States suffers from a mental disorder in any 6-month period, and that 1 of every 3 persons suffers a disorder in his or her lifetime. Fewer than 20 percent of those with a recent mental disorder seek help for their problem, according to the survey. High rates of co-morbid (the occurrence of more than one disorder in the same person at the same time) substance abuse and mental disorders were found, particularly among those who had sought treatment for their disorders. The survey also reported that 29 percent of persons with mental disorders also have a history of either drug or alcohol abuse.

The following list shows lifetime prevalence of mental disorders in the United States and percent of affected adults aged 18 and older by specific disorder in rank order.

Diagnoses are based on the criteria in the *Diagnostic and Statistical Manual of Mental Disorders,* third edition, and were obtained in five communities in the

United States through lay-interviewer administration of the National Institute of Mental Health Diagnostic Interview Schedule.

Disorder	*Percent*
1. Substance use disorders	16.7
2. Anxiety disorders	14.6
3. Alcohol abuse/dependence	13.5
4. Phobia	12.6
5. Depressive (affective) disorders	8.3
6. Drug abuse/dependence	6.1
7. Major depression	5.9
8. Dysthymia	3.3
9. Antisocial personality disorder	2.6
10. Obsessive-compulsive	2.5
11. Severe cognitive impairment	1.7
12. Panic disorder	1.6
13. Schizophrenia/schizophreniform disorders	1.5
14. Bipolar (manic episode)	0.8
15. Somatization disorder	0.1

Source: Public Health Reports, vol. 107 (Nov.–Dec. 1992), 663–68. U.S. Department of Health and Human Services, Public Health Service.

Glossary of Psychiatric Terms and Diagnoses

Acute treatment—formally defined procedures used to reduce and remove the signs and symptoms of depression and to restore psychosocial function.

Adequate treatment analysis—analysis of data in terms of the relationship between the number of patients who received a predetermined minimum amount of treatment and the number who responded.

Agoraphobia—a disorder characterized by a fear of open, public places or of situations where crowds are found.

Anhedonia—an absence of or the inability to experience a sense of pleasure from any activity.

Behavioral therapy—a form of psychotherapy that focuses on modifying observable problematic behaviors by systematic manipulation of the environment.

Bipolar disorder—a major mood disorder characterized by episodes of major depression and mania or hypomania, formerly called manic-depressive psychosis, circular type. The diagnosis of bipolar I disorder requires one or more episodes of mania. The diagnosis of bipolar II disorder requires one or more episodes of hypomania and is excluded by the history or presence of a manic episode. Current episode may be manic, depressed, hypomanic, or mixed manic type.

Clinical management—education of and discussion with patients and, when appropriate, their families about the nature of depression, its course, and the relative costs and benefits of treatment options. It also includes assessment and management of the patient while in treatment, along with resolution of obstacles to treatment adherence, monitoring and management of treatment side effects, and assessment of outcome.

Cognitive therapy—a treatment method that focuses on revising a person's maladaptive processes of thinking, perceptions, attitudes, and beliefs. Cognitive therapy has been developed for different specific disorders, including depression.

Completer analysis—analysis of data in terms of the relationship between the number of patients whose conditions improved and the number who completed the treatment episode.

Cyclothymic disorder—a mood disorder of at least two years' duration characterized by numerous periods of mild depressive symptoms not sufficient in duration or severity to meet criteria for major depressive episodes, interspersed with periods of hypomania. Some view this condition as a mild variant of bipolar disorder.

Dementia—a group of mental disorders involving a general loss of intellectual abilities, including memory, judgment, and abstract thinking. There may be associated poor impulse control and/or personality change. Dementias may be progressive, reversible, or static and have a variety of causes.

Dysthymia—a mood disorder characterized by depressed mood and loss of interest or pleasure in customary activities, with some additional signs and symptoms of depression, that is present most of the time for at least two years. Many patients with dysthymia go on to develop major depressive episodes.

Electroconvulsive therapy—a treatment method usually reserved for very severe or psychotic depressions or manic states that often are not responsive to medication treatment. A low-voltage alternating current is sent to the brain to induce a convulsion or seizure, which accounts for the therapeutic effect.

Hypomania—an episode of illness that resembles mania, but is less intense and less disabling. The state is characterized by a euphoric mood, unrealistic optimism, increased speech and activity, and a decreased need for sleep. For some, there is increased creativity, while others evidence poor judgment and impaired function.

Intent-to-treat analysis—analysis of data in terms of the relationship between the number of patients randomized to treatment and the number whose conditions improved.

Interpersonal psychotherapy—a time-limited psychotherapeutic approach that aims at clarification and resolution of one or more of the following interpersonal difficulties: role disputes, social isolation, prolonged grief reaction, and role transition. The patient and therapist define the nature of the difficulty and work to its resolution.

Maintenance treatment—treatment designed to prevent a new mood episode (e.g., depression, mania, hypomania).

Major depressive disorder—a major mood disorder characterized by one (single) or more (recurrent) episodes of major depression, with or without full recovery between episodes.

Mania—an episode of illness usually seen in the course of bipolar I disorder and characterized by hyperexcitability, euphoria, and hyperactivity. Rapid thinking and speaking, agitation, a decreased need for sleep, and a marked increase in energy are nearly always present. During manic episodes, some patients also experience hallucinations or delusions. Manic episodes can also be caused by selected general medical disorders.

Melancholic features—symptoms usually found in severe major depressive episodes, including marked loss of pleasure, psychomotor retardation or agitation, weight loss, and insomnia.

Mood disorders—a grouping of psychiatric conditions that has as a central feature a disturbance in mood (usually profound sadness or apathy, euphoria, or irritability). These disorders may be episodic or chronic.

Obsessive-compulsive disorder—a condition that is characterized by the presence of obsessions and/or compulsions. Obsessions are recurrent, intrusive thoughts—usually irrational worries—that often necessitate behaviors to prevent untoward consequences (e.g., fears of contamination from dirt requiring the individual to wear gloves at all times).

Compulsions are recurrent behaviors beyond the normal range that the individual feels compelled to undertake, usually to preserve personal safety, to avoid embarrassment, or to perform adequately (e.g., checking multiple times to see that the gas is turned off before leaving home). The disorder affects 1 to 2 percent of the population.

Open trial—a trial of a treatment in which both patient and practitioner are aware of the treatment being used.

Panic disorder—an anxiety disorder characterized by discrete intense periods of fear and associated symptoms. Panic disorder may be accompanied by agoraphobia.

Remission—a return to the asymptomatic state, usually accompanied by a return to the usual level of psychosocial functioning.

Somatization disorder—a disorder characterized by multiple, often long-standing somatic complaints of bodily dysfunction (e.g., pain complaints, gastrointestinal disturbances). The disorder usually begins before the age of 30 and has a chronic, albeit fluctuating, course.

Supportive therapy—psychotherapy that focuses on the management and resolution of current difficulties and life decisions, using the patient's strengths and available resources.

Symptom breakthrough—the return of symptoms in the course of either continuation or maintenance phase treatment.

Vegetative symptoms—a group of symptoms that refers to sleep, appetite, and/or weight regulation.

Source: Depression in Primary Care: Volume 1, Detection and Diagnosis (Apr. 1993). U.S. Department of Health and Human Services, Public Health Service, Agency for Health Care Policy and Research, Rockville, Maryland.

Rare Disorders and Orphan Drugs

RARE DISORDERS

A rare disorder or orphan disease is one that affects fewer than 200,000 people. It can strike any age, race, sex, or ethnic background. Many rare disorders are genetic, while others are caused by the environment. However, most rare disorders fall into a category the medical profession calls idiopathic, which means "of unknown causation." Not only are the causes unknown, but many physicians have little, if any, experience diagnosing and treating rare disorders.

Twenty million Americans are affected by any one of the 5,000 known rare disorders. While this may appear to be a sizable number of people, the relative rarity of these diseases can be put in proper perspective when one considers that diabetes *alone* afflicts some 12 million Americans, and 37 million have arthritis.

One-third of people with rare disorders take between one and five years to be properly diagnosed, and 15 percent remain undiagnosed for more than five years. This unfortunate state of affairs is due to the relative scarcity of diagnostic tests for specific rare disorders, especially if the disorder is a neurological one. Instead, in the absence of such tests, physicians must rely on a physical examination and the patient's medical history. Compounding the problem is the fact that rare-disease experts are often located at university-affiliated hospitals, to which patients must be referred by local physicians prior to further examination.

Some examples of orphan diseases most often misunderstood or misdiagnosed are Tourette syndrome, narcolepsy, Ehlers-Danlos syndrome, and Marfan syndrome.

Tourette syndrome is a neurological disorder characterized by involuntary repetitive "tic" movements or vocalizations, such as rapid eye blinking, shoulder shrugging, head jerking, facial twitches, sniffing, throat clearing, grunting, barking, or outbursts of inappropriate words. These tics usually begin during elementary school years and are often mistaken for nervous habits, because they tend to get worse under stress. Since most children with Tourette syndrome also have problems with hyperactivity, their symptoms are often dismissed as behavioral problems. Tourette syndrome is treatable with several medications.

Narcolepsy, a sleep disorder often mistaken for laziness, generally develops during teenage years, and is characterized by the tendency to fall asleep at inappropriate times. Relaxing environments can result in short, irresistible naps. Complications of narcolepsy may cause the person to suddenly fall to the floor in a dream state and/or to lose muscle control during episodes of instant dreaming. Narcolepsy is treatable with stimulant drugs.

Ehlers-Danlos syndrome and *Marfan syndrome* are congenital hereditary connective-tissue diseases. People with Ehlers-Danlos syndrome appear incredibly flexible. Their ability to bend and flex their joints is so great, in fact, that it should be apparent that something is wrong. Other symptoms include fragile skin that easily bruises and a tendency to experience poor healing of wounds.

Similarly, people with Marfan syndrome appear unusually tall, with unusually long hands and feet, and ocular, skeletal, and cardiovascular abnormalities. They may otherwise appear to be perfectly healthy; therefore, the disorder may go undiagnosed, until complications such as a ruptured aorta arise, at which time diagnosis is too late.

THE ORPHAN DRUG ACT

For many people, being diagnosed with a rare disorder can be tragic; however, for too long a factor compounding this tragedy was the unavailability of medications to treat these conditions. While medical researchers discovered drugs that could provide effective treatment, the pharmaceutical industry was reluctant to develop these products. Medications developed for these illnesses are considered "drugs of little commercial value" and cost between $50 million and $80 million to produce and bring to the market. Faced with the prospects of high development costs and little, if any, profit, pharmaceutical companies required some sort of incentive to produce these drugs.

Through the efforts of the families of those affected by rare disorders and the encouragement of others, Congress responded by passing the Orphan Drug Act, which became law on January 4, 1983. Funding, in the form of grants from the Food and Drug Administration (FDA), is made available to drug companies to cover the cost of research and development of otherwise unprofitable drugs for rare disorders. Drug companies are also permitted to recoup a portion of the costs incurred to conduct the FDA-mandated clinical trials (a phase of development that includes testing the medication on animals and humans). Without clinical trials, new medications would never make it onto the market.

The Orphan Drug Act, as amended in 1992, gives pharmaceutical companies further incentives to produce orphan drugs. For one thing, the government guarantees the company $200 million in sales or a nine-year monopoly on the drug, whichever comes first.

With these types of incentives, pharmaceutical companies in many cases can profit from producing orphan drugs, and people with rare diseases can final-

ly be treated. Since the passage of the Orphan Drug Act, some 90 drugs have been developed and approved, with another 400 currently in some stage of development.

One example of an orphan drug developed as a result of this program is Ceredase (alglucerase), used to treat Gaucher disease, which is an inherited illness that deprives the patient of an enzyme that normally dissolves a certain kind of fatty material in the body. An estimated 2,000 to 3,000 people suffer from this lifelong disease.

Another orphan drug available is Erythropoietin (epoetin alfa), used to treat anemia caused by kidney failure. More than 50,000 people suffer from this lifelong condition.

A third orphan drug available is Protropin (somatrem). This is a growth hormone used to treat short stature caused by lack of a brain hormone. Approximately 12,000 patients suffer from this.

The Orphan Drug Act, however, has not put an end to the pain suffered by patients with rare disorders. It only enables these people to obtain needed medications, which in many cases treat rather than cure the illnesses.

THE NATIONAL ORGANIZATION FOR RARE DISORDERS

The National Organization for Rare Disorders (NORD) was created by voluntary health agencies and people affected by rare diseases to help get the Orphan Drug Act passed. NORD aids in the needs and concerns of people with rare diseases and provides information to the public about rare diseases and orphan drugs. It also links people who are affected by the same diseases and encourages the formation of support groups between them. NORD also links patients with doctors who are researching their diseases, as well as provides funding for small clinical research groups. Treatment information may be obtained from NORD's database available on the CompuServe network. Or you can write for information to the following address.

National Organization for Rare Disorders (NORD)
P.O. Box 8923
New Fairfield, CT 06812
800-447-6673
203-746-6518

Sexually Transmitted Diseases and Sexual Problems

Venereal disease or sexually transmitted diseases (STDs) is the general name given to a group of diseases caused by organisms that are spread from person to person during sexual intercourse or genital contact. Syphilis, gonorrhea, genital herpes, and AIDS are major STDs, because they are the most prevalent and do the most damage. But there are over fifteen diseases and related disorders that can be spread sexually. (See the beginning of this section for a discussion of AIDS.)

SYPHILIS

Syphilis is a sexually carried disease caused by a type of bacteria and marked by three stages over a period of years. A person catches syphilis by direct contact with an infectious lesion on the mouth, penis, or in the vagina of an infected person.

As soon as a person is infected with syphilis, a painless, bloodless ulcer (called a chancre)—an infectious lesion—will develop on the place of infection. It may be unnoticeable and will disappear in about 4 weeks.

In the secondary stage, skin rashes may develop. The rash may be raised, flat, spreading, moist or dry. Rashes may appear on the palms of the hands, on the arms, in the scalp, in the lining of the mouth, between the toes, or anywhere else on the body. The person may have a general feeling of illness with headaches, fever, swollen glands, or a sore throat. During this stage a person with syphilis is highly infectious.

During the latent stage of syphilis, the rashes may have disappeared, but they may be replaced by a fast-growing large tumor that invades and destroys tissues and organs. Sometimes patients will develop paresis, or brain damage brought on by the destruction of brain tissue, causing such symptoms as paranoia. Destruction of the knee joints, lightning pains, vomiting, loss of bladder and bowel control, heart disease, and difficulty in walking are also signs of late syphilis.

The symptoms of congenital syphilis, syphilis that is passed on to a child, may develop before the child is 2 years of age. These symptoms include skin sores, lesions of the mucous membranes, anemia, complications in bone development, and an enlarged spleen or liver. Later symptoms include blindness, poorly formed teeth, depression or paranoia, a deformed face or skeleton, or a malformed heart.

Although there is no cure for syphilis, penicillin is used in treatment. For people who are allergic to penicillin, tetracycline and erythromycin are effective treatments.

GONORRHEA

Gonorrhea is another disease that can only be spread through sexual contact. For a man, symptoms of infection include a burning sensation, frequent urination, and a discharge of pus from the penis. If this stage remains untreated, secondary stages may develop, including consequences such as sterility, brain damage, heart disease, and arthritis.

For females, the symptoms are mild urinary discomfort, mild burning, and frequent urination, along with a discharge of pus from the vagina. These mild symptoms may go unnoticed, however. If untreated, the disease will move into the secondary stage, which may include infection of fallopian tubes and ovaries, inflammation of the abdomen, and sterility in some cases. In rare cases, a rupture may occur in the reproductive organs of the female, which may cause sudden shock and death. Arthritis and heart disease may also be present in a female.

A mother who is infected with gonorrhea could possibly pass the disease on to her child during delivery of the baby. The baby's eyes may become infected, causing permanent blindness. This can be prevented, however, if a doctor uses antibiotic eyedrops on the baby's eyes immediately after the baby is born.

Penicillin is an effective treatment for gonnorhea. One type of gonorrhea is resistant to penicillin, however. For this type, two other medications, called spectinomycin and cefoxitin, may be used.

One other complication of gonorrhea possible in women is *pelvic inflammatory disease* (PID). It is an infection that extends from the cervix up into the fallopian tubes. Signs of PID are fever, chills, listlessness, loss of appetite, nausea, indigestion, vomiting, vaginal discharge, painful urination, and abdominal pain. Sometimes severe pain may prevent a woman from carrying out normal daily activities. Complications of PID include repeated infections, pain in the pelvic region, ectopic pregnancy, and sterility. Risks for PID are higher in women who use intrauterine devices (IUDs) for birth control. PID is treated by penicillin or tetracycline.

GENITAL HERPES

Genital herpes spreads through direct contact of the lips, eyes, or genitals with those infected areas of a partner. A person need not have vaginal intercourse to contract herpes; oral-genital sex, anal intercourse, and even the skin-to-skin rubbing of the genitalia can transmit herpes. Although a condom may help prevent herpes, the disease may have spread to uncovered areas such as the thighs and buttocks.

The first symptoms of herpes include a general feeling of discomfort or uneasiness, headache, swollen glands, muscle aches, fever, pain in the genital areas, painful urination, painful intercourse, a stiff neck, and a rash on the genital organs, on the buttocks, thighs, or in the rectal area. Depression may also set in.

Once a person has herpes, it never leaves the body. There is also strong evidence that herpes can lead to cancer, especially cervical cancer in women.

Recurrences of genital herpes can be triggered by emotional stress, lack of sleep, fever, sexual intercourse, masturbation, friction from tight-fitting clothes, and extended exposure to the sun and wind.

A person with herpes may use the following tips: Don't touch, pick, or puncture blisters. Wash hands more frequently than usual. Keep lesions dry with talcum powder or cornstarch. Wear loose-fitting cotton undergarments. Apply ice to severe pain. Avoid prolonged or frequent bathing and keep the water warm. And minimize stress.

Although there is no cure for genital herpes, an ointment called Zovirax (acyclovir) can minimize the pain of blisters of herpes.

OTHER STDS

Trichomoniasis causes inflammation of the vagina, resulting in a grayish, frothy, foul-smelling discharge and sometimes sores in the vagina and possible abdominal pain. The infection usually causes little distress in males. Trichomoniasis is usually treated with metronidazole.

Genital *chlamydial infections* are caused by bacteria transmitted by either vaginal or anal sex. The particular bacterium, *Chlamydia trachomatis,* is the most prevalent cause of blindness worldwide. Touching an eye with a hand that has infectious secretions on it can cause an eye infection; furthermore, a mother can transmit the infection to her child during delivery. In many cases, especially in women, there may be no symptoms. When present, symptoms are similar to those of gonorrhea but milder. In men, the infection sometimes causes a burning sensation during urination and a discharge from the urethra. Antibiotics are generally prescribed for chlamydial infections.

Venereal warts (condylomata acuminatum) resemble warts on other parts of the body, and they are most likely caused by the same virus, papilloma. Females with the virus may develop warts on the hymen and on the vulva, while males develop them on the head and shaft of the penis. Mild cases can be treated with an antiwart chemical, while severe cases may require surgical removal. In some cases the warts may become cancerous.

Crab lice (pediculosis pubis) are bloodsucking lice that are transmitted through pubic hair contact. They cause itching and rash in the pubic area. The treatment is simply the use of soap and water.

Scabies can be transmitted through sexual and nonsexual contact. The mite burrows into the skin and deposits eggs. One to three months later, itchy bumps develop on the skin. Benzyl benzoate lotion applied to skin is the treatment for scabies.

Monilial vaginitis (yeast infection) is a fungal infection of the vagina. The vagina becomes inflamed and produces a thick discharge. Pain and itching of the vulva are also symptoms. A male who acquires this condition will probably develop a painful and itchy inflammation of the penis. Treatment involves the use of antifungal drugs, careful cleansing of the skin, boiling of underwear, and frequent changes of clothing.

Nonspecific urethritis is an infection of the urethra, although it is not known exactly what causes the infection. The symptoms for men include a strong discharge from the urethra and painful urination. In a woman, symptoms are urinary pain, burning, and a thick vaginal discharge. Tetracycline antibiotics are used in treatment.

Hepatitis is a viral infection of the liver. It begins with fever and shaking chills. Other symptoms are loss of appetite, headache, muscle pain, pain in the abdomen, joint pains, skin rashes, discolored urine, yellowing skin, nausea, vomiting, and extreme fatigue, irritability, and despondency. Although this disease does not specifically affect the genitals, it can be sexually transmitted. Recovery from hepatitis may take several months.

Sleep and Sleep Disorders

Sleep, a bodily function that takes up about one-third of a person's life, is an essential process of the human body. It is not fully understood exactly why we sleep, what the function of sleep is, or what precise chemical processes cause us to sleep, but it is known that without sleep humans would not be able to function efficiently.

Humans suffering from sleep deprivation may develop irritability, paranoia, impaired memory and judgment, short attention span, visual and auditory hallucinations, and even an impaired immune system. The process of sleep allows the brain and other metabolic processes of the body to rest and replenish themselves. This is not to say that the brain is inactive during sleep. Brain activity, measured by an electroencephalogram (EEG), persists in sleep, and, in some areas of the brain, brain activity even surpasses that during wakefulness.

NREM AND REM SLEEP

There are two kinds of sleep: NREM (non–rapid eye movement) sleep and REM (rapid eye movement) sleep. Through the course of a sleep period, NREM and REM sleep states alternate three to five times.

NREM sleep consists of four stages, each a progressively deeper stage of sleep in which the heart and respiration slow, muscles relax, and blood pressure falls, and all of which have a characteristic brain wave pattern as shown by an EEG. *Stage 1* NREM sleep, a transitional stage between a wakeful state and a sleeping one, is the "lightest" stage of sleep and brain activity displays alpha wave patterns and vertex sharp wave patterns. Stage 1 NREM sleep, or the onset of sleep, lasts about 10 to 15 minutes and is characterized by slow, rolling eye movements, hypnic jerks (muscular twitches), and dreamlike thoughts. *Stage 2* sleep is characterized by an EEG pattern of two kinds of alternating waveforms: sleep spindle waves and K-complex waves. *Stages 3 and 4,* deeper stages of NREM sleep called slow-wave sleep, display delta waves and waveforms that change in amplitude and in frequency.

REM sleep, characterized by a sawtooth wave pattern of brain activity, follows the deeper stages of NREM sleep and is the sleep state in which vivid dreaming takes place. REM sleep, named for the rapid eye movements that herald the arrival and accompany this kind of sleep, is a state in which much of the brain is intensely active. It occupies about 90 to 100 minutes of the total night's sleep period. REM sleep, sometimes called paradoxical sleep, is marked by a complete absence of muscle tone (though may be interrupted by occasional twitches), irregular respiration and blood pressure, and intense levels of brain activity. Again, the exact function of REM sleep is unknown, but it is thought that REM sleep helps to preserve long-term memory and healthy immune system function.

CHEMISTRY OF SLEEP

Sleep involves the communication of brain cells, which release chemicals called neurotransmitters. Sleep and wakefulness are controlled by the chemical reactions of neurotransmitters found in the brain stem, concentrated in an area known as the reticular activating system (RAS). Here, nerve impulses carried by neurotransmitters such as acetylcholine, serotonin, adenosine, and glutamate move through the brain to the cerebral cortex, where processes of sleeping and waking are activated. Also involved in the process of sleep are elements known as sleep factors, which include muramyl peptides and interleukin-1 and other sleep-controlling mechanisms such as prostaglandins. However, the exact role these sleep factors play in the entire process is still not fully understood.

CIRCADIAN RHYTHMS

Sleep, specifically the sleep/wake cycle, is also regulated by an internal body clock called a circadian rhythm. Just as other physiological functions in the body are controlled in some way by a daily rhythmic pattern, so too is sleep. Human circadian rhythms are set (entrained) by sunlight and basically maintain a clock that runs slightly longer than 24 hours. The precise location for the internal body clock is a cluster of neurons in the hypothalamus called the suprachiasmatic nuclei. Without the circadian rhythm functioning properly, a person may not be able to fall asleep or awaken at desired normal times. This is what the body experiences most commonly in jet lag or in shift work (occupational jet lag), where the body's clock is advanced or delayed by traveling across time zones or keeping an irregular sleep pattern.

SLEEP DISORDERS

Sleep disorders are not as uncommon as one would think: There is probably not one single person who has not had difficulty in sleeping at least a few times in his or her life. There are 222 known sleep disorders, which can be lumped into four basic categories: difficulty in falling/staying asleep; difficulty in staying awake; difficulty in maintaining a proper sleep/wake cycle; and difficulty with various types of disruptive behavior during sleep.

Common sleep disorders include insomnia, narcolepsy, and parasomnias, including sleep apnea and RBD (REM behavior disorder). Even though sleep disorder medicine is a relatively new field, there are growing numbers of sleep clinics and doctors who concern themselves with sleep research and study.

Insomnia

Insomnia, the most common sleep disorder, is the inability to fall asleep or stay asleep. A person with insomnia cannot get the proper amount of rest needed for daily functioning. (Sleep requirements vary from person to person, but an average length of a nightly sleep period is 7 to 8 hours.) The insomniac experiences fatigue, irritability, and a lack of alertness the following day which may interfere with one's daily tasks.

Insomnia is classified according to the frequency with which one is unable to sleep: transient insomnia (several nights, usually due to excitement or stress), short-term insomnia (2 to 3 weeks, due to stress or illness), and chronic insomnia (frequent insomnia, due to a variety of factors). Causes of insomnia can stem from a physical illness or the medications to treat that illness (usually illnesses that produce pain), a psychological illness (depression, anxiety disorders), behavioral factors (habits in lifestyle that are not conducive to healthful sleep), a circadian rhythm disorder, or other sleep disorders (PLMS—periodic leg movements syndrome; sleep apnea). Older people frequently suffer from insomnia because the quality of sleep and the body's ability to maintain a healthful, sound sleep have been diminished.

Treatment of insomnia involves identifying the underlying problem of the sleeplessness, administering benzodiazepines (medications that act on the central nervous system) to induce sleep, or changing certain behavioral habits (maintaining good sleep hygiene).

Narcolepsy

Narcolepsy is a disease in which a person uncontrollably falls into REM sleep during a state of total wakefulness. Sleep attacks may occur several times a day and endanger the individual's safety (for example, when the person is driving a car). It begins in adolescence and young adulthood—with the most common narcoleptic symptom, excessive daytime sleepiness—and continues throughout life. Its cause is unknown.

The four symptoms associated with narcolepsy, called the narcolepsy tetrad, are excessive daytime sleepiness (EDS), sleep paralysis (temporary paralysis of muscles), cataplexy (short episodes of sudden muscular weakness and tone), and hypnagogic hallucinations (visual, auditory, tactile, or kinetic hallucinations). Other symptoms include restless sleep, impaired memory and eyesight, and vivid dreams. Treatment of narcolepsy includes following good sleep hygiene and the use of central nervous system stimulants such as methylphenidate and pemoline (for sleepiness) and tricyclic antidepressants (for other symptoms such as cataplexy).

Parasomnias

Parasomnias are those disorders not associated with the processes responsible for sleep, but instead involve the respiratory system, the motor system, or the cognitive system during sleep. There are four categories of parasomnias: arousal disorders (sleepwalking and sleep terrors); disorders during the transition between sleeping and waking (hypnic jerks); disorders associated with REM sleep (nightmares, REM behavior disorder, sleep paralysis); and other parasomnias, including snoring, sudden infant death syndrome, bed-wetting, and sleep apnea.

Sleep Apnea

Sleep apnea, a potentially life-threatening condition, is a sleep disorder characterized by loud snoring and by periodic lapses in breathing. Because of an obstruction or some kind of abnormality in the upper airway of the body (obstructive sleep apnea) or because of a failure in autonomic breathing control (central sleep apnea), the individual ceases to breathe. Obstructive sleep apnea is the most common of the two types of apnea and results in a cessation of

Sleep Hygiene

Good sleep hygiene entails adopting certain types of behavior that are favorable to good sleep and avoiding those activities and substances that contribute to poor sleep. Sleep hygiene includes keeping a regular sleep schedule, maintaining a comfortable sleep environment just for the purpose of sleep, avoiding late-day caffeine and nicotine intake, limiting daytime naps, and avoiding late-night exercise and ingestion of alcohol or sleeping pills. Sleeping pills and alcohol may be an effective short-term solution for sleeplessness; however, these substances can produce side effects and possibly drug dependence.

breathing due to an obstruction: The airway becomes blocked and collapses. In central sleep apnea, the mechanisms that automatically control breathing do not function properly and, even though the airway remains open, the individual cannot breathe. In both types of apnea, the body rouses itself in order to restart the breathing process. The cessation of breathing may last 10 seconds or longer, and arousals recur, unremembered by the individual, several times within one sleep period.

Sleep apnea commonly affects older males and obese people. Individuals with sleep apnea experience fatigue, headaches, restless sleep, impaired concentration and memory, and excessive daytime sleepiness. Apnea may even lead to cardiovascular difficulties, hypertension, and stroke. Treatment of sleep apnea can be surgical (removing obstructive tissue, tonsillectomy, trachea realignment) or nonsurgical (using medications—respiratory stimulants and nasal decongestants—reducing weight, changing sleeping habits, or using mechanical devices that aid in maintaining airflow). CPAP, or continuous positive airway pressure, provides the individual with constant airflow pressure through a facial mask, ensuring that the airway does not collapse.

REM Behavior Disorder

REM behavior disorder (RBD) is a behavioral parasomnia disorder where, during REM sleep, an individual (mostly males) exhibits violent behavior, locomotion, or acts out nightmares or dreams or other movements (grasping, punching, looking around). The cause of RBD is not known and RBD worsens over time. Whereas skeletal muscles are normally inactive (a condition called muscle atonia) during REM sleep, in RBD, neuronal pathways malfunc-

tion and carry signals to motor cells, which then activate muscular activity. Luckily, RBD can be controlled with medication, specifically a benzodiazepine anticonvulsant called clonazepam. This drug controls the violent behavior and quells the nightmarish dreams.

RESOURCES FOR SLEEP DISORDERS

The following are organizations involved in sleep disorder research and study who may provide more information on specific topics.

American Narcolepsy Association
P.O. Box 26230
San Francisco, CA 94126-6230
800-222-6085
415-788-4793

American Sleep Apnea Association
P.O. Box 3893
Charlottesville, VA 22903

American Sleep Disorders Association
1610 14th Street N.W., Suite 300
Rochester, MN 55901-2200
507-287-6006

Better Sleep Council
P.O. Box 13
Washington, DC 20044
800-827-5337

National Sleep Foundation
122 S. Robertson Boulevard, Suite 201
Los Angeles, CA 90048
310-288-0466

The Narcolepsy Network
P.O. Box 1365, FDR Station
New York, NY 10150

Special Problems and Medical Conditions of Children

Children with special medical conditions and disorders need special care from their doctors and families. Diagnosis of these conditions can be upsetting to parents as well as to the children. But with a better understanding of these conditions and their treatments, along with the care and support of local self-help groups, these children and their families can achieve healthier, happier lives.

Many disorders are passed on genetically, meaning that they are inherited from the parents, just as eye color, height, and other physical characteristics are inherited. Each human cell contains forty-six chromosomes, a genetic code that determines physical appearance and biochemical makeup as well as the traits that will be passed on to children. Unequal division of the reproductive cells may cause many consequences, such as Down syndrome (a birth defect marked by mental retardation and many physical defects); however, it is important to keep an appropriate perspective on the actual odds. The truth is that 14 out of 15 infants are born without birth defects. It is also important to note that many birth defects or disorders are caused by environmental factors, or by a combination of genetic and environmental factors.

DIAGNOSIS

In order to prescribe the correct treatment for any illness, a doctor must first diagnose the cause of the illness. Often, the diagnosis can be determined after a discussion with parents of all of the child's symptoms, along with a complete physical examination of the child. The physician will then decide whether further diagnostic testing is necessary.

Diagnostic testing is avoided by most pediatricians whenever possible because many of these tests can cause discomfort and unnecessary side effects in the child. However, sometimes further testing is necessary to obtain proper diagnosis and to prescribe the correct treatment.

LIFE-LIMITING OR LIFE-THREATENING ILLNESSES OR CONDITIONS

Autism

Autism is a severe communication and behavior disorder usually present at birth or fully diagnosed by the child's third birthday. In most instances, it is diagnosed within the first year of life. It is characterized by self-absorption and the inability to form relationships with others. It is a rare disorder, occurring about 2 to 4 times in 10,000 births. While there is no identifiable cause, there is reason to believe that some form of brain damage has occurred, since some children with autism also experience epileptic seizures. For as yet unexplained reasons, autism affects three times more boys than girls.

Other symptoms include unresponsiveness to parents or others, resistance to change, preoccupation with objects, severe tantrums, and ritual play. It is very difficult to teach the autistic child new skills because he or she has a strong resistance to any change in established patterns. Speech development, too, is seriously impaired because the autistic child exhibits little interest in learning speech necessary for normal communication. When a child does attempt speech, it is usually rote based upon something the child heard, as opposed to a cognitive thought process.

Other bizarre behavior, such as self-inflicted injuries from knives, razor blades, or matches or sudden fits of screaming, is not unusual in the autistic child. While there's no specific treatment for autism, special schools, support groups, and an understanding family may enable the autistic child to eventually modify his or her behavior.

Medication is prescribed to control any epileptic seizures an autistic child has; however, there are no medical interventions capable of treating autism itself. Although the outlook for most autistic children is not promising, there are instances where a child may exhibit an unusual talent for art, music or mathematics.

Cerebral Palsy

Cerebral palsy is a nonprogressive—which means that it does not worsen with time—neurological disorder, present at birth or shortly thereafter, that affects the arm and leg muscles of the newborn and is usually the result of brain damage. While it may be diagnosed at birth, most cases of cerebral palsy are fully diagnosed by the age of 3; however, some milder forms may not be detected for years after birth.

The most likely cause of cerebral palsy is brain damage due to cerebral hypoxia (loss of oxygen to the brain), although a maternal infection, while the baby is in utero, may be responsible in some cases. When cerebral palsy occurs after birth, it may be caused by encephalitis (inflammation of the brain), meningitis (inflammation of the covering of the brain), or head injury.

Symptoms in newborns include stiffness, particularly on one side, or involuntary kicking with only one leg. Later signs may include walking or crawling with one leg trailing behind, always standing on tiptoe, or loss of balance and coordination.

Later consequences of this disease include the inability to control some muscles and/or mental impairment, and severity varies. Some children affected with cerebral palsy may also be hearing-impaired or suffer from seizures. In rare cases the symptoms of cerebral palsy disappear gradually. The incidence rate of cerebral palsy in the U.S. is about 4 per 1,000 live births.

There is no medical treatment for cerebral palsy that will reverse the symptoms of the condition; however, medication to control seizures may be prescribed. Nonmedical adaptive therapies such as physical therapy, speech therapy, and special education enable some people with cerebral palsy to lead a relatively full and independent life.

Cystic Fibrosis

Cystic fibrosis is an inherited genetic disease that leads to chronic lung infections and interferes with the body's ability to absorb fats and other nutrients from food. In order to develop cystic fibrosis, a person must inherit the recessive gene from both parents. Inheriting one gene would make the person a carrier, which means that he or she would not develop any symptoms but is capable of passing along the gene to offspring (if the gene is matched with another such recessive gene in the other parent). Until the development of antibiotics, most children diagnosed with cystic fibrosis died in childhood.

Cystic fibrosis is characterized by the production of thickened mucus that clogs the bronchi, making breathing difficult and creating an environment in which infections can develop. It affects the pancreas by interfering with the production of enzymes essential for the breakdown of fats and their absorption in the intestines.

Until the development of antibiotics, there was very little that could be done to treat cystic fibrosis. Today, antibiotics are used to control and eliminate lung infections, and replacement enzyme therapy aids in digestion of essential nutrients. While there is no medication that can reverse the condition, heart and lung transplants have been tried with varying degrees

of success, and hold out great promise for the future. Even though these developments have enabled children with cystic fibrosis to live longer, they experience more illness and generally have shorter lives.

Down Syndrome

Down syndrome is a genetic disorder in which the child has decreased muscle tone, short stature, mental retardation, small nose and low nasal bridge, upward slant to the eyes, and short stubby fingers. The cause of Down syndrome is an extra chromosome in the body resulting in forty-seven instead of the normal forty-six (a child receives twenty-three chromosomes from each parent).

The incidence of Down syndrome is 1 in 650 births; however, when the maternal age is over 40 the incidence jumps to 1 in 40 births. Genetic testing using amniocentesis (sampling the fluid surrounding the fetus) or chorionic villus sampling (testing a portion of the placenta) can help determine whether or not the fetus is carrying the extra chromosome responsible for Down syndrome.

In addition to the physical characteristics of babies with Down syndrome, these children are also born with congenital heart defects, narrowing of the intestines, and hearing problems. While there is no medical cure for Down syndrome, improved medical care and surgical correction of life-threatening birth defects have made survival to early middle age a possibility.

Children with Down syndrome can generally be taught basic skills, such as reading and elementary arithmetic. In addition, sheltered workshops and special education classes have enabled some adults with Down syndrome to obtain jobs and enjoy a form of independence while living in group homes.

Fetal Alcohol Syndrome

Fetal alcohol syndrome is a birth defect that results when the mother consumes excessive amounts (defined as two mixed drinks or up to three glasses of beer or wine per day) of alcohol during pregnancy. However, it should be remembered that there is no such thing as a "safe" amount of alcohol, since all alcohol affects fetal growth.

Consuming alcohol not only risks birth defects but has also been linked to an increase in the rate of miscarriages.

Infants diagnosed with fetal alcohol syndrome are born unusually small, suffer mild to moderate mental retardation, congenital heart defects, droopy eyelids, a cleft palate, microcephaly (small head), and/or joint abnormalities. Mortality within the first few weeks following birth is quite high at 20 percent.

An infant with fetal alcohol syndrome is treated the same as an alcoholic going through detoxification. Once the baby has been detoxified, then an evaluation can be made as to corrective surgery for other physical defects.

Mental Retardation

Mental retardation is the term used to describe a subnormal ability to learn, a substantially low IQ, and impaired social adjustment. With proper care and training, some mentally retarded people have enough intellectual ability to function reasonably well as adults. These people hold jobs, interact with their community, and even marry. At one time, many of these same people were confined to institutions; however, today they are able to live on their own or in the familylike setting of a group home.

The many causes of mental retardation include congenital or chromosomal abnormalities, infections, birth injuries, toxic substances, accidents, metabolic or hormonal disorders, and nutritional deficiencies. In most cases, however, the cause is unknown. The degree of retardation based on IQ varies a great deal, from mild to profound. Mild is defined as an IQ of 50 to 70; moderate, 35 to 49; severe, 20 to 34; and profound, under 20. Mental retardation is difficult to diagnose in infancy and early childhood. Since infants develop at different rates, many doctors are reluctant to diagnose before the second or third year of development, depending on the child.

Although in most cases there is no cure for many of these conditions, mentally retarded children should be helped to reach their full potential. Special education classes in the school system offer many of the courses that help them with speech, dress, care for basic needs, reading, etc. Love, attention, and parental support are also very important in achieving this. Parents may contact national and local support groups as well as advocates for the mentally retarded for more information on specific programs available in their area.

Muscular Dystrophy

Muscular dystrophy is a family of inherited genetic conditions, affecting only males, characterized by the gradual wasting of the muscles. It is a term that describes several muscle diseases, the most common type being Duchenne's muscular dystrophy. This condition, which is usually not diagnosed before the age of 3, is characterized by slow development of basic movement skills, much later than those of most normal children. As the condition progresses, the children walk with a waddling gait and have difficulty climbing stairs. Deterioration is rapid, with the child becoming wheelchair-bound usually by the time he or she is a teenager. Other problems also develop quickly, such as enlargement of the thighs (as fat replaces muscle tissue), respiratory difficulty (leading to chest infections), heart failure, and mild mental retardation.

Although there is no effective treatment, genetic counseling is suggested for women whose brothers or maternal uncles suffered from the disorder.

Spina Bifida

Spina bifida, the incomplete formation of the spinal column, can lead to significant disabilities. Spina bifida occurs in about 3 of every 1,000 births. In this condition, part of the spinal cord protrudes through the spinal column and can result in impairment of walking and bowel and bladder control. Hydrocephalus, or enlargement of the head due to abnormal accumulation of cerebrospinal fluid in the brain, can occur because the open spine allows the lower portion of the brain to slip into the spinal column, disrupting the normal flow of spinal fluid.

Surgery to repair the opening in the spinal canal can be a very effective form of treatment if performed a few days following birth. When hydrocephalus is present, a shunt, or tube, is inserted in the brain to drain excess fluids. A urinary catheter (a tube inserted in the bladder) may be used to relieve urinary retention or incontinence.

Physically Handicapped Infants

From the time of birth of an infant who is handicapped, regardless of the handicap, parents can adjust the child's environment with stimulants for the maximum potential for development.

Overprotection of a handicapped child is often a problem because, in many cases, the child is not taught to care for him- or herself. Another problem is social isolation, which also may have negative results for a handicapped child. When separated from their parents, these children can fall victim to insensitive statements from others. Parents should seek out play groups in which the child can develop as normally as possible.

Blindness
Blind children can be at risk of being raised with the idea that they lack potential. Parents may delay in giving the child solid foods, in toilet training the child, or in teaching the child to dress, which denies the child early learning. Positive stimulation can be learned by parents very early on so that the child can be raised to reach his or her full potential.

Deafness
Similarly, deaf children are often treated as retarded because they lack a sense that is important for learning, and therefore develop slowly. Early recognition of deafness is helpful for parents in order that they substitute other stimuli to boost development.

When selecting a pediatrician for handicapped children, make sure that the doctor shows the child the proper care and attention he or she deserves. Family counseling is also helpful to parents and siblings of handicapped children

Stress
A recent poll reports that Americans are working more hours per week than ever before. Just between 1977 and 1988, the average workweek jumped from under 41 hours to almost 47 hours; during that same period, leisure time shrank 37 percent. A recent survey reports that more than 50 percent of CEOs expect their middle and top managers to work at least 50 to 59 hours a week.

With this added emphasis on work, and leisure time that is often rushed, it's not surprising that many Americans feel "stressed-out" much of the time.

Feeling stressed actually refers to the physical response the body mounts to a perceived threat (whether the threat is real or imagined, physical or psychological). When the nervous system senses danger, it prepares the body for the "fight or flight" response. Muscles tense, blood pressure and heart rate rise, and adrenaline and other stress-triggered hormones that increase the level of alertness are released.

Unless the stress response is followed by a relaxation period, a number of physical and mental health problems can result: Stress has long been associated with heart disease and often is a factor in chronic low-back pain and types of depression and anxiety disorders. When stress leads to loss of sleep, the body loses its ability to fight off infection and disease and the individual becomes more accident-prone.

Stress can also manifest itself in other ills, such as stroke, stomach ulcers, asthma, gastritis, menstrual disorders, ulcerative colitis, angina, irritable colon, increased blood pressure, duodenal ulcers, and headaches.

The short-term effects of the mind-body connection are obvious. It should be no surprise, then, that your everyday frame of thinking can have a profound impact on your physical life over the long haul, too. Indeed, researchers are building a mountain of evidence showing that mental well-being can improve your health and add years to your life. Here are more examples:

- People who don't reach out to others in times of stress and who withdraw into themselves suffer a greater incidence of cancer and suicide, according to a long-running Johns Hopkins University study begun in 1946.
- One in 7 people who let severe depression go untreated commits suicide. Suicide is the eighth leading cause of death in the United States, claiming more than 30,000 lives per year.
- People with an angry and hostile personality run a higher risk of heart attack, according to research at Duke University Medical Center.
- Optimists develop fewer chronic diseases of middle age than pessimists, according to a study of graduates of the Harvard University class of '42.
- People who don't have close friends, are unmarried, and who avoid community involvement are twice as likely to die than more sociable folks, according to Yale and University of California at Berkeley researchers.

This research is only the tip of the iceberg. Here's how you can tap your brain and think yourself to a long life:

1. Recognize that stress is a killer.
2. Learn to identify sources of excess stress in your life.
3. Eliminate or modify the stressors in your life.
4. Learn to cope with stressors that can't be changed.
5. Deal with chronic hostility and anger, the blood brothers of stress.

How Stressful Events Affect Your Life

To rate how much stress you are experiencing in your life, add up the numbers listed for life events you have undergone within the last year. If you score more than 200, you have a 50 percent chance of becoming seriously ill from stress; a score of 300 or more raises your chances of illness to 80 percent.

Life Event	Score
1. Death of spouse	100
2. Divorce	73
3. Marital separation	65
4. Jail term	63
5. Death of close family member	63
6. Personal injury or illness	53
7. Marriage	50
8. Being fired	47
9. Marital reconciliation	45
10. Retirement	45
11. Change in health of family member	44
12. Pregnancy	40
13. Sex difficulties	39
14. Having a baby	39
15. Business readjustment	39
16. Change in financial state	38
17. Death of close friend	37
18. Change to different line of work	36
19. Change in number of arguments with spouse	35
20. Mortgage large in relation to income	31
21. Foreclosure of mortgage or loan	30
22. Change in responsibilities at work	29
23. Son or daughter leaving home	29
24. Trouble with in-laws	29
25. Outstanding personal achievement	28
26. Spouse begins or stops work	26
27. Begin or end school	26
28. Change in living conditions	25
29. Change in personal habits	24
30. Trouble with boss	23
31. Change in work hours or conditions	20
32. Change in residence	20
33. Change in schools	20
34. Change in church activities	19
35. Change in recreation	19
36. Change in social activities	18
37. Small mortgage in relation to income	17
38. Change in sleeping habits	16
39. Change in number of family get-togethers	15
40. Change in eating habits	13
41. Vacation	13
42. Christmas	12
43. Minor violations of the law	11

Source: Holmes and Rahe, "Social Readjustment Rating Scale." Reprinted from *Journal of Psychosomatic Research,* vol. 11, 1967. Headington Hill Hall, Oxford: Pergamon Press Ltd.

Suicide

Suicide, the deliberate taking of one's life, accounts for approximately 30,000 deaths each year in the U.S. A total of 30,906 people committed suicide in the U.S. in 1990. Of that number, 20.7 percent of the victims were older than 65, while 15.8 percent were 15 to 24 years of age. Men are two to six times more likely than women to take their lives, depending on age.

Most successful suicide attempts are by people suffering from depression; 5 to 15 percent of such patients eventually take their lives.

Suicide has become the third leading cause of death among 15-to-24-year-olds, after accidents and homicide, and is the fastest-growing cause of death among that age group.

Approximately 60 percent of suicides are committed with firearms. The second leading method of suicide is hanging (14 percent), followed by the use of gas or the ingestion of solid or liquid poison.

Statistics for attempted suicide, or parasuicide, are not as firm as those for suicide. An estimated 4 to 5 percent of Americans attempt suicide at some point in their lives. It is also believed that for every suicide, there are eight to twenty attempts. Studies show that four times as many men as women die of suicide, but that there are three female attempts for every male attempt. White men commit suicide more often than do women or black men.

CAUSES

No single cause or set of causes leads to a suicide, just as no typical profile exists of suicide victims. In general, however, family disruption, through divorce, desertion or death of a parent, is frequently a contributing factor to young suicides. Stable community structure has been found to help prevent suicides.

Young suicides or parasuicides are more likely than their peers to suffer from psychiatric disorders or to have parents who do. But some researchers believe that adolescent suicide and parasuicide are more likely to represent a reaction to external circumstances, while adult suicide is a response to feelings of hopelessness and despair arising from psychiatric disorders.

Suicide is indirectly related to religion and culture, occurring with greater incidence in such countries as Japan, where it has historically been considered an acceptable option, and occurring less frequently in Catholic, Orthodox Jewish, and Muslim communities.

Consumption of alcohol has been found to weaken inhibitions against suicide, and also to lead to the long-term pattern of thoughts that precede a suicide or an attempt. Maltreatment of a small child by parents may also contribute to the adolescent's suicide or attempt.

The term "cluster phenomenon" has been coined to describe communities in which five or six suicides, usually by adolescents, occur within a short period of time. Evidence exists that extensive media publicity can lead to clusters of suicides.

Adults over 65 have the highest rate of suicide of any age group in the U.S. Theories of causes include depression, the desire to end a terminal illness, and the alienation, loss of control, status, and influence that are often associated with aging.

WARNING SIGNS

Warning signs that a young person may be contemplating suicide include direct statements such as "I wish I were dead" or "I don't want to go on living," and indirect statements like "How do you leave your body to science?" or "Soon you won't have to worry about me anymore." Such statements must be taken seriously and the person making them should be questioned directly by a friend, family member, or professional.

Depression is another warning sign. Symptoms of depression include sleep disturbances, loss or increase in appetite, lack of energy, abrupt behavior changes, and feelings of hopelessness, low esteem, and despair.

Another warning sign of suicide is the sudden setting in order of one's affairs, including the giving away of prized possessions. Other clues include such erratic behavior as excessive irritability, crying, guilt, and inability to concentrate.

The most serious sign of impending suicide is a suicide attempt. No matter how weakly it may have been undertaken, any suicide attempt must be regarded as a cry for attention that, if ignored, might become more lethal in the future.

PREVENTION AND THERAPY

Prevention of suicide includes:

1. Hospitalization and other medical treatment after an attempted suicide
2. Establishment of agencies to befriend or help potential victims, such as the Samaritan organization started in 1953 in Great Britain

3. Restricting access by potential victims to the means of suicide, such as firearms, poisons, and drugs
4. School courses in coping, problem solving, and suicide awareness
5. Establishment of crisis centers

Family management and therapy for suicide attempters seeks to do the following:

1. Analyze the events and reasons leading up to the attempt
2. Measure the seriousness of the attempt
3. Determine if the person suffers from a psychiatric disorder
4. Examine the family's history of suicide and psychiatric disorders
5. Evaluate the attempter's coping mechanisms
6. Establish a peer support group or a relationship between the attempter and a trusted adult
7. Measure the risk of another attempt

Therapy can be provided in several forms. In individual counseling, a mental health professional collaborates with the attempter to identify and solve his or her problems. Between counseling sessions, the patient takes small steps to work on the problems.

In family counseling, a professional seeks to change the interactions and improve communication among family members. In group interactive therapy, a patient discusses his or her attempted suicide and the reasons for it with members of a peer group.

Finally, medication is given to suicide attempters, usually for the treatment of depression or other psychiatric disorders.

U.S. Suicides in 1990

	Number	Per Day	Rate*	% of Deaths
Nation	30,906	84.7	12.4	1.4
Males	24,724	67.7	20.4	2.2
Females	6,182	16.9	4.8	0.6
Whites	28,086	76.9	13.5	1.5
Nonwhites	2,820	7.7	7.0	1.0
Blacks	2,111	5.8	6.9	0.8
Elderly†	6,394	17.5	20.5	0.4
Young‡	4,869	13.3	13.2	13.3

* Per 100,000 population.
† 65 years and older.
‡ 15–24 years.

101 Major Medical Conditions

The following is a listing and descriptions of 101 medical conditions that occur most commonly or receive the most publicity in the United States. Not included are diseases that once were common but that have been largely eradicated. Newer diseases and conditions such as Lyme disease, AIDS, and chronic fatigue syndrome are included.

Adrenal gland diseases. Located atop each kidney, but not directly related to the kidneys, the two adrenal glands consist of a cortex and a medulla and secrete hormones that influence such body functions as sugar metabolism, heart contractions, and blood pressure.

Adrenal insufficiency, or Addison's disease, can result from damage to the adrenal cortex by a deficiency of adrenocorticotropic hormone (ACTH) from the pituitary gland. *Symptoms* include weakness, lack of energy, lethargy, mental depression, light-headedness, an inability to think clearly, and mottled skin. Salt may be lost into the urine, causing the victim to eat extra salt and develop low blood sugar (hypoglycemia). Catastrophic symptoms result from acute adrenal insufficiency; these include shock and cardiovascular collapse.

The disease is treated by taking supplemental cortisol or cortisone. The patient must carry a supply of the medication with him in the event that stress causes acute adrenal in sufficiency.

AIDS (acquired immune deficiency syndrome). Virtually unknown in the United States before 1981, AIDS has killed tens of thousands of people and infected millions worldwide. Thought to have originated in Africa, the disease has spread to every continent. It is usually diagnosed through blood testing.

Cause. AIDS is caused by the human immunodeficiency virus (HIV), which attacks the T cell lymphocytes of the immune system and renders the body vulnerable to illnesses that a healthy immune system would otherwise overcome. HIV is transmitted through blood and body fluids, especially semen. No known cases exist of transmission through handshakes, hugs, embraces, insect bites, or exchange of tears or saliva.

Risk population. People most at risk of contracting AIDS include promiscuous homosexual or bisexual men, intravenous drug users who share needles, sex partners of HIV-infected individuals, and hemophili-acs and others who receive transfusions of tainted blood. Infected mothers can transmit AIDS to infants at birth.

Signs. Signs of AIDS include enlarged lymph nodes, fatigue, fever, loss of appetite or weight, and night sweats. The two major illnesses that result from an AIDS-weakened immune system are a parasitic lung infection and a cancer called Karposi's sarcoma. Symptoms of the first are cough, fever, and breathing difficulty; symptoms of the second are bluish or brown spots. Some AIDS patients experience visual impairment and blindness or neurological complica-tions to the brain.

Treatment. Some drugs appear to slow the progress of AIDS, but none can restore the immune system. Other drugs slow, but do not cure, the accom-panying infections. Some victims die within months of diagnosis; others have lived for more than a decade.

Prevention. Public health campaigns in the United States have urged people to abstain from promiscuous sex or to use condoms, and to use clean needles when taking drugs.

Alcoholism. Society has long debated whether alco-holism, which affects an estimated 10 million adult Americans, or 7 percent of the population, is a med-ical illness, a social illness, or a moral handicap.

Early signs. Early signs of alcoholism include gulping of alcoholic drinks, early-morning drinking, surreptitious drinking, increased absence from work, loss of interest in nondrinking activities, a desire to "outdrink" peers, financial difficulties, family disrup-tions, and frequent changes in family, social, and business relationships.

Later signs. Later signs can include increased ca-pacity for alcohol (blood-alcohol content of 150 mg per deciliter without evident intoxication), physiolog-ical dependency (evidenced by withdrawal symptoms such as tremors or seizures), and continued drinking despite the loss of control over one's behavior.

Consequences. About 100,000 people die each year in the U.S. from alcohol-related causes, includ-ing traffic fatalities and other accidents. Alcoholics are more likely to commit acts of violence and often suffer loss of memory and ability to concentrate. They are more likely than nonalcoholics to injure themselves, to commit suicide, and to contract cancer, heart disease, lung disease, and liver disease. Women

who drink during pregnancy can give birth to babies afflicted with fetal alcohol syndrome.

Treatment of alcoholism includes hospitalization, dietary assistance, psychiatric counseling, religious counseling, and group therapy. The most effective re-covery program is offered by Alcoholics Anonymous (AA), a worldwide organization of recovering alco-holics who advocate sobriety, adherence to a twelve-step program, mutual support, and public sharing of experiences.

Allergies. People who react abnormally to everyday stimuli (allergens), such as dust mites, pollens, milk, or cat hairs, suffer from allergies. Common allergies include hay fever, eczema, rashes, upset stomach, breathing difficulties, and asthma.

The *allergic reaction* is triggered when an allergen enters the body, usually through the nose or mouth, and affects the mucous membranes of the nose, throat, respiratory system, or digestive system. There, the allergen combines with immunoglobulin E (IgE), which is attached to small mast cells, causing the cells to release histamine and other substances. These substances cause surrounding blood vessels to dilate and leak fluid, resulting in sneezing, hives, rashes, and other allergic symptoms.

Common allergens include *foods,* especially milk, cheese, egg whites, nuts, tomatoes, shellfish, straw-berries, and fish; *pollens,* especially ragweed, which causes hay fever; *molds* from plants and foods, which are more likely than pollens to cause asthma; *house dust,* which contains dust mites and other in-sects, food particles, fibers, hair from house pets; and *medications,* especially penicillin. Also *venom* from the stings of such insects as bees and wasps, and *plant oils,* especially those from the Rhus family, which include poison ivy, poison oak, and poison sumac.

Diagnosis. Allergies can be distinguished in sever-al ways from respiratory illnesses. An allergic illness is less likely to be accompanied by pain, fever, sore throat, or cough, except in cases of postnasal drip. It is more likely to occur seasonally. Diagnosis is also done by examination of patient history, by allergy skin testing, and by a radioimmunoassay procedure called radioallergosorbent test (RAST), which uses serum to detect IgE antibodies.

Prevention and treatment of allergies include avoidance of the allergen; medication, especially an-tihistamines; and allergy shots (immunotherapy).

Alzheimer's disease, once referred to as senile dementia, is a pattern of forgetfulness, disorientation, and loss of memory that usually afflicts the elderly but is not an inevitable part of the aging process. The causes are not known, but research on deceased patients has found abnormal nerve fibers, deposits of abnormal protein, and loss of an abnormal number of brain cells. Some researchers suspect a deficit of an enzyme needed to manufacture a chemical vital to memory formation. Others suspect a virus, aluminum and other environmental toxins, and genetics.

Early symptoms include loss of memory, especially of recent events and the names and faces of familiar people. Later symptoms include confusion of time and place, incontinence, wandering, and a tendency to lose things.

Treatment. No effective treatment has been found to reverse the process or relieve the symptoms.

Amyotrophic lateral sclerosis, better known as Lou Gehrig's disease, after the baseball player, is a fatal disease of the nervous system caused by degeneration of the motor cells of the brain and spinal cord. *Symptoms* are muscular weakness of the hands and arms, followed by progressive paralysis and wasting of the muscles used for breathing and swallowing. There is no cure. Physical therapy can slow muscle atrophy.

Angina pectoris, which means "strangling in the chest," is the chest pain that is the most common symptom of heart disease. It results when the amount of blood flowing to the heart is insufficient to accomplish the work demanded of the heart. Angina can be caused by increased exertion or sudden deep-felt emotions, or by a spasm that clamps one of the arteries leading to the heart.

Angina is often brought on by walking and relieved by resting. It can strike anywhere in the upper half of the body, but is felt most often in the center of the chest. It can occur as the patient first lies down at night and can be accompanied by shortness of breath, nausea, and sweating.

Treatment. Nitroglycerin and other blood vessel expanders relieve angina by increasing coronary circulation. Other drugs, such as calcium blockers and beta-blocking agents, relieve angina by impairing the strength of the heart contraction, slowing pulse rate, decreasing blood pressure, and otherwise decreasing the work of the heart.

Appendicitis is an inflammation of the appendix, the seemingly useless organ protruding from the cecum, or upper end of the large intestine. *Symptoms,* which often occur suddenly, include shifting pain, nausea, vomiting, tenderness, and fever. *Treatment* is relatively simple surgical removal.

Arteriosclerosis, or hardening of the arteries, is the most common disease of the arteries and one of the major causes of heart disease. It is caused when deposits (called plaques) of fats (especially cholesterol), calcium, and smooth muscle cells restrict the flow of blood and facilitate the forming of blood clots. Obstruction in an artery leading to the heart can cause chest pain or a heart attack. In an artery leading to the brain, it can cause a stroke. Obstructions in leg arteries can cause walking to become painful and result in gangrene.

Causes. Heredity appears to play a major role in arteriosclerosis. The female hormone estrogen appears to provide protection, before menopause. Other causes are a diet heavy in saturated fat and cholesterol, smoking, drinking, high blood pressure, diabetes, emotional stress, inactivity, and obesity.

Early symptoms include pain, cramping, limping or weakness in the legs during walking. Symptoms are felt in the arch of the foot, the calf, the thigh, the buttocks, or the arms. *Later symptoms* include skin ulcers and gangrene.

Treatment includes exercise to promote circulation, loss of excess weight, and angioplasty, or the surgical opening of clogged arteries accomplished through lasers or the inflation of a tiny balloon.

Arthritis is inflammation of one or more joints due to infectious, metabolic, or constitutional causes. Arthritis affects more than 37 million Americans, according to the Arthritis Foundation. Types of arthritis include rheumatic fever, which affects children; gonococcal arthritis, a venereal disease that primarily afflicts young adults; rheumatoid arthritis, which afflicts young to middle-aged adults; and gout, which affects the middle-aged and older.

Degenerative arthritis, or osteoarthritis, develops over many years. It begins when cartilage cushioning the bone softens and cracks, intruding upon the fluid capsule that lubricates the joint. New bone growth narrows the capsule further and causes it to fill with bits of cartilage and bone. Later, cysts develop and bone spurs distort the capsule, restricting or immobilizing the joint.

Rheumatoid arthritis, a chronic inflammatory condition of the joints and some internal organs, strikes between ages 20 and 45. It begins with stiffness of the hands and feet, making fine finger movements, such as buttoning, difficult.

Symptoms of arthritis include pain, stiffness, weakness and disability, swelling, tenderness, and deformities.

Diagnostic tests include X rays, radioisotopic scanning, electromyography (examination of electrical impulses emitted by muscles and nerves), arthroscopy, analysis of the joint fluid, biopsy, and other laboratory tests.

Treatments include anti-inflammatory drugs such as aspirin, ibuprofen, and cortisone; remittive agents such as gold salts and penicillamine, which can restore joints; exercise and physical therapy; joint replacement; acupuncture; special diets; relocation to a drier climate; and the application of heat, cold, and mineralized water, including spas.

Asthma is an obstructive lung disease characterized by sudden attacks of coughing, breathlessness, and wheezing that can sometimes result in suffocation. Asthma sufferers often carry inhalers with them; these handheld devices spray medication directly into the lungs.

Extrinsic asthma is provoked by dust or allergens in the air, which enter the lungs, react with the surfaces of cells, causing the cells to release chemicals that contract bronchial muscles, cause secretions, and swell tissues.

Intrinsic asthma occurs without external irritants. Sufferers are more likely to be adults than children, and sometimes have polyps in their nasal passages.

Treatments include drugs, called bronchodilators, that relax air passages and can be administered orally or, during severe attacks, intravenously. Sufferers are also advised to avoid pollens or other allergens known to trigger attacks, or to take hyposensitization injections.

Atherosclerosis is the thickening and decreased elasticity of the arteries accompanied by formation of fatty deposits (plaque) on the insides of artery walls. Causes include smoking, drinking, stress, and high-fat-content diets. When the plaque blocks blood flow in the arteries leading to the brain or heart, it can cause a stroke or heart attack. Kidney failure and gangrene in the leg can also result.

Backache, sometimes called lumbago, is triggered by strain on the muscles near the spine and can sometimes be remedied with exercise and proper shoes, weight, mattress, and posture. Causes include stress, osteoporosis, arthritis, kidney disease, premenstrual pressure, or the spending of too much time seated in a chair.

Bladder inflammation (cystitis) can be caused by drugs, radiation, foreign objects, or bacterial infections. *Symptoms* include burning on urination, frequent urination, pain in the lower abdomen over the bladder, and cloudy or bloody urine. Antibiotics are prescribed to treat infections.

Breast cancer is the second leading cancer killer among women. Suspected causes include family history, early start of periods, late menopause, late first pregnancy or no pregnancy, diet, alcohol, smoking, and local radiation. Signs include nipple discharge, scaling, or bleeding; change in nipple direction; change in breast contour; skin dimpling; and persistent lumps. Monthly self-examination and regular exams by a doctor are recommended. Detection is made by a mammography. *Treatment* is surgical removal of a lump, a part of the breast, or the entire breast, often followed by chemotherapy or radiation therapy in the event of spreading to surrounding lymph nodes.

Bronchitis, a common inflammation of the bronchial tubes, or air passages, of the lungs, is caused by infection or by exterior irritation, often including cigarette smoke. *Symptoms* include coughing and expectorating, or spitting of phlegm, and may last one or two months. Chemicals are common irritants causing bronchitis, but cigarette smoke is the overwhelming culprit.

Bronchitis results when the irritated bronchial wall linings thicken and secrete mucus, rendering the patient vulnerable to bacterial infection. Patients experience shortness of breath. *Treatment* consists of rest, fluids, and antibiotics.

Like emphysema, bronchitis is sometimes called a chronic obstructive lung disease.

Cataracts, a common eye problem among older adults and one of the leading causes of vision loss, can almost always be corrected by surgery. Cataracts occur when the normally clear eye lens hardens and clouds with age, blocking light waves to the retina and obstructing vision.

Early symptoms of cataracts include hazy vision or poor night vision. The clouded lens often scatters light, especially in bright sunlight, causing a dazzling effect.

Treatment is a surgical operation, often performed on an outpatient basis, in which an ophthalmologist removes the old lens using ultrasound or aspiration and replaces it with a tiny plastic lens that is clipped into place with tiny hooks. Vision returns to normal in a few days or weeks. More than 98 percent of operations are successful.

Cerebral palsy is a neuromuscular disorder, caused by damage to the brain during pregnancy or shortly after birth. Signs include inability to control arms and legs, speech impairment, and jerky head and torso movements. Intelligence is not often affected. *Treatment* includes physical therapy, muscle-relaxing drugs and surgery to correct uncontrolled muscle contractions.

Cervical cancer—one of the most common female cancers—is a cancerous tumor of the uterine cervix. Early cancer is usually without symptoms; however, a watery vaginal discharge or spotting of blood may be present. Advanced tumors may cause a dark, foul-smelling vaginal discharge, weight loss, back and leg pains, and general ill health. *Symptoms* include polyps, bleeding, and lesions. *Treatments* include radiation and radical hysterectomy, or removal of the uterus, adjoining tissue and lymph nodes, and ovaries. Early detection, which is accomplished by regular Pap smear examinations, is crucial.

Chicken pox (also called varicella) is a highly contagious viral disease caused by a herpes virus and mainly occurring in children 5 to 10 years old. It is marked by a rash of pink spots on the face and abdomen. Spots blister and dry, and cause itching. Scratching can cause skin infections and scars. The disease is spread by direct contact with the blisters or by droplets spread from the upper respiratory tract of infected persons, usually early in the disease. *Treatment* is rest, fluids, medication to reduce fever, and compresses and topical medication to ease itching. When the virus attacks adults, it can cause shingles.

Chlamydial infections, caused by microorganisms (neither virus nor bacteria) that attack the urogenital tracts and anuses of males and females, are the most prevalent sexually transmitted disease, afflicting 3 to 10 million Americans. *Symptoms,* including burning and frequency of urination, often do not appear until infection is advanced. Chlamydia can cause sterility in adults, and scarring and blindness to infants born to infected mothers. *Treatment* is tetracycline and other antibiotics.

Chronic fatigue syndrome, also called chronic fatigue immune dysfunction syndrome, is defined by the U.S. Centers for Disease Control and Prevention as a variety of at least eight unexplained symptoms that cause a 50 percent reduction in activity for at least six months. *Symptoms* can include sore throat, muscle pain, muscle weakness, tender lymph nodes, chills or low-grade fever, headaches, extreme fatigue, joint pain (no swelling), neurological problems, and sleep disorders. Cause is unknown. The disease is not contagious or fatal.

Cirrhosis, a degenerative disease of the liver, is usually associated with alcoholics and affects 15 percent of heavy drinkers. Hepatitis and overconsumption of salt can also cause cirrhosis. *Symptoms,* which often do not appear until irreversible damage has been done, include abdominal swelling, soreness under the rib cage, swollen ankles, weight loss, and fatigue. *Treatment* includes abstention from alcohol, rest, supplementary vitamins, and a protein-rich diet.

Colon cancer is the second biggest cancer killer in the United States, after lung cancer. Twenty percent of cases are thought to be traceable to genetic predisposition. Other causes include a diet high in fat and red meat and low in fiber. Further, people who have long-term ulcerative colitis and polyps of the colon are thought to have a greater risk of developing this kind of cancer. *Symptoms* include dark, sticky stools containing blood and a change in bowel habits. *Treatment* includes surgery and chemotherapy.

Common colds are generally mild infections of the upper respiratory tract that are caused by any of more than two hundred different viruses and can afflict otherwise healthy individuals several times a year. *Symptoms* last three or four days and include runny nose, sore throat, sneezing, partial loss of sense of taste and smell, mild headache, teary eyes; and somewhat labored breathing. There is no effective treatment besides bed rest and alleviation of symptoms. Vitamin C is believed by some to help prevent colds.

Conjunctivitis is inflammation of the thin membrane lining the eyelid and covering the front of the eye. Commonly called pinkeye, conjunctivitis can be caused by bacteria or virus, by an allergic reaction, or by an ingrown eyelash in the lower lid. *Treatment* includes antibiotic ointment, or corticosteroids (to reduce the swelling).

Constipation is a condition in which bowels become too hard to eliminate easily or when bowel movements become infrequent. Causes include faulty diet, especially a lack of fiber, lack of exercise, anxiety, overdependence on laxatives, and use of certain drugs, such as antacids. The body requires 24 to 48 hours to turn food into waste, and frequency of elimination may vary from once or twice a day to once a week. *Treatment* is consumption of fruits, vegetables, fiber, and lots of water, and daily exercise. Metamucil may be prescribed to increase bulk content of stool.

Croup is a common ailment affecting small children that occurs when inflammation of the larynx causes difficulty in breathing and a harsh croaking sound. Hospitalization may be necessary if the gap between the vocal cords closes, obstructing breathing. In this case, it will need to be opened. While cold, damp conditions encourage respiratory infections, hot dry air seems to encourage croup.

Cyst is an abnormal closed sac or pouch inside or under the skin that is usually filled with fluid or solid material. Cysts can occur when the duct of an organ or gland becomes blocked, causing accumulation of a secreted material. Treatment is not necessary unless a cyst is causing other symptoms. Cysts are surgically removed if they are unsightly, are putting pressure on surrounding structures, or are suspected of originating in a tumor.

Cystic fibrosis, often diagnosed in infancy or early childhood, is caused by an inherited defect of the glands affecting the respiratory and digestive systems.

Symptoms, which usually show up soon after birth, include chronic infection, shortness of breath, coughing, wheezing, and intestinal problems. The lungs secrete a mucus that is too thick to be cleared and that breeds infections. Digestive glands secrete insufficient amounts of digestive enzymes.

Treatment includes breathing support and has improved so that more and more patients survive. In past years, most patients died in infancy from infection or respiratory failure.

Depression is a chronic psychiatric disorder characterized by feelings of helplessness, hopelessness, diminished self-worth, and guilt, and a loss of pleasure from usual activities. Victims may find it difficult to concentrate or make decisions. Causes may be genetic or environmental—for instance, loss of a loved one or loss of a job. Five percent or more of depressed people commit suicide. *Treatment* includes psychoanalysis and psychotherapy, antidepressant medications, and sometimes hospitalization.

Diabetes mellitus, a chronic disease marked by excess glucose in the blood and urine, is caused by the failure of the pancreas to release enough insulin (or any at all) into the body. It may also be caused by a defect in the parts of cells that accept the insulin. Insulin metabolizes glucose into energy. Major *symptoms* include frequent urination, chronic thirst, excessive hunger, and weight loss. *Treatment* includes administering of insulin. Patients must monitor and control medication, diet, and energy output.

Diarrhea is the frequent passage of loose, watery stool. Diarrhea can be chronic or acute. Acute diarrhea can be caused by ingestion of a protozoa or toxic bacteria, by traveling, or by a sudden change in diet. Chronic diarrhea can occur as a symptom of another disease, such as colitis (inflammation of the large intestine), diverticulitis (inflammation of one or more pouches in the wall of the large intestine), or cancer, or as a sign of irritable bowel syndrome. Blood in the stool during diarrhea can signal dysentery or typhoid fever. Diarrhea can occur as a side effect of antibiotics. Untreated diarrhea may lead to dehydration.

Diverticulitis is an inflammation of the diverticula, or small, mucus-lined sacs that form in the wall of the large intestine. *Symptoms* are attacks of pain in the left, lower abdomen, often recurring over a period of years and associated with constipation or diarrhea. Diverticulitis can cause narrowing of the colon, perforation of the colon wall (peritonitis), hemorrhaging, and inflammation of nearby organs. *Treatment* is laxatives and antispasmodic drugs, rest, and surgery for hemorrhaging and peritonitis.

Down syndrome, the most common form of inherited mental retardation, is caused by defective chromosome development in the embryo. Many physical defects are also present, including—in addition to certain physical and facial characteristics—bowel defects, inborn heart disease, long-term respiratory infections, and vision problems. Incidence of Down syndrome, once called mongolism because of the shape of the patient's eyelids, rises with the age of the mother at the time of pregnancy. Today, people with Down syndrome can learn language skills with computers and are more likely to live in private homes than in institutions.

Earache is pain in the ear caused by teething (in small children); by the eruption of wisdom teeth (in adults); by dental disease; by infection or congestion of the nose, throat, and jaw; or by the blocking of the eustachian tube (which joins the nose-throat cavity and the inner ear). *Treatment* includes antibiotic eardrops, removal of excess earwax, and dental assessment.

Eczema is a noninfectious and usually chronic inflammatory skin disease that causes blistering and scaling. Eczema can run in families prone to hay fever and asthma and can also be caused by food allergies and exposure to mineral oils, detergents, and degreasing agents. Symptoms can be confused with dermatitis, which technically refers to a more acute skin inflammation.

Emphysema, Greek for "inflation," is a lung disease that mostly afflicts men but is becoming more common among women as the rate of female smokers increases. Emphysema is characterized by enlargement of the lungs and progressively worsening breathlessness. Coughing is another symptom, but wheezing is less typical and there is little sputum. Enlargement is caused by overinflation and breakdown of the air cells in the lung (alveoli) where gas is exchanged. Scarring and destruction can occur to the alveolar sacs and to bronchial tissue.

Treatment consists of bronchodilators and antibiotics to ease breathing. Smoking must be stopped. Exercise may be prescribed as a means of slowing the respiratory rate.

Epilepsy, characterized by seizures lasting from a few seconds to 15 or 20 minutes, is a symptom of overactive brain impulses and excitability of the brain. Suspected causes include heredity factors and injuries or illnesses that leave scars on the brain surface, or cortex.

Diagnosis is done with electroencephalography (EEG), computerized axial tomography (CAT scan), magnetic resonance imaging (MRI), and video EEG monitoring.

Treatment includes anticonvulsant drugs, which block brain overactivity. These drugs include barbiturates, hydantoins, carbamazepine, valproic acid, suximides, benzodiazepines, and phenacemide. Most have side effects. All need to be monitored so that proper levels of the drug are maintained. In rare cases, surgery is performed.

Seizure management. During a seizure, an epileptic's head should be placed on a soft surface and the clothing around his neck should be loosened. As the person relaxes after the rigid portion of the attack, his head should be turned sideways to prevent swallowing of saliva, and his throat opened to allow breathing.

Food poisoning is an acute illness, usually gastrointestinal, caused by eating contaminated or poisonous food. *Symptoms* include nausea, vomiting, diarrhea, and abdominal cramps. Agents include bacteria, parasites, viruses, chemicals, and poisons. Foods likely to cause poisoning include undercooked poultry or eggs and poorly refrigerated or preserved foods. *Botulism,* found usually in poorly canned foods, attacks the central nervous system and can cause death. *Symptoms* of botulism include double vision, puffy or drooping eyelids, and paralysis. Victims must be hospitalized.

Gallstones (also called biliary calculi) are solid masses that form in the gallbladder or bile ducts. The gallbladder drains and stores bile from the liver. Gallstones may be a combination of calcium, bile pigments, and cholesterol; or pure cholesterol; or bile pigments only. Some stones can be medically dissolved; others must be removed surgically. Gallstones can cause jaundice and inflammation of the gallbladder.

Gastroenteritis is an inflammation to the stomach and intestinal lining that is caused by infection. *Symptoms* are general discomfort, loss of appetite, abdominal cramps, diarrhea, and vomiting. *Treatment* is rest, fluids, and a bland diet. The illness usually runs its course in 48 hours, but can cause dehydration in severe cases, especially in infants. Other causes include food poisoning, harsh laxatives, and some antibiotics.

Glaucoma, one of the leading causes of blindness, is a painless illness that is often not noticed until some vision has been lost. Glaucoma results when fluid pressure inside the eye presses on and damages the optic nerve. The pressure may result from abnormal fluid production, blockage of fluid inside the eye, or other problems or injuries.

Prevention and treatment are made easier by the regular checking of intraocular pressure and peripheral vision, especially among middle-aged and older adults. Eyedrops and pills can be administered in an effort to reduce pressure. If unsuccessful, laser surgery can be performed to improve the eye's drainage system. If this fails, direct surgery can be performed to make a small opening through which fluid can drain.

Gonorrhea, one of the most common sexually transmitted diseases, is an infection of the genitals and urinary tract. *Symptoms in men* include the frequent desire to urinate, severe pain during urination, and the discharge of pus from the penis. *Symptoms in women* are less noticeable and often are not felt until the disease has spread to the reproductive organs. They can include more frequent urination, pain during urination, pus discharge, and abscesses. *Treatment* includes penicillin and other antibiotics. Infected persons should notify their sexual partners. Condoms are not always a reliable means of protection.

Gout is a form of arthritis that causes swelling of one or more joints and is caused by accumulation in the blood of uric acid, a waste product. *Symptoms* are sudden and severe pain and swelling in one joint, often starting with the big toe. Gout is more common in men than in women. *Treatment* includes anti-inflammatory drugs and drugs to stimulate the elimination of uric acid and reduce its production.

Headaches afflict an estimated two-thirds of the world's current population at one time or another. About 1 percent of headaches are caused by an accompanying disease. Other headaches result from

stress or tension, and others are thought to result from the swelling of scalp blood vessels. Kinds of headaches include cluster headaches, sinus infection headaches, tension headaches, and migraine headaches—the latter two being some of the most common forms of chronic headaches.

Physicians generally categorize headaches into two broad types: muscle contraction headaches and blood vessel (vascular) headaches. The person's description of the quality of pain can help the physician diagnose the type of headache. Throbbing pain, for instance, usually denotes a vascular headache. And a tension headache is usually felt as an intense pain across the top of the head or the back of the neck.

Treatment usually includes nonnarcotic analgesics, and sometimes, depending upon the type of headache and its frequency, antidepressants may be prescribed. Often, again depending upon the specific type of headache, avoidance of factors that trigger the headache—such as food, stress, tobacco, or alcohol—may be recommended.

Heart attack, or myocardial infarction, results when blood supply to the heart is blocked by a clot or plaque in one or more coronary arteries. The part of the heart that is deprived of blood dies, or infarcts. Causes are smoking, obesity, diabetes, hypertension, high blood cholesterol, fatty diet, and emotional stress.

Symptoms include sudden, severe pain in the center of the chest that radiates into the arms, shoulders, and back; pallor, nausea, sweating, and shortness of breath.

Treatment is most effective when administered immediately and in a hospital; in sudden heart attacks, treatment includes oxygen, heart drugs, and anticoagulants. Painkillers and sleeping pills are also given. Bypass surgery may be recommended.

Heat exhaustion is the accumulation of large amounts of blood near the skin, in an attempt to cool it, and the simultaneous deprivation of blood to interior organs. *Symptoms* include pale skin, heavy perspiration, rapid breathing and pulse, dizziness, and vomiting—but not high temperature. *Treatment* includes lowering the head to improve circulation to the brain, placing the victim in shade, drinking salt water, elevating the feet and loosening clothing, and applying wet compresses.

Heatstroke is an emergency condition in which blockages of the sweat glands result in body temperatures as high as 106°. Other signs are hot, dry, and red skin. The condition often follows heavy exertion. Victims are more likely to be older males, especially alcoholics. Consequences include brain or kidney damage and circulatory collapse. *Treatment* includes stripping the clothes, applying a cool (not cold) water sponge to the body, drying and cooling with fans. Hospitalization is usually recommended.

Hemophilia is an incurable, sex-linked genetic blood disorder in which the blood is unable to clot. The gene is carried by females, but contracted nearly always only by males. Bleeding can be controlled with an infusion of clotting agents. Aspirin must be avoided. Hemophiliacs run a high risk of contracting hepatitis B and AIDS through transfusions of tainted blood.

Hemorrhoids are dilated, irritated veins covered by folds of skin that lie within or protrude from the anal canal. They result from inflammation of the anus that can be caused by hard bowel movements or straining during a bowel movement.

Symptoms include pain, itchiness, and occasionally bloody stools. *Treatment* includes sitz baths (sitting in warm baths), suppositories, and external application of medicine. In cases where blood clots form in a hemorrhoid, or the hemorrhoids form a bulky ring around the anus, the hemorrhoid may be surgically removed or sealed off using a laser.

Hepatitis, characterized by inflammation of the liver, involving yellowing of the skin, stomach discomfort, abnormal liver functioning, and dark urine, may be caused by a virus and/or bacteria, parasites, alcohol, drugs, poison, or transfusions of problematic blood. Type A hepatitis is spread by fecal matter. *Symptoms* include nausea, vomiting, loss of appetite, jaundice, fatigue. Type B hepatitis is transmitted through the blood and is more severe, persisting for several weeks or months and sometimes scarring the liver. A vaccine for Type B hepatitis is recommended for homosexually active males and drug users.

Hernia is the protrusion of all or part of an organ through a weak spot in the surrounding muscular wall. Hernias can occur in the groin, near a surgical incision, and in the diaphragm. *Symptoms*, depending upon the hernia's location, include pain, heartburn, indigestion, breathing difficulties, and regurgitation of food. *Treatment* ranges from resting on the side and sleeping propped on pillows to surgery. Some hernias self-correct.

Herpes is any of a group of recurring viral illnesses marked by outbreaks of blisters in the genitals, anus, cornea, mouth, or brain. Herpes simplex causes the cold sore (fever blister) and the highly contagious genital herpes. Herpes zoster causes chicken pox and shingles. The virus lies dormant in the body and the blister outbreaks recur. There is no cure. *Treatment* includes painkillers and antibiotics.

Hodgkin's disease is a chronic, malignant cancer of the lymph nodes that usually strikes people between ages 15 and 35, and between 50 and 60. *Symptoms* include enlarged lymph nodes in the neck, armpit, or groin; fever and night sweats; weight loss; and uncontrollable itching. Depending on the severity of the disease, it can involve a single node or region of nodes, two regions of nodes either above or below the diaphragm, nodes both above and below the diaphragm, and cancers that have spread beyond the lymph nodes to other organs. *Treatment* includes radiation and chemotherapy.

Hypertension, or high blood pressure, is a common disorder (often without symptoms) that is characterized by high blood pressure consistently exceeding 140/90. Blood pressure is the pressure exerted against arterial walls. The most common type of hypertension is essential hypertension, which has no known cure, although the risk for it is increased by being overweight, having high sodium and cholesterol levels in the blood, and having a family history of high blood pressure. The condition can be controlled by regular exercise, a low-salt diet, weight loss, stopping smoking, moderating alcohol intake, and medications such as beta blockers (which reduce the activity of the heart), diuretics, and vasodilators.

Hypoglycemia is an abnormally low level of blood sugar which can signal the sudden onset of diabetes or another disease, or which can afflict a diabetic with too much insulin. *Symptoms* include sweating, palpitations, and trembling hands. Left untreated, hypoglycemia can lead to confusion, sleepiness, and sometimes unconsciousness.

Infertility, estimated to afflict 1 in 7 married couples, can be caused in men by low sperm count in the semen or by poor quality sperm. *Treatment in men* consists of small doses of two hormones—testosterone or chorionic gonadotropin. In women, infertility can be caused by lack of ovulation or inability of the fertilized egg to implant in the uterine lining. *Treatment in women* is surgery to clear blocked fallopian tubes, drugs to induce ovulation, and hormone therapy to prepare the lining of the uterus for implantation.

Influenza, also called flu or grippe, is a contagious respiratory disease caused by one of a group of airborne viruses, spread by coughs, sneezes, and exhaled breath and sometimes occurring in epidemics. *Symptoms* usually run their course in ten days and include runny nose, sore throat, mucus congestion and coughing, aching joints, and appetite loss. *Treatment* includes fluids, bed rest, and aspirin or another painkiller. Vaccines have been developed but cause adverse reactions.

Insomnia, or sleeplessness, can be caused by a variety of physical and psychological factors, including eating rich foods, drinking caffeinated beverages 2 hours or less before bedtime, poor ventilation, uncomfortable mattress, or becoming overly excited before bedtime. Insomnia can result from depression or anxiety. *Treatment* includes daytime exercise, warm evening baths, and drinking warm milk, as well as sedatives, tranquilizers, and psychotherapy.

Kidney disorders include pyelonephritis (infection of the urine-collecting ducts), nephrosis (leakage of protein into the urine), and cysts, stones (usually of calcium), and other abnormalities that impair drainage. *Symptoms* include lower-back pain, change in urine color, discomfort during urination, and puffiness of body parts, especially the eyes. Kidney failure leads to uremia, or the accumulation of urea nitrogen in the blood.

Laryngitis is inflammation of the mucous membranes lining the larynx, characterized by the swelling of the vocal cords and hoarseness or loss of voice. Acute laryngitis results from infection and is accompanied by fever and cough. *Treatment* includes steam inhalation, cough suppressants, and occasionally antibiotics. Chronic laryngitis, usually from abuse or overuse of the voice, must be treated with complete rest of the voice.

Leukemia is any of a group of diseases characterized by a proliferation of white blood cells in the bone marrow that impedes the manufacture of red blood cells. Males are affected twice as frequently as females. *Symptoms* are unexplained weight loss, low energy, fever, subcutaneous hemorrhaging, anemia, and lowered resistance to infection. Once fatal, leukemia can now be treated successfully in some cases with radiation and chemotherapy, anticancer drugs, antibiotics, steroids, and transfusions. Possible causes include exposure to radioactivity, industrial pollution, and food contamination.

Lung cancer, which has surpassed breast cancer as the leading cancer killer of women, kills more than twenty-five times as many men as it did in 1930. Cigarette smoking is the primary cause of lung cancer—only 10 percent of patients are nonsmokers—but other risks include exposure to industrial substances, such as asbestos, nickel, chromium, arsenic, radon, and halogenated ethers. Lung cancer often invades neighboring lymph nodes and spreads to other parts of the body.

Symptoms include weight loss, general fatigue, chest pain, coughing of blood, and a tumor that can be discovered by X rays.

Treatment includes surgical removal of the tumor, a lobe of the lung, or the whole lung, depending on the extent to which the disease has spread. Drug therapy and radiotherapy (administration of X rays) are also prescribed for patients whose tumors have spread.

Lyme disease, named for the town in Connecticut where it first appeared in 1975, is transmitted by the bite of the tiny deer tick, which is usually found in wooded areas. *Symptoms,* which may disappear on their own, include a rash at the site of the bite, red spots elsewhere on the body, and flulike symptoms such as fatigue, headache, aching joints, sore throat, and fever. About half of victims develop arthritis; some are immobilized. Pain and inflammation can subside but recur. The *treatment,* antibiotics, is most effective when administered early.

Measles is a highly contagious viral disease common to children and characterized by a rash of dark red spots on the face, trunk, and limbs. *Symptoms* include fever, cough, runny nose, watery eyes, and irritability. Complications can include bronchitis, pneumonia, and, in rare cases, encephalitis. Vaccination with a measles live-virus vaccine is recommended for those considered susceptible; however, the combined measles, mumps, rubella vaccine (MMR) is the vaccine of choice for those likely to be susceptible to mumps and/or rubella.

Meningitis, inflammation of the membranes covering the brain and spinal cord, can be serious but is treatable when caused by bacteria. It is also caused by virus and can occur in epidemics and in isolated cases.

Symptoms include fever, sleepiness, inability to wake up, irritability, and stiffness and pain in the neck. Patients are often unable to touch their chin to their chest. A rash of tiny red spots may occur on the trunk and buttocks, and pain may be felt in the back and leg muscles.

Treatment. A vaccine is available for children aged 18 months to 4 years, the period of greatest risk for one type of bacterial meningitis. Antibiotics are prescribed for bacterial meningitis. An examination of spinal fluid extracted by a needle can determine which type of bacteria is involved. Muscle weakness or brain damage may result if the disease is not promptly and thoroughly treated.

Menopause is the end of menstruation, and is commonly described as the end of the female reproductive phase of life. Menstruation stops naturally with the decline of monthly hormonal cycles, somewhere between 45 and 60 years of age. However, menses may end earlier in the woman's life, usually the result of illness or the surgical removal of the uterus or both ovaries. Menstrual periods become irregular, and production of the female hormone estrogen decreases.

There is growing controversy over the designation of menopause as a medical condition, one, that is, distinct from a natural passage. However, it is included here, simply because of the many manifestations from woman to woman and because of the inordinate amount of attention paid in the medical and popular press to symptoms and treatment.

General *symptoms* differ among women, although the most common signs include hot flashes and shrinking of the genital organs. Inability to sleep, irritability, and depression may also be experienced. Estrogen replacement therapy (ERT) helps relieve

symptoms and stabilizes osteoporosis, but is not without its own controversy.

Mononucleosis, a viral infection, causes swelling and tenderness of the lymph glands in the armpits, groin, elbow, and neck. Jaundice may develop. *Symptoms* include sore throat, fever, headache, and aching joints. Recovery requires several days to several weeks. Bed rest is prescribed, but no other treatment is effective.

Multiple sclerosis (MS) is a nonfatal disease of undetermined cause that strikes when nerve cells lose myelin, the fatty substance essential for normal conduction of electrical impulses. Because MS is concentrated in temperate climates and seldom occurs in arctic or tropic regions, researchers suspect an environmental or climactic influence. MS strikes suddenly, in one or more parts of the central nervous system, between the teen years and age 35.

Symptoms include visual abnormalities, unsteady gait, tremors, sensory impairment, bladder disturbance, paralysis, and slurring of speech. The nerve cells heal in two to three weeks, but not completely, resulting in partial loss of function. The disorder recurs in a year or two, resulting in greater loss of function.

Treatment includes corticosteroids, avoidance of heat, physical therapy, and experimental immunosuppressive drugs.

Mumps is a contagious viral disease common to children that attacks the parotid gland in front of the ear. *Symptoms* include fever, swelling in front of the ears, difficulty swallowing and chewing, headache, and sore throat. Mumps is more serious if contracted after puberty, when it can cause swelling of the testes and ovaries. Vaccination with a mumps live-virus vaccine is recommended for those considered susceptible; however, the combined measles, mumps, rubella vaccine (MMR) is the vaccine of choice for those likely to be susceptible to measles and/or rubella.

Muscular dystrophy is a neuromuscular disease in which the muscles enlarge, then begin to separate, with muscular tissue being replaced by fat and connective tissue. It appears to be caused by a defect in the enzyme that regulates muscle metabolism. The disease is painless but progressive, leading possibly to the inability to walk and even cardiac and respiratory failure.

Symptoms include localized weakness and the inability of one part of the body to perform its function. *Treatment* is not usually effective, but can include physical therapy.

Duchenne's muscular dystrophy is a sex-linked disease affecting mainly males and usually confined to the muscles of the trunk and legs. Since it is marked by progressive wasting of the muscles in the legs and pelvis, affected children are usually confined to wheelchairs by age 12.

Osteoporosis, a degenerative disease characterized by increasing brittleness of the bones, afflicts an estimated 15 million Americans, most of them older women. The disease is caused by postmenopausal estrogen deficiency and is aggravated by smoking, drinking, and physical inactivity. *Symptoms* include compression of the spine, loss of height, and broken bones. *Treatments* include estrogen, calcium supplements, and exercise.

Parkinson's disease, or parkinsonism, is a disease commonly occurring after age 50 that is caused by the loss of cells that produce the neurotransmitter chemical dopamine in the basal ganglia of the brain.

Symptoms include tremors in the hands, head, and feet, stiffness of the limbs, slowing of movements, and stooped posture. The disease is not genetic, but its cause is unknown. Researchers suspect an environmental cause.

Treatment includes administration of levodopa to substitute for dopamine, administration of Actane, and an operation, still in the experimental stages, that transplants dopamine-producing cells from the adrenal medulla to the brain.

Periodontal diseases of the gums and other tissues surrounding the teeth can cause gums to recede and teeth to loosen and fall out. Regular dental checkups are advised, as are daily brushing and flossing of teeth to prevent breeding of bacteria that thrive in dental plaque.

Phlebitis is the swelling of a vein, often with the formation of a clot, especially in the legs and in areas afflicted with varicose veins. *Symptoms* include tenderness, redness, and swelling. Causes include injury, being overweight, atherosclerosis, and extended bed rest. Anticoagulants (medication to decrease blood clotting) and surgery are often recommended when phlebitis occurs in a large vein and causes clotting, causing the entire leg to swell and become painful.

Pneumonia is a swelling of the lungs, caused by a bacteria or virus. Bacterial pneumonia is most often caused by the pneumococcus bacterium, which is inhaled into the lungs. Viral pneumonia, which is usually less serious, often follows a viral infection that has lowered resistance.

Symptoms include severe chills, chest pain, cough, fever, and shortness of breath, and also, in the case of viral pneumonia, stuffy nose, sore throat, watery eyes, headache, muscle aches, and severe fatigue.

Treatment for bacterial pneumonia consists of antibiotics. Viral pneumonia is not cured by antibiotics. Bed rest, fluids, and analgesics (aspirin) are also advised, and oxygen, if needed.

Some severe types of pneumonia can cause death, especially among children and the elderly. Vaccines for several types of bacterial pneumonia have been developed and are still being evaluated.

Poliomyelitis, a viral infection of the nervous system, was greatly feared until vaccines developed in the 1950s virtually eradicated it from the United States.

Symptoms include fever, headache, vomiting, sore throat, and later, pain in the muscles and sometimes permanent paralysis. The virus is swallowed, multiplies in the intestinal tract, and sometimes spreads to the nervous system. Vaccines are taken orally. One, consisting of a weakened, live virus, is used more commonly in the United States than elsewhere. The other vaccine consists of a killed virus.

Premenstrual syndrome (PMS) is the feeling of mental tension, irritability and depression, the headaches and bloatedness (edema, or the swelling of body tissues due to retention of fluid) that occur in women in the week before menstruation. Several ideas attempt to place the cause on hormonal changes or imbalances, stress, and poor eating.

Prostate cancer, the second most common cancer among American men, is almost always a primary cancer, meaning that it originates in the prostate, rather than traveling there from another part of the body. Typically it begins in the outer part of the prostate. As the tumor grows, it may spread to the inner part of the prostate. Like other cancers, prostate cancer can then metastasize, or spread, to other parts of the body. As with any cancer, cure depends on what stage the cancer has reached, whether the tumors are still confined to the prostate or have escaped the prostatic capsule. In many cases, prostatic cancer is a very slow-growing malignancy. Autopsy studies have shown that about one-third of men over the age of 50 have microscopic evidence of prostate cancer, yet the vast majority of these cancers grow so slowly they never become a threat to life.

Detection is usually through a rectal examination—done by a doctor with a gloved finger to check for tumors—or a blood test to test the level of prostate-specific antigen (an enzyme that rises in men with prostate cancer), and infrequently through transrectal ultrasound.

Psoriasis, a scaly inflammation of the skin caused by overproduction of outer skin cells, affects 1 to 2 percent of Americans. Scaly red patches appear and are covered with a silvery scale; they may appear anywhere but are most common on the scalp, ears, arms, and pubic area. The scales fall off, leaving red spots. Itching may occur. The condition can be chronic or intermittent. Arthritis sometimes accompanies the condition. There is no cure. *Treatment* includes special soaps, creams, and shampoos; hormone creams; and ultraviolet light.

Retinal breaks and detachments occur when the liquid portion of the eye (the vitreous gel) pulls away from the retina (the light-sensing nerve in the back of the eye). As a person ages, the gel begins to shrink and pulls away from the retina. If there's enough shrinkage, the force of the gel pulling away from the retina may cause a break at a weak spot. Sometimes this may occur without causing symptoms; other times you may notice flashes of light, "floaters," or smoke or cobweblike formations in your field of vision. When the retina detaches, you may experience a general darkening in your field of vision as though viewing something in a shadow. Any of these symptoms should prompt an immediate call to an eye care professional for a thorough examination.

Retinal breaks may be treated with cryotherapy (cold treatment) or laser (light energy). Cryotherapy uses a probe to freeze the tissue where the break occurred. As the frozen area heals, scar tissue forms and attaches the retinal layers together. The end result is something like putting a patch on an inner tube.

Laser therapy uses a light beam to generate heat and seal the break. The light of the laser strikes the retina, causing the blood to congeal and form a seal. You may think of this as a sort of spot welding of the retina.

Retinal detachments are treated using a combination of cryotherapy and surgery. A cold probe is used to freeze the tissue or repair any breaks, then a silicone band, much like a rubber band, is placed around the eye and sutured in place. The band causes the eye to indent inward, pushing the vitreous gel into the retina, allowing the layers to reattach.

Reye's syndrome is a childhood degenerative disease of the brain and liver that usually follows a viral disease such as influenza or chicken pox. It often affects people under 18 years of age, causing a rash, vomiting, and confusion, and starts about one week after the beginning of an illness. Because doctors suspect that aspirin triggers the disease, they usually prescribe nonaspirin medication, such as acetaminophen, to control fever during infections. There is no specific treatment.

Rheumatic fever, a bacterial inflammation of the throat usually affecting children, can sometimes be triggered by untreated streptococcus infections. Symptoms include swelling and soreness of the joints. Antibiotics are prescribed and usually prevent the development of rheumatic heart disease that was more common earlier in the twentieth century.

Rubella, also called German measles, is an acute viral infection and common contagious disease of childhood. *Symptoms* are fever and rash. Women who contract the disease when pregnant subject their unborn baby to high risk of brain damage, heart defects, blindness, and other deformities. Vaccination with a rubella live-virus vaccine is recommended for those considered susceptible; however, the combined measles, mumps, rubella vaccine (MMR) is the vaccine of choice for those likely to be susceptible to measles and/or mumps.

Schizophrenia is a category of psychosis characterized by severely disturbed patterns of thinking that cause bizarre behavior. Schizophrenia usually strikes young adults. Its cause is unknown. *Symptoms* include hallucinations, delusions of grandeur or persecution, obsessive-compulsive behavior, mood swings, personality changes, and loss of control over fantasies. *Treatment* includes psychotropic drugs, psychotherapy, and, in extreme cases, hospitalization.

Sexually transmitted diseases (STDs), formerly called venereal disease (VD), are contracted during the act of sex. They include AIDS, hepatitis B, chlamydial infections, gonorrhea, syphilis, genital herpes, and genital warts. Millions of new cases, especially of chlamydia and herpes, are reported each year. Prevalence is attributed to increased promiscuity among the young, new resistant strains of bacteria, increased travel, and the fact that many carriers experience no symptoms.

Sickle-cell anemia is an inherited disease of African-Americans, occurring in about 1 in 400 births. Ninety to 100 percent of normal hemoglobin is replaced by abnormal hemoglobin whose red blood cells take on the shape of a sickle and are destroyed more rapidly than normal red blood cells. The sickle cells can block blood vessels, restricting oxygen supply to body cells. Fever, dehydration, and acid imbalance can result. Treatment is difficult. Patients typically require extra water, supplementary oxygen, and occasionally transfusions.

Sinusitis is an inflammation of one or more of the four nasal sinus cavities. *Symptoms* include pain and tenderness, and a thick nasal discharge. Sinusitis usually occurs as a complication to the common cold. *Treatment* includes antibiotics, steam inhalation, and, in extreme cases, surgery to drain sinuses or remove the inner lining.

Skin cancer is the most common and easiest to diagnose of all the cancers. *Symptoms* include growths or nodules on the skin that break and bleed. Melanoma usually begins as a brown spot on the skin; the lesion gradually forms an irregular border, variations in color, and an irregular surface. Basal cell carcinoma and squamous cell carcinoma are the two most common types of skin cancer and are easily cured in most cases. *Treatment* includes surgery or topical medication.

Malignant melanoma is the most serious form of skin cancer but also the rarest. An estimated 5,500 Americans die of this disease yearly. Radiation and chemotherapy offer little help in combating malignant melanoma. Prolonged exposure to sun increases the chances of contracting skin cancer. People who sunburn easily are especially susceptible.

Slipped disk is the dislocation or herniation (bulging) of one of the cartilaginous rings that separate the spinal vertebrae. The disks absorb shocks to the vertebrae that result from lifting and bending and other activities. Causes include injury and degeneration of the disk due to age. The spinal nerve most often impacted is the sciatic nerve. *Symptoms* include a pain that radiates from the lower back to the buttock, thigh, and even the feet. *Treatment* includes bed rest on a firm mattress, painkillers, back support, acupuncture, and exercises. Prevention includes exercises to strengthen the lower back, maintenance of proper body weight, avoidance of high-heeled shoes, and the lifting of heavy objects from the knees.

Streptococcus infection is a category of common bacterial diseases, including pharyngitis (strep throat), scarlet fever, puerperal fever, and some pneumonias. Antibiotics are prescribed, and a full course must be taken to prevent development of rheumatic fever or glomerulonephritis. *Symptoms* include fever, severe sore throat, difficulty swallowing, swollen lymph glands in the neck, and, in the case of scarlet fever, a rash.

Strokes are sudden brain disturbances resulting from an interruption in the flow of blood to the brain. The attacks are usually caused by a disease of the arteries supplying the brain. There are three types of strokes. In a *cerebral hemorrhage,* a blood vessel ruptures and bleeds into the brain or its membranes. In a *cerebral thrombosis,* a blood clot in a cerebral blood vessel blocks the flow of blood. In a *cerebral embolism,* a blood clot or foreign body migrates from another part of the body to block circulation to the brain. Strokes can result in temporary or permanent loss of speech, paralysis, and loss of coordination and sensation. They can also be fatal.

Prevention. The risk of strokes is increased by smoking, diabetes, high blood pressure, high fat content in the blood, obesity, and heart disease. Steps should be taken to alleviate these conditions. Also, many major strokes are preceded by minor strokes from which complete recovery is possible.

Treatment includes bed rest, restriction of fluids, potassium, and drugs, such as aspirin, that inhibit clot formation. Physical therapy may be prescribed for those suffering paralysis or loss of function.

Sudden infant death syndrome (SIDS) is the most common cause of death for infants 1 to 12 months old in the United States, accounting for 30 percent of all deaths in that age group. Also called crib death, SIDS is an unexpected death in which an autopsy fails to find a cause. The immediate cause of death is cessation of breathing during sleep (sleep apnea). Contributing causes appear to include premature birth and narcotic addiction or alcoholism of parents. Some researchers believe SIDS results from a transient, or temporary, disorder of the nervous system that regulates breathing and heartbeat.

Syphilis is one of the most serious of the sexually transmitted diseases, caused by a bacterium, whose first sign is a hard painless ulcer that appears on the genitals, lips, tongue, or finger two to six weeks after contact with an infected person. A secondary stage one month later is marked by fever, rash, lymph node swelling, and sore throat. Months or years later, a third stage features lesions that can damage heart valves, blood vessels, the brain, the spinal cord, or other major organs. The disease can be diagnosed by a blood test and treated with penicillin.

Tonsillitis is an infection or inflammation of a tonsil (a small mass of lymphoid tissue in the throat). *Symptoms* of tonsillitis include sore throat, high fever, earache, difficult swallowing, and swollen lymph nodes in the neck. Breathing difficulty may be experienced. Antibiotics, painkillers, and warm irrigations of the throat are usually successful. Surgery is recommended only in severe and recurring cases.

Tuberculosis (TB) is a long-term grainy tumorous infection caused by a rod-shaped bacterium. Once prevalent in the United States, it poses much less of a threat than it once did, although it is making a comeback among AIDS victims and some homeless people. Tuberculosis is usually spread by inhalation or ingestion of infected droplets and develops over a period of years. It can affect any organ of the body, but is most common in the lungs.

Symptoms include a cough, listlessness, weight loss, fever, and night sweats, but these do not manifest themselves until the disease is established. *Diagnosis* is done by injecting a small amount of extract of tu-berculosis organisms into the skin of the forearm. Inflammation indicates previous infection. Lung damage does not occur until the later stages of the disease.

Treatment includes several weeks of hospitalization and antibiotics, which achieve a cure rate of almost 100 percent, but must be taken for months or years.

Ulcers of the stomach and small intestine are called peptic ulcers and include duodenal (intestine) and gastric (stomach) ulcers. Ulcers occur when acid secreted for digestion burns a hole in the mucous membrane and, in the case of bleeding ulcers, in a blood vessel. Signs include a burning pain a few hours after eating. Causes include the untimely secretion of hydrochloric acid, bacterial agents, stress, spicy diets, coffee, and cigarette smoking. Drugs that suppress or neutralize acid and create a coating gel are generally considered more effective treatment than diet.

Urinary incontinence, the involuntary leaking of urine, often occurs in women when the supporting tissue of the bladder is damaged by childbirth or when estrogen levels drop after menopause. Incontinence in children may result from psychogenic factors or even allergies. Sedatives, diuretics, insomnia drugs, decongestants, alcohol, coffee, and tea can aggravate the condition. Drugs, exercises, psychotherapy, and special underwear can alleviate the problem. Surgery is recommended only in serious cases.

Varicose veins are veins, usually in the back and inner side of the calf, that are swollen and enlarged and visible through the skin as a bluish-red network of lines. More common among women than men, varicose veins are caused by obesity and frequent standing in one place. Treatment consists of physical exercise, use of elastic stockings, elevating the feet, and, in serious cases, surgery.

Vertigo (also called dizziness) is the sensation of loss of balance and the irregular and whirling motion of oneself or of nearby objects. Vertigo can be brought on by watching objects in rapid motion or by moving rapidly in a circular motion. It can also serve as a symptom of a disease that affects the portion of the middle ear that controls balance.

Whooping cough (pertussis) is an infectious disease of the mucous membranes lining the air passages that mainly affects children. Whooping cough is characterized by convulsive bouts of coughing followed by a noisy "whoop" or inhalation of air. Treatment consists of bed rest and medication to control coughing. Vaccination for pertussis is usually given in conjunction with diphtheria and tetanus as the DPT vaccine.

Common Pathogens

Pathogens are microorganisms—bacteria and viruses—that are able to cause disease. The most lethal of the pathogens are capable of producing an effect that is 700,000 times more powerful than strychnine.

There are literally billions and billions of microorganisms that live in the air, soil, our bodies, and so forth. Without some of them life would be impossible, or at least a little more difficult. We need the helpful bacteria in our digestive tracts to aid in breaking down food in order to supply the body with nutrients it requires. Other, less friendly organisms can have a devastating effect on the body by causing serious illness.

BACTERIA

About 2,000 different varieties of bacteria have been classified, and most of these are harmless—in fact, some are beneficial—to humans. Bacteria come in one of four general shapes. These are: rod-shaped, or bacilli; spherical, or cocci; spiral, or spirilla; and curved, or vibrios. A single bacterium can reproduce itself in 20 to 30 minutes; in 15 hours, one bacterium can generate 1 million descendants.

Pathogenic (disease-producing) bacteria attack their host by breaking through the skin or through the mucous membranes that cover internal surfaces. Where they attack the host is specific to the type of bacteria. For example, diphtheria bacillus attacks the tonsils, and Salmonella typhi (typhoid fever) attacks the intestines. The chief danger comes from the poisons (toxins) the bacteria release: Exotoxins are poisons released while the bacteria grow; endotoxins are those released as the bacteria die. Fortunately, however, with the use of antibiotics, many bacterial diseases that were once notorious killers have been tamed.

Bacteria cannot survive high temperature combined with moisture. This is why surgical instruments are boiled and why milk is pasteurized before drinking.

10 Bacteria and the Diseases They Cause

Bordetella pertussis. This coccobacillus infects the mucous membranes lining the air passages and can lead to whooping cough, or pertussis. It is a disease that affects children, especially those under age 1, and is marked by convulsive bouts of coughing followed by noisy breathing. It can be prevented by vaccination.

Clostridium botulinum. Botulism, a life-threatening form of food poisoning, is caused by this bacterium. The disease results from eating undercooked foods or canned foods that have not been properly sterilized: Home-preserved vegetables are the leading cause of botulism in the United States.

The toxin attacks the nervous system, resulting in blurred vision, difficulty in swallowing, and muscular weakness. Antitoxins can counter botulism's lethal effects.

Clostridium tetani. This microorganism causes tetanus. Like the related botulism-causing bacterium, this bacterium produces spores that become activated in the absence of oxygen—the bacteria reproduce only in dirty wounds or in the bloodless tissue surrounding deep wounds. Toxins enter the nerves and reach the spinal column where they cause muscle spasm and convulsions. An early symptom is a stiffness of the jaw (thus the common name for tetanus, lockjaw). Tetanus is entirely preventable by immunization.

Corynebacterium diphtheriae. Diphtheria is an acute contagious disease in children. Its early symptoms are a sore throat and fever followed by the appearance of a gray membrane that forms over the tonsils, palate, and back of the mouth. Toxins enter the bloodstream and attack the heart, muscles, and nerves. Fortunately, diphtheria is extremely rare in developed countries, thanks to immunization. The immunization for diphtheria, along with those for tetanus and pertussis, is the DPT shots familiar to parents of young children.

Neisseria meningitidis. This is one species of bacteria that can cause bacterial meningitis; the others are *Diplococcus pneumoniae* and *Hemophilus influenzae*. When any of these bacteria attack the lining of the brain, the meninges (membranes that envelope the brain and spinal cord) can become inflamed and the space between membranes fill with pus. Headache, high fever, and stiffness of the neck are common symptoms. If untreated, the illness can lead to coma and death. All three forms are sensitive to antibiotics.

Pneumococcus. Before the age of antibiotics, the most common form of pneumonia was lobar pneumonia caused by the bacterium pneumococcus. This disease is confined to one lung or one lobe of a lung. Lobar pneumonia causes a high fever (often with delirium), chills, coughing, rapid shallow breathing, and inflammation of the covering of the lungs.

Shigella. Four different bacteria from the genus *Shigella* are responsible for several types of bacterial dysentery. *Shigella sonnei* usually leads to a mild infection; however, *S. boydii, S. dysenteriae,* and *S. flexneri* are responsible for the more virulent forms found in tropical and subtropical countries. The infection is spread by food contaminated by feces, the result of poor standards of hygiene and sanitation. Symptoms can include severe and bloody diarrhea with abdominal pain. Bacterial dysentery should not be confused with amoebic dysentery.

Staphylococcus. Some kinds of this bacterium are usually found on the skin and in the throat; other kinds cause severe infections or produce a poison, which may cause nausea, vomiting, and diarrhea. Life-threatening "staph" infections may originate in hospitals. Another kind, *Staphylococcus aureus,* is responsible for toxic shock syndrome (TSS), a sudden, sometimes fatal infection affecting menstruating women. Tampon use appears to elevate the risk of this disease, whose toxins can invade almost any body part.

Streptococcus. This group of bacteria is responsible for rheumatic fever, scarlet fever, and strep throat. Rheumatic fever can arise when a case of strep throat goes untreated with antibiotics. It occurs in 1 in 50,000 children and affects the joints, heart, skin, and, in some cases, brain.

Scarlet fever is caused by those strep throat toxins that create a scarlet rash on the skin. It is most often seen among schoolchildren. Symptoms include fever, rapid pulse, headache, and sore throat, followed by the rash a day or two later. Its importance has lessened with the advent of antibiotics.

Strep throat is an infection of the throat and tonsils that causes chills, fever, and swollen lymph nodes in the neck. Symptoms usually appear suddenly after exposure to the germs through either airborne droplets or direct contact with an infected person.

Streptococcus pyogenes. Erysipelas (St. Anthony's fire) is a serious skin disease that can result from infection following a scratch or a surgical wound not properly cared for. Its symptom is a red, glistening swelling of the skin. Antibiotics are highly effective.

VIRUSES

Viruses are tiny organisms that can only grow in the cells of another animal and are composed of DNA or RNA. They differ from bacteria in a few important ways: Viruses are smaller than bacteria, they grow only in living tissue (not in an artificial culture), and many are subject to mutations that change the properties of the virus and its virulence.

Viruses that cause human influenza periodically undergo mutations: A particularly virulent mutant strain killed 20 million people worldwide during the Spanish flu epidemic of 1918.

Changes in human behavior play a role in viral transference. Epidemiologists report new viral epidemics following human intrusion into virus-infested areas of the world where no one previously traveled, such as remote areas of the Amazon. In a related example, the worldwide trade in used tires from Asia has led to the introduction of mosquitoes that carry yellow fever and other tropical diseases into new lands.

Viruses can be transferred in four ways: through direct contact (inhaling droplets from sneezes and coughs); via insects; through water, milk, and food; and through blood transfusions and organ transplantation.

Viruses affect the cells they inhabit in the following ways: They may kill the cell; change the cell from normal to cancerous; or produce a latent infection—in the latter case the virus lies dormant until triggered into action at a later date. An example of a latent infection is shingles, in which dormant cells left over from a childhood case of chicken pox become activated.

Viruses are classified by the type of nucleic acid they have at their core as well as by their appearance. Some viruses have nucleic acid composed of DNA (double helix), while others have a single strand called RNA. The main groups of viruses that are important medically are: adenoviruses (respiratory and eye infections), arborviruses (yellow fever), arenaviruses (Lassa fever), coronaviruses (common cold), enteroviruses, herpesviruses (cold sores, genital herpes, chicken pox), paramyxoviruses (measles, mumps, rubella), papovaviruses (warts), picornaviruses (polio, throat infections), poxviruses (cowpox, smallpox), reoviruses (upper respiratory tract infections), retroviruses (AIDS), and rhabdoviruses (rabies).

Unlike bacteria, viruses do not respond to antibiotics. The body's immune system deals with viruses by producing antibodies to combat the invading agents. Once the immune system produces antibodies against a virus, it will recognize the virus the next time it tries to invade the body. There is, however, ongoing research into developing antiviral agents. Some successes have been reported.

3. Healing Arts

INTRODUCTION

It used to be simple. You got sick and went to the doctor. Today, however, it is not so easy. Modern health care is made up of a myriad of providers, many practicing forms, or specialties, of medicine completely alien to your own experience.

The age of the lone general practitioner, the one who handled all that was wrong with you, is gone. The medical landscape is now filled with practitioners who specialize, some who subspecialize, and even some who only consult with subspecialists. Consumers have a mind-boggling choice of different specialists and alternative practitioners from which to choose. While each has a place in the health care system, the important issue is to find the one that is appropriate to your needs or problems.

In this section, you will find not only a complete explanation of the range of medical specialists and alternative practitioners available, but you will also learn what criteria to consider when making a selection. You will also find a complete listing, including addresses, of major resources that can help you in the process. In addition, the most common medical abbreviations and medical terms are defined and explained so that you and your practitioner can speak on an even plane.

Knowing and understanding the education and medical viewpoint of different health care professionals helps you make choices that may ultimately ensure better health care for you and your family.

Doctors and the Consumer Criteria for Selecting One

Aside from the life-and-death issues and the fact that your doctor may someday hold your life in his or her hands, there are obvious economic advantages for the consumer to shop carefully for a doctor. In 1992 Americans spent $2,868 per capita on health care expenses, and the annual bill is expected to top $3,380 by year end 1993. But the reality of the matter is that most consumers spend more time selecting a roofer than they do choosing someone to look after their health. True, with the growth of consumerism in medicine over the past few years, this is changing, but there is still more progress to be made.

Choosing a doctor isn't easy. It's a process filled with questions, both for the prospective doctor and for yourself, but the right choice can save you money. After all, bad medical care costs a lot more than good care and takes its toll on your health and your family as well as your pocketbook.

The time to find the right practitioner is *before* you need one. Don't wait until you have a medical problem or, worse yet, a medical emergency. Not always the best choices, spur-of-the-moment decisions can be costly, too.

Begin your search by getting a few good recommendations from family members, friends, and neighbors. Word of mouth is still one of the best methods of finding out which doctors are taking new patients and what others think of these doctors. The old adage "If you want to find a good doctor, ask a nurse" is probably a good one, but may not always be practical.

Don't overlook recommendations from your present doctor, especially if your relationship with this doctor is ending because he or she is leaving practice or retiring. Other sources to consider are:

- Doctor referral services operated by the local medical society (usually county-based) and local hospitals. Not necessarily our first choice, such services will refer only those doctors who are members of the society or are on the hospital staff. Lest you attach altruistic motives to the physician referral services that two-thirds of all community hospitals run, according to a *Medical Economics* article, just remember that hospitals, now more than ever, need doctors to fill their beds. And a big chunk of hospitals' ever-growing marketing budgets (according to the American Hospital Association, an average of $407,000 per hospital, with almost 1 in 5 going over the $1-million mark) is spent on this marketing strategy. Another major drawback to these services is that they will not comment on the ability of physicians other than to perhaps mention their board certifications.
- Newspaper advertisements of doctors announcing the opening of a new practice. A *caveat emptor* is appropriate here, too—ask yourself why the doctor is advertising. To attract patients because he is just out of medical school? Or

because he's in a highly competitive and glutted market? Or has he just moved in from a state where his license was revoked?

- Your company personnel office. Companies sometimes use certain doctors for employment physicals and disability claims.
- Your health insurance company, which can sometimes be helpful when you require a specialist for a second opinion.
- Listings in the telephone directory. Doctors' names are usually arranged according to practice or specialty, but again be wary. Just because a doctor says he or she specializes in a certain area of medicine does not mean the doctor actually took any advanced training in it; a doctor can practice in any specialty area he or she chooses. Look for board certification. We have more to say on this later.
- Senior centers. Some have lists of doctors either affiliated with or recommended by the center. Other senior citizens who have had good or bad experiences with doctors can also pass along that information to you.

Before we explore the procedures and questions to ask in shopping for a doctor, there is another important matter to discuss.

WHEN SHOULD YOU SWITCH DOCTORS?

The ready answer to this question is when you are no longer getting the best care for your dollar, but that's not easy to evaluate. Sure, every once in a while something goes so wrong with the doctor-patient relationship that it comes to an abrupt end, but more often than not the relationship drags out until you've spent too much time and money and received too little in return.

In order to prevent a protracted but inevitable farewell, first know the legal aspects of the doctor-patient relationship. Once established, this relationship becomes a legal arrangement, which only four conditions can end:

- If both parties agree to end the relationship
- If it is ended by the patient
- If the doctor is no longer needed
- If the doctor gives reasonable notice that he/she is withdrawing from the relationship

If these procedures are not followed, a patient could make a case for abandonment by the doctor.

When things are going wrong with the doctor-patient relationship, certain signs should serve as warnings to you that all is not well:

- Overcrowded waiting rooms. Certainly doctors should be allowed some deviance from scheduled appointments due to emergencies, but habitual overbooking is another matter. Besides, the doctor who crowds too many appointments into the day is going to leave at least one person waiting too long and/or have to whisk people in and out of examinations/consultations.
- Excessive waiting time. You should be willing to accept the explanation that the doctor had an emergency, but not if it happens every time. (To save you time and money, try telephoning ahead to ask if the doctor is on schedule or what the approximate wait is.)
- Hurries through appointment. A doctor who does not permit you sufficient time to explain your symptoms or complaints and ask questions and who eyes the door or jiggles the doorknob as he/she talks with you may not be providing the best of care.
- Unavailability. You want to ask the doctor some questions but don't want to schedule an appointment. Will the doctor accept your telephone call? If he/she does not set aside a "telephone hour" once or twice a week to take calls, it may be time to switch to a doctor who does. After all, if the question can be answered briefly at such a time, you have saved yourself the time and expense of an office visit. Be aware, however, that it is not uncommon—or even unreasonable—for a doctor to charge for a telephone consultation, but the fee should be less than that of a regular office visit.
- Lack of communication. How well does the doctor explain the medical problem and any proposed tests and/or treatments? If the doctor does not engage in effective dialogue with you, preferring instead to issue orders or pronouncements, and if he/she shows little interest in what you have to say or shows annoyance when you raise questions, then you may want to shop around.
- Fee increases. If you're like most people, you can accept an increase in fees when the increase is justified by better service or a legitimate claim of higher overhead. But paying more money for

the same old service does not sit well with you, a problem that may be compounded by your insurance company's unwillingness to pay the higher fee. In this case, you're stuck with an out-of-pocket expense.

• Refuses access to medical records. Treating your medical record with confidentiality is one thing; denying you rightful access is another. How can you develop an equal partnership with a doctor who does not trust you enough to share copies of *your own* health history and medical record with you? Laws and regulations in many states allow patient access to doctors' records, and even in the absence of specific laws there are ways to obtain your record. Of course, all states allow patients (or at least their attorneys) access to their medical records in the context of a lawsuit. We have more to say about this under "The Importance of Your Medical Record" in section 10, "Consumer Protection: Your Legal and Medical Rights."

THE GET-ACQUAINTED VISIT

Doctor-shopping should include a get-acquainted visit, the object of which is to determine if you and the doctor are right for each other. Many problems do not arise until the first face-to-face encounter with the practitioner, the office, and the office staff.

When you telephone for an appointment, be sure to tell the receptionist that you want to arrange a get-acquainted visit. If the doctor refuses, go on to the next doctor on your list. You should be aware that some doctors charge for a get-acquainted visit and some do not. For instance, some busy, established doctors prefer not to give their time away, while other doctors are eager for new business and willing to waive even a nominal charge for a get-acquainted visit. As competition continues to heat up between doctors and other health plans, the get-acquainted visit becomes even more of a selling point.

On the other hand, the doctor who agrees to a get-acquainted visit may be more consumer-oriented than other doctors, but you should not let this gesture completely color your view of the doctor, since he or she may also be motivated solely by economic considerations.

The first thing you want to notice is the doctor's office and staff. Most offices will have a receptionist who will greet you and ask you to complete a few forms for their records. Ask the receptionist to orient you to the particulars regarding making appointments, telephoning the doctor, getting prescription refills, and obtaining copies of your medical records. Be sure to let them know, especially the doctor, that you have not yet decided on becoming a patient.

A first-time visit will probably run 10 to 15 minutes, so you need to have your questions ready and make the minutes count. When you meet the doctor, concentrate on his or her credentials—medical degree, board certification, and other specialized and/or postgraduate education—and hospital affiliations. If the doctor is not on staff of any hospital, or at least the hospital of your choosing, then the doctor may not be able to serve you when you need him or her most. Ask about the doctor's fee schedule and payment plans. A doctor who will openly discuss fees may be more willing to discuss other aspects of your medical care. If you are on Medicare, find out if the doctor accepts assignment. If not, ask if he/she will in your case; it's negotiable.

Determine what importance the doctor places on preventive health measures and what the doctor's philosophy of practice is—whether he/she sees the patient as a full partner in health care. An excellent point of reference is the People's Medical Society Code of Practice (see sidebar).

Pay particular attention to the doctor's manner and attitude as he/she answers your questions. Is the doctor addressing the heart of your questions and answering in a forthright manner?

You should also notice a few other things:

• Is the practice solo or group? The lone practice is almost a vanishing breed. While a group practice offers the advantage of someone always covering the office even during weekends, the possible downside is an overcrowded waiting room and the feeling that you are receiving assembly-line medical care. The doctor may be a part of a one-specialty group or a multispecialty group where there is a mix of primary care doctors and specialists. The latter can be helpful when, needing a second opinion and having to find a specialist, you can be referred to another doctor in the group. But the multispecialty group works against your best interests when the doctors refer only to the specialists in the group and not necessarily to the best specialist for you.

In 1983 the People's Medical Society created the Code of Practice as a statement we believe each doctor should subscribe to. Ask your doctor to review it and tell you whether he or she will apply it to your care.

The People's Medical Society Code of Practice

I will assist you in finding information resources, support groups, and health care providers to help you maintain and improve your health. When you seek my care for specific problems, I will abide by the following Code of Practice:

Office Procedures

1. I will post or provide a printed schedule of my fees for office visits, procedures, tests, and surgery, and provide itemized bills.
2. I will provide certain hours each week when I will be available for nonemergency telephone consultation.
3. I will schedule appointments to allow the necessary time to see you with minimal waiting. I will promptly report test results to you and return phone calls.
4. I will allow and encourage you to bring a friend or relative into the examining room with you.
5. I will facilitate your getting your medical and hospital records, and will provide you with copies of your test results.

Choice in Diagnosis and Treatment

6. I will let you know your prognosis, including whether your condition is terminal or will cause disability or pain, and will explain why I believe further diagnostic activity or treatment is necessary.
7. I will discuss with you diagnostic, treatment, and medication options for your particular problem (including the option of no treatment), and describe in understandable terms the risk of each alternative, the chances of success, the possibility of pain, the effect on your functioning, the number of visits each would entail, and the cost of each alternative.
8. I will describe my qualifications to perform the proposed diagnostic measures or treatments.
9. I will let you know of organizations, support groups, and medical and lay publications that can assist you in understanding, monitoring, and treating your problem.
10. I will not proceed until you are satisfied that you understand the benefits and risks of each alternative and I have your agreement on a particular course of action.

- Does the office appear neat and clean? Patient-friendly? Are there modern magazines? A telephone for patient use?
- Does the staff maintain a professional, friendly attitude?
- Is your insurance coverage accepted?
- Was your appointment kept on time?

GENERALIST VS. SPECIALIST

Years ago the problem of generalist versus specialist did not even come up in the search for a good doctor. Doctors were generalists—able to deliver babies, set broken bones, and perform surgeries—and that was that. Kindly Marcus Welby, the popular representation of an old-time general practitioner, or G.P., was a man who moved confidently from examining room to operating room to his patients' living rooms as he cared for entire families. But that warm and glowing picture began to change by the 1950s with the decline of general practice. Since then, the numbers of all-around physicians have been decreasing and specialists proliferating.

Although there is a bewildering array of medical specialists administering to every nook and cranny of the human body, the primary need of each and every one of us remains the same: a personal physician for self and family who can provide routine care for a wide range of medical problems—if for no other reason than that a primary physician generally comes cheaper than a specialist. Using a gynecologist or cardiologist for basic medical care will cost you a whole lot more than having your family physician handle the problem. That's not to say that specialists are not needed, just that the first line of defense is what's called a primary care physician.

Adults have three types of primary care physicians from which to choose:

General practitioners. Though dwindling in numbers, some G.P.'s still practice today. The *University of California, Berkeley, Wellness Letter* describes them as "usually older men who went into practice after only a year of postgraduate residency, and who often make up in clinical experience what they lack in formal training." They usually treat a whole range of medical problems.

Family practitioners. Unlike the general practitioner of old who began to practice as soon as he finished his internship, doctors today who intend to become family practitioners take additional training beyond medical school. Since 1969 when the American Medical Association recognized family practice as a specialty, any doctor wishing to qualify must take a three-year residency that covers certain aspects of internal medicine, gynecology, minor surgery, obstetrics, pediatrics, orthopedics, and preventive medicine, plus pass a comprehensive examination.

Internists. Like family practitioners, these specialists in internal medicine complete a three-year residency and must pass a comprehensive examination. Unlike family practitioners, however, these doctors do not normally take training in pediatrics, orthopedics, and child delivery, but instead have more advanced training in the diagnosis and management of problems involving such areas as the gastrointestinal system, heart, kidney, liver, and endocrine system. While internists may set up practices in which they act as highly trained family doctors, they often subspecialize in other areas, such as any of the ones listed above.

For children, add one more primary care provider, the *pediatrician.* Pediatricians, who provide the bulk of primary medical care for children in the United States, are physicians who have acquired knowledge of the physical, emotional, and social health needs of children from birth to young adulthood. They have graduated from medical school and fulfilled a three-year residency in general pediatrics; some may also have completed an additional two-year fellowship in a pediatric subspecialty.

WHAT IS A SPECIALIST?

A specialist is a doctor who concentrates on a specific body system, age group, or disorder. After obtaining an M.D. or D.O. degree, a doctor then undergoes two to three years of supervised specialty training (called a residency). Many specialists also take one or more years of additional training (called a fellowship) in a specific area of their specialty, called a subspecialty.

How can you tell if a doctor is a trained specialist? A doctor who has taken extra training in his or her field often chooses to become what is called board-certified. In addition to the extra training, the doctor must pass a rigorous examination administered by a specialty board, a national board of professionals in that specialty field. A doctor who passes the board examination is given the status of Diplomate. Most board-certified doctors also become members of their medical specialty societies, and any doctor who meets the full requirements for membership is called a Fellow of the society and may use the designation. For instance, the title "FACOG" after a doctor's name denotes that he is a Fellow of the American College of Obstetricians.

In its most basic sense, board certification indicates that a physician has completed a course of study in accordance with the established educational standards of one or more of the twenty-three member boards of the American Board of Medical Specialties, a Chicago-based independent regulatory body. Board certification has been called a minimum standard of excellence and nothing more. Paper certification does not produce professional excellence. On the other hand, although there are some inferior doctors who somehow manage to become board-certified, and there are some excellent doctors without board certification, board certification is a good sign that the person is up-to-date on the procedures, theories, and success-failure rates in the specialty.

Just bear in mind that specialization profoundly influences the way medicine is practiced. Patients are referred from doctor to doctor to be reassured that nothing is wrong with the organ system that is the doctor's field of interest/specialty. Although not all bad, the proliferation of specialists has become confusing and expensive. Therefore, the choice of the type of doctor to consult requires understanding the training, orientation, and special skills of each type of physician.

Glossary of Medical Specialties

Below is the list of what the American Medical Association calls "self-designated [medical] specialty classifications." Translated, this means that these specialties are those the physicians use to describe themselves and their primary and secondary fields of practice. The American Medical Association is quick to point out that this list does not imply "endorsement" or "recognition" (quotes theirs) by the AMA; it is merely a catalog of the myriad of possible areas of "expertise" a physician may claim.

You should be aware that a licensed physician may practice any specialty and call himself/herself a specialist in a particular field, whether or not the physician is actually board-certified in that specialty.

Abdominal Surgery—subspecialty of surgery involving the abdominal organs

Adolescent Medicine—subspecialty of pediatrics dealing with the medical needs of young people between the ages of 14 and 19

Allergy and Immunology—subspecialty of internal medicine or pediatrics involving the diagnosis and treatment of all forms of allergy and allergic disease and other disorders potentially involving the immune system.

Anesthesiology—involves the administration of drugs (anesthetics) to prevent pain or induce unconsciousness during surgical operations or diagnostic procedures. Anesthesiologists may further specialize in critical care medicine as practiced in critical care and intensive care units, postanesthesia recovery rooms, and other settings.

Cardiovascular Diseases (Cardiology)—subspecialty of internal medicine that deals with the heart and blood vessels

Cardiovascular Surgery—subspecialty of cardiology involving surgery on the heart and associated vascular system. Cardiovascular surgeons perform open-heart surgery, which may include heart transplants.

Child Neurology—branch of psychiatry and neurology involving the diagnosis and treatment of nervous system disorders in children

Child Psychiatry—subspecialty of psychiatry that deals with emotional problems of children

Colon and Rectal Surgery (Proctology)—diagnosis and treatment of diseases of the intestinal tract, rectum, and anus

Cosmetic Surgery—surgery to reshape normal structures of the body in order to improve a person's appearance and self-esteem

Dermatology—diagnosis and treatment of benign and malignant disorders of the skin and related tissues. The dermatologist also diagnoses and treats a number of diseases transmitted through sexual activity.

Diagnostic Radiology—subspecialty of radiology employing the use of ionizing, electromagnetic, or sound wave imaging devices to diagnose medical problems

Emergency Medicine—focuses on the immediate decision making and action necessary to prevent death or further disability. It is primarily hospital emergency department based.

Endocrinology—subspecialty of internal medicine that deals with disorders of the internal (or endocrine) glands such as the thyroid and adrenal glands. Endocrinology also deals with disorders such as diabetes, pituitary diseases, and menstrual and sexual problems.

Family Practice/General Practice—concerned with total health care of the individual and the family. The scope of family practice is not limited by age, sex, organ system, or disease entity.

Gastroenterology—subspecialty of internal medicine that involves disorders of the digestive tract: stomach, bowels, liver, gallbladder, and related organs

General Surgery—surgery of the parts of the body that are not in the domain of specific surgical specialties (some areas do overlap, however)

Geriatrics—subspecialty of family practice and internal medicine that deals with the diseases of the elderly and problems associated with aging

Gynecology—diagnosis and treatment of problems associated with the female reproductive organs

Hand Surgery—subspecialty of orthopedic surgery, general surgery, or plastic surgery that is limited to the musculoskeletal structure of the hands, including bone, muscle, and ligaments

Head and Neck Surgery—subspecialty of otolaryngology that deals with surgery of the head and neck, excluding the brain and eyes

Hematology—diagnosis and treatment of diseases and disorders of the blood and blood-forming parts of the body

Immunology—study and treatment of problems of the body's immune system, which may include allergies, infections, and life-threatening diseases such as AIDS

Infectious Diseases—subspecialty of internal medicine involving the diagnosis and treatment of life-threatening infectious illnesses

Internal Medicine—diagnosis and nonsurgical treatment of diseases, especially those of adults. While internists may set up practices in which they act as highly trained family doctors, they often subspecialize in many other areas.

Laryngology—branch of medicine that involves the throat, pharynx, larynx, nasopharynx, and tracheobronchial tree

Maxillofacial Surgery—subspecialty of dentistry that deals with problems of the mouth and jaw

Neonatal-Perinatal Medicine—subspecialty of pediatrics that deals with disorders of newborn infants, including premature ones

Nephrology—subspecialty of internal medicine concerned with disorders of the kidney

Neurological Surgery (Neurosurgery)—diagnosis and surgical treatment of diseases of the brain, spinal cord, and nerves

Neurology—diagnosis and nonsurgical treatment of diseases of the brain, spinal cord, and nerves

Nuclear Medicine—use of radioactive substances for diagnosis and treatment

Nuclear Radiology—subspecialty of radiology that involves the use of radioactive materials in the diagnosis and treatment of disease.

Obstetrics and Gynecology—care of pregnant women and treatment of disorders of the female reproductive system.

Occupational Medicine—subspecialty of preventive medicine that deals with the special physical and psychological risks in industry

Oncology—subspecialty of internal medicine concerned with the diagnosis and treatment of all types of cancer and other benign and malignant tumors

Ophthalmology—diagnosis, monitoring, and medical/surgical treatment of vision problems and other disorders of the eye, including the prescription of glasses/contact lenses

Orthopedic Surgery (Orthopedics)—care of diseases of the muscles, and diseases, fractures, and deformities of the bones and joints

Otolaryngology—medical and surgical care of patients with diseases and disorders that affect the ears, respiratory and upper alimentary systems, and related structures: in general, the head and neck

Otology—subspecialty of otolaryngology that deals with the medical treatment of and surgery on the ear

Pathology—examination and diagnosis of organs, tissues, body fluids, and excrement

Pediatrics—concerned with the physical, emotional, and social health of children from birth to young adulthood

Pediatric Allergy—subspecialty of pediatrics that involves the diagnosis and treatment of allergies in children

Pediatric Cardiology—subspecialty of pediatrics that deals with diseases of the heart

Pediatric Endocrinology—subspecialty of pediatrics that deals with diseases resulting from an abnormality in the endocrine glands (glands that secrete hormones)

Pediatric Hematology-Oncology—subspecialty of pediatrics that treats blood disorders and cancers

Pediatric Nephrology—subspecialty of pediatrics that deals with kidney disorders

Pediatric Pulmonology—subspecialty of pediatrics that deals with the prevention, diagnosis, and treatment of all respiratory diseases affecting infants, children, and adolescents

Pediatric Radiology—subspecialty of pediatrics that utilizes radiant energy to diagnose and treat childhood diseases

Pediatric Surgery—subspecialty of surgery that deals with the surgical problems of premature and newborn infants, children, and adolescents

Physical Medicine and Rehabilitation (Physiatry)—diagnosis, evaluation, and treatment of patients with impairments and/or disabilities involving musculoskeletal, neurologic, cardiovascular, or other body systems

Preventive Medicine—focuses on the health of individuals and the prevention of disease through immunization, good health practice, and concern with environmental and occupational factors

Psychiatry—diagnosis, treatment, and prevention of mental, emotional and/or behavioral disorders. (Do not confuse the psychiatrist with the non-physician psychologist.)

Psychosomatic Medicine—more a way of practicing medicine than a specialty as such; a concept of total medical care that considers the emotional needs of the patient by taking into account the mind-body interactions of the patient

Public Health—branch of medicine that deals with the protection and improvement of community health by organized community effort, and includes the monitoring and screening of populations to prevent the spread of communicable diseases. Many consider public health to be allied with, if not actually a subspecialty of, preventive medicine.

Pulmonary Diseases—subspecialty of internal medicine concerned with diseases of the lungs and other chest tissues, including pneumonia, cancer, occupational diseases, bronchitis, emphysema, and other complex disorders of the lungs

Radiology—study and use of various types of radiation, including X rays, in the diagnosis and treatment of disease

Reconstructive Surgery—surgery on abnormal structures of the body, caused by congenital defects, developmental abnormalities, trauma, infection, tumors, or disease, and generally performed to improve function but may also be done to approximate a normal appearance

Rheumatology—subspecialty of internal medicine that deals with diseases of the joints, muscles, and tendons, including arthritis

Rhinology—see Otolaryngology

Surgical Critical Care (Traumatic Surgery)—subspecialty of surgery that deals with the treatment of the critically ill patient, particularly the trauma victim, and the postoperative patient in the emergency department, intensive care unit, trauma unit, burn unit, and other similar settings

Therapeutic Radiology (Radiation Oncology)—subspecialty of radiology that deals with the therapeutic applications of radiant energy, especially in the treatment of malignant tumors

Thoracic Surgery—operative, peri-operative, and critical care of patients with disease-causing conditions within the chest, including coronary artery disease, cancers of the lung, esophagus, and chest wall, abnormalities of the great vessels and heart valves, and injuries to the airway and chest

Urological Surgery—subspecialty of urology that deals with the surgical treatments of the adrenal gland and genitourinary system

Urology—diagnosis and treatment of diseases of the urinary system as well as the organs of reproduction in men, such as the prostate

Vascular Surgery—subspecialty of surgery that deals with medical disorders affecting the blood vessels, excluding those of the heart, lungs, and brain

Where to Turn for More Information

The important question is, how can you determine if a physician is a certified specialist or sub-specialist? The American Board of Medical Specialties has a toll-free number you can call to verify certification status: 800-776-2378.

QUESTIONS TO ASK YOUR DOCTOR BEFORE YOU SEE A SPECIALIST

You usually encounter a specialist when your primary care doctor wants to confirm a diagnosis or wants a second opinion. *If your family physician recommends a specialist or you seek one on your own, here are questions that need to be answered:*

• "Why do I have to see a specialist?" Or, put another way, "I'd like a good explanation of what you think is wrong with me." Ask your doctor to furnish you a complete and understandable, point-by-point diagnostic portrait. Going to a specialist should not be a casual next step routinely taken in every medical situation.

• "Why this kind of specialist?" Again, it's information you're after. You need to know about the specialist's areas of expertise, and what is involved with the performance of that specialty. Knowing this will help you determine whether you want to see the specialist at all. That is an option. You don't have to see a specialist (or see that particular specialist) immediately if you are not convinced that consultation is justified. Let your doctor know that he or she must make a very good case for every step taken in your medical care.

• "Why this particular specialist?" Why Dr. Jones and not Dr. Smith? Is Dr. Jones the best person for the job? Are you being sent to Dr. Jones because she is an excellent representative of her profession? Or is it because Dr. Jones and your doctor are friends who have an arrangement, each recommending the other? While there is nothing wrong with friends referring patients to each other, you want to feel confident that competence is the basic reason for the referral.

U.S. Medical Schools: Allopaths

The following schools grant M.D. (doctor of medicine) degrees.

Alabama

University of Alabama at Birmingham
School of Medicine
University Station
Birmingham, AL 35294

University of South Alabama
College of Medicine
307 University Boulevard
Mobile, AL 36688

Arizona

University of Arizona
College of Medicine
Arizona Health Sciences Center
1501 N. Campbell Avenue
Tucson, AZ 85724

Arkansas

University of Arkansas at Little Rock
College of Medicine
4301 W. Markham Street
Little Rock, AR 72205

California

Loma Linda University
School of Medicine
Loma Linda, CA 92350

Stanford University
School of Medicine
300 Pasteur Drive
Stanford, CA 94305

University of California at Davis
School of Medicine
Davis, CA 92616

University of California at Irvine
College of Medicine
Irvine, CA 92717

University of California at Los Angeles
School of Medicine
UCLA Center for Health Sciences
Los Angeles, CA 90024

University of California at San Diego
School of Medicine
La Jolla, CA 92093

University of California at San Francisco
School of Medicine
513 Parnassus Avenue
San Francisco, CA 94143-0410

University of Southern California
School of Medicine
1975 Zonal Avenue
Los Angeles, CA 90033

Colorado

University of Colorado at Denver
School of Medicine
4200 E. 9th Avenue
Denver, CO 80262

Connecticut

University of Connecticut
School of Medicine
263 Farmington Avenue
Farmington, CT 06032

Yale University
School of Medicine
333 Cedar Street
P.O. Box 3333
New Haven, CT 06510

District of Columbia
George Washington University
School of Medicine and Health Sciences
2300 I Street N.W.
Washington, DC 20037

Georgetown University
School of Medicine
3900 Reservoir Road N.W.
Washington, DC 20007

Howard University
College of Medicine
520 W Street N.W.
Washington, DC 20059

Florida
University of Florida
College of Medicine
J. Hillis Miller Health Center
Box J-215
Gainesville, FL 32610

University of Miami
School of Medicine
1600 N.W. 10th Avenue
P.O. Box 016099
Miami, FL 33101

University of South Florida
College of Medicine
12901 Bruce B. Downs Boulevard
Tampa, FL 33612-4799

Georgia
Emory University
School of Medicine
Woodruff Health Sciences Center
1440 Clifton Road N.E.
Atlanta, GA 30322

Medical College of Georgia
School of Medicine
1120 15th Street
Augusta, GA 30912

Mercer University
School of Medicine
1550 College Street
Macon, GA 31207

Morehouse School of Medicine
720 Westview Drive S.W.
Atlanta, GA 30310-1495

Hawaii
University of Hawaii at Manoa
John A. Burns School of Medicine
1960 East-West Road
Honolulu, HI 96822

Illinois
Loyola University of Chicago
Stritch School of Medicine
2160 S. First Avenue
Maywood, IL 60153

Northwestern University
Medical School
303 E. Chicago Avenue
Chicago, IL 60611-3008

Rush University
Rush Medical College
600 S. Paulina Street
Chicago, IL 60612

Southern Illinois University at Springfield
School of Medicine
801 N. Rutledge
P.O. Box 19230
Springfield, IL 62794-9230

University of Chicago
Pritzker School of Medicine
5841 S. Maryland Avenue
Chicago, IL 60637

University of Health Sciences/Chicago
Medical School
3333 Green Bay Road
North Chicago, IL 60064

University of Illinois at Chicago
College of Medicine
1853 W. Polk Street
P.O. Box 6998 (M/C 784)
Chicago, IL 60680

University of Illinois
College of Medicine at Peoria
One Illini Drive
P.O. Box 1649
Peoria, IL 61656

University of Illinois
College of Medicine at Rockford
1601 Parkview Avenue
Rockford, IL 61107

University of Illinois
College of Medicine at Urbana-Champaign
190 Medical Sciences Building
506 S. Mathews
Urbana, IL 61801

Indiana

**Indiana University
School of Medicine**
1120 South Drive
Indianapolis, IN 46202-5114

Iowa

**University of Iowa
College of Medicine**
200 Eckstein Medical Research Building
Iowa City, IA 52242

Kansas

**University of Kansas
School of Medicine**
39th Street and Rainbow Boulevard
Kansas City, KS 66103

**University of Kansas
School of Medicine at Wichita**
1010 N. Kansas
Wichita, KS 67214

Kentucky

**University of Kentucky
College of Medicine**
800 Rose Street
Lexington, KY 40536-0084

**University of Louisville
School of Medicine**
Health Sciences Center
Louisville, KY 40292

Louisiana

**Louisiana State University
School of Medicine in New Orleans**
1542 Tulane Avenue
New Orleans, LA 70112-2822

**Louisiana State University
School of Medicine in Shreveport**
P.O. Box 33932
Shreveport, LA 71130-3932

**Tulane University
School of Medicine**
1430 Tulane Avenue
New Orleans, LA 70112

Maryland

**Johns Hopkins University
School of Medicine**
720 Rutland Avenue
Baltimore, MD 21205

**Uniformed Services University of the Health Sciences
F. Edward Hebert School of Medicine**
4301 Jones Bridge Road
Bethesda, MD 20814-4799

**University of Maryland
School of Medicine**
655 W. Baltimore Street
Baltimore, MD 21201

Massachusetts

**Boston University
School of Medicine**
80 E. Concord Street
Boston, MA 02118

Harvard Medical School
25 Shattuck Street
Boston, MA 02115

**Tufts University
School of Medicine**
136 Harrison Avenue
Boston, MA 02111

**University of Massachusetts
Medical Center at Worcester**
55 Lake Avenue N.
Worcester, MA 01655

Michigan

**Michigan State University
College of Human Medicine**
A-110 E. Fee Hall
East Lansing, MI 48824

University of Michigan Medical School
1301 Catherine Road, Building I
Ann Arbor, MI 48109-0624

**Wayne State University
School of Medicine**
540 E. Canfield Avenue
Detroit, MI 48201

Minnesota

Mayo Medical School
200 First Street S.W.
Rochester, MN 55905

**University of Minnesota at Duluth
School of Medicine**
10 University Drive
Duluth, MN 55812

**University of Minnesota
School of Medicine**
420 Delaware Street S.E.
UMHC Box 293
Minneapolis, MN 55455

Mississippi

**University of Mississippi
School of Medicine**
2500 N. State Street
Jackson, MS 39216

Missouri

St. Louis University
School of Medicine
1402 S. Grand Boulevard
St. Louis, MO 63104

University of Missouri at Columbia
School of Medicine
1 Hospital Drive
Columbia, MO 65203

University of Missouri at Kansas City
School of Medicine
2411 Holmes Street
Kansas City, MO 64108

Washington University
School of Medicine
660 S. Euclid Avenue
St. Louis, MO 63110

Nebraska

Creighton University
School of Medicine
California Street at 24th Street
Omaha, NE 68178

University of Nebraska at Omaha
College of Medicine
600 S. 42nd Street
Omaha, NE 68198

Nevada

University of Nevada at Reno
School of Medicine
Savitt Medical Sciences Building
Reno, NV 89557-0046

New Hampshire

Dartmouth College
Medical School
Hanover, NH 03756

New Jersey

University of Medicine and Dentistry of New Jersey
New Jersey Medical School
185 S. Orange Avenue
Newark, NJ 07103-2757

University of Medicine and Dentistry of New Jersey
Robert Wood Johnson Medical School at Camden
401 Haddon Avenue
Camden, NJ 08103

University of Medicine and Dentistry of New Jersey
Robert Wood Johnson Medical School
675 Hoes Lane
Piscataway, NJ 08854-5635

New Mexico

University of New Mexico
School of Medicine
Albuquerque, NM 87131

New York

City University of New York
Mt. Sinai School of Medicine
1 Gustave L. Levy Place
New York, NY 10029-6574

Columbia University
College of Physicians and Surgeons
630 W. 168th Street
New York, NY 10032

Cornell University
Medical College
1300 York Avenue
New York, NY 10021

New York Medical College
Sunshine Cottage
Valhalla, NY 10595

New York University
School of Medicine
550 First Avenue
New York, NY 10016

State University of New York
Health Science Center at Brooklyn
College of Medicine
450 Clarkson Avenue
Brooklyn, NY 11203

State University of New York at Buffalo
School of Medicine and Biomedical Sciences
3435 Main Street
Buffalo, NY 14214

State University of New York at Stony Brook
School of Medicine
Stony Brook, NY 11794

State University of New York
Health Science Center at Syracuse
College of Medicine
750 E. Adams Street
Syracuse, NY 13210

Union University
Albany Medical College
47 New Scotland Avenue
Albany, NY 12208

University of Rochester
School of Medicine and Dentistry
601 Elmwood Avenue
Rochester, NY 14642

Yeshiva University
Albert Einstein College of Medicine
1300 Morris Park Avenue
Bronx, NY 10461

North Carolina

Duke University
School of Medicine
P.O. Box 3005
Durham, NC 27710

East Carolina University
School of Medicine
Greenville, NC 27858-4354

University of North Carolina at Chapel Hill
School of Medicine
Chapel Hill, NC 27599

Wake Forest University
Bowman Gray School of Medicine
300 S. Hawthorne Road
Winston-Salem, NC 27103

North Dakota
University of North Dakota
School of Medicine
501 N. Columbia Road
Grand Forks, ND 58203

Ohio
Case Western Reserve University
School of Medicine
2119 Abington Road
Cleveland, OH 44106-2333

Medical College of Ohio
P.O. Box 10008
Toledo, OH 43699

Northeastern Ohio Universities
College of Medicine
4209 State Route 44
P.O. Box 95
Rootstown, OH 44272

Ohio State University
College of Medicine
370 W. 9th Avenue
Columbus, OH 43210

University of Cincinnati
College of Medicine
231 Bethesda Avenue
Cincinnati, OH 45267-0555

Wright State University
School of Medicine
P.O. Box 927
Dayton, OH 45401-0927

Oklahoma
University of Oklahoma
College of Medicine
P.O. Box 26901
Oklahoma City, OK 73190

University of Oklahoma
Tulsa Medical College
2808 S. Sheridan
Tulsa, OK 74129

Oregon
Oregon Health Sciences University
School of Medicine
3181 S.W. Sam Jackson Park Road
Portland, OR 97201-3098

Pennsylvania
Hahnemann University
School of Medicine
Mail Stop 440
Broad and Vine Streets
Philadelphia, PA 19102-1192

Medical College of Pennsylvania
3300 Henry Avenue
Philadelphia, PA 19129

Pennsylvania State University
College of Medicine
500 University Drive
P.O. Box 850
Hershey, PA 17033

Temple University
School of Medicine
3400 N. Broad Street
Philadelphia, PA 19140

Thomas Jefferson University
Jefferson Medical College
1025 Walnut Street
Philadelphia, PA 19107

University of Pennsylvania
School of Medicine
36th and Hamilton Walk
Philadelphia, PA 19104-6015

University of Pittsburgh
School of Medicine
Alan Magee Scaife Hall of the Health Professions
Pittsburgh, PA 15261

Puerto Rico
Ponce School of Medicine
P.O. Box 7004
Ponce, PR 00732

Universidad Central del Caribe
School of Medicine
Call Box 60-327
Bayamón, PR 00621-6032

University of Puerto Rico
School of Medicine
Medical Sciences Campus
GPO Box 5067
San Juan, PR 00936

Rhode Island
Brown University
Program in Medicine
97 Waterman Street
Providence, RI 02912

South Carolina

Medical University of South Carolina
College of Medicine
171 Ashley Avenue
Charleston, SC 29425

University of South Carolina
School of Medicine
Columbia, SC 29208

South Dakota

University of South Dakota
School of Medicine
2501 W. 22nd Street
Sioux Falls, SD 57117-5046

Tennessee

East Tennessee State University
Quillen College of Medicine
P.O. Box 23320-A
Johnson City, TN 37614

Meharry Medical College
School of Medicine
1005 D. B. Todd Jr. Boulevard
Nashville, TN 37208

University of Tennessee at Memphis
College of Medicine
800 Madison Avenue
Memphis, TN 38163

Vanderbilt University
School of Medicine
21st Avenue S. at Garland Avenue
Nashville, TN 37232

Texas

Baylor College of Medicine
1 Baylor Plaza
Houston, TX 77030

Texas A&M University
College of Medicine
147 Medical Sciences Building
College Station, TX 77843-1114

Texas Tech University
Health Sciences Center
School of Medicine
3601 4th Street
Lubbock, TX 79430

University of Texas Health Science Center at Houston
School of Medicine
P.O. Box 20708
Houston, TX 77225

University of Texas Health Science Center
at San Antonio
School of Medicine
7703 Floyd Curl Drive
San Antonio, TX 78284-7790

University of Texas Medical Branch at Galveston
School of Medicine
301 University Boulevard
Galveston, TX 77550

University of Texas Southwestern Medical Center
at Dallas
Southwestern Medical School
5323 Harry Hines Boulevard
Dallas, TX 75235

Utah

University of Utah
School of Medicine
50 N. Medical Drive
Salt Lake City, UT 84132

Vermont

University of Vermont
College of Medicine
Burlington, VT 05405

Virginia

Medical College of Hampton Roads
Eastern Virginia Medical School
P.O. Box 1980
Norfolk, VA 23501

University of Virginia
School of Medicine
Box 395, Medical Center
Charlottesville, VA 22908

Virginia Commonwealth University
Medical College of Virginia
School of Medicine
Box 565, MCV Station
Richmond, VA 23298

Washington

University of Washington
School of Medicine
Seattle, WA 98195

West Virginia

Marshall University
School of Medicine
1801 6th Avenue
Huntington, WV 25755-9000

West Virginia University
School of Medicine
Morgantown, WV 26506

Wisconsin

Medical College of Wisconsin
8701 Watertown Plank Road
Milwaukee, WI 53226

University of Wisconsin at Madison
Medical School
1300 University Avenue
Madison, WI 53706

Osteopathic Medicine

In brief, D.O.'s, or doctors of osteopathic medicine, are fully licensed and recognized physicians and surgeons who stress the unity of all body systems. They also emphasize the musculoskeletal system, holistic medicine, and proper nutrition and environmental factors. And they view manipulation or palpation as an aid to the diagnosis and treatment of various illnesses.

Osteopathic medicine was founded on the Missouri frontier in 1874 by Dr. Andrew Taylor Still, who was dissatisfied with the ineffectiveness of nineteenth-century medicine. He decried the rudimentary drugs and surgery of the day and saw many people, including his own three children, die from serious diseases. Concepts such as anesthesia, sterile surgery, antiseptics, antibiotics, and X rays were not imagined in the 1870s. Consequently, he identified palpation and the human touch as vital to gaining patient confidence and providing effective medical care. And he stressed manipulation as a less intrusive form of diagnosis and treatment.

Certain essential concepts are found throughout osteopathic medicine.

- The human body is a unified organism. Osteopathic physicians emphasize that all body systems, including the musculoskeletal system, operate in unison, and disturbances in one system can alter the functions of other systems.
- D.O.'s follow a holistic, commonsense approach to health care delivery that views each patient in his or her entirety. Some 52 percent of graduating D.O.'s enter primary care. In addition, two-thirds of today's osteopathic physicians practice in smaller towns and rural areas—where the need for primary health care is greatest. Even when a D.O. becomes a specialist, such as a surgeon, cardiologist, anesthesiologist, or psychiatrist, he or she still sees each patient as a whole person and stresses that illness can have its origin in any part of the body.
- The body's musculoskeletal system is central to the patient's well-being. This system includes the bones, muscles, tendons, tissues, nerves, and spinal column—about 60 percent of the body mass. D.O.'s point out that the musculoskeletal framework is far more than an anatomical rack on which the other organs are hung. It works in concert with all other organs. It responds—properly or improperly—every time a breath is drawn or any other body movement occurs. Besides being prone to mechanical disorders, the musculoskeletal system reflects many internal illnesses and may aggravate or accelerate the process of disease in the circulatory, lymphatic, nervous, and other body systems.
- Osteopathic manipulation of the musculoskeletal system is a viable and proven technique for many hands-on diagnoses and treatments. Often it can provide an alternative to more intrusive therapies involving drugs and/or surgery.

Osteopathic physicians utilize all of the recognized procedures and modern technologies for prevention, diagnosis, and treatment of disease, including drugs, radiation, and surgery. But the D.O. also has another pair of tools that enables him or her to accurately diagnose areas of dysfunction and treat them effectively. These tools are his or her hands.

Manipulation brings an added dimension to the osteopathic physician's diagnostic and therapeutic armamentarium. Following are some of the manipulation procedures most commonly used by osteopathic physicians to diagnose and treat somatic (body) dysfunctions.

Hands-on contact. The value of the placing of hands on a patient is universally acknowledged by health professionals. When the D.O. examines a patient by auscultation of the chest or palpation of the abdomen or spine, treatment already has begun, in the osteopathic view.

Soft tissue technique. This procedure is commonly applied to the musculature surrounding the spine, and consists of a rhythmic linear stretching, deep pressure, and traction. Its purpose is to move tissue fluids (edema) and to relax hypertonic muscles and myofascial (fibrous tissue) layers associated with somatic dysfunction.

Lymphatic technique. This method promotes circulation of the lymphatic fluids and can be used to relieve upper and lower respiratory infections. Pressure is applied with the physician's hands to the prone patient's upper anterior chest wall. When the force applied to the chest reaches its maximum on expiration, the physician's hands are removed suddenly. This increases negative pressure of the chest to assist the body's respiratory mechanism to move lymphatic fluids.

Thrust technique. In this form of manipulation, the physician applies a high-velocity/low-amplitude thrust to restore motion to a joint. With such a technique, the joint regains its normal range of motion and breaks abnormal neural reflexes.

Muscle energy technique. Here the patient is directed to use his or her muscles from a precise position and in a specific direction against a counterforce applied by the physician. The purpose is to mobilize a particular somatic dysfunction.

Counterstrain. With the counterstrain technique, the patient is moved passively away from the restricted motion barrier, toward planes of easy motion, searching for the position of greatest comfort. At this point, passive, asymptomatic strain is induced. This technique is indicated for relief of somatic dysfunctions that are too acute or too delicate to treat in other ways.

Contact the American Osteopathic Association for more information on osteopathic medicine.

Public Relations Department
American Osteopathic Association
142 E. Ontario Street
Chicago, IL 60611
312-280-5854

M.D.'s and D.O.'s
What's the Difference to You and Your Health?

Osteopathy is a sometimes forgotten branch of mainstream medical care. By no means insignificant in numbers of practitioners—28,200 in this country alone—osteopathy nevertheless is overshadowed by allopathic medicine and its half million practitioners, and in part ignored as a result of the public perception that the M.D. is the sole torchbearer for traditional medicine. This is simply not true. Both osteopathy and allopathy claim scientifically accepted methods of diagnosis and treatment as their basis. Except for a notable difference in philosophy and, to a lesser extent, practice habits, D.O.'s and M.D.'s are essentially the same.

If traditional medicine can be neatly categorized into two basic approaches—focus on the patient versus focus on the patient's disease—osteopathy stresses the former. In brief, D.O.'s, or doctors of osteopathic medicine, are fully licensed physicians and surgeons who

hold that the body is an interrelated system. The practitioners are called *osteopaths* because they emphasize the role of bones, muscles, and joints of the body—the musculoskeletal system—in a person's well-being.

Consequently, manipulation and hands-on diagnosis and treatment are mainstays of osteopathic practice and, in short, what distinguish D.O.'s from M.D.'s. In fact, whether such manipulations, used alone or in conjunction with other therapies, are indeed of any value is the crux of what remains of a once virulent M.D.-D.O. squabble.

As a general rule, compared to M.D.'s, D.O's *tend* to be more holistic in their approach to care, *tend*—at least at first—not to order a full battery of tests for diagnostic purposes but instead rely on a more selective range, and *tend* to utilize manipulation before drugs and surgery. D.O.'s employ two forms of hands-on contact, or manipulation:

U.S. Medical Schools: Osteopaths

The following schools grant D.O. (doctor of osteopathy) degrees.

California
College of Osteopathic Medicine of the Pacific
College Plaza
Pomona, CA 91766-1889

Florida
Southeastern University of Health Sciences
College of Osteopathic Medicine
1750 N.E. 168th Street
North Miami Beach, FL 33162-3097

Illinois
Chicago College of Osteopathic Medicine
555 31st Street
Downers Grove, IL 60615-1235

Iowa
University of Osteopathic Medicine
and Health Sciences
Colleges of Osteopathic Medicine and Surgery
3200 Grand Avenue
Des Moines, IA 50312

Maine
University of New England
College of Osteopathic Medicine
11 Hills Beach Road
Biddeford, ME 04005

Michigan
Michigan State University
College of Osteopathic Medicine
E. Fee Hall
East Lansing, MI 48824

One is palpation (touch), literally a hands-on diagnostic procedure to detect soft tissue changes or structural asymmetries. D.O.'s also use manipulative therapy, whereby muscles, bones, joints, nerves, and tissue are in some way manipulated or have pressure applied to them in order to effect some beneficial change in a patient's condition.

Let us say here that, while it is true that D.O.'s underscore the body's natural ability to heal itself (called *vis medicatrix naturae*, an ancient philosophy virtually banished from allopathy), they also utilize all the recognized procedures and modern technologies, including drugs, radiation, and surgery.

Whether one becomes a D.O. or an M.D., the route of complete medical training is basically the same. In matters of licensing, D.O.'s hold the same unlimited practice rights as M.D.'s in all fifty states and the District of Columbia and can admit and treat patients in both osteopathic and allopathic hospitals and clinics. (There are nearly 200 designated osteopathic hospitals in the United States, which provide special osteopathic care in addition to general medical/surgical services. But more likely than not, D.O.'s practice alongside M.D.'s in allopathic facilities, with referrals between the two professions common.) Osteopaths also participate in federal Medicare and Medicaid programs on an equal basis with their allopathic counterparts.

Most D.O.'s are generalists, but some have additional training and qualifications and work in specialized fields. Except insofar as the basic approach to care differs, osteopathic specialties resemble allopathic ones. The American Osteopathic Association (AOA), a trade organization similar to the American Medical Association, recognizes seventeen areas of certification: anesthesiology, dermatology, emergency medicine, general practice, internal medicine, neurology and psychiatry, nuclear medicine, obstetrics and gynecology, ophthalmology, orthopedic surgery, pathology, pediatrics, preventive medicine/public health, proctology, radiology, rehabilitation medicine, and surgery.

Missouri

Kirksville College of Osteopathic Medicine
800 W. Jefferson Street
Kirksville, MO 63501

University of Health Sciences
College of Osteopathic Medicine
2105 Independence Avenue
Kansas City, MO 64124

New Jersey

University of Medicine and Dentistry of New Jersey
School of Osteopathic Medicine
40 E. Laurel Road, Suite 100
Stradford, NJ 08084

New York

New York Institute of Technology
New York College of Osteopathic Medicine
Old Westbury, NY 11568

Ohio

Ohio University
College of Osteopathic Medicine
Grosvenor and Irvine Halls
Athens, OH 45701

Oklahoma

Oklahoma State University
College of Osteopathic Medicine
1111 W. 17th Street
Tulsa, OK 74107

Pennsylvania

Philadelphia College of Osteopathic Medicine
4150 City Avenue
Philadelphia, PA 19131

Texas

Texas College of Osteopathic Medicine
3500 Camp Bowie Boulevard
Ft. Worth, TX 76107

West Virginia

West Virginia School of Osteopathic Medicine
400 N. Lee Street
Lewisburg, WV 24901

Medical Abbreviations and Medical Term Derivatives

MEDICAL ABBREVIATIONS: THE 200+ MOST COMMON AND HOW TO DECIPHER THEM

Doctors, nurses, and other health care professionals have a long-established habit of using abbreviated medical terms and everyday words, especially in charts and medical records. They have been trained to think that no one except another doctor or nurse will look at what is scribbled there, and they have all learned the code in the course of their training. But patients do not know it, and when you look at your chart and records (something you ought to do regularly), you are at a loss and have no hint of what your doctor is thinking about you, about your condition, and about your prognosis. It is a major obstacle blocking your participation in your own care.

The following list can change all that. It is a collection from many sources of abbreviations frequently used in records, on forms and prescriptions, and even in everyday conversation. (If something you see or hear doesn't appear on this list, ask your doctor, nurse, hospital patients' representative, or some other person in the know to translate.)

One reason doctors or hospital personnel might not want you to know what they've written may be that they fear that the message could be misunderstood and even be embarrassing for them if interpreted accurately. Sometimes descriptive terms medical people use in referring to their patients and their patients' conditions are derogatory and are couched in a colorful code purposely indecipherable to the uninitiated. For example, if "LOL" is noted next to your name on your chart, and you ask your nurse what it means, she might turn a couple shades of crimson. "LOL" is medicode for "little old lady." This signals those reading the record that you are a nice, perhaps cheery, certainly passive, unquestioning female senior citizen.

If you hear that the patient next door "boxed," that means he or she died. A "gork" is a brain-damaged person, a vegetable. A "gomer" is the acronym for "Get out of my emergency room"—a patient whom no one wants to treat.

And what about the abbreviations that pertain directly to your state of health or medical care? If you see "FBS," followed by numbers, this is the results of your test for "fasting blood sugar." Same with "BMR." That means "basal metabolic rate."

In medicode, a "delightful" patient is one who does anything anybody tells him or her to do and never asks questions. The same goes for those patients described as "pleasant."

A "turkey" is something quite different. A turkey is a patient who asks a lot of questions, demands respect, knows his or her rights, and won't stop wanting to be a part of his or her own healing care. In other words, a smart and careful medical consumer. This is somebody many doctors and nurses happily could do without. Turkeys of the world, we salute you!

Here are abbreviations you are likely to encounter in medical records, on forms or prescriptions, or overhear in hospital rooms and corridors:

a = before
aa = of each
a.c. = before meals
Ad. = to, up to
ADL = activities of daily living
ad lib = as needed, as desired
A.F. = auricular fibrillation
agit = shake, stir
AMA = against medical advice
Ap. = appendicitis
Aq. = water
A.S.H.D. = arteriosclerotic heart
B.E. = barium enema
b.i.d. = twice a day
Bl. time = bleeding time
B.M. = bowel movement
B.M.R. = basal metabolic rate
BP = blood pressure
BRP = bathroom privileges
Bx = biopsy
C = centigrade
$\bar{c}$ = with
CA = cancer
CAD = coronary artery disease
cap(s) = capsule(s)
CBC = complete blood count
CBD = common bile duct
cc = cubic centimeter
CC = chief complaint
CCU = coronary care unit
CHD = coronary heart disease; or congenital heart
    disease

CHF = congestive heart disease failure
Chol = cholesterol
Cl. time = clotting time
CNS = central nervous system
comp = compound
cont rem = continue the medicine
COPD = chronic obstructive pulmonary disease
CSF = cerebrospinal fluid
CV = cardiovascular
CVA = cerebrovascular accident
CVP = central venous pressure
CXR = chest X ray
d = give
D&C = dilation and curettage
dd in d = from day to day
dec = pour off
dexter = the right
dil = dilute
Disp. = dispense
div = divide
DM = diabetes mellitus
dos = dose
dur dolor - while pain lasts
D/W = dextrose in water
Dx = diagnosis
ECG or EKG = electrocardiogram
EEG = electroencephalogram
emp = as directed
ER = emergency room
F = Fahrenheit
FBS = fasting blood sugar
febris = fever
FH = family history
Fx = fracture
GA = general anesthesia
garg = gargle
GB = gallbladder
GC = gonorrhea
GI = gastrointestinal
GL = glaucoma
gm = grams
"gomer" = "Get out of my emergency room"
        (a patient no one wants to treat)
"gork" = a brain-damaged person
gr. = grains
grad = by degrees
gravida = pregnancies
gtt. = drops
GTT = glucose tolerance test
GU = genitourinary

GYN = gynecology

h = hour

HASHD = hypertensive arteriosclerotic
heart disease

Hb or Hgb = hemoglobin

HCT = hematocrit

HHD = hypertensive heart disease

HOB = head of bed

h.s. = at bedtime, before retiring

Hx = history

ICU = intensive care unit

I&D = incision and drainage

IM = intramuscular

I.M. = infectious mononucleosis

ind = daily

I&O = intake and output (measure fluids going into
and out of body)

IPPB = intermittent positive pressure breathing

IV = intravenous

IVP = intravenous pyelogram

L = left

liq = liquid

LLE = left lower extremity

LLQ = left lower quadrant

LMP = last menstrual period

LOL = "little old lady" (a passive, unquestioning female senior citizen)

LP = lumbar puncture

LUE = left upper extremity

LUQ = left upper quadrant

(m) = murmur

M = mix

m et n = morning and night

mg = milligrams

MI = heart attack (myocardial infarction)

mor dict = in the manner directed

M.S. = morphine sulfate

neg. = negative

N-G = nasogastric

no. = number

non rep; nr = do not repeat

NPO = non per os (nothing by mouth)

NS = normal saline

NSR = normal heart rate

N&V = nausea and vomiting

o = none

O = oxygen

OD = right eye

O.D. = once a day

OL = left eye

OOB = out of bed

OPD = outpatient department

OR = operating room

OS = left eye

OT = occupational therapy

OU = both eyes

P;$\overline{P}$ = after

Para = number of births

Path. = pathology

pc = after meals

PE = physical examination; rotic heart disease or pulmonary embolus

PI = present illness

pil = pill

P.O. = per os (by mouth)

Post. = posterior

post-op = postoperative, after the operation

PR = pulse rate; or rectally

prn = as needed, as often as necessary

Prog. = prognosis

pt = patient

PT = physical therapy

PTA = prior to admission

Px = prognosis

q = every

q.h. = every hour (q4h = every 4 hours; q8h = every
8 hours; and so on)

qid = four times a day

qn = every night

qod = every other day

qs = proper amount, quantity sufficient

qv = as much as desired

R = right

rbc = red blood cells

RBC = red blood cell count

rep = repeat

RHD = rheumatic heart disease

RLQ = right lower quadrant

RN = registered nurse

ROM = range of motion

RR = respiratory rate; or recovery room

RT = radiation therapy

rub = red

RUQ = right upper quadrant

Rx = prescription; or therapy

$\overline{s}$ = without

S&A = sugar and acetone (a urine test)

SC = subcutaneous

scop. = scopolamine

SH = social history

SICU = surgical intensive care unit
sig = write, let it be imprinted
sing = of each
SOB = shortness of breath
sol = solution
solv = dissolve
SOP = standard operating procedure
SOS = can repeat in emergency
ss = half
S&S = signs and symptoms
SSE = soapsuds enema
stat = right away, immediately
sub Q = subcutaneous
suppos = suppository
Sx = symptoms
T&A = tonsillectomy and adenoidectomy
tab = tablet
TAT = tetanus antitoxin
tere = rub
TIA = transient ischemic attacks
tid = three times a day
tinc. or tinct. = tincture
TPR = temperature, pulse, and respiration
Tx = treatment
ung = ointment
URI = upper respiratory infection
ut dict = as directed
UTI = urinary tract infection
VD = venereal disease
VS = vital signs
WBC = white blood cell count
WC = wheelchair
YO = year old
↑ = increase
↗ = increasing
↓ = decrease
↙ = decreasing
→ = leads to
← = resulting from
♂ = male
♀ = female

MEDICAL TERM DERIVATIVES... IT DOESN'T HAVE TO BE GREEK TO YOU

As the medical world becomes more specialized and technical (and as new medical "cures" are invented yearly), medical terms appear to multiply overnight. To unlock the code, all you need is the key to translating the terms.

As a rule, medical terms are built from three blocks—the prefixes, roots, and suffixes. Each block doesn't mean much on its own. But when interlocked, these blocks form an infinite number of long and mysterious medical words much favored by white-coated professionals. Fortunately, you don't need the degree of *medicinae doctor* to decode these terms. Just refer to the following translation table to locate the meaning of the blocks and convert them into understandable words and phrases.

First, the *prefixes*, the blocks that sit at the front of words to indicate the wheres, ifs, and how muches.

a, an = not, without
ab = away from
acid = sour
ad = near (*d* changes to *c, f, g, p, s,* or *t* when it precedes roots that begin with those letters)
alb = white
amph(i) = both, twice as much
ante = before
anti = against
ap(o) = detached
brady = slow
contra = against, counter to
cry = cold
dia = through or passing through, going apart, between, across
dys = painful, difficult
e = out from
ecto = outside of, outer, exterior
endo = within
epi = upon, on, over
erythr = red
eso = inside
exo = outside of
hemi = half
hyper = increased, excessive, above
hypo = under, below, deficient
in = not (*n* changes to *l, m,* or *r* when it precedes roots that begin with those letters)
infra = below
inter = between
intra = within
leuco, leuko = white
macro = large
mal = bad, ill, wrongful, disordered
meta = after, beyond, changing
micro = small
para = beyond, beside

peri = around
poly = many, multiple
post = after
pre = before, in front of
pseud(o) = false
re = again
retro = backward, behind
sub = under, below
super = above, beyond, over
supra = above
syn (sy, syl, sym) = with, together
tachy = fast

The next group of blocks, which are called the *roots,* are at the center of the words. When used in medical terms, the roots usually indicate the body parts affected by a condition.

abdomin = abdomen, stomach
adeno = gland
adip = fat
angi(o) = vessel (blood, lymph)
aph = sense of touch
arteri(o) = artery
arthr(o) = joint
aur = ear
blephar = eyelid
brachi = arm
bronch = windpipe
cardi(o) = heart
cephal = head
cervic = neck
chole, cholo = bile, gall
cholecyst = gallbladder
chondr = cartilage
col(o) = colon
colpo = vagina
crani(o) = skull
cut = skin
cystido, cysto = bladder, sac, cyst
cyto = cell
dent = tooth
enter = intestine
fasci = face
gastr(o) = stomach
glyco = sugar
gnath = jaw
hema, hemato, hemo = blood
hepat(o) = liver
hyster(o) = uterus

ile, ili = intestines, lower abdomen
labi = lip
lact = milk
lapar = loin, flank, abdomen
laryng = windpipe
lipo = fat
lumbar = loin
mast = breast
meno = menstruation
ment = mind
myel = marrow
myelo = spinal cord
myo = muscle
nephro(o) = kidney
neur(o) = nerve
ocul = eye
odont = teeth
oophor = ovary
ophthalm = eye
orchii(o) = testicle
os = mouth, opening
oss, oste(o) = bone
ot(o) = ear
ov = egg
pharyng = throat
phleb = vein
pleur = rib
pneuma, pneumato, pneumo = air, gas, lung
pod = foot
procto = anus, rectum
pulmo = lung
ren = kidney
rhino = nose
salping = fallopian tube
sperm, spermato = semen
splen = spleen
staphyl = uvula
stear = fat
tact = touch
teno = tendon
thorac(o) = chest
thromb = clot, lump
tracheo = windpipe
ur = urine
ureter(o) = tube from kidney to bladder,
            carrying urine
urethra = tube from bladder to the exterior
vas = vessel, duct
veno = vein
vesic = bladder

Finally, there are the *suffixes*, the linguistic cabooses that specify what has gone wrong with—or what will be done to—the part of the body designated by a medical word's prefix and root.

algia = pain
blast = a growth in its early stages
cele = tumor, hernia
cente = puncture
desis = fusion
dynia = pain
ectomy = excision of, surgical removal
hydr = water
itis = inflammation
lysis = freeing of
megaly = very large
oma = tumor, swelling
oscopy = looking at an organ or internal part
osis = disease, abnormal condition or process
ostomy = creation of an artificial opening
otomy = incision, cutting into
pathy = disease of, abnormality
pexy = fix, sew
plasty = reconstruct, formation of
pnea = breathing
ptosis = falling, drooping
rhage, rhagia, rrhage, rrhagis = bursting forth, bleeding
rhea, rrhea = flow, discharge
scler(osis) = hard, hardening
uria = urine (condition of, presence in)

Put the blocks together, and they form a medical term. For example, suppose your doctor says that you are suffering from endocarditis. Just consult the lists: prefix "endo" means within; "cardio" has to do with the heart; and "itis" means inflammation. Endocarditis: inflammation of the inside of the heart (more or less). Certainly not a cheery diagnosis, but at least you have the information you need to ask more intelligent questions about what is going to happen to you next.

Getting a Second Opinion

A second opinion is another doctor's advice or thoughts on a diagnosis of a condition, method of treatment, or the necessity of treatment. It is becoming common practice, not only among doctors but also among many medical insurers who have made it mandatory before they will agree to pay for a procedure. It is important for any consumer to realize that he or she has a right to a second opinion.

A consumer wishing to obtain a second opinion may ask another doctor—in other words, not his or her regular practitioner—for additional information and advice. A second opinion may be initiated by the regular doctor himself and may come in the form of a doctor's referral to another doctor or specialist. Or the patient may decide to seek another doctor's opinion on the diagnosis, treatment, and cost of treatment.

WHY ASK FOR A SECOND OPINION?

A second opinion is often useful because not all doctors agree on medical problems—what they are, how to diagnose them, and how (or even whether) to treat them. And too often people accept the opinion of their family doctors or surgeons and undergo a lot of pain, financial hardship, and perhaps complications and doctor-caused mishaps because of procedures that might not have been necessary in the first place.

A second opinion is vitally important, especially if a trip to the hospital looms in your near future. Even a good doctor, convinced that the benefits of surgery outweigh more conservative and less costly treatment, can be eager to rush you into the operating room. True, a second opinion might confirm the original diagnosis (and perhaps the need for hospitalization), but it could also contradict the first doctor's conclusions and thus precipitate some doubt about the need for hospitalization. You may even require a third, tie-breaking opinion.

But don't limit the search for a second opinion merely to procedures that involve surgery. Many types of therapy performed in a hospital are risky or invasive even though not surgical. Ask another doctor for assurance about the need for any procedure that concerns you.

WHOM DO YOU ASK?

A lot of second-opinion doctors recommended by first-opinion doctors turn out to be not that valuable in terms of independent judgments. This is true in part because surgeons are the doctors most often asked for second opinions, and they generally recommend surgery over less invasive procedures. The other, more prevalent problem is that second-opinion doctors may be reluctant to disagree with the friend who recommended them. The truth is that doctors depend on each other for referrals, and too many non-confirming second opinions may lead to a loss of referrals. Therefore, you should consider finding yourself a doctor for a fair and original second opinion.

HOW DO YOU BEGIN?

First, check the *Directory of Medical Specialists* in your local library's reference section. In addition, check with your employer's benefits department or ask your insurance company to provide you with a list of physicians it uses for its second-opinion program. New York Hospital–Cornell Medical Center's Health Benefits Research Center also sponsors a toll-free referral service called the National Second Opinion Program. The number there is 800-522-0036.

A Medicare beneficiary may contact the local Social Security Administration office for a directory of doctors who participate in the Medicare second-opinion program.

Academies

The following academies represent medical professionals who are interested in the scientific aspects of their particular specialty, especially where matters of quality of care are concerned.

American Academy of Allergy and Immunology (AAAI)
611 E. Wells Street
Milwaukee, WI 53202

American Academy for Cerebral Palsy and Developmental Medicine (AACPDM)
1910 Byrd Avenue, #118
P.O. Box 11086
Richmond, VA 23230-1086

American Academy of Child and Adolescent Psychiatry (AACAP)
3615 Wisconsin Avenue N.W.
Washington, DC 20016

American Academy of Cosmetic Surgery (AACS)
159 E. Live Oak Avenue, Suite 204
Arcadia, CA 91006

American Academy of Craniomandibular Disorders (AACD)
10 Joplin Court
Lafayette, CA 94549

American Academy of Crown and Bridge Prosthodontics (AACBP)
3302 Gaston Avenue, Room 330
Dallas, TX 75246

American Academy of Dental Electrosurgery (AADE)
P.O. Box 374, Planetarium Station
New York, NY 10024

American Academy of Dental Radiology (AADR)
P.O. Box 31162
Aurora, CO 80041

American Academy of Dermatology (AAD)
1567 Maple Avenue
P.O. Box 3116
Evanston, IL 60201-3116

American Academy of Environmental Medicine (AAEM)
P.O. Box 16106
Denver, CO 80216

American Academy of Esthetic Dentistry (AAED)
500 N. Michigan Avenue, Suite 1400
Chicago, IL 60611

American Academy of Facial Plastic and Reconstructive Surgery (AAFPRS)
1110 Vermont Avenue N.W., Suite 220
Washington, DC 20005

American Academy of Family Physicians (AAFP)
8880 Ward Parkway
Kansas City, MO 64114

American Academy of Gnathologic Orthopedics (AAGO)
1723 N. Hearthside Court
Richmond, TX 77469

American Academy of Head, Facial and Neck Pain and TMJ Orthopedics (AAHFNPTO)
Atlantic Building, Suite 1310
260 S. Broad Street
Philadelphia, PA 19102

American Academy of Implant Dentistry (AAID)
6900 Grove Road
Thorofare, NJ 08086

American Academy of Implant Prosthodontics (AAIP)
5555 Peachtree-Dunwoody Road N.E., Suite 140
Atlanta, GA 30342

American Academy of Maxillofacial Prosthetics (AAMP)
MCG/School of Dentistry
Department of Prosthodontics
Augusta, GA 30912

American Academy of Medical Hypnoanalysts (AAMH)
5587 Murray Road
Memphis, TN 38119

American Academy of Neurological and Orthopaedic Surgeons (FAANAOS)
2320 Rancho Drive, Suite 108
Las Vegas, NV 89102

American Academy of Neurological Surgery
Department of Neurosurgery
Temple University Hospital
3401 N. Broad Street
Philadelphia, PA 19140

American Academy of Neurology (AAN)
2221 University Avenue S.E., Suite 335
Minneapolis, MN 55414

American Academy of Nurse Practitioners (AANP)
Capitol Station, LBJ Building
P.O. Box 12846
Austin, TX 78711

American Academy of Ophthalmology (AAO)
655 Beach Street
San Francisco, CA 94109

American Academy of Optometry (AAO)
5530 Wisconsin Avenue N.W., Suite 1149
Washington, DC 20815

American Academy of Oral Medicine (AAOM)
4143 Mischive
Houston, TX 77025

American Academy of Orthodontics for the General Practitioner (AAOGP)
3953 N. 76th Street
Milwaukee, WI 53222

American Academy of Orthopaedic Surgeons (AAOS)
222 S. Prospect Avenue
Park Ridge, IL 60068-4058

American Academy of Orthotists and Prosthetists
717 Pendleton Street
Alexandria, VA 22314

American Academy of Osteopathy (AAO)
P.O. Box 750
1127 Mt. Vernon Road
Newark, OH 43055

American Academy of Otolaryngic Allergy (AAOA)
8455 Colesville Road, Suite 745
Silver Spring, MD 20910-9998

American Academy of Otolaryngology—Head and Neck Surgery (AAO—HNS)
1 Prince Street
Alexandria, VA 22314

American Academy of Pediatric Dentistry (AAPD)
211 E. Chicago Avenue, Suite 1036
Chicago, IL 60611

American Academy of Pediatrics (AAP)
141 Northwest Point Boulevard
P.O. Box 927
Elk Grove Village, IL 60009-0927

American Academy of Periodontology (AAP)
211 E. Chicago Avenue, Suite 1400
Chicago, IL 60611

American Academy of Physical Medicine and Rehabilitation (AAPMR)
122 S. Michigan Avenue, Suite 1300
Chicago, IL 60603

American Academy of Physician Assistants (AAPA)
950 N. Washington Street
Alexandria, VA 22314

American Academy of Podiatric Sports Medicine (AAPSM)
1729 Glastonberry Road
Potomac, MD 20854

American Academy of Psychotherapists (AAP)
P.O. Box 607
Decatur, GA 30031

American Academy of Restorative Dentistry (AARD)
P.O. Box 247
Marshfield, WI 54449

American Academy of Somnology (AAS)
P.O. Box 29124
Las Vegas, NV 89126

American Academy of Spinal Surgeons (AASS)
2320 Rancho Drive, Suite 108
Las Vegas, NV 89102-4592

American Academy of Sports Physicians (AASP)
17113 Gledhill Street
Northridge, CA 91325

American Academy of Thermology (AAT)
138 Church Street N.E.
Vienna, VA 22180

American Academy of Tropical Medicine (AATM)
16126 E. Warren
Detroit, MI 48224

Source: Medical and Health Information Directory, 1992–93.

Associations

The following associations promote the professional, economic, and political interests of their members by disseminating information to members and the general public.

American Association for Acupuncture and Oriental Medicine
1424 16th Street N.W., Suite 501
Washington, DC 20036

American Association of Ayurvedic Medicine
P.O. Box 541
Lancaster, MA 01523

American Association of Behavioral Therapists
P.O. Box 767156
Roswell, GA 30076-7156

American Association of Cardiovascular and Pulmonary Rehabilitation
7611 Elmwood Avenue, Suite 201
Middleton, WI 53562

American Association of Certified Allergists
800 E. Northwest Highway, Suite 1080
Palatine, IL 60067

American Association of Certified Orthoptists
Hermann Eye Center
6411 Fannin
Houston, TX 77030-1697

American Association of Community Psychiatrists
P.O. Box 5372
Arlington, VA 22205

American Association for Counseling and Development
5999 Stevenson Avenue
Alexandria, VA 22304

American Association of Critical-Care Nurses
1 Civic Plaza
Newport Beach, CA 92660

American Association of Electrodiagnostic Medicine
21 2nd Street S.W., Suite 306
Rochester, MN 55902

American Association of Endodontists
211 E. Chicago Avenue, Suite 1501
Chicago, IL 60611

American Association of Foot Specialists
P.O. Box 54
Union, NJ 07083

American Association for Functional Orthodontics
106 S. Kent Street
Winchester, VA 22601

American Association of Genito-Urinary Surgeons
Baylor College of Medicine
6560 Fannin, Suite 1004
Houston, TX 77030

American Association for Geriatric Psychiatry
P.O. Box 376-A
Greenbelt, MD 20768

American Association of Gynecological Laparoscopists
13021 E. Florence Avenue
Santa Fe Springs, CA 90670

American Association for Hand Surgery
2934 Fish Hatchery Road, Suite 210
Madison, WI 53713

American Association of Homeopathic Pharmacists
P.O. Box 2273
Falls Church, VA 22042

American Association of Immunologists
9650 Rockville Pike
Bethesda, MD 20014

American Association of Neurological Surgeons
22 S. Washington Street, Suite 100
Park Ridge, IL 60068

American Association of Neuropathologists
204 Farber Hall
Department of Pathology
Buffalo Medical School, State University of New York
Buffalo, NY 14214

American Association of Neuroscience Nurses
218 N. Jefferson Street, #204
Chicago, IL 60606

American Association of Nurse Anesthetists
216 W. Higgins Road
Park Ridge, IL 60068-5790

American Association of Nutritional Consultants
1641 E. Sunset Road, B117
Las Vegas, NV 89119

American Association of Occupational Health Nurses
50 Lenox Pointe
Atlanta, GA 30324

American Association of Oral and Maxillofacial Surgeons
9700 W. Bryn Mawr
Rosemont, IL 60018

American Association of Oriental Healing Arts
P.O. Box 718
Jamaica Plain, MA 02130

American Association of Orthodontists
460 N. Lindbergh Boulevard
St. Louis, MO 63141-7883

American Association of Orthomolecular Medicine
900 N. Federal Highway, Suite 330
Boca Raton, FL 33432

American Association of Orthopedic Medicine
5147 Lewiston Road
Lewiston, NY 14092

American Association of Osteopathic Specialists
804 Main Street, Suite D
Forest Park, GA 30050

American Association of Plastic Surgeons
10666 N. Torrey Pines Road
La Jolla, CA 92037

American Association of Podiatric Physicians and Surgeons
603 Griswold Street
Port Huron, MI 48060

American Association for Rehabilitation Therapy
P.O. Box 93
North Little Rock, AR 72115

American Association for Respiratory Care
11030 Ables Lane
Dallas, TX 75229

American Association of Sex Educators, Counselors and Therapists
435 N. Michigan Avenue, Suite 1717
Chicago, IL 60611

American Association of Spinal Cord Injury Nurses
75-20 Astoria Boulevard
Jackson Heights, NY 11370-1178

American Association for the Surgery of Trauma
New York Burn Center
525 E. 68th Street, L-706
New York, NY 10021

American Association for Thoracic Surgery
13 Elm Street
P.O. Box 1565
Manchester, MA 01944

American Association of Women Dentists
111 E. Wacker Drive, Suite 600
Chicago, IL 60601

American Association of Women Radiologists
1891 Preston White Drive
Reston, VA 22091

Colleges

The following colleges represent physicians, researchers, and educators interested in advancing the practice of their particular specialty by establishing educational programs and promoting professional standards.

American College of Advancement in Medicine (ACAM)
23121 Verdugo Drive, Suite 204
Laguna Hills, CA 92653

American College of Allergy and Immunology (ACAI)
800 E. Northwest Highway, Suite 1080
Palatine, IL 60067

American College of Cardiology (ACC)
9111 Old Georgetown Road
Bethesda, MD 20814

American College of Chest Physicians (ACCP)
330 Dundee Road
Northbrook, IL 60062

American College of Chiropractic Orthopedists (ACCO)
1030 Broadway, Suite 101
El Centro, CA 92243

American College of Cryosurgery (ACC)
P.O. Box 3116
Evanston, IL 60204

American College of Dentists (ACD)
7315 Wisconsin Avenue, Suite 352N
Bethesda, MD 20814

American College of Emergency Physicians (ACEP)
P.O. Box 619911
Dallas, TX 75261-9911

American College of Foot Orthopedists (ACFO)
108 Orange Street, Suite 6
Redlands, CA 92373

American College of Foot Surgeons (ACFS)
444 N. Northwest Highway, Suite 155
Park Ridge, IL 60068

American College of Gastroenterology (ACG)
4222 King Street
Alexandria, VA 22302

American College of General Practitioners in Osteopathic Medicine and Surgery (ACGPOMS)
330 E. Algonquin
Arlington Heights, IL 60005

American College of Home Obstetrics (ACHO)
P.O. Box 508
Oak Park, IL 60303

American College of Mohs Micrographic Surgery and Cutaneous Oncology (ACMMSCO)
P.O. Box 3116
Evanston, IL 60204

American College of Neuropsychiatrists (ACN)
28595 Orchard Lake Road, Suite 200
Farmington Hills, MI 48334

American College of Neuropsychopharmacology (ACNP)
Vanderbilt University
Box 1823, Station B
Nashville, TN 37235

American College of Nuclear Medicine (ACNM)
P.O. Box 5887
Columbus, GA 31906

American College of Nuclear Physicians (ACNP)
1101 Connecticut Avenue N.W., Suite 700
Washington, DC 20036

American College of Nurse-Midwives (ACNM)
1522 K Street N.W., Suite 1000
Washington, DC 20005

American College of Nutrition (ACN)
722 Robert E. Lee Drive
Wilmington, NC 28412-0927

American College of Obstetricians and Gynecologists (ACOG)
409 12th Street S.W.
Washington, DC 20024

American College of Occupational Medicine (ACOM)
55 W. Seegers Road
Arlington Heights, IL 60005

American College of Oral and Maxillofacial Surgeons (ACOMS)
1100 N.W. Loop 410, Suite 500
San Antonio, TX 78213-2266

American College of Orgonomy (ACO)
P.O. Box 490
Princeton, NJ 08542

American College of Osteopathic Emergency Physicians (ACOEP)
5200 S. Ellis Avenue
Chicago, IL 60615

American College of Osteopathic Internists (ACOI)
300 5th Street N.E.
Washington, DC 20002

American College of Osteopathic Obstetricians and Gynecologists (ACOOG)
900 Auburn Road
Pontiac, MI 48342

American College of Osteopathic Pediatricians (ACOP)
172 W. State Street, Suite 303
Trenton, NJ 08608

American College of Osteopathic Surgeons (ACOS)
123 N. Henry Street
Alexandria, VA 22314

American College of Physicians (ACP)
Independence Mall W.
6th Street at Race
Philadelphia, PA 19106

American College of Podiatric Radiologists (ACPR)
169 Lincoln Road, #308
Miami Beach, FL 33139

American College of Podopediatrics (ACP)
10515 Carnegie Avenue
Cleveland, OH 44106

American College of Preventive Medicine (ACPM)
1015 15th Street N.W., Suite 403
Washington, DC 20005

American College of Prosthodontists (ACP)
1777 N.E. Loop 410, Suite 904
San Antonio, TX 78217

American College of Psychiatrists (ACP)
P.O. Box 365
Greenbelt, MD 20768

American College of Psychoanalysts (ACPA)
2006 Dwight Way, #304
Berkeley, CA 94704

American College of Radiology (ACR)
1891 Preston White Drive
Reston, VA 22091

American College of Rheumatology (ACR)
17 Executive Park Drive N.E., Suite 480
Atlanta, GA 30329

American College of Sports Medicine (ACSM)
P.O. Box 1440
Indianapolis, IN 46206-1440

American College of Surgeons (ACS)
55 E. Erie Street
Chicago, IL 60611

Medical Societies

Medical societies are trade groups that represent the professional, educational, legislative, and economic interests of their members. In addition to the national organization, these societies have affiliated groups in each state. The following list contains the national and state organizations for allopathic (M.D.) and osteopathic (D.O.) physicians.

Allopathic Medicine

American Medical Association
515 N. State Street
Chicago, IL 60610
312-464-5000

State-Affiliated Societies

Medical Association of the State of Alabama
19 S. Jackson Street
Montgomery, AL 36104
205-263-6441

Alaska State Medical Association
4107 Laurel
Anchorage, AK 99508
907-562-2662

Arizona Medical Association
810 W. Bethany Home Road
Phoenix, AZ 85013
602-246-8901

Arkansas Medical Society
10 Corporate Hill Drive
Little Rock, AR 72205
501-224-8967

California Medical Association
221 Main Street
San Francisco, CA 94120
415-541-0900

Colorado Medical Society
P.O. Box 17550
Denver, CO 80217
303-779-5455

Connecticut State Medical Society
160 St. Ronan Street
New Haven, CT 06511
203-865-0587

Medical Society of Delaware
1925 Lovering Avenue
Wilmington, DE 19806
302-658-7596

Medical Society of the District of Columbia
1707 L Street N.W., Suite 400
Washington, DC 20036
202-466-1800

Florida Medical Association
760 Riverside Avenue
Jacksonville, FL 32204
904-356-1571

Medical Association of Georgia
938 Peachtree Street N.E.
Atlanta, GA 30309
404-876-7535

Hawaii Medical Association
1360 S. Beretania
Honolulu, HI 96814
808-536-7702

Idaho Medical Association
305 W. Jefferson
P.O. Box 2668
Boise, ID 83701
208-344-7888

Illinois State Medical Society
20 N. Michigan, Suite 700
Chicago, IL 60602
312-782-1654

Indiana State Medical Association
3935 N. Meridian Street
Indianapolis, IN 46208
317-925-7545

Iowa Medical Society
1001 Grand Avenue
West Des Moines, IA 50265
515-223-1401

Kansas Medical Society
1300 Topeka Avenue
Topeka, KS 66612
913-235-2383

Kentucky Medical Association
3532 Ephraim McDowell Drive
Louisville, KY 40205
502-459-9790

Louisiana State Medical Society
1700 Josephine Street
New Orleans, LA 70113
504-561-1033

Maine Medical Association
P.O. Box 190
Manchester, ME 04351
207-622-3374

Medical and Chirurgical Faculty of the State of Maryland
1211 Cathedral Street
Baltimore, MD 21201
410-539-0872

Massachusetts Medical Society
1440 Main Street
Waltham, MA 02154
617-893-4610

Michigan State Medical Society
120 W. Saginaw
East Lansing, MI 48826
517-337-1351

Minnesota Medical Association
2221 University Avenue S.E., Suite 400
Minneapolis, MN 55414
612-378-1875

Mississippi State Medical Association
P.O. Box 5229
Jackson, MS 39216
601-354-5433

Missouri State Medical Association
P.O. Box 1028
Jefferson City, MO 65102
314-636-5151

Montana Medical Association
2021 11th Avenue, Suite 1
Helena, MT 59601
406-443-4000

Nebraska Medical Association
1512 FirsTier Bank Building
Lincoln, NE 68508
402-474-4472

Nevada State Medical Association
3660 Baker Lane
Reno, NV 89509
702-825-6788

New Hampshire Medical Society
7 N. State Street
Concord, NH 03301
603-224-1909

Medical Society of New Jersey
2 Princess Road
Lawrenceville, NJ 08648
609-896-1766

New Mexico Medical Society
7770 Jefferson N.E.
Albuquerque, NM 87109
505-828-0237

Medical Society of the State of New York
420 Lakeville Road
Lake Success, NY 11042
516-488-6100

North Carolina Medical Society
222 N. Person Street
Raleigh, NC 27601
919-833-3836

North Dakota Medical Association
204 W. Thayer Avenue
Bismarck, ND 58501
701-223-9475

Ohio State Medical Association
1500 Lake Shore Drive
Columbus, OH 43204
614-486-2401

Oklahoma State Medical Association
601 Northwest Expressway
Oklahoma City, OK 73118
405-843-9571

Oregon Medical Association
5210 S.W. Corbett
Portland, OR 97201
503-226-1555

Pennsylvania Medical Society
777 E. Park Drive
P.O. Box 8820
Harrisburg, PA 17105-8820
717-558-7750

Puerto Rico Medical Association
1305 Fernández Juncos Avenue
Santurce, PR 00908
809-721-6969

Rhode Island Medical Society
106 Francis Street
Providence, RI 02903
401-331-3207

South Carolina Medical Association
P.O. Box 11188
Columbia, SC 29211
803-798-6207

South Dakota State Medical Association
1323 S. Minnesota Avenue
Sioux Falls, SD 57105
605-336-1965

Tennessee Medical Association
P.O. Box 120909
Nashville, TN 37212
615-385-2100

Texas Medical Association
401 W. 15th Street
Austin, TX 78701
512-370-1300

Utah Medical Association
540 E. 500 S.
Salt Lake City, UT 84102
801-355-7477

Vermont State Medical Society
136 Main Street
P.O. Box H
Montpelier, VT 05601
802-223-7898

Virgin Islands Medical Society
P.O. Box 520
St. Croix, VI 00820

Medical Society of Virginia
4205 Dover Road
Richmond, VA 23221
804-353-2721

Washington State Medical Association
2033 6th Avenue, Suite 900
Seattle, WA 98121
206-441-9762

West Virginia State Medical Association
P.O. Box 4106
Charleston, WV 25364
304-925-0342

State Medical Society of Wisconsin
P.O. Box 1109
Madison, WI 53701
608-257-6781

Wyoming Medical Society
P.O. Drawer 4009
Cheyenne, WY 82003
307-635-2424

Osteopathic Medicine

American Osteopathic Association
142 E. Ontario Street
Chicago, IL 60611
312-280-5800
800-621-1773

State-Affiliated Societies

Alabama Osteopathic Medical Association
800 W. Memorial Drive
Piedmont, AL 36272
205-272-1002

Alaska Osteopathic Medical Association
10928 Eagle River Road, Suite 130
Eagle River, AK 99577
907-248-2400

Arizona Osteopathic Medical Association
5057 E. Thomas Road
Phoenix, AZ 85018
602-840-0460

Arkansas Osteopathic Medical Association
101 Windwood Drive, Suite 5
Beebe, AR 72012
501-882-7540

Osteopathic Physicians and Surgeons of California
1010 11th Street, Suite 220
Sacramento, CA 95814
916-447-2004
800-638-6772

Colorado Society of Osteopathic Medicine
50 S. Steele Street, Suite 440
Denver, CO 80209
303-322-1752

Connecticut Osteopathic Medical Society
225 Main Street
Manchester, CT 06040
203-646-8534

Delaware State Osteopathic Medical Society
P.O. Box 845
Wilmington, DE 19899
302-764-6120

Osteopathic Association of the District of Columbia
4001 N. 9th Street, Suite 216
Arlington, VA 22203
703-522-8404

Association of Military Osteopathic Physicians and Surgeons
P.O. Box 273294
Boca Raton, FL 33427
407-368-5971

Florida Osteopathic Medical Association
2007 Apalachee Parkway
Tallahassee, FL 32301
904-878-7364

Georgia Osteopathic Medical Association
1900 The Exchange, Suite 160
Atlanta, GA 30338
404-953-0801

Hawaii Association of Osteopathic Physicians and Surgeons
122 Oneawa Street
Kailua, HI 96734
808-261-6105

Idaho Osteopathic Medical Association
522 W. Main Street
Grangeville, ID 83530
208-376-2522

Illinois Association of Osteopathic Physicians and Surgeons
P.O. Box 1037
Ottawa, IL 61350
815-434-5576

Indiana Association of Osteopathic Physicians and Surgeons
3520 Guion Road, #106
Indianapolis, IN 46222
317-926-3009

Iowa Osteopathic Medical Association
1113 Locust Street, Suite 2-B
Des Moines, IA 50309
515-283-0002

Kansas Association of Osteopathic Medicine
1260 S.W. Topeka Boulevard
Topeka, KS 66612
913-234-5563

Kentucky Osteopathic Medical Association
796 Shamrock Drive
Madisonville, KY 42431
502-223-5322

Louisiana Association of Osteopathic Physicians
6018 Colbert Street
New Orleans, LA 70124
504-488-6743

Maine Osteopathic Association
R.R. 5, Box 140
Augusta, ME 04330
207-623-1101

Maryland Osteopathic Association
Routes 32 and 144
West Friendship, MD 21794
301-489-7272

Massachusetts Osteopathic Society
237 Main Street
P.O. Box 147
Reading, MA 01867
508-896-7247

Michigan Association of Osteopathic Physicians and Surgeons
33100 Freedom Road
Farmington, MI 48366
313-476-2800
800-543-2136

Minnesota Osteopathic Medical Society
Hoffman Clinic
Hoffman, MN 56339-0206
612-986-2038

Mississippi Osteopathic Medical Association
89 Jeff Street
Oxford, MS 38655
601-482-9695

Missouri Association of Osteopathic Physicians and Surgeons
1423 Randy Lane
P.O. Box 748
Jefferson City, MO 65102
314-634-3415

Montana Osteopathic Association
Box 2004
Phillipsburg, MT 59858
602-242-1701

Nebraska Association of Osteopathic Physicians and Surgeons
Box 24744, West Omaha Station
Omaha, NE 68124
913-234-5563 (Calls taken by Kansas Association.)

Nevada Osteopathic Medical Association
2300 S. Rancho Road
Las Vegas, NV 89102
702-255-6665

New Hampshire Osteopathic Association
RFD 2, Bible Hill Lane
Warner, NH 03278-1333
603-456-2178

New Jersey Association of Osteopathic Physicians and Surgeons
1212 Stuyvesant Avenue
Trenton, NJ 08618
609-393-8114

New Mexico Osteopathic Medical Association
P.O. Box 3096
Albuquerque, NM 87190
505-828-1905

New York State Osteopathic Medical Society
87 S. Lake Avenue
Albany, NY 12203
518-663-8812
800-841-4131

North Carolina Medical Association
207 Viking Drive
Fayetteville, NC 28303
919-864-7515

North Dakota Association of Osteopathic Physicians and Surgeons
737 Broadway
Fargo, ND 58123
701-293-7262

Ohio Osteopathic Association
53 W. 3rd Street
P.O. Box 8130
Columbus, OH 43201
614-299-2107

Oklahoma Osteopathic Association
4848 N. Lincoln Boulevard
Oklahoma City, OK 73105-3321
405-528-4848
800-522-8379

Osteopathic Physicians and Surgeons of Oregon
9221 S.W. Barbur Boulevard, Suite 310
Portland, OR 97219
503-244-7592

Pennsylvania Osteopathic Medical Association
1330 Eisenhower Boulevard
Harrisburg, PA 17111
717-939-9318
800-544-7662

Rhode Island Society of Osteopathic Physicians and Surgeons
1763 Broad Street
Cranston, RI 02905
401-781-3940

South Carolina Osteopathic Association
P.O. Box 31433
Charleston, SC 29407
803-871-8533

South Dakota Society of Osteopathic Physicians and Surgeons
c/o MASSA-Berry Clinic
Sturgis, SD 57785
605-347-3616

Tennessee Osteopathic Medical Association
1900 The Exchange
Atlanta, GA 30339
404-955-5538

Texas Osteopathic Medical Association
226 Bailey Avenue
Ft. Worth, TX 76107
817-336-0549
800-444-8662

Utah Osteopathic Medical Association
2230 N. University Avenue, Suite 2B
Provo, UT 84604
801-379-7190

Vermont State Association of Osteopathic Physicians and Surgeons
28 School Street
Montpelier, VT 05602
802-229-9418

Virginia Osteopathic Medical Association
2004 Bremo Road, Suite 201
Richmond, VA 23226
804-827-7997
800-452-4244

Washington Osteopathic Medical Association
P.O. Box 16486
Seattle, WA 98116-0486
206-937-5358

West Virginia Society of Osteopathic Medicine
P.O. Box 5266
Charleston, WV 25361
304-345-9836

Wisconsin Association of Osteopathic Physicians and Surgeons
34615 Road E.
Oconomowoc, WI 53066
414-567-0520

Wyoming Association of Osteopathic Physicians and Surgeons
1805 E. 19th Street, Suite 202
Cheyenne, WY 82001
307-635-4362

Medical Specialty Boards (M.D.)

The following certifying boards are recognized by the American Board of Medical Specialties and have jurisdiction over particular specialties and subspecialties. They are responsible for establishing requirements for certification and administering certifying examinations.

American Board of Allergy and Immunology
University City Science Center
3624 Market Street
Philadelphia, PA 19104
215-349-9466

American Board of Anesthesiology
100 Constitution Plaza, Room 1668
Hartford, CT 06103
203-522-9857

American Board of Colon and Rectal Surgery
8750 Telegraph Road, Suite 410
Taylor, MI 48180
313-295-1740

American Board of Dermatology
Henry Ford Hospital
Detroit, MI 48202
313-871-8739

American Board of Emergency Medicine
200 Woodland Pass, Suite D
East Lansing, MI 48823
517-332-4800

American Board of Family Practice
2228 Young Drive
Lexington, KY 40505
606-269-5626

American Board of Internal Medicine
University City Science Center
3624 Market Street
Philadelphia, PA 19104
215-243-1500

American Board of Neurological Surgery
Smith Tower
6550 Fannin Street, Suite 2139
Houston, TX 77030-2701
713-790-6015

American Board of Nuclear Medicine
900 Veteran Avenue, Room 12-200
Los Angeles, CA 90024
213-825-6787

American Board of Obstetrics and Gynecology
4225 Roosevelt Way N.E., Suite 305
Seattle, WA 98105
206-547-4884

American Board of Ophthalmology
111 Presidential Boulevard, Suite 241
Bala Cynwyd, PA 19004
215-664-1175

American Board of Orthopedic Surgery
737 N. Michigan Avenue, Suite 1150
Chicago, IL 60611
312-664-9444

American Board of Otolaryngology
5615 Kirby Drive, Suite 936
Houston, TX 77005
713-528-6200

American Board of Pathology
5401 W. Kennedy Boulevard, Suite 780
P.O. Box 25915
Tampa, FL 33622
813-286-2444

American Board of Pediatrics
111 Silver Cedar Court
Chapel Hill, NC 27514
919-929-0461

American Board of Physical Medicine and Rehabilitation
Norwest Center, Suite 674
21 First Street S.W.
Rochester, MN 55902
507-282-1776

American Board of Plastic Surgery
7 Penn Center
1635 Market Street
Philadelphia, PA 19103-2204
215-587-9322

American Board of Preventive Medicine
Department of Community Medicine
Wright State University School of Medicine
P.O. Box 927
Dayton, OH 45401
513-278-6915

American Board of Psychiatry and Neurology
500 Lake Cook Road, Suite 335
Deerfield, IL 60015
312-945-7900

American Board of Radiology
300 Park, Suite 440
Birmingham, MI 48009
313-645-0600

American Board of Surgery
1617 John F. Kennedy Boulevard, Suite 860
Philadelphia, PA 19103-1847
215-568-4000

American Board of Thoracic Surgery
One Rotary Center, Suite 803
Evanston, IL 60201
312-475-1520

American Board of Urology
31700 Telegraph Road, Suite 150
Birmingham, MI 48010
313-646-9720

Osteopathic Specialty Boards (D.O.)

The following osteopathic certifying boards have jurisdiction over particular specialties and subspecialties and are responsible for establishing requirements for certification and administering certifying examinations.

American Osteopathic Board of General Practice
2474 Dempster Street, Suite 217
Des Plaines, IL 60016
312-635-8477

American Osteopathic Board of Anesthesiology
17201 E. 40 Highway, Suite 204
Independence, MO 64055
816-373-4700

American Osteopathic Board of Dermatology
25510 Plymouth Road
Detroit, MI 48239
313-937-1200

American Osteopathic Board of Emergency Medicine
Philadelphia Osteopathic Medical Center
4190 City Avenue
Philadelphia, PA 19131
215-871-2811

American Osteopathic Board of Internal Medicine
5200 S. Ellis Avenue
Chicago, IL 60615
312-947-4880

American Osteopathic Board of Neurology and Psychiatry
Department of Psychiatry
401 Haddon Avenue
Camden, NJ 08103-1505
609-757-7765

American Osteopathic Board of Nuclear Medicine
5200 S. Ellis Avenue
Chicago, IL 60615
312-947-4490

American Osteopathic Board of Obstetrics and Gynecology
Ohio University College of Osteopathic Medicine
Grosvenor Hall, West 064
Athens, OH 45701
614-593-2239

American Osteopathic Board of Ophthalmology and Otorhinolaryngology
405 Grand Avenue
Dayton, OH 45405
513-222-4213

American Osteopathic Board of Orthopedic Surgery
5155 Raytown Road, Suite 103
Kansas City, MO 64133
816-353-6400

American Osteopathic Board of Pathology
13355 E. Ten Mile Road
Warren, MI 48089
313-759-7565

American Osteopathic Board of Pediatrics
2700 River Road, Suite 407
Des Plaines, IL 60018
312-635-0201

American Osteopathic Board of Preventive Medicine
12535 Lt. Nichols Road
Fairfax, VA 22033
703-648-3834

American Osteopathic Board of Proctology
75 Skylark Road
Springfield, NJ 07081
201-687-2062

American Osteopathic Board of Radiology
Route 2, Box 75
Milan, MO 63556
816-265-4991

American Osteopathic Board of Rehabilitation Medicine
9058 W. Church
Des Plaines, IL 60016
312-699-0048

American Osteopathic Board of Surgery
405 Grand Avenue
Dayton, OH 45405
513-226-2656

State Medical Licensing Boards (M.D.)

The following state boards are responsible for regulating the medical profession, including the issuance of licenses, enforcement of the medical practice act, investigation of complaints against doctors, and imposition of fines, suspensions, and license revocations against doctors who violate the law.

Alabama
Alabama Medical Licensure Commission
P.O. Box 887
Montgomery, AL 36101
205-261-4116

Alaska

Alaska Department of Commerce and Economic Development
State Medical Board
P.O. Box D-LIC
Juneau, AK 99811
907-465-2541

Arizona

Arizona Board of Medical Examiners
2001 W. Camelback Road, Suite 300
Phoenix, AZ 85015
602-255-3751

Arkansas

Arkansas Board of Medical Examiners
P.O. Box 102
Harrisburg, AR 72432
501-578-2448

California

California Board of Medical Quality Assurance
1430 Howe Avenue
Sacramento, CA 95825
916-920-6393

Colorado

Colorado Board of Medical Examiners
1525 Sherman Street, #132
Denver, CO 80203
303-866-2468

Connecticut

Connecticut Board of Medical Examiners
150 Washington Street
Hartford, CT 06106
203-566-1035

Delaware

Delaware Board of Medical Practice
Margaret O'Neill Building, 2nd Floor
Dover, DE 19903
302-736-4522

District Of Columbia

District of Columbia Occupational and Professional Licensing Division
614 H Street N.W., Room 904
Washington, DC 20001
202-727-7480

Florida

Florida Board of Medical Examiners
1940 N. Monroe Street
Tallahassee, FL 32399-0750
904-488-0595

Georgia

Georgia Composite State Board of Medical Examiners
166 Pryor Street S.W.
Atlanta, GA 30303
404-656-3913

Hawaii

Hawaii Board of Medical Examiners
P.O. Box 3469
Honolulu, HI 96801
808-548-4100

Idaho

Idaho State Board of Medicine
500 S. 10th Street, Suite 103
Boise, ID 83720
208-334-2822

Illinois

Illinois Department of Registration and Education
320 W. Washington Street
Springfield, IL 62786
217-785-0800

Indiana

Indiana Consumer Protection Division
219 Statehouse
Indianapolis, IN 46204
317-232-6330
800-382-5516

Iowa

Iowa State Board of Medical Examiners
Executive Hills W.
1209 E. Court Avenue
Des Moines, IA 50319
515-281-5171

Kansas

Kansas State Board of Healing Arts
900 S.W. Jackson, Suite 553
Topeka, KS 66612
913-296-7413

Kentucky

Kentucky Board of Medical Licensure
400 Sherburn Lane, Suite 2222
Louisville, KY 40207
502-896-1516

Louisiana

Louisiana State Board of Medical Examiners
830 Union Street, Suite 100
New Orleans, LA 70112
504-524-6763

Maine

Maine Board of Registration in Medicine
Statehouse Station 137
Augusta, ME 04333
207-289-3601

Maryland

Maryland Physician Quality Assurance
P.O. Box 2571
Baltimore, MD 21215-0095
410-764-4777

Massachusetts

Massachusetts Board of Registration in Medicine
10 West Street
Boston, MA 02111
617-727-3086

Michigan

Michigan Board of Medicine
P.O. Box 30192
Lansing, MI 48909
517-373-1870

Minnesota

Minnesota State Board of Medical Examiners
2700 University Avenue W., Room 106
St. Paul, MN 55114
612-642-0538

Mississippi

Mississippi State Board of Medical Licensure
2688-D Insurance Center Drive
Jackson, MS 39216
601-354-6645

Missouri

**Missouri State Board of Registration
for the Healing Arts**
P.O. Box 4
Jefferson City, MO 65102
314-751-2334 ext. 151

Montana

Montana Board of Medical Examiners
1424 9th Avenue
Helena, MT 59620
406-444-4284

Nebraska

Nebraska Board of Medical Examiners
301 Centennial Mall S.
Box 95007
Lincoln, NE 68509
402-471-2115

Nevada

Nevada State Board of Medical Examiners
P.O. Box 7238
Reno, NV 89510
702-329-2559

New Hampshire

New Hampshire Board of Registration in Medicine
Health And Welfare Building
6 Hazen Drive
Concord, NH 03301
603-271-1203

New Jersey

New Jersey State Board of Medical Examiners
28 W. State Street
Trenton, NJ 08608
609-292-4843

New Mexico

New Mexico Board of Medical Examiners
P.O. Box 20001
Santa Fe, NM 87504
505-827-9933

New York

New York State Department of Health
Office of Professional Medical Conduct
Corning Tower Building
Empire State Plaza
Albany, NY 12237
518-474-8357

North Carolina

North Carolina Board of Medical Examiners
P.O. Box 26808
Raleigh, NC 27611
919-876-3885

North Dakota

North Dakota State Board of Medical Examiners
City Center Plaza, Suite C-10
418 E. Broadway Avenue
Bismarck, ND 58501
701-223-9485

Ohio

Ohio State Medical Board
77 S. High Street, 17th Floor
Columbus, OH 43215
614-466-3938

Oklahoma

Oklahoma State Board of Medical Examiners
5104 N. Francis, Suite C
Oklahoma City, OK 73118
405-848-6841

Oregon
Oregon State Board of Medical Examiners
1500 S.W. First Avenue, Room 620
Portland, OR 97201
503-229-5770

Pennsylvania
Pennsylvania State Board of Medical Education and Licensure
P.O. Box 2649
Harrisburg, PA 17105
717-787-2381

Puerto Rico
Puerto Rico Board of Medical Examiners
Call Box 10200
Santurce, PR 00908
809-725-7903

Rhode Island
Rhode Island Division of Professional Regulation
3 Capitol Hill
Providence, RI 02908
401-277-2827

South Carolina
South Carolina State Board of Medical Examiners
1220 Pickins Street
Columbia, SC 29201
803-734-8901

South Dakota
South Dakota State Board of Medical and Osteopathic Examiners
1323 S. Minnesota Avenue
Sioux Falls, SD 57105
605-336-1965

Tennessee
Tennessee Board of Medical Examiners
283 Plus Park Boulevard
Nashville, TN 37217
615-367-6231

Texas
Texas Board of Medical Examiners
P.O. Box 13562, Capitol Station
Austin, TX 78711
512-452-1078

Utah
Utah Department of Commerce
Medical Licensing
160 East 300 South, 4th Floor
P.O. Box 45802
Salt Lake City, UT 84145
801-530-6628

Vermont
Vermont Board of Medical Practice
Secretary of State's Office
Pavilion Office Building
Montpelier, VT 05602
802-828-2673

Virgin Islands
Virgin Islands Department of Health
Attn: Licensure
St. Thomas Hospital
St. Thomas, VI 00801
809-774-0117

Virginia
Virginia State Board of Medicine
1601 Rolling Hills Drive
Richmond, VA 23229
804-662-9908

Washington
Washington State Medical Boards
Division of Professional Licensing
P.O. Box 9012
Olympia, WA 98504
206-753-2205

West Virginia
West Virginia Board of Medicine
101 Dee Drive
Charleston, WV 25311
304-558-2921

Wisconsin
Wisconsin Medical Examining Board
1400 E. Washington Avenue
P.O. Box 8935
Madison, WI 53708-8935
608-266-2811

Wyoming
Wyoming Board of Medical Examiners
Barrett Building, 3rd Floor
Cheyenne, WY 82002
307-777-6463

State Osteopathic Licensing Boards (D.O.)

The following state boards are responsible for regulating the osteopathic medical profession, including the issuance of licenses, enforcement of the medical practice act, investigation of complaints against osteopathic doctors, and imposition of fines, suspensions, and license revocations against doctors who violate the law.

Alabama

Alabama Medical Licensure Commission
P.O. Box 887
Montgomery, AL 36101
205-261-4153

Alaska

Alaska Osteopathic Medical Board
Department of Commerce and Economic Development
Division of Occupational Licensing
P.O. Box D
Juneau, AK 99811
907-465-2541

Arizona

**Arizona Osteopathic Examiners in Medicine
and Surgery**
1830 W. Colter Street, Suite 104
Phoenix, AZ 85015
602-255-1747

Arkansas

Arkansas Board of Medical Examiners
P.O. Box 102
Harrisburg, AR 72432
501-578-2448

California

California Board of Osteopathic Examiners
921 11th Street, Suite 1201
Sacramento, CA 95814
916-322-4306

Colorado

Colorado Board of Medical Examiners
1525 Sherman Street
Denver, CO 80203
303-866-2468

Connecticut

Connecticut Osteopathic Medical Board
Department of Health Services
Division of Medical Quality Assurance
79 Elm Street
Hartford, CT 06106
203-566-1039

Delaware

Delaware Board of Medical Practice
O'Neill Building
P.O. Box 1401
Dover, DE 19903
302-736-4522

District of Columbia

**District of Columbia Commission on Licensure to
Practice the Healing Art**
605 G Street N.W.
Washington, DC 20001
202-727-5365

Florida

Florida Board of Osteopathic Medical Examiners
1940 N. Monroe Street
Tallahassee, FL 32399-0775
904-488-7546

Georgia

Georgia Composite State Board of Medical Examiners
166 Pryor Street S.W.
Atlanta, GA 30303
404-656-3913

Hawaii

Hawaii Board of Osteopathic Examiners
P.O. Box 3469
Honolulu, HI 96801
808-548-3952

Idaho

Idaho State Board of Medicine
Statehouse
Boise, ID 83720
208-334-2822

Illinois

Illinois Department of Professional Regulation
320 W. Washington, 3rd Floor
Springfield, IL 62786
217-782-0458

Indiana

Indiana Medical Licensing Board
One American Square, Suite 1020
Box 82067
Indianapolis, IN 46282
317-232-2960

Iowa

Iowa State Board of Medical Examiners
Executive Hills W.
1209 E. Court Avenue
Des Moines, IA 50319
515-281-5171

Kansas

Kansas Board of Healing Arts
900 S.W. Jackson, Suite 553
Topeka, KS 66612
913-296-7413

Kentucky
Kentucky Board of Medical Licensure
400 Sherburn Lane, Suite 222
Louisville, KY 40207
502-896-1516

Louisiana
Louisiana State Board of Medical Examiners
830 Union Street
New Orleans, LA 70112
504-524-6763

Maine
**Maine Board of Osteopathic Examination
and Registration**
Statehouse Station 142
Augusta, ME 04333
207-289-2480

Maryland
Maryland Physician Quality Assurance
4201 Patterson Avenue
P.O. Box 2571
Baltimore, MD 21215-0002
410-764-4777

Massachusetts
Massachusetts Board of Registration in Medicine
10 West Street
Boston, MA 02111
617-727-3086

Michigan
Michigan Board of Osteopathic Medicine and Surgery
P.O. Box 30018
Lansing, MI 48909
517-373-6650

Minnesota
Minnesota State Board of Medical Examiners
2700 University Avenue W., Suite 106
St. Paul, MN 55114-1080
612-642-0538

Mississippi
Mississippi State Board of Medical Licensure
2688-D Insurance Center Drive
Jackson, MS 39216
601-354-6645

Missouri
Missouri Board of Registration for the Healing Arts
P.O. Box 4
Jefferson City, MO 65102
314-751-2334

Montana
Montana Board of Medical Examiners
1424 9th Avenue
Helena, MT 59620-0407
406-444-4284

Nebraska
Nebraska Board of Examiners in Medicine and Surgery
P.O. Box 95007
Lincoln, NE 68509
402-471-2115

Nevada
Nevada Board Of Osteopathic Examiners
1198 Sweetwater Drive
Reno, NV 89509
702-826-8383

New Hampshire
New Hampshire Board of Registration in Medicine
Health and Welfare Building
Hazen Drive
Concord, NH 03301
603-271-1203

New Jersey
New Jersey Board of Medical Examiners
28 W. State Street, Room 602
Trenton, NJ 08608
609-292-4843

New Mexico
New Mexico Board of Osteopathic Medical Examiners
725 St. Michaels Drive
P.O. Box 25101
Santa Fe, NM 87504
505-827-7171

New York
New York Board for Medicine
New York State Education Department
Cultural Education Center
New York State Plaza, Room 3023
Albany, NY 12230
518-474-3841

North Carolina
North Carolina Board of Medical Examiners
1313 Navaho Drive
Raleigh, NC 27609
919-876-3885

North Dakota
North Dakota Board of Medical Examiners
City Center Plaza, Suite C-10
418 E. Broadway
Bismarck, ND 58501
701-223-9485

Ohio
Ohio State Medical Board
77 S. High Street, 17th Floor
Columbus, OH 43266-0315
614-466-3934

Oklahoma
Oklahoma Board of Osteopathic Examiners
4848 N. Lincoln Boulevard, Suite 100
Oklahoma City, OK 73105
405-528-8625

Oregon
Oregon State Board of Medical Examiners
1500 S.W. First Avenue, Room 620
Portland, OR 97201
503-229-5770

Pennsylvania
Pennsylvania Board of Osteopathic Medical Examiners
P.O. Box 2649
Harrisburg, PA 17105
717-783-7156

Puerto Rico
Puerto Rico Board of Medical Examiners
Call Box 10200
Santurce, PR 00908
809-725-7903

Rhode Island
Rhode Island Board of Medical Licensure and Discipline
Department of Health
Cannon Building, Room 205
3 Capitol Hill
Providence, RI 20908-5097
401-277-3855

South Carolina
South Carolina Board of Medical Examiners
1220 Pickens Street
P.O. Box 12245
Columbia, SC 29201
803-734-8901

South Dakota
South Dakota Board of Medical and Osteopathic Examiners
1323 S. Minnesota Avenue
Sioux Falls, SD 57105
605-336-1965

Tennessee
Tennessee Board of Osteopathic Examination
283 Plus Park Boulevard
Nashville, TN 37219-5407
615-367-6393

Texas
Texas Board of Medical Examiners
P.O. Box 13562, Capitol Station
Austin, TX 78711
512-452-1078

Utah
Utah Department of Commerce
Division of Occupational and Professional Licensure
160 East 300 South
P.O. Box 45802
Salt Lake City, UT 84145-0802
801-530-6628

Vermont
Vermont Board of Osteopathic Examination and Registration
Secretary of State's Office
Pavilion Office Building
Montpelier, VT 05602
802-828-2673

Virgin Islands
Virgin Islands Department of Health
Attn: Licensing
St. Thomas Hospital
St. Thomas, VI 00801
809-774-0117

Virginia
Virginia State Board of Medicine
Department of Health Professionals
1601 Rolling Hills Drive
Richmond, VA 23229-5005
804-662-9908

Washington
Washington Division of Professional Licensing
P.O. Box 9012
Olympia, WA 98504
206-753-3095

West Virginia
West Virginia Board of Osteopathy
334 Penco Road
Weirton, WV 26062
304-723-4638

Wisconsin
Wisconsin Medical Examining Board
P.O. Box 8935
Madison, WI 53708
608-266-2811

Wyoming
Wyoming Board of Medical Examiners
Barrett Building, 3rd Floor
Cheyenne, WY 82002
307-777-6463

Dentists

Whether you desire it or not, it's a good bet that at least once in your life you will find yourself in the dentist's chair. However, you should not allow old images of painful procedures to deter your resolve to practice proper oral care. The use of anesthesia practically eliminates pain once associated with dental procedures. In addition, dentistry now emphasizes prevention of tooth and mouth problems as well as restorative procedures.

One of the first things to know about dentistry is that very few dentists are all things to all patients. Just as doctors have gradually developed specialties, so have dentists. There's the orthodontist who straightens crooked teeth, the endodontist who performs root canals, and the pedodontist who takes care of children's teeth.

These days the dentist is not the only professional found in the office. Another is the dental hygienist, a specialist in oral hygiene. Hygienists clean your teeth and make notes on the general health status of your mouth, gums, and teeth. They also take X rays, apply fluoride treatments, administer topical anesthesia, and apply tooth sealants.

D.D.S. vs. D.M.D.

Some dentists affix the initials *D.D.S.* after their names and others have *D.M.D.* What's the difference? And should you be impressed with one over the other?

Currently, the majority of dental schools in the United States award their graduates the D.D.S. degree, which stands for doctor of dental surgery. But more and more schools are adopting the other designation—the doctor of medical dentistry degree, abbreviated D.M.D. The schools that award the D.M.D. degree claim that their curriculums are more "medically oriented," and no doubt believe that the consumer will have more respect and reverence for the practitioner by giving the impression that he/she has a medical degree. But, in actuality, *there is no difference between the two.*

According to the American Dental Association, all dental schools in the U.S. are accredited, with clearly stated requirements, and there is no difference in what is taught. D.D.S. or D.M.D.—one is just as good as the other, or just as bad, depending on the individual dentist.

DENTISTS AND DONTISTS— WHO'S WHO?

According to the American Dental Association (ADA), a specialist must have certain qualifications:

- Two years of education beyond the general degree at an accredited dental school, and/or
- Certification by an ADA-recognized certifying organization

What is certification? Dentists who have continued their studies in depth in their chosen field may choose to become "board-certified." They must pass qualifying examinations administered by specialty boards before they are granted board certification, which is an achievement awarded by their colleagues. Certification is not necessarily an indicator of higher quality or skill, but it does indicate additional education. And you can contact these specialty boards directly in order to verify the specialist's credentials (see later in this section).

The American Dental Association has approved eight special areas of dental practice:

Endodontics. An *endodontist* does root canals. Although a general practitioner can perform root canals, a particularly complicated case may be referred to the specialist, whom you can reasonably expect to be more proficient and expert—and more expensive. One thing to bear in mind, however, is that with a successful root canal you have avoided the expense of having the tooth extracted and a false tooth put in its place.

Oral and Maxillofacial Surgery. Sometimes called an *exodontist,* an *oral and maxillofacial surgeon* extracts teeth as well as performs surgery on the mouth, jaws, and related structures. While the general practitioner can perform simple extractions, problem extractions are usually referred to the specialist—complications such as an impacted wisdom tooth (embedded in the bone under the gum far back in the mouth) or the tip of a broken root. The "maxillofacial" designation, referring to the jaw and the face, is relatively recent, and requires some skilled surgical techniques such as are involved in cosmetic surgery and surgery on the temporomandibular joints.

Oral Pathology. The *oral pathologist* is involved in the diagnosis of disease through biopsy and other methods. Only when your general dentist or specialist

These Commonly Used Dental Terms Will Help You Increase Your Dental IQ

Amalgam—silver/mercury alloy used to fill teeth.

Anteriors—front teeth.

Bitewing X rays—X rays of upper and lower back teeth.

Bonding—new tooth-restoring process in which the tooth surface is mildly etched to create microscopic voids for receiving a plastic material that will change the tooth shape or improve its appearance.

Bridge (either fixed or removable)—a replacement for a missing tooth or missing teeth, to "bridge" the gap.

Calculus (also called tartar)—plaque hardened into crusty deposits.

Caries—the disease that causes cavities.

Crown—(1) part of the tooth above the gum line; (2) also called cap or jacket: an artificial tooth-shaped cap put over the natural crown of a tooth after some of it has been ground away to make space, as a cover-up for a broken tooth, a way to save a tooth so full of filling that it's crumbling away, or a necessary support for a fixed bridge.

Fluoride—mineral that protects teeth from decay.

Full mouth X rays—a series of sixteen to eighteen X rays.

Gingiva—gum tissue.

Gingivitis—inflammation of the gums, an early form of gum disease.

Malocclusion—a bad bite caused by the upper and lower teeth not meeting properly when they are brought together.

Nitrous Oxide (laughing gas)—used as a dental analgesic to reduce anxiety.

---

is stymied by a particularly tricky problem would you be referred to an oral pathologist.

Orthodontics. The *orthodontist* corrects malocclusion (the improper position of the teeth) by wiring the teeth so that they move into the correct and most attractive positions. Although it was once true that older children and teenagers were the orthodontist's only customers, lately more adults are getting braces. The general practitioner usually does not do orthodontics, referring patients instead to the specialist. Of course, you can choose that specialist yourself—preferably someone whose "success stories" you have seen personally. Considering that the therapy takes around two years, on the average, it pays to find an orthodontist you can stand for that length of time, not to mention one you can afford and who is willing to make financial arrangements you can live with.

Pedodontics. The *pedodontist* looks after children's teeth—not that the general practitioner cannot or does not, but the specialist is supposed to know more about the psychological and emotional aspects of working with children. Usually children with behavioral problems, handicapped children, and children with unusual dental problems are sent to the pedodontist. Some pedodontists even do orthodontic work, and you may end up saving money by having both phases of your child's dental work done by one specialist. Check into it. Selecting such a practitioner for your child is different from selecting one for yourself, since the process often relies on tuning into the child's impressions of the practitioner, which are not always easy to discover, as well as determining such a vague quality as the pedodontist's attitude toward children.

Periodontics. Probably known best for the treatment of gum problems, the *periodontist* also looks after the bones and supportive tissue that surround the teeth. Although the general dentist can treat some gum disease, only the periodontist does gum surgery, which involves various procedures including the recontouring, tightening, or grafting of gum tissue. If your dental problems require this specialist's services, again choose carefully, because much of the

Novocaine—a local anesthetic.

Operatory—dental treatment room.

Periodontitis (also called **pyorrhea**)—an advanced form of gum disease in which the underlying bone is attacked.

Plaque—bacterial substance that causes dental decay.

Pocket—a space between the tooth and the gum where food can be trapped, usually associated with gum disease.

Posteriors—back teeth.

Primary teeth (baby teeth)—a child's first teeth.

Prophylaxis—professional teeth cleaning.

Root—part of the tooth anchored to the jaw.

Root canal therapy—a process involving drilling down to the nerve of the tooth, removing it and other dead material, then sealing up the tooth, as a way to save it rather than extract it.

Scaling—the removal of calculus, stains, and other deposits from the tooth surface by dental instruments, including ultrasonic scaling machines.

Sealant—plastic coating to protect teeth from decay.

Temporomandibular joints—the joints that connect the jawbone to the skull near the ear, and that allow the mouth to move.

Temporomandibular joint disorder (TMJ; also called myofascial pain dysfunction)—a catchall phrase to describe a variety of head and neck pains, and other symptoms related to the temporomandibular joints.

Third molars—wisdom teeth.

Five surfaces to a tooth:

occlusal: the biting side

mesial: the side toward the midline

distal: the side away from the midline

facial: the side toward the face

lingual: the side toward the tongue

---

treatment calls for multiple visits and an extended series of checkups.

Prosthodontics. The *prosthodontist* replaces missing teeth with prosthetic (artificial) ones: caps, bridges, and dentures. Most general dentists do some prosthodontic work in their practices, so the specialist is reserved for the truly difficult cases that the dentist does not want to undertake.

Dental Public Health. The *public health dentist* is involved in community dental education, community/school screening programs, and fluoridation issues.

Although not recognized by the American Dental Association as a separate specialty, cosmetic dentistry is getting more and more popular. *Cosmetic dentistry* is the "artistic" side of the profession, in which new techniques such as bleaching, bonding, veneering, and resculpting have been developed to "brighten the smiles" of people with chronically stained, broken, or malformed teeth. A word of caution: Since cosmetic dentistry is not an approved specialty, and has no certifying board, there are no criteria, standards, and

qualifications to be a cosmetic dentist. So ask the dentist if he/she has taken classes in this—where and when. And, if you can, see the dentist's work. Check and double-check before entrusting your smile to major cosmetic renovation.

THE DENTAL HYGIENIST

Almost as important as knowing who does what and when in the dental office is knowing what's going on these days between dentists and dental hygienists. There's a move afoot to let hygienists have their own practices in which they can perform limited procedures. Currently, Colorado is the only state that allows hygienists to practice independently, unsupervised by dentists. And California is the only state now considering legislation that would permit hygienists to practice in health care facilities, such as hospitals, nursing homes, and clinics, but not own their own practices.

Much of the controversy revolves around the difference of opinion between the two factions as to the

Choosing a Dentist for Your Child

Choosing a dentist for your child is not easy. If you're like a lot of people, you may find it an even trickier process than choosing a dentist for yourself. Why? Because as a parent you are attempting to judge a quality that's not easy to describe and not easy to pin down: the practitioner's attitude toward children. In short, *does he or she enjoy working on children?* This is something only you can determine, and something you and your child will have to work on together. But certainly there are specific clues you can find, even in the dentist's waiting room, and questions you can ask so that your child's relationship with his or her dentist starts out right. Better that the foundation be a positive experience than the basis for future dental fears and anxieties.

The first questions most parents ask is "When should my child's first visit to the dentist take place?" Most dentists recommend that a child see a dentist anytime after all twenty of the child's primary teeth are in—that is, sometime between the ages of 2 and 4. Of course, a toothache or an injury might land your child in the dentist's chair even sooner, but it's a good idea not to wait until it hurts or until an emergency before you look for somebody.

For basic care most parents choose the general practitioner, although a child's dental care may involve specialists as well. The *pedodontist* specializes in children's dental treatment and has postgraduate training in the dental problems of children and in the principles of child psychology. And there's the

orthodontist, whose practice typically has more children than adults, and who accordingly is supposed to know the unique features of working with young patients. Regardless of the practitioner you're shopping for, whether a family dentist or a specialist, the tips to help you make the right choice are pretty much the same:

• Ask friends about the practitioner who treats their children, and what they like about that practitioner. You may even want to ask your child's pediatrician or physician. While it's helpful to look in the yellow pages or call the local dental society for some names of family dentists and pedodontists, that's all they are—names, and not personal references. But if you're new in town and that's the only way for you to even get names, then do it, but be especially alert and shop around.

• Just because your child is just that, a child, there's no need to believe he or she must go to a pedodontist. For one thing, such specialists are hard to find in some parts of the country, and for another, as specialists they're likely to charge more for the same services that general practitioners can do. Sure, pedodontists have specially designed waiting rooms and operatories to attract and please the kids, but a family dentist should incorporate these elements into his or her practice, too, to some degree. So look around the waiting room: Is there an area set aside for children, with games, toys, and books? A practice that fails to cater to children with even such rudimentary items is likely to ignore their needs (and perhaps their comfort and safety) in more substantive ways.

• Other than looking for a dentist who enjoys working with children, that hard-to-define quality we mentioned before, you're looking for a prevention-oriented dentist. You want one who is not just worried about repair work, but who is oriented to teaching the child good dental health habits and is concerned with the whole child. Sound familiar? These qualities should—they make for a good dentist for the adult, too. Look around the waiting room and operatory: Are there educational books and pamphlets geared to children's developmental levels? Are there educational tools, such as a model tooth and toothbrush, and take-home "starter kits"? You can find out about these things during your get-acquainted visit, which we strongly recommend.

• Does the dentist make it a practice to give the "first-timer" an orientation to and tour of the dental office, preferably before doing any work on the child?

• Some of the knowledge that the dentist should know and be able and willing to impart to children is the role of diet, eating habits, and food substitutions. Ask the dentist if and what nutritional advice is part of the program. Also ask if he or she knows about the applications of sealants, which are coatings of plastic material applied to the biting surfaces of teeth. If done correctly, these protective layers assure that plaque and bacteria won't penetrate the plastic and cause cavities, and they're especially useful for a child's six-year molars, the first permanent teeth.

• Can you accompany your child into the operatory? Even before you ask, you should know that most dentists usually want to see the child alone. They say it's easier for the dentist-patient relationship and that kids are more cooperative on a one-to-one basis. However, some parents do not want their child in the operatory alone, without them there to intervene, interpret, and perhaps even protect. Find out if the dentist can accommodate you. Just remember, though, that your child may not be afraid, and you may unknowingly transfer your fears by being too aggressive.

• What about X rays? How often, and when for the first time? Initial X rays around the age of 3 or 4 is the recommendation of the American Society of Dentistry for Children and the American Academy of Pediatric Dentistry. But how often after that will depend upon the dental and oral health of the child, says the American Academy of Pediatric Dentistry. So, obviously, this is an important issue to discuss with your child's dental practitioner all along the way.

• What is the charge for your child's dental visit? To the nondentist, a fair price would be less than the cost of the same service performed on an adult patient, but the philosophy in the dental business is that treating children requires much time—usually more than the same procedure would take on an adult—and much patience. So be prepared to pay more. This is another good reason to shop around; you may find great differences in prices.

educational qualifications of hygienists. Generally, here's how a person becomes a practicing hygienist:

- Completes a two-year program at a community college, technical institute, school of dentistry, or a college/university and receives a certificate or associate degree; *or*
- Completes some courses at a college-level, then enters a two-year dental hygiene program and receives a degree there; *or*
- Completes four years of college work and receives a baccalaureate (bachelor of science) degree in dental hygiene; *and*
- Passes regional and state board licensing examinations.

The American Dental Association holds that hygienists with two-year associate degrees—that the majority of hygienists have, although increasing numbers are going for the baccalaureate degree—are not trained to practice in unsupervised settings, a concept that calls for hygienists to detect problems and refer patients to dentists when necessary. Hygienists say they are prevention specialists, with many claiming training in that area superior to that of the dentists.

Other than cleaning and polishing teeth, what services do dental hygienists provide? Again, that depends on the state. Some states permit the administration of local anesthesia: Alaska, Arizona, California, Colorado, Hawaii, Idaho, Kansas, Missouri, Montana, Nevada, New Mexico, Oklahoma, Oregon, South Dakota, Utah, Washington, and Wyoming. In Oklahoma, hygienists can administer nitrous oxide, and a few states even have a hygienist on the state dental licensing board.

WHEN THINGS GO WRONG

Your teeth, jaw, or gums have been damaged by your dentist. What do you do? Not pleasant to think about, but it can happen. And, rather than waiting until you're plunged into the rigmarole and trauma—and have to resort to the quick fix because you're too distraught to think straight—why not get the facts now?

At the very least, try talking to the dentist about the problem. You may even want to seek a second opinion on the existence and extent of harm done. Then, if this face-to-face communication doesn't resolve the problem, you have two avenues open to you.

First, contact your local, or county, dental society and request a peer review or grievance resolution. If your request is granted, a panel of dentists will look at the work

in your mouth, evaluate your complaint, and decide what action to take. Possible solutions? The panel may refund your money, advise that you have the work redone, or determine that the dentist was not at fault. A word of warning: Local dental and medical societies are trade associations, and as such have primarily the dentist's best interests at heart—not the consumer's.

Thus, we advise instead that you file a formal complaint with the dental licensing board in your state (see "State Dental Licensing Boards" in this section). Since, by filing this complaint, you are starting an administrative review process, you should be willing to see it through to the end. Here's how to do it:

1. Put your complaint in writing.
2. Include the name of the dentist.
3. Describe the nature of your complaint.
4. Indicate where it occurred (place).
5. Indicate when it occurred (time and date).
6. Obtain statements from witnesses, if any.
7. Include copies of bills or other items.

Remember: The information presented here should not be considered as formal legal advice. Furthermore, you should be willing and able to provide additional documentation if requested. For your own protection, it would be wise to retain legal counsel.

DENTAL HEALTH RESOURCES

American Dental Association
Bureau of Communications
211 E. Chicago Avenue
Chicago, IL 60611
312-440-2806
The American Dental Association does not diagnose specific cases or recommend particular treatments. It does, however, answer general questions about dentistry and dental health.

American Dental Hygienist Association
444 N. Michigan Avenue, Suite 3400
Chicago, IL 60611
312-440-8900

American Society for Dentistry for Children
211 E. Chicago Avenue, Suite 1430
Chicago, IL 60611
312-943-1244
The American Society of Dentistry for Children will provide the names of dentists who specialize in children's dentistry; the request must be put in writing.

AIDS Alert

The year 1987 saw the first known case of a dentist's catching the AIDS virus through apparent on-the-job exposure to patients' blood and saliva. According to researchers from the Montefiore Medical Center in New York, the dentist jabbed himself with dental instruments up to ten times a year, rarely wore gloves, and practiced with cuts on his hands. While there have been other reported cases in which nurses have gotten AIDS infections through contact with AIDS patients' blood, this was the first documented case involving a dental professional and, as such, deserves the close attention of any consumer shopping around for a dentist.

While much of the early attention focused on the transmission of the AIDS virus from patient to practitioner, an event occurred in December 1989 that would forever change all this. In that month, a young woman by the name of Kimberly Bergalis was diagnosed as being HIV positive. What made this discovery so shocking was that Ms. Bergalis did not fit into any of the recognized high-risk categories for HIV.

At first, researchers from the Centers for Disease Control and Prevention (CDC) were baffled, until they learned that she had dental surgery in 1987 to remove wisdom teeth. Using a form of DNA fingerprinting, CDC researchers determined that Ms. Bergalis could have contracted the AIDS virus only from her dentist, David Acer.

He died shortly after Ms. Bergalis was diagnosed with AIDS, and since then five more of his patients have been diagnosed as HIV positive. Dr. Acer, reportedly a bisexual and thus in a high-risk category, did not reveal his HIV status to any of his patients. Ms. Bergalis died in December 1991, two years after being diagnosed with AIDS. Compounding this tragedy is the fact that dentists are still not required to disclose their HIV status, even though the American Dental Association has a policy to this effect.

The fact is that even the experts do not agree on the exact manner in which an infected dentist can spread the virus to his or her patients. So, to be safe, as always our advice is to find out exactly what precautions the dentist is taking against all infections, including AIDS. As a final precaution, you can always ask your dentist about his or her HIV status.

INFECTION CONTROL IN THE DENTAL OFFICE

The dental office can be a high-risk setting for infectious disease transmission. Not only do the dental procedures involve sharp instruments, but the dentist is working in an environment of blood and saliva that may be contaminated with any number of infectious diseases. In the past, the hepatitis B virus in particular has been the culprit spread from patient to dentist and dentist to patient because of lax or nonexistent infection control practices. But the disease getting the most attention of late has been the AIDS virus (see accompanying box). Today, more than ever before, finding a safe dental office is absolutely imperative.

How do you do that? You ask a lot of questions—about the specific infection control measures being used to protect you as well as the dentist. Find out exactly what the day-to-day approach to effective infection control is in that dental office. Here are some important pointers:

• The American Dental Society strongly recommends that dentists, and any of their staff who come in direct contact with patients, wear gloves, masks, and eyeglasses. These items are the first line of defense, so make sure the dentist you choose follows this advice to the letter and does not waver. Refuse to be treated by anyone who doesn't.

- All dentists and the appropriate office staff should be vaccinated against hepatitis B—and, according to an infection control consultant with the American Dental Association, it wouldn't hurt if they were vaccinated against other potentially disabling diseases such as measles, rubella, and influenza. Ask if your dentist has been.
- Not even dental equipment and materials are immune to infection control measures. If you want to delve more deeply into the infection control practices in your dentist's office, you need to know the key recommendations from experts in the field. Effective infection control includes:
  - Heat sterilization for all instruments and items that can withstand exposure to heat
  - Routine use of "wraps" for instrument sterilization (These sterilized packets ensure sterility during storage)
  - Use of disposable items whenever possible
  - Periodic check of all sterilization units to see if they're functioning and sterilizing properly
- Even the seemingly innocuous handpiece (the device at the end of the tube that holds the attached drill or polisher) can be a troublemaker. A retraction valve within the handpiece is designed to prevent the inconvenient drip of water onto the patient's lap every time the handpiece is removed from the mouth. Because of the mechanism of this valve, microorganisms from the patient's saliva are sucked back into the handpiece and the equipment's water lines. Ask if the dentist flushes water from the dental unit into a sink or container 20 to 30 seconds before and between each patient—and also flushes the water for several minutes before the first patient of the day.
- Of course, there's the old standby, handwashing—which, along with an antimicrobial antiseptic, is of invaluable benefit in preventing the transmission of germs. Don't let your dentist's hands, unwashed and now ungloved, anywhere near your mouth. It's as simple as that.

DENTISTS, ANESTHESIA, AND EMERGENCY PREPAREDNESS

The use of anesthetic techniques and sedation in the dentist's office is somewhat different from their use in

the hospital. Dental procedures are usually shorter, the depth of anesthesia or sedation often less, and rather than the nature of the procedure it's the fear and apprehension of the dental patient that dictates the use of these techniques.

In an effort to make dental treatment less fearful and anxiety-producing, some dentists may use drugs to premedicate, especially for long procedures and with particularly apprehensive patients. Some drugs commonly used for dental premedication are barbiturates, antihistamines, and Valium. And, of course, there's "laughing gas" (nitrous oxide), an inhalant that produces a euphoric state in which a person's pain threshold is altered without loss of consciousness.

Conscious sedation (often intravenously administered) produces a slightly depressed level of consciousness in which the person remains awake and capable of carrying on a conversation. The same drugs used to effect conscious sedation are administered in general anesthesia, only in smaller amounts. When administered properly, conscious sedation holds little risk; however, on rare occasions, a person may descend by degrees into a state of deeper sedation, general anesthesia, or even death. And dentists with inadequate training may not be equipped to save a life in the case of an overdose.

General anesthesia is a controlled state of unconsciousness accompanied by a partial or complete loss of protective reflexes, including the inability to respond to verbal commands. In other words, the person is completely "asleep" for the procedure. The American Society for the Advancement of Anesthesia in Dentistry says that general anesthesia is no longer encouraged in the dental office, and its use should be carefully and seriously considered by both the patient and the dentist. According to many experts, most dental procedures requiring general anesthesia should be performed in the hospital, with the benefit of competent anesthesiologists, or in a specialist's office.

While generally the record of safety for anesthetic techniques is good, problems have occurred and questions have been raised concerning the training necessary for the safe and effective use of sedation and general anesthesia and the proper monitoring of the patient. To be able to ask questions concerning your own safety in the dental office, first you must determine what forms of anesthesia and sedation are used, then find out what the dentist's policies are concerning administration of the drugs and emergency preparedness.

- Make sure the dentist has credentialed training in the anesthetic procedure he or she uses. All states regulate the use of general anesthesia in the dental office, which means that the dentist who uses this technique must present his or her educational qualifications to the state board of dental examiners before a permit is issued. Ask to see the dentist's permit.

- Conscious sedation is regulated in more than half of the states, with more states usually adding some sort of regulatory guidelines each year. Call the state board of dental examiners or the state dental association and ask whether your state has such regulations. If not, be certain that the dentist who uses conscious sedation techniques is amply qualified with as much as two years' training. Ask for proof.

- Ask how many people are involved in the administration of the drugs and the monitoring of the patient in all anesthetic and sedation techniques. In 1985, a national conference on the issue recommended the following: For conscious sedation, the minimum number should be two—the dentist or other licensed professional, and an assistant trained to monitor. For deep sedation or general anesthesia, at least three appropriately trained persons are required.

- Most states regulate the use of nitrous oxide and, as such, demand that the dentist have a permit. In the case of any of these permits, there is no general requirement that the permit be displayed, so again your best bet is to ask the dentist to show you the permit. Also ask how many people are usually present during administration of laughing gas. Because some people experience strange dreams and hallucinations when under the drug's influence, it's often recommended that a third person be present to stop the patient from harming himself/herself and others. And one more thing: The gas-delivery machine should have a fail-safe mechanism that will not allow the patient to go completely "to sleep."

- The safe dental office has monitoring devices, emergency drugs, and equipment capable of delivering oxygen under positive pressure. A plan for dealing with emergencies should be developed, and emergency drills carried out periodically. Finally, determine that there is someone in the dental office who knows how to do cardiopulmonary resuscitation (CPR). Not too long ago the *Journal of the American Dental Association* reported that only a little more than half of dental practitioners questioned were certified in CPR. For your own safety, choose one who is.

State Dental Licensing Boards

State dental boards are responsible for policing the dental profession, including enforcement of the state dental practice act, administration of licensing examinations, investigations of complaints against dentists, and imposition of fines, suspensions, and license revocations.

Alabama

Alabama State Board of Dental Examiners
2308-B Starmount Circle
Huntsville, AL 35801
205-533-4638

Alaska

Alaska State Board of Dental Examiners
Department of Commerce
Division of Occupational Licensing
P.O. Box D-LIC
Juneau, AK 99811-0800
907-465-2544

Arizona

Arizona State Board of Dental Examiners
5060 N. 19th Avenue, Suite 406
Phoenix, AZ 85015
602-255-3696

Arkansas

Arkansas State Board of Dental Examiners
Tower Building, Suite 1200
4th and Center Streets
Little Rock, AR 72201
501-682-2085

California

California State Board of Dental Examiners
1430 Howe Avenue, Suite 85B
Sacramento, CA 95825
916-920-7451

Colorado

Colorado State Board of Dental Examiners
1525 Sherman, Room 132
Denver, CO 80203
303-866-5807

Connecticut

Connecticut Department of Health Services
Medical Quality Assurance—Dental
150 Washington Street
Hartford, CT 06106
203-566-1027

Delaware

Delaware State Board of Dental Examiners
O'Neill Building
P.O. Box 1401
Dover, DE 19903
302-736-3029

District of Columbia

**District of Columbia Department of Consumer and
Regulatory Affairs**
614 H Street N.W., Room 910
Washington, DC 20001
202-727-7823

Florida

Florida Department of Professional Regulation
1940 N. Monroe Street
Tallahassee, FL 32399-0750
904-488-6015

Georgia

Georgia Board of Dentistry
166 Pryor Street S.W.
Atlanta, GA 30303
404-656-3925

Hawaii

Hawaii State Professional and Vocational Licensing
P.O. Box 3469
Honolulu, HI 96801
808-548-4100

Idaho

Idaho State Board of Dentistry
Statehouse
Boise, ID 83720
208-334-2369

Illinois

Illinois State Department of Professional Regulation
Attn: Dental Unit
100 W. Randolph Street, Suite 9-300
Chicago, IL 60601
312-917-4481

Indiana

Indiana Consumer Protection Division
Health Professions Bureau
One American Square, Suite 1020
Box 82067
Indianapolis, IN 46282
317-232-2960

Iowa

Iowa State Board of Dental Examiners
Executive Hills W.
1209 E. Court
Des Moines, IA 50319
515-281-5157

Kansas

Kansas State Board of Dental Examiners
4301 Huntoon, Suite 4, Lower Level
Topeka, KS 66604
913-273-0780

Kentucky

Kentucky State Board of Dentistry
2106 Bardstown Road
Louisville, KY 40205
502-451-6832

Louisiana

Louisiana State Board of Dental Examiners
1515 Poydras Street, Suite 2240
New Orleans, LA 70112
504-568-8574

Maine

Maine State Board of Dental Examiners
Statehouse Station 143
Augusta, ME 04333
207-289-3333

Maryland

Maryland State Board of Dental Examiners
4201 Patterson Avenue
Baltimore, MD 21215-2299
410-764-4730

Massachusetts

**Massachussetts State Board of Registration
in Dentistry**
Investigative Unit
100 Cambridge Street, Room 1509
Boston, MA 02202
617-727-7406

Michigan

Michigan Department of Licensing and Regulation
Bureau of Health Services
Licensing Division
P.O. Box 30018
Lansing, MI 48909
517-373-6650
To file a complaint 517-373-9196

Minnesota

Minnesota Board of Dentistry
2700 University Avenue W., Suite 109
St. Paul, MN 55114
612-642-0579

Mississippi
Mississippi State Board of Dental Examiners
P.O. Box 1960
Clinton, MS 39060
601-924-9622

Missouri
Missouri Dental Board
P.O. Box 1367
Jefferson City, MO 65102
314-751-2334

Montana
Montana Department of Commerce
1424 9th Avenue
Helena, MT 59620-0407
406-444-3745

Nebraska
Nebraska State Board of Dental Examiners
Bureau of Examining Boards
P.O. Box 95007
Lincoln, NE 68509-5007
402-471-2115

Nevada
Nevada State Board of Dental Examiners
P.O. Box 80360
Las Vegas, NV 89180
702-258-4230

New Hampshire
New Hampshire State Board of Dental Examiners
Health and Welfare Building
6 Hazen Drive
Concord, NH 03301
603-271-4561

New Jersey
New Jersey State Board of Dental Examiners
1100 Raymond Boulevard, Room 321
Newark, NJ 07102
201-648-7087

New Mexico
New Mexico State Board of Dental Examiners
P.O. Box 25101
Sante Fe, NM 87504
505-827-6207

New York
New York State Education Department
Office of Professional Discipline
622 3rd Avenue
New York, NY 10017
212-557-2100
800-442-8106

North Carolina
North Carolina State Board of Dental Examiners
P.O. Box 32270
Raleigh, NC 27622
919-781-4901

North Dakota
North Dakota State Board of Dental Examiners
P.O. Box 179
Valley City, ND 58072
701-845-3708

Ohio
Ohio State Dental Board
77 S. High Street, 18th Floor
Columbus, OH 43266-0306
614-466-2580

Oklahoma
Oklahoma State Board of Governors of Registered Dentists
2726 N. Oklahoma
Oklahoma City, OK 73105
405-521-2350

Oregon
Oregon Board of Dentistry
1515 S.W. 5th Avenue, Suite 400
Portland, OR 97201
503-229-5520

Pennsylvania
Pennsylvania Department of State
Bureau of Professional Occupational Affairs
Dental Board, Complaint Department
P.O. Box 2649
Harrisburg, PA 17105
717-787-8503
800-922-2113

Puerto Rico
Puerto Rico Board of Dental Examiners
Department of Health
Call Box 10200
Santurce, PR 00908
809-723-1617

Rhode Island
Rhode Island Department of Health
Division of Professional Regulation
3 Capitol Hill
Providence, RI 02908
401-277-2827

South Carolina
South Carolina State Board of Dental Examiners
1315 Blanding Street
Columbia, SC 29201
803-734-8904

South Dakota

South Dakota State Board of Dentistry
1708 Space Court
Rapid City, SD 57702
605-342-3026

Tennessee

Tennessee State Board of Dental Examiners
283 Plus Park Boulevard
Nashville, TN 37219-5407
615-367-6228

Texas

Texas State Board of Dental Examiners
P.O. Box 13165, Capitol Station
Austin, TX 78711
512-834-6021

Utah

Utah Department of Commerce
160 East 300 South
P.O. Box 45802
Salt Lake City, UT 84145
801-530-6628

Vermont

Vermont Secretary of State Office
Attn: Complaint Department
Pavilion Office Building
Montpelier, VT 05602
802-828-2390

Virgin Islands

Virgin Islands Department of Health
48 Sugar Estates
St. Thomas, VI 00802
809-774-0117

Virginia

Virginia State Board of Dental Examiners
1601 Rolling Hills Drive
Richmond, VA 23229
804-662-9906

Washington

Washington State Dental Disciplinary Board
Department of Licensing, Program
Management Division
P.O. Box 9012
Olympia, WA 98504-8001
206-753-1156

West Virginia

West Virginia Board of Dental Examiners
P.O. Drawer 1459
Beckley, WV 25802-1459
304-252-8266

Wisconsin

Wisconsin State Board of Dental Examiners
Department of Regulation and Licensing
P.O. Box 8935
Madison, WI 53708
608-266-1396

Wyoming

Wyoming State Board of Dental Examiners
P.O. Box 1024
Powell, WY 82435
307-754-3476

Dental Specialty Boards

These organizations have been approved by the Commission on Dental Accreditation of the American Dental Association to administer examinations and certify dentists in the following specialties. To be eligible for certification in a particular specialty, a dentist must have completed two years of education beyond the general degree and must have successfully passed the certification examination.

American Board of Endodontics
211 E. Chicago Avenue, Suite 1501
Chicago, IL 60611
312-266-7310

American Board of Oral and Maxillofacial Surgery
625 N. Michigan Avenue, Suite 1820
Chicago, IL 60611
312-642-0070

American Board of Oral Pathology
5401 W. Kennedy Boulevard
P.O. Box 25915
Tampa, FL 33622
813-286-2444

American Board of Orthodontics
225 S. Meramec Avenue, Room 310
St. Louis, MO 63105
314-727-5039

American Board of Pediatric Dentistry
Indiana University School of Dentistry
1193 Woodgate Drive
Carmel, IN 46032
317-573-0877

American Board of Periodontology
University of Southern California
School of Dentistry
925 W. 34th Street
Los Angeles, CA 90089
213-743-2800

American Board of Prosthodontics
4707 Olley Lane
Fairfax, VA 22032
703-273-7323

Mental Health Practitioners

Generally, mental health practitioners can be divided into psychiatrists (who are physicians, M.D. or D.O.), psychologists (Ph.D. in psychology), mental health social workers, and family, marriage, or pastoral counselors. In addition, there are psychiatric nurses, who are usually found in psychiatric hospitals, general hospitals, or mental health clinics. In short, the mental health field is full of many different titles for and types of counselors. You must very carefully check the credentials and practices of mental health practitioners, especially in states with little or no regulation.

A *psychiatrist* is a medical doctor who specializes in the prevention, diagnosis, and treatment of mental and emotional disorders. Following medical school, a doctor completes four years of specialized training in psychiatry. This training enables the psychiatrist to understand the biological, psychological, and social components of mental illness. Psychiatrists employ both medical and nonmedical treatment methods, including medication and psychoanalysis (counseling). After completing their specialized area of study, many psychiatrists choose to become board-certified by the American Board of Psychiatry and Neurology, which means that they have passed a written and oral examination administered by a panel of their peers. Board certification, while no guarantee of competence, does indicate additional education and training.

A *psychologist* is trained to deal with the emotional problems of people, but cannot prescribe medications. Psychologists perform psychological testing on patients and practice psychotherapy (counseling) in a one-on-one or group setting. Most psychologists hold an advanced degree—doctor of philosophy (Ph.D.), doctor of psychology (Psy.D.), or doctor of education (Ed.D). Along with the degree requirements, psychologists are required to complete a one-year internship or postdoctoral supervised work experience.

Some states license psychologists who hold master's degrees and meet certain other work-related experience requirements. However, this is not the case in every state, as standards for practice and licensure vary from state to state. Some psychologists may seek voluntary accreditation by the American Board of Professional Psychology.

A *mental health social worker* generally holds a master's degree in social work (M.S.W.) and has special training in the area of psychology and, as such, participates in providing mental health services.

Many mental health social workers work in social services agencies as well as crisis centers, where they are often the first contacts for people seeking mental health services.

Mental health social workers may be employed by general and psychiatric hospitals, long-term care facilities, adolescent residence centers, community mental health centers, and local governments. Mental health social workers may or may not be licensed, since there is no uniformity among state laws.

Family, marriage, or pastoral counselors are the general terms given to people who advertise themselves to be specialists in these areas. In some cases these people are psychologists, in other cases they are social workers or even registered nurses, and in other cases they are not specifically educated and trained in any counseling field. In some states these practitioners are licensed, while in other states anyone may use the title "counselor" and attach one of these terms: family, marriage, or pastoral.

Clergy are generally recognized as counselors (and are exempt from licensing), even though they may not have completed any specific courses in counseling.

A *psychiatric nurse* is an RN with special education and training in the area of psychiatry. Psychiatric nurses may be found in general and acute care hospitals with psychiatric departments and in dedicated psychiatric hospitals. They carry out treatment plans designed by doctors, and are responsible for administering and monitoring medications given to patients. In addition, they may also participate in patient therapy sessions, or help ensure that patients are attending their therapy sessions.

For information on resources, see "Mental Health and Mental Disorders" in section 2, "Medical Conditions."

Healing Arts: Options in Providers

ACUPUNCTURE

Acupuncture is the ancient Chinese healing art in which very thin needles are inserted under the skin in order to treat illness and restore good health. A practitioner of this art is an *acupuncturist*.

Acupuncture reportedly dates from 1600 to 1500 B.C. It attracted renewed attention and interest in the West after the opening of China in the early 1970s.

A key element in understanding acupuncture is an acceptance of the Eastern belief in the poles or extremes of yin and yang (roughly corresponding to our ideas of negative and positive, or female and male, forces) and the flow of a life force known as chi. Chinese medicine teaches that in order to remain healthy the yin and yang forces must be perfectly balanced and that it is necessary to have a flow of chi throughout the body. The chi flows along paths known as meridians (sets of invisible lines) and covers the body in set patterns. While meridians are not identical to the nervous system or circulatory system, they are thought to resemble them. Each meridian has its own pulse, and these pulses provide information about any meridians that need to have their energy balance restored.

When illness occurs, the acupuncturist examines the meridians and carefully selects acupuncture sites. It is at these sites that acupuncture treatment is given.

Extremely thin needles made from gold, silver, or copper are placed in carefully selected sites just below the skin by the acupuncturist. A gentle twisting of the needle helps to ensure that it is properly placed and will correct the flow of chi along the meridians.

Acupuncturists believe that currents, or impulses, begin to flow along the meridians where the needles are placed. This current travels through the nervous system and goes to the organ that is out of balance. Once the obstruction or hindrance is removed, the life forces are free to circulate once again, and balance is restored.

Reports from China indicate that major surgery has been performed while using acupuncture as the only anesthetic. Acupuncture also includes herbal medicine, disease-specific and preventive nutritional measures, relaxation skills, exercise, and specific advice on health behaviors.

Western medicine, with its foundations in the scientific method, has been slow to show interest in acupuncture, but some physicians now use it, and their numbers are growing.

For more information, contact:

Traditional Acupuncture Institute
American City Building, Suite 108
Columbia, MD 21044
301-596-6006

ALLOPATHIC MEDICINE

Allopathic medicine is a healing art founded on scientific principles in which diseases are treated with medications that produce conditions incompatible with the disease-causing agent. It is based on the philosophy that the physician must actively intervene to combat illness. An *allopathic physician* is a practitioner who has completed the prescribed course of study leading to the degree of doctor of medicine (M.D.) and who has a license to practice. Most physicians also complete a residency program in a specialty or subspecialty of their choosing.

Historically, allopaths trace their origins to Hippocrates, and to the surgeon-barbers of the Middle Ages who were known for their bloodletting technique. It was also during this latter period that the three so-called heroic remedies—bleeding, blistering, and purging—were developed. Often these cures were worse than the condition that prompted the need for treatment.

Allopathic medicine has been the dominant medical philosophy in the United States since the early 1900s. Its rise to predominance was hastened by the scientific discoveries that were made in the areas of bacteriology, pathology, organic chemistry, and surgery. During this time the scientific principle of double-blind study was introduced, a technique that enables doctors and medical researchers to evaluate the effectiveness of their methods using an experimental group and a control group.

Allopathic medicine has proven to be very effective against the acute infectious diseases that once ravaged humankind, such as smallpox, polio, pneumonia, whooping cough, and plague. Advances in surgery now permit transplantation of organs, reattachment of limbs, replacement of joints, and cosmetic applications.

An allopathic physician begins by taking a complete medical history and conducting a physical examination, often including a battery of diagnostic tests that may involve blood work, analysis of body specimens, X rays, ultrasound, or other sophisticated scanning devices. Once a diagnosis has been determined, the physician may administer medications, each selected on the basis of how well it combats or counteracts what is going on within the body. Other treatment modalities include chemotherapy, surgery, and ionizing radiation.

For more information, contact:

American Medical Association
515 N. State Street
Chicago, IL 60610
312-464-5000

Ayurvedic Medicine

Ayurveda is a system of holistic medicine that originated in India and is among the oldest of the healing arts. Ayurvedic medicine combines the mysticism of Eastern religion with the science of healing and serves as the basis for many of the Oriental healing methods.

Ayurveda is holistic in nature and views the person in terms of body, mind, and spirit. The *Ayurvedic physician* believes that disease is caused by imbalances in the body's five basic elements and the forces in those elements. Earth, fire, water, air, and ether are the basic elements, and they combine into three principles, or humors, known as the tridosha.

The first of these is vata, which is formed by air and ether, and the second is pitta, formed by fire and water. The third and last is kapha, formed by earth and water. These elements govern all the biological, psychological, and physiological functions of the body, mind, and spirit. When these elements are out of balance, disease occurs.

An Ayurvedic physician will take a complete history from the patient and conduct a thorough physical examination before determining what caused the particular imbalance. Fasting, baths, diets, and applications to the skin are used to cleanse the body before a specific treatment is recommended. A complete pharmacopoeia is consulted, and drugs to restore normal health and balance are given in the form of jellies, tinctures, powders, pills, or oils.

Other branches of Ayurvedic medicine include surgery, obstetrics, gynecology, pediatrics, and psychology.

For more information, contact:

Ayurvedic Institute
11311 Menaul N.E., Suite A
Albuquerque, NM 87112
505-291-9698

Bach Flower Remedies

Bach flower remedies are a form of herbal medicine devised in the early 1930s by Dr. Edward Bach, a British bacteriologist who later became a pathologist. The doctor's interest in the healing powers of trees and plants had produced thirty-eight herbal remedies by the time of his death in 1936.

Bach's formula for devising a particular remedy involved collecting the flowering heads of wild plants, placing them in water, and then filtering the solution before bottling. Basically, he believed that the solutions he prepared contained the physical properties of the derivative plants. Much of what Bach devised depends upon discovering the emotional state of the person, and the remedies are supposed to quiet the disharmonies within the person and thus restore health.

Bach's remedies, best used for emotional rather than physical complaints, are divided into seven groups that cover the negative states of mind that affect most people: fear, uncertainty, lack of interest, despondency, overcare for others, loneliness, and oversensitivity. He was never able to fully describe how his solutions worked; rather, he claimed they had "the power to elevate our vibrations, and thus draw down the spiritual power which cleanses mind and body, and heals."

Although a few practitioners limit themselves exclusively to Bach remedies, most remedies are employed as complements to natural healing, especially in herbal medicine.

For more information, contact:

Westbrook University
404 N. Mesa Verde
Aztec, NM 87410
800-447-6496

Chinese Medicine

Chinese medicine consists of acupuncture, massage, and herbal medicine and includes an acceptance of the poles or extremes of yin and yang (roughly corresponding to our ideas of negative and positive, or female and male, forces) and the flow of a life force known as chi. Chinese medicine teaches that in order to remain healthy the yin and yang forces must be perfectly balanced and that it is necessary to have a flow of chi throughout the body.

In place of highly technological diagnostic and treatment equipment, practitioners of Chinese medicine rely upon looking, listening, smelling, asking, and touching to make their diagnosis.

Another theory in Chinese medicine, one basic to determining a particular illness and the prescribed treatment, is called Five Elements. The five elements are fire, wood, earth, metal, and water, which practitioners of Chinese medicine use when evaluating bodily functions, organs, acupuncture meridians, emotions, and external influences. As always, they are seeking to discover some disturbance in the flow of chi throughout the body.

As we said, touching is an important aspect of Chinese medicine, much more so than in Western medicine. By carefully taking the pulses of the body, the practitioner can detect slight imbalances that may indicate a condition of disease. These pulses flow along the meridians of the body, and since they connect to every organ system, it is possible to determine which organ or body part is affected.

When a diagnosis is made, the practitioner will decide upon one or all of the treatment methods available, specifically acupuncture, the manipulative therapy acupressure, and herbal medicine. (See our discussions of each of these elsewhere in this section.)

For more information, contact:

American Association of Acupuncture and Oriental Medicine
1424 16th Street N.W., Suite 501
Washington, DC 20036
202-265-2287

CHRISTIAN HEALING

Christian healing is a paranormal therapy centered on the belief that a healer has the power to cure physical illnesses through the laying-on of hands. It is also called faith healing or therapeutic touch.

Healing without medicines and surgery has always been viewed skepticism, not only by traditional medicine but also by mainstream religions. Many people find it hard to believe that someone who claims to possess an energy field can actually cure illness.

Miracles were always the province of religion, and their occurrences have been duly recorded in scripture. It was believed that only simpleminded people with limited education would have any interest in faith healing, and it was not until parapsychologists began investigating the claims of faith healers that serious attention was paid to this practice.

Christian healing involves belief, and specifically belief that a particular person for whatever reason is tuned into a source of power not of this world. The effectiveness of Christian healing depends upon the willpower of the person being healed. Research into

the powers of the mind indicates that humans have the capacity to will physical changes, but it is necessary that the person wishing to be healed believe in the healing process.

In some medical schools today, medical students are being taught that touching patients may be just as important as writing a prescription or performing surgery. Some religiously affiliated medical centers are now permitting lay ministers to visit the sick and pray with them if the patient has no objections.

For further information, contact:

New Life Clinic
Mt. Washington United Methodist Church
Falls Road
Baltimore, MD 21209
410-561-0428

Healing Light Center
204 E. Wilson
Glendale, CA 91206
818-244-8607

DENTISTRY

Dentistry is the healing art concerned with the care and treatment of teeth and the surrounding tissue and bone structure of the oral cavity. A *dentist* is a professional who has completed the prescribed course of study leading to the degree of doctor of dental surgery (D.D.S.) or doctor of dental medicine (D.M.D.) and who has a license to practice.

Early dentists were more tradesmen than professionals, since there really was not much available in the way of formal training. Aside from a few herbal remedies, the only treatment for an aching tooth was to remove it. The concept of modern dentistry, with its emphasis on prevention and restoration, was still many centuries away.

Today dentists treat tooth and gum problems with a wide array of materials and techniques. The filling of cavities can be done almost painlessly, and high-speed drills and improved anesthetics make it possible to save teeth that otherwise might be lost.

Cosmetic dentistry is the newest direction in the profession and is becoming so popular that an array of cosmetic techniques—bleaching, bonding, veneering, and resculpting—is available to brighten the smiles of people with chronically stained, broken, or malformed teeth. These cosmetic techniques account for more than half of all dental restorative work currently being done.

For more information, contact:

American Dental Association
211 E. Chicago Avenue
Chicago, IL 60611
312-440-2500

American Academy of Esthetic Dentistry
500 N. Michigan Avenue, Suite 1400
Chicago, IL 60611
312-661-1700

American Academy of Restorative Dentistry
P.O. Box 247
Marshfield, WI 54449
715-384-4224

HERBAL MEDICINE

Herbal medicine is a healing art that uses plants to prevent and cure illnesses. A person skilled in the art of herbal medicine who can compound herbal mixtures made from the various plants is an *herbalist.*

Herbology, the use of plants as medicine, is probably as old as humankind. According to historians, many ancient peoples, including the Chinese, Egyptians, Babylonians, and Aztecs, practiced herbal medicine. Some of the herbs used were elderberry, pomegranate bark, cinnamon, mustard, gentian, and rhubarb.

Humans probably learned how to use herbs to treat illnesses by watching animals and noting what plants they ate when they were sick. Herbalists claim that their remedies do not have the harmful side effects that are so common with modern medicines.

Before scientific medicine gained the upper hand early in this century, both herbology and allopathy existed side by side. Once the scientific faction won out, however, herbology was relegated to the status of folk medicine or just plain quackery. But the fact of the matter is that all early medicines were vegetable in origin, since the elaborate process of making synthetic compounds did not exist. Once the use of organic and inorganic chemicals became dominant, the need for plant-derived medicines waned.

Herbs can be used as astringents, tonics, laxatives, and acidifiers. Nervines are another class of herbs that can either relax or excite the nervous system. Some people brew herbal teas to help them relax or sleep, with camomile being the most popular herb for this. Garlic is another herb receiving renewed interest as an adjunct to traditional medications.

As with medications, the key to using herbs is to carefully research the claims for each one. Libraries and health food stores usually have books on herbal medicine.

For more information, contact:

American Botanical Council
P.O. Box 201660
Austin, TX 78720
512-331-8868

HOMEOPATHIC MEDICINE

Homeopathic medicine treats illnesses by using safe natural medicines that stimulate a person's own healing powers while avoiding harmful side effects. A practitioner skilled in the art of homeopathic medicine is a *homeopathic physician.* Most homeopathic physicians in practice today are M.D.'s or D.O.'s who have additional training in homeopathic principles.

The concept of homeopathy dates to Hippocrates, but it was a German physician, Samuel Hahnemann, who provided the scientific foundation. In 1810 he published the *Organon of Medicine,* which set forth the principles of homeopathy as he saw them.

Homeopathic medicine believes that like cures like and that medicines that cause symptoms of diseases in healthy people will bring about cures in sick people. Another basic tenet of homeopathy is that the whole person must be treated and not just the disease.

Allopaths treat the symptoms of diseases, for instance fever, with medication that will produce the opposite effect. The homeopath views the symptoms as indicating an imbalance in the person's life forces and strives to restore balance to the body, mind, and spirit.

Aside from the principle that like cures like, homeopathic medicine also believes in the use of a single remedy. Homeopaths will administer only one medicine at a time, and if the condition persists, then a second medication is used but never a combination of medications. Finally, because it is concerned with the body's ability to absorb the medication, homeopathic medicine encourages the smallest dose possible in order to prevent outright rejection or reactions from strong doses.

Homeopathic medications are extracted from naturally occurring substances such as plants, animal material, and natural chemicals. These preparations are distinctive in that they are taken by mouth, tend to be tasteless, can be stored for periods of time, and do not produce toxic side effects.

Homeopathic remedies usually indicate how many times they have been diluted from the original material, although a basic belief of homeopathy is that no matter how many times a solution has been diluted it will remain effective.

While homeopathic medical schools have been absorbed by their allopathic counterparts, many physicians today still abide by homeopathic principles.

For more information, contact:

National Center for Homeopathy
801 N. Fairfax Street, Suite 306
Alexandria, VA 22314
703-548-7790

HYDROTHERAPY

Hydrotherapy uses water, either internally or externally, to treat certain illnesses and bodily injuries. Hydrotherapy is most often associated with physical therapy.

Archaeological records suggest that ancient civilizations made great use of water as a healing therapy. Public baths were commonplace in the Roman Empire, with most early baths located adjacent to hot mineral springs whose therapeutic powers were widely known.

You may have used hydrotherapy already and not realized it. Have you ever soaked your aching feet in a basin of hot water? That's hydrotherapy.

Athletic trainers make extensive use of whirlpool baths to treat athletes who have strained or sore muscles. Water therapy has become so popular that many people have installed "hot tubs" in their homes. Not too long ago hydrotherapy was used for polio victims as a method to help them regain some use of their crippled limbs. Swimming, by far the most popular form of hydrotherapy, is done by millions of people around the world. In hydrotherapy the water may be hot, cold, or tepid, depending upon the particular need, and may be used in any one of three states: liquid, solid (ice), or gas (steam). Ice packs are a form of hydrotherapy used to prevent swelling associated with injuries.

Some other popular hydrotherapy techniques are:

Sitz bath. A sitting bath used to treat many abdominal and pelvic conditions.

Contrast baths. The alternative application of hot and cold to the body, which results in dilation and contraction of blood vessels to improve circulation.

Cold mitten friction. A mitten made from Turkish towel material is dipped in cold water, wrung out lightly, and then rubbed briskly across the body.

Epsom salts bath. Magnesium sulfate is added to very hot bath water, which causes profuse sweating. After an Epsom salts bath, the person showers and receives a brisk rubdown.

Colonic. The internal applications of water to flush waste products and toxins from the body and cleanse the lower digestive tract.

MANIPULATIVE THERAPIES

Acupressure
Acupressure is a form of therapy in which the fingertips are used to apply pressure along meridians found on the body. By stimulating the acupressure points along the meridians, life forces are permitted to flow to various parts of the body. A practitioner skilled in the application of acupressure is an *acupressurist.*

Acupressure originated at about the same time as acupuncture and is an integral part of Chinese medicine. The major difference between acupressure and acupuncture is the use of the fingertips as opposed to very fine needles.

The fingers are used to rub or massage specific acupressure points along the body's meridians (invisible lines that crisscross the body) in order to promote the even flow of the life forces known as chi. In a healthy person, chi flows evenly, maintaining a balance between the vigorous yang and the restraining yin elements. Practitioners of acupressure or any other Chinese therapy aim to correct any imbalances and encourage chi to flow freely again.

The acupressurist studies the meridians of the body and locates the acupressure points along these meridians. It is thought that all life force flows along these pathways. If there is some blockage or deficiency along the pathways, then the vital force cannot reach the organs or other parts of the body.

Through proper stimulation of the acupressure points, the flow of vital energy is restored and good health returns. Conversely, it is also possible to have too much life force or energy flowing in a particular organ or body part. Once again, the acupressurist would stimulate the correct acupressure points and redistribute the life force.

There's really nothing strange about rubbing a sore or aching spot, since most of us do it naturally. Acupressure may be an ancient healing method originating in traditional Chinese medicine, but it appears to have a place in today's world.

For more information, contact:

Acupressure Institute
1533 Shattuck Avenue
Berkeley, CA 94709
510-845-1059

Alexander Technique

The Alexander technique is classified as a manipulative therapy because it attempts to correct a range of disorders by improving posture. The technique was developed in the late 1800s by F. Matthias Alexander, an Australian actor who had experienced problems with his voice. In his efforts to discover the cause, he hit upon the idea of postural changes. By studying what he was doing with his posture when the problems arose, he learned that he was pulling his head downward and backward.

Alexander borrowed the theory of spinal integrity from chiropractic and osteopathy, but with two important distinctions: He believed that if the vertebrae were out of alignment, it was due to misuse. And he believed that the way we use our bodies, and the habits we develop—such as slumping, tensing, and slouching—influence function.

The Alexander technique is really one of relearning or learning what not to do. There are no formal exercises, so the technique will vary with the individual. The basic approach is for a teacher to evaluate and determine where postural changes are needed and where reconditioning must begin. Then the teacher manipulates various parts of the body, such as the head, neck, limbs, or pelvis, and the person is told to focus on the instructions given—for example, "neck free, head forward and out." Alexander believed very strongly in the mind and body con-

nection. This technique is repeated until the problem is corrected.

For more information, contact:

American Center for the Alexander Technique
Abraham Goodman House
129 W. 67th Street
New York, NY 10023
212-799-0468

Applied Kinesiology/Touch for Health

Applied kinesiology/Touch for Health is a form of healing that uses therapeutic touch to correct imbalances in the body's energy system and to restore health. A practitioner who employs the principles of kinesiology and is trained in the proper functioning of the body's muscle systems is a *kinesiologist*. (Chiropractors and massage therapists also may use the principles of kinesiology in their practices.)

Applied kinesiology/Touch for Health is a branch of natural healing that applies touch to transmit and arouse the healing forces. It combines some of the manipulative practices of chiropractic and massage with the concept of energy flow found in acupuncture and shiatsu. At the core of applied kinesiology is a system of muscle testing that enables the practitioner to identify the weaknesses in the body's energy system. Once these weaknesses are corrected, the body is restored to balance and good health.

A chiropractor, George Goodheart, established the basis for applied kinesiology while he was attempting to determine the cause of taut muscles or muscles in spasm. During his investigation, he determined that the tautness or spasms were caused by weak muscles on the opposite side of the body. He reasoned that the energy flow to the muscles must be disrupted. By applying chiropractic techniques and Eastern ideas of energy flow, he devised a system for restoring muscle balance.

A practitioner looks for symptoms of muscle weakness by examining the person's posture and testing specific muscles. The patient lies flat on the examining table while the practitioner rotates and flexes the arms and legs. The meridians of acupuncture are used as reference points and to determine where energy is restricted or excessive. For example, a practitioner will test the relative strength of the hamstring muscles if he or she suspects an intestinal problem. Treatment is started if these muscles are found to be weak.

For more information, contact:

Touch for Health Foundation
1174 N. Lake Avenue
Pasadena, CA 91104
818-794-1181

Chiropractic

Chiropractic is a healing art that emphasizes manipulation of the spinal vertebrae as a method of restoring bodily health. A *chiropractor* is a practitioner of the art of chiropractic who holds the degree of doctor of chiropractic (D.C.) and is licensed to provide chiropractic treatments.

Chiropractic in the United States can be traced to Daniel David Palmer, who in 1895 reportedly manipulated the spine of a deaf man and restored his hearing. Chiropractic is based upon the principle that the spinal column is central to a person's entire sense of well-being because it is instrumental in maintaining the health of the nervous system. Through chiropractic adjustments, or the manipulation of the vertebrae by a chiropractor, the nervous system is kept in or returned to good health.

Chiropractic is considered a drugless therapy, since chiropractors generally believe the body's own healing forces can be utilized to combat disease. This view of health care requires acceptance of the flow of life forces through the body and the use of those forces to maintain health. Hence, if something interferes with the flow of these forces, illness will occur.

Since chiropractors are concerned with the structure of the body, they are required to study anatomy, physiology, neurophysiology, biomechanics, and kinesiology. This training, as well as the use of certain diagnostic procedures, permits chiropractors to consider the body's entire neuromusculoskeletal system when making a diagnosis.

Diagnostic procedures used by chiropractors include treadmills, temperature sensing, stationary bicycles, and devices to measure the distribution of the body weight. The X ray remains the staple for examination of the spinal column and its twenty-four vertebrae.

Chiropractic treatment generally consists of spinal adjustments in which the chiropractor pushes on the vertebrae to reposition them. When a chiropractor is making an adjustment, the patient may hear a "pop" or "click" sound as the vertebra goes back into place.

Other joints also are manipulated and returned to their normal positions.

There are two main schools of thought in the practice of chiropractic today: One emphasizes traditional spinal manipulation and is called the straight school. Chiropractors from this school adhere to the principles first set down by Dr. Palmer and, as such, do not use any adjunctive therapies, such as heat, ultrasound, traction, vitamins, minerals, and exercise. On the other hand, chiropractors who supplement traditional spinal manipulation with adjunctive therapies are said to be from the mixed school, which accounts for the majority of chiropractors in practice today.

Chiropractic adjustments have been successful for a number of people; however, chiropractors point out that adjustments may not work in every case. When a chiropractor detects a condition that is beyond his or her scope of practice, a referral is made to the proper medical specialists.

For more information, contact:

International Chiropractors Association
["straight school"]
1110 N. Glebe Road
Arlington, VA 22201
800-423-4690

American Chiropractic Association
["mixed school"]
1701 Clarendon Boulevard
Arlington, VA 22209
703-276-8800

Listed below are colleges approved by the Commission on Accreditation of the Council on Chiropractic Education, in West Des Moines, Iowa.

California
Cleveland Chiropractic College
590 N. Vermont Avenue
Los Angeles, CA 90004

Life Chiropractic College, West
2005 Via Barrett
P.O. Box 367
San Lorenzo, CA 94580

Los Angeles College of Chiropractic
P.O. Box 1166
Whittier, CA 90609-1166

Palmer College of Chiropractic, West
1095 Dunford Way
Sunnyvale, CA 94087

Georgia
Life College
1269 Barclay Circle
Marietta, GA 30060

Illinois
National College of Chiropractic
200 E. Roosevelt Road
Lombard, IL 60148

Iowa
Palmer College of Chiropractic
1000 Brady Street
Davenport, IA 52803

Minnesota
Northwestern College of Chiropractic
2501 W. 84th Street
Bloomington, MN 55431

Missouri
Cleveland Chiropractic College
6401 Rockhill Road
Kansas City, MO 64131

Logan College of Chiropractic
P.O. Box 1065
Chesterfield, MO 63006-1065

New York
New York Chiropractic College
P.O. Box 167
Glen Head, NY 11545

Oregon
Western States Chiropractic College
2900 N.E. 132nd Avenue
Portland, OR 97230

Texas
Parker College of Chiropractic
2500 Walnut Hill Lane
Dallas, TX 75229

Texas Chiropractic College
5912 Spencer Highway
Pasadena, TX 77505

Feldenkrais Technique

The Feldenkrais technique was designed by Dr. Moshe Feldenkrais after World War II for the purpose of improving posture and general health. In some respects Feldenkrais owes his concept to the work done by F. Matthias Alexander in the development of the Alexander technique.

There are two facets to the Feldenkrais technique: awareness through movement, and private manipulative treatment. The first involves group-based classes where various exercises are performed while lying down in order to lessen the effects of gravity on the body. The purpose is to gently exercise the muscles and joints with as little strain as possible. A Feldenkrais teacher instructs pupils on the proper way to completely relax until they feel that "the body is hanging lightly from the head, the feet do not stomp on the ground, and the body glides when moving."

The second foundation of the Feldenkrais technique is private manipulative therapy, referred to as "functional integration." This is the person-to-person phase of the technique in which the teacher works with the pupil by using a series of gentle manipulative movements, but does not work directly on a problem in the belief that this could add to the pain and discomfort. For example, the legs and pelvis may be manipulated in order to relieve a problem in the shoulders.

Like the Alexander technique, the Feldenkrais technique strives to correct posture and break bad habits that lead to muscular and joint discomfort.

While there are Feldenkrais teachers, the most likely place to find the technique practiced is in other types of massage therapy.

For more information, contact:

Feldenkrais Center for Learning
48 N. Pleasant Street, Suite 204
Amherst, MA 01002
413-253-3550

Feldenkrais Guild
14 Corporate Woods
8717 W. 100th, Suite 140
Overland Park, KS 66210
913-492-1444

Massage Therapy

Massage therapy is the healing art in which hand manipulation of the body is employed to create a feeling of relaxation, ease mental and physical tensions, alleviate aches and pains, improve circulation, and generally reinvigorate and stimulate the body's systems. A *massage therapist* is trained in one or more of the following forms of massage therapy: Swedish massage, shiatsu, acupressure, Rolfing, reflexology, polarity, and bioenergetics.

The philosophy of massage is rooted in Eastern medicine and is based upon the balance point of the human body. It is believed that when this balance is tipped, one way or the other, illness can occur. Massage therapy can relax the body and improve circulation, which enables the body to regain its balance point and return to good health.

While an integral part of Chinese medicine, massage therapy generally has been avoided in Western medicine. When it is utilized, it is usually in connection with the conditioning of athletes and primarily to limber up joints and relieve aches and pains. However, today there is more interest in the use of massage therapy for a myriad of health care problems. In fact, two groups of medical practitioners already use a form of manipulation as part of their treatment. Osteopaths and chiropractors manipulate joints of the body to treat certain conditions.

Massage therapists claim it is effective in treating stress and fatigue, headaches, insomnia, lower back pain, muscle fatigue, and pregnancy and postpartum problems, as well as in aiding digestion and circulation.

Most massages begin at the head or feet, then gradually work toward the heart, since this is believed to be the body's natural circulatory path. Each massage is composed of a series of strokes or movements done with different pressure. The basic massage strokes are kneading, tapping or striking, and gliding. Swedish massage makes use of two additional motions: vibration and friction.

Since massage therapy is noninvasive and involves no drugs, just about anyone can enjoy its benefits. And, if nothing else, massage makes you feel good.

For more information, contact:

American Massage Therapy Association
1130 W. North Shore Avenue
Chicago, IL 60626
312-761-2682

Myotherapy

Myotherapy is a method of pain relief that is based upon locating "trigger points" in muscles that cause the muscles to go into spasm. Using the fingers, knuckles, or elbows, pressure is applied to these trigger points. A person certified in the use of myotherapy techniques is a *myotherapist.*

Trigger points are difficult to explain, but can best be described as sensitive spots that contribute to pain. The pain occurs when these points "fire," thus causing the muscles to react.

Trigger points occur because muscles are subjected to bumps, sprains, blows, and strains. Many of these points can be located in a single muscle, and during a lifetime it's possible to accumulate a large number of them. Not limited only to the large muscles of the body—legs, back, shoulders, chest, and so on—trigger points also occur in the muscles of the face, hands, and feet.

Very familiar with anatomy and the complete muscle structure of the body, a myotherapist searches for trigger points by pushing on or putting pressure on the muscles. Since myotherapy is a drugless therapy, the only tools are fingers, knuckles, and elbows, and something called a bodo. Basically, this is a wooden dowel used to apply pressure.

The whole point of myotherapy is that trigger points can be released or neutralized by applying pressure for at least 7 seconds, a rule that works fine for most muscles; however, smaller muscles respond to as little as 4 seconds of pressure. Myotherapists also go easier when working with children or the elderly.

While there is no scientific basis per se for myotherapy, it has received favorable notice from the media and is looked upon as a form of physical therapy.

For more information, contact:

Bonnie Prudden Workshops
7800 East Speedway
Tuscon, AZ 85710
602-529-3979

Reflexology

Reflexology is the practice of stimulating certain areas of the feet that correspond to various organs and other parts of the body. Proper stimulation of these points can aid in maintaining good health. The person who practices reflexology is a *reflexologist.* Some reflexologists are also certified, which indicates they have completed a formal course of instruction in reflexology.

Reflexology has its proponents as well as its detractors. With origins in Chinese medicine, reflexology is considered a cousin of acupuncture but uses the hands to massage the toes and bottom of the feet. Both approaches believe in the flow of life force to every part of the body, and both attempt to improve that flow as a way to ward off disease.

The first known writings on reflexology in the United States were done by Eunice D. Ingham in the

1930s. A booklet entitled "Stories the Feet Can Tell" sets forth the principles of reflexology and described how various organs and body parts correspond to specific locations on the feet.

Surprisingly complex, the foot contains twenty-six bones, fifty-six ligaments, and thirty-eight muscles. Reflexologists knead, rub, stroke, and pry at the muscles and toes of the feet to improve circulation of the life force to the organs and joints in the body.

A reflexologist will "read" the foot for symptoms of illness, which usually are indicated by a gritty or sandy feeling. These are often referred to as crystals, which represent waste products that are impeding normal circulation. The location of these crystals enables the reflexologist to determine which organ or body system is experiencing a problem. The reflexologist uses the thumb and fingers to break up the crystals and thus restore normal circulation.

Reflexologists seldom claim that their therapy cures. Rather, reflexology is looked upon as a preventive method for maintaining good health. Some sources indicate that reflexology can be effective in helping to relieve headaches, stress, sinus problems, constipation, and other functional disorders.

There is still considerable debate as to how or why reflexology works. To Western medicine the concepts of life forces and energy fields are difficult to comprehend, so it has not readily accepted the philosophy of its Eastern counterpart.

For more information, contact:

International Institute of Reflexology
P.O. Box 12642
St. Petersburg, FL 33733
813-343-4811

Rolfing

Rolfing is a therapy in which very deep massage is used to correct improper structural or postural positions. A practitioner skilled in the use of this deep muscle massage to bring about structural balances is a *Rolfer*.

Rolfing was developed in the 1930s by Ida Rolf and grew in popularity when people began exploring healing methods outside of traditional medicine. As with any manipulative therapy, Rolfing owes its philosophical and physical tenets to healing methods developed in the East, such as acupressure.

Rolfing involves the manipulation of muscles and fascia (connective tissue of the body, including ten-

dons, lymph nodes, and ligaments) to permit freer movement of the body. As the muscles and fascia are manipulated, the body returns to its natural posture. Rolfing usually consists of ten sessions conducted over a 5 or 10 week period. These sessions are divided into three distinct parts in which the Rolfer has very specific objectives to achieve.

Rolfers are interested in freeing the body from the constraints imposed by stress, poor living habits, and bad posture. Since part of the problem is related to breathing, the Rolfer first works to loosen the chest and pelvic muscles. The second group of sessions concentrates on the ankles and feet.

The final sessions concentrate on establishing new patterns of movement, and once these are developed, the person should notice an improvement in both physical and mental energies.

Some massage therapists, kinesiologists, and chiropractors may be familiar with the technique of Rolfing.

For more information, contact:

Rolf Institute
P.O. Box 1868
Boulder, CO 80306
303-449-5903

Shiatsu

Shiatsu is a form of Japanese massage in which the fingers are used to apply pressure to specific points on the body known as meridians. The philosophy behind shiatsu is to promote better health by stimulating the meridians and improving the flow of chi energy throughout the body.

MIDWIFERY

Midwifery is the practice of assisting in childbirth. A person who practices midwifery is a *midwife*, usually a certified nurse-midwife.

In large measure due to changes in conventional medicine and the desire of women to control the circumstances of giving birth, midwifery has reemerged as a force in maternity care.

Having supplanted the lay midwife, the certified nurse-midwife is the predominant practitioner. This is a registered nurse who has taken additional training in obstetrics and gynecology and newborn care and who has passed an extensive credentialing examination administered by the American College of Nurse-Midwives.

Nurse-midwives practice in a variety of settings: hospitals, birthing centers, health maintenance organizations, public health departments, and public and private health clinics. Although nurse-midwives independently manage maternity and newborn care, they are affiliated with physicians—an aspect of independent practice recognized by many insurance companies that now reimburse for nurse-midwife services.

Nurse-midwives provide care before, during, and after pregnancy. Women are advised of family-planning methods, normal gynecological care, diet and nutrition, birthing methods, and newborn care. During labor the nurse-midwife monitors progress and offers emotional and physical support, and also monitors the presence or absence of fetal distress and whether physician services are required. At birth the nurse-midwife assists the delivery and examines the newborn.

For more information, contact:

American College of Nurse-Midwives
1522 K Street N.W., Suite 1120
Washington, DC 20005
202-347-5445

NATUROPATHIC MEDICINE

Naturopathic medicine is a healing art that emphasizes the body's natural healing forces. It is a drugless therapy that makes use of massage, light, heat, air, and water. A person schooled in the art of naturopathic medicine who has earned the degree of doctor of naturopathic medicine (N.D.) is a *naturopathic physician*. Students enrolled in naturopathic medical schools complete courses that are a balance of traditional naturopathic philosophy, medical science, and the effectiveness of natural therapeutics.

Naturopathic medicine is rooted in the concept of *vis medicatrix naturae*, the healing power of nature. Naturopaths trace their origins to Hippocrates, who is said to have believed in the ability of nature to cure illnesses. One explanation given for the emergence of naturopathic medicine was disenchantment with the heroic remedies of orthodox medicine: bleeding, blistering, and purging. Very often they proved worse than the illness and did little to relieve the underlying health problem.

Naturopathy is practiced throughout the world, yet little is known in the West because of the bias against any healing art that is not founded in allo-pathic philosophy. Naturopathy is concerned with removing the root cause of disease, whether it be psychological, chemical (faulty eating, drinking, breathing, or elimination), or mechanical (bad posture or muscular tension).

To the naturopath, a person's medical history is the most important piece of information used to make a diagnosis. Naturopaths also rely on laboratory tests and other diagnostic techniques, such as X rays, scans, physicals, and so on. Once the diagnosis is made, the naturopath sets about restoring health by taking the whole person into account and not just the symptoms.

Naturopaths consider diet and nutrition essential to good health, and will advise patients on proper nutrition, including the types of food that should be eaten as well as those to avoid. In some cases, naturopaths will recommend fasting as one method for detoxifying the body before beginning a new regimen of diet and nutrition. The fasting process is not designed to be starvation; rather, it is an attempt to permit the body's metabolic functions to rest, thus enabling the body to eliminate waste and toxic products and thereby cleanse itself.

Naturopathic medical colleges are four-year post-graduate schools with admissions requirements comparable to those of conventional medical schools. The doctor of naturopathic medicine degree requires four years of graduate-level study in the medical sciences.

For more information, contact:

Bastyr University
144 N.E. 54th Street
Seattle, WA 98105
206-523-9585

National College of Naturopathic Medicine
11231 S.E. Market Street
Portland, OR 97216
503-255-4860

OPTOMETRY

Optometry is the practice of examining, diagnosing, and treating visual defects through the use of lenses, other visual aids, and visual therapies. A professional who practices optometry, an *optometrist*, must complete a four-year course of study before receiving the degree of doctor of optometry (O.D.), and must obtain a license before opening a practice.

Vision is one of the most important senses that humans possess. It is estimated that over 90 percent of all we know and learn has been acquired through the visual sense. When vision problems do arise, a visit to any eye care specialist is usually in order.

Optometrists study the manner in which the eyes receive light rays and the way the lenses focus that light upon the retina. They are concerned with the general health of the eye and the surrounding structure, including the eyelids, eyelashes, tear ducts, muscles, and so forth.

Optometrists measure the visual power of the eyes by using various instruments. They also test for color blindness, glaucoma, and other eye disorders.

Optometrists use lenses to correct the two more common visual problems: myopia (nearsightedness) and hyperopia (farsightedness). Optometry also makes use of prisms and other visual aids to correct other eye disorders such as crossed eyes (strabismus) and "lazy eye" (amblyopia).

Optometrists also do vision therapy, exercises, and other techniques that enable people to maintain or improve their vision without the use of mechanical aids such as eyeglasses or contact lenses.

When optometrists detect conditions beyond their scope, such as a disorder that may require surgery, they refer the patient to an ophthalmologist, an M.D. who specializes in the medical or surgical treatment of eye diseases.

For more information, contact:

American Optometric Association
243 N. Lindbergh Boulevard
St. Louis, MO 63141
314-991-4100

OSTEOPATHIC MEDICINE

Osteopathic medicine is a healing art founded by Dr. Andrew Taylor Sill, based on the theory that the entire body must be considered when treating disease. An essential part of osteopathic practice is the belief in the relationship between disease and the body's structure. One schooled in the art of osteopathic medicine is an *osteopathic physician* or *osteopath*. To be granted the degree of doctor of osteopathy (D.O.), a person must complete four years of study at an approved school of osteopathic medicine.

Osteopathy has much the same scientific foundations as allopathic medicine, but does have certain philosophical differences. Osteopaths believe in treating the whole person and not just the symptoms of a particular illness. Another major difference is that osteopaths use manipulative therapy to reposition joints in the body or the vertebrae of the spine. Otherwise, they use the same methods of diagnosis and treatment as allopathic practitioners—examinations, tests, X rays, medications, and surgery.

Because of the osteopathic philosophy of treating the whole person, many practitioners are in general or family practice. However, osteopaths also have developed specialties and are board-certified by the American Osteopathic Association (AOA). Specialties currently certified by the AOA include anesthesiology, dermatology, internal medicine, neurology, obstetrics-gynecology, ophthalmology, pathology, pediatrics, physical medicine, proctology, psychiatry, radiology, and various surgical specialties.

To be certified in a specialty, an osteopath must complete a residency program that usually requires an additional two to five years of study.

Because of past biases, osteopaths were forced to establish their own hospitals, since they were not permitted in the M.D.-dominated hospitals. However, as osteopathy has gained acceptance, some hospitals now grant privileges to both M.D.'s and D.O.'s.

For more information, contact:

American Osteopathic Association
142 E. Ontario Street
Chicago, IL 60611
312-280-5800

PODIATRY

Podiatry is the field of medical care that deals with the diagnosis and treatment of diseases, injuries, deformities, and other conditions of the foot. A *podiatrist* is a practitioner of podiatry who has completed a four-year course of study for the degree of doctor of podiatric medicine (D.P.M.). Licensure is required before a practice can be established.

Once known as chiropodists and considered tradesmen as opposed to medical professionals, podiatrists now treat foot conditions ranging from simple corns to infectious diseases. They also perform surgery to correct deformities of the foot and toes, including the removal of bone spurs, warts, and tumors. Podiatrists set fractures and prepare orthoses (devices to rearrange the weight-bearing structure of the foot).

Preventing injuries is also a major concern of podiatrists. Many athletes consult with podiatrists to determine the best methods for preventing injuries to the foot, ankle, and connective muscles and tendons. Podiatrists rely upon physical examinations, tests, and X rays to aid in making a diagnosis.

Treatment modalities include medications; surgery on bones, muscles, and tendons; ultrasound; diathermy; and physical therapy.

For problems of the feet, the most obvious choice is between a podiatrist and an orthopedic specialist (an M.D. who specializes in bone disorders). Many people choose podiatrists because they believe this practitioner is more likely to recommend a conservative approach.

Podiatrists are becoming more involved with screening the lower extremities for signs of other systemic disorders such as diabetes and hardening of the arteries. When such problems are found, podiatrists will make referrals to the appropriate medical specialists. While there is still some controversy over the proper role of the podiatrist in the medical world, organized medicine has not been able to prevent podiatrists from gaining hospital admitting privileges.

For more information, contact:

American Podiatric Medical Association
9312 Old Georgetown Road
Bethesda, MD 20814
301-571-9200

PSYCHOLOGICAL THERAPIES

Biofeedback

Biofeedback uses the conscious mind to control the involuntary body functions, such as respiration, heartbeat, and body temperature. It can be learned by anyone and utilized when needed for specific conditions.

While there may not be a precise definition of biofeedback, the following example demonstrates how we all use biofeedback at one time or another.

You may not have given much thought to how you learned to ride a bicycle, yet you employed a form of biofeedback in the learning process. If you had to think consciously of all the steps it takes to ride a bicycle, you may not have gotten past the first one. As you pedaled the first few shaky feet, your brain was processing the feedback it was getting from your body as it sought to make automatic adjustments to

achieve the balance necessary for you to keep pedaling and stay on the bike.

The application of biofeedback to health disorders is not new. For many years, especially in Eastern cultures, yogis have been able to control involuntary body reflexes such as respiration and heartbeat. By slowing down body functions, they are able to induce many conditions that a more active or conscious body cannot.

Biofeedback has found acceptance in the psychological profession as practitioners seek alternative methods to drug therapies. For many people, living with pain and stress has become the price for living in the modern world. And while drug therapy may be effective, many people are concerned about drug side effects. Biofeedback holds some promise as being one way to help people cope with chronic pain and deal with stress. It should be pointed out, however, that biofeedback is not a cure, but is a method of dealing with symptoms.

The techniques used to train someone in the use of biofeedback have become very sophisticated. It is now possible to monitor brain impulses and make them audible to the person who is using biofeedback. By monitoring this electrical activity and listening to the series of "beeps," the person will learn how to control the situation.

Some people use biofeedback to control their body temperature or increase the flow of blood to certain body parts. Biofeedback has also been employed for stress headaches, migraine headaches, back pain, temporomandibular joint pain, and nerve damage.

The concept of using biofeedback to control the involuntary workings of the body is new to Western medical thought; therefore, you may not find every practitioner open to discussing its use. A good starting point is a certified biofeedback instructor.

For more information, contact:

Biofeedback Society of America
10200 W. 44th Avenue
Wheat Ridge, CO 80033
303-422-8436

Hypnotherapy

Hypnotherapy is the use of hypnosis as an adjunctive therapy in the treatment of physical and mental disorders. A professional who is schooled in the art of hypnosis and who uses hypnosis as a healing method is a *hypnotherapist*.

Ever since Franz Mesmer told his first patient,

"You are getting very sleepy," there has been skepticism about the effectiveness of hypnosis. Most of the skeptics have been practitioners of orthodox medicine whose rigid adherence to scientific dogma precluded the belief in anything as theatrical as hypnosis.

Some evidence suggests that hypnosis, or the induction of a trancelike state, was known in ancient times, when the Druids were said to be able to induce a "magic sleep." Certain Egyptian writings also referred to hypnosis.

However, today the use of hypnosis is gaining additional respectability as both psychiatrists and psychologists employ a form of it in their practices.

Although not exactly asleep, a person in a hypnotic state is not fully awake either. The state is, if nothing else, an altered one wherein the subject is more responsive to the power of suggestion. A person who is hypnotized may have incredible powers of concentration and be able to accomplish things not necessarily possible in a more conscious state.

Contrary to popular myth, you cannot be hypnotized against your will or forced to do something you do not want to do. If you can be hypnotized, you may be able to use the power of your subconscious to focus all your mind's energy on one problem. The ability to focus on one problem is a result of being insulated from the distractions of the outside world. Among orthodox medical practitioners, hypnotherapy has gained some respectability based on the results of trials conducted on burn victims. It seems that when hypnotized they were better able to deal with the pain associated with the deep burn wounds. Other practitioners have used hypnotherapy to help patients deal with pain from migraine headaches, chronic pain, stress, stomach problems, arthritis, colitis, and hemophilia, to name just a few. Hypnosis may also be self-administered.

Learning to break an old habit or establish a new healthy habit can be accomplished through hypnosis. People wishing to quit smoking often use hypnosis, and there have also been reports of success in helping people to lose weight and adhere to a new diet. Some therapists, especially those in pediatric hospitals, use hypnosis to help patients overcome their fears of hospitalization.

For more information, contact:

American Society of Clinical Hypnosis
2200 E. Devon, Suite 291
Des Plaines, IL 60018
708-297-3317

Psychotherapy

Psychotherapy is a healing art that approaches the treatment of disorders with mental rather than physical methods. Forms of psychotherapy include suggestion, dialogue, reeducation, confidence building, and moral support. A person who uses any of the various forms of psychotherapy to treat mental disorders and behavioral disturbances is a *psychotherapist*. Practitioners include psychiatrists, psychologists, psychiatric social workers, psychiatric nurses, psychoanalysts, and pastoral counselors.

Psychotherapy seeks to help people overcome life's problems, which may or may not be rooted in deep emotional conflicts. Often the pressures of daily life create situations in which a person feels as though he or she can no longer cope. The emphasis in psychotherapy is in the cognitive arena, where dialogue is more important than drug therapy. Building a relationship with a therapist is one of the keys to making psychotherapy work. Another factor is the commitment the person has to making the therapy work.

The list of psychotherapies available is rather extensive and includes the following: Freudian, Jungian, Gestalt, Adlerian, Rogerian, group, reality, cognitive, integrity, shock, primal scream, hypnotherapy, behavior modification, biofeedback, Erhard Seminars Training (est), orthomolecular psychiatry, rebirthing, and Rolfing.

However, most types of psychotherapy can be grouped into a few broad categories: traditional psychotherapies (Freudian, Jungian, and Adlerian), human potential therapies (client-centered, Gestalt, and bioenergetics), group therapies (psychodrama, family therapy, and transactional analysis), and cognitive-behavior therapies (behavior therapy and biofeedback).

Psychotherapy is intended to help people deal with reality, take charge of situations, and regain control of their lives. Those suffering from phobias may be helped by various therapies designed to free them from their fears, or at least to recognize what is frightening them. Group therapy is sometimes used to help people overcome feelings of loneliness and become more involved in society. Behavior modification can be utilized to correct behavior that is self-destructive by teaching adaptive skills.

The two most popular psychotherapists are the psychiatrist (an M.D. specializing in psychiatry) and the psychologist (a Ph.D. in psychology). Both have certifying organizations to help ensure that only qualified professionals are permitted to practice. Some of the other types of practitioners, such as counselors and social workers, have their own certifying organization, the American Board of Professional Psychology, which issues diplomas to candidates who have met both education and experience criteria. And there's a movement in many states toward the licensing of social workers and family counselors.

For more information, contact:

American Psychological Association
1200 17th Street N.W.
Washington, DC 20036
202-955-7600

American Board of Professional Psychology
2100 E. Broadway, Suite 313
Columbia, MO 65201
314-875-1267

American Board of Psychiatry and Neurology
500 Lake Cook Road, Suite 335
Deerfield, IL 60015
708-945-7900

YOGA

Yoga is a philosophy of life that originated in India and espouses the uniting of body, mind, and spirit in order to achieve a higher self-realization; it has been practiced for some 6,000 years. A person who practices yoga, follows its philosophy, or teaches yoga is a *yogi*.

As with all mystical philosophies, yoga requires the acceptance of a world in which disharmonies and interferences restrict an individual's spiritual growth. Some people see yoga as a religion, while others view it as a philosophy intended to help them achieve their goals.

According to legend, yoga exercises were designed by Lord Shiva at the beginning of time and have remained the same since then. The first codified yoga system is believed to have been written in the second century B.C. by the Indian sage Pantanjali. To this day yoga utilizes eighty-four of the postures handed down by Pantanjali.

Yoga is deeply rooted in Eastern mysticism and the belief in some formless god who creates and arranges all matter. The yogi attempts to unite with this force and reach a state of consciousness and awareness in which harmony exists. But before reaching this state, the yogi must perform a series of exercises involving breathing and posture. This is hatha yoga.

Other forms of yoga include:

Mantra yoga. A mantra is a word or phrase that is repeated thousands of times. The mind focuses on the vibrations of the mantra and thus increases concentration.

Bhakti yoga. This is the yoga of faith, devotion, and worship. Yogis chant to help increase their spiritual bliss.

Jnana yoga. This is the yoga of knowledge or intellect. It requires the yogi to focus on those things that have occurred and to learn from them.

Karma yoga. This is cause and effect, with good deeds producing good karma and bad deeds producing bad karma.

Raja yoga. This is the ultimate state of superconsciousness, or deep meditation, that yogis strive to attain. This form of perfect mind control permits the yogi to control all thought processes and keep them free from distractions.

Laya yoga. This yoga explores the seven energy centers of the body known as the chakras. It requires a person to still the mind and awaken the inner force, called kundalini.

The practice of yoga in the West has been increasing as more people seek alternative methods for achieving a feeling of well-being and seek to improve their self-discipline, concentration, and positive thinking.

For further information, contact:

Integral Yoga Institute
227 W. 13th Street
New York, NY 10011
212-929-0585

Himalayan International Institute of Yoga Science and Philosophy
R.R. 1, P.O. Box 400
Honesdale, PA 18431
717-253-5551

Nuclear Medicine: A Medical Specialty

Nuclear medicine is the medical specialty that employs the nuclear properties of radioactive and stable nuclides in diagnosis, therapy, and research.

A specialist in nuclear medicine is a physician who has been awarded a medical degree from an approved medical or osteopathic school and has satisfactorily completed two or more years of residency training in a general medical specialty and two additional years of nuclear medicine residency in an accredited residency program. He or she has satisfactorily passed a written examination encompassing the diagnostic and therapeutic uses of radioactive materials and in the related physical and biological sciences.

The X-ray technician is an allied professional who prepares patients for X-ray examinations, takes and develops X-ray pictures, and assists with other imaging techniques. As the field of nuclear medicine expands, a growing number of these technicians are themselves specializing in specialized X-ray exams, specifically radionuclide scanning. They are commonly called nuclear medicine technicians.

Nuclear Medicine and Common Nuclear Scans

In nuclear medicine, radioactive materials are introduced into the body to help in the diagnosis and treatment of certain diseases. (The more important application of nuclear medicine is in diagnosis.) A very small amount of the radioactive substance is swallowed, injected, or inhaled. Isotopes of iodine, iron, and indium are the ones most often used: They have short half-lives—meaning that isotopes lose half of their radioactivity within minutes or hours and therefore minimize possible radiation damage—and they emit enough gamma radiation to enable a camera outside the body to detect the isotope within the body. Nuclear scanning is an important tool, since it can reveal abnormalities that ordinary X-ray film is unable to detect.

Most radioisotopes are used as "tags." This means they are combined with another molecule, either a biological one that's present in the body or a nonbiological one. For example, when the dye Rose Bengal is tagged with radioiodine and injected into the body, it travels to the liver. The gamma camera picture will show the presence of the dye in the liver, and any area of the liver where the dye is not present is most likely the site of an abnormality, such as a tumor or cyst.

As with X rays, certain risk factors must be taken into account. If a nuclear scan is ordered, inform your doctor if you are pregnant, or suspect you may be, or if you are breast-feeding.

PET AND SPECT

Like the more commonly known and performed imaging techniques—computed axial tomography (CAT) and magnetic resonance imaging (MRI)—positron emission tomography (PET) and single photon emission computed tomography (SPECT) use computer technology to enable your doctor to view the inside of your body "sliced" into multiple planes: front-to-front, side-to-side, and up and down.

But unlike CAT scans and MRIs, which can only reveal anatomy, PET and SPECT can also look at physiology, or how various organs and systems are actually working. PET and SPECT images also show the inside of organs, not just the surfaces.

The difference between these two high-tech systems is in the type of atomic particle used. The positrons used in PET systems have a very short half-life and, for this reason, need to be produced on site in a small, low-energy cyclotron (a device that smashes atoms and releases gamma rays). For this reason, PET is very expensive and available only at university research centers. However, research conducted on PET systems can be adapted to the less expensive SPECT systems that use commercially prepared radioisotopes and are more readily available at hospitals across the United States.

PET research has made advances in the understanding of how the brain and heart function, including how the brain uses oxygen. SPECT systems are helpful in diagnosing problems with the liver, kidneys, skeletal system, cardiac function and some brain abnormalities.

COMMON NUCLEAR SCANS AND WHY THEY ARE PERFORMED

Bone scan. Frequently done to see if a known cancer has spread or when suspicion of skeletal pathology is not revealed by X-ray; monitors the effectiveness of cancer therapy; evaluates unexplained bone pain; and may reveal cause for elevated blood level of alkaline phosphate (an enzyme that affects bone metabolism). A scan called absorptiometry is used to evaluate bone density to check for osteoporosis.

Brain scan. Performed when there is suspicion of a mass or other abnormality; monitors response of a brain tumor to surgery. See earlier explanation of PET and SPECT.

Gallbladder and biliary tract scans (cholescintigraphy). Evaluates suspected gallbladder and biliary tract disease; evaluates pain in the upper right side of abdomen, jaundice and abdominal trauma when injury to liver is suspected.

Gallium scan (body scan). Detects primary cancers, cancers that have spread, or inflammations and abscesses; monitors response of tumors to radiation and chemotherapy; detects hidden infections; and evaluates unexplained masses.

Liver/spleen scan. Determines if a known cancer has spread to the liver or spleen; may also be used to detect enlarged liver and spleen or check for abdominal masses. Both organs are examined at once, using one intravenous injection.

Lung scans. Performed when a blood clot is suspected (pulmonary embolism); determines severity of chronic lung disease. There are two types of lung scans: *Perfusion scans* detect the distribution of blood to a body part. This test images the blood flow in each lung following an injection of radioactive material; areas not receiving adequate blood could indicate a possible blockage. *Ventilation scans* measure airflow in and out of the lungs. A mask is placed over the nose and mouth and the patient inhales the isotope xenon in gaseous form; the patient then rebreathes the

gas for several minutes while sitting in front of a gamma camera that is measuring the radioactivity in the patient's lungs. In the normal lung, air is distributed evenly; if air distribution is not even, it could mean pneumonia or a tumor is present.

Renal scans (renogram, renal scintigraphy, renography, and kidney scan). Evaluate kidney function, renal blood flow, kidney transplants, kidney disease, and suspected kidney masses, stones, or injury; detect narrowing of arteries supplying kidneys.

Thyroid scan and radioactive iodine (RAI) uptake test. Evaluates swelling of the neck, enlarged thyroid or lump in thyroid; detects excessive thyroid hormone production (hyperthyroidism); checks for thyroid cancer.

Gynecology and Obstetrics

Gynecology is a branch of medicine that deals exclusively with the health of women, specifically the health and proper functioning of the female reproductive system. The reproductive system consists of organs that allow a woman to conceive, house a developing fetus, and eventually give birth.

Female reproductive organs include two ovaries (which produce ova for fertilization), fallopian tubes (tubes that connect the ovaries and the uterus), uterus (muscular organ where the fetus develops and which is the site for menstruation), cervix (opening of the uterus that leads to the vagina), vagina (muscular organ that serves as the birth canal, the site where sperm is collected, and connects the uterus to the external genitals).

The external female genitalia, or vulva, consists of the mons pubis (fat tissue covering the pelvic bones), labia majora and minora (folds of skin and muscle that protect other organs), clitoris (an erectile mass of tissue), and the vestibule (opening of the vagina). The area of tissue between the vagina and anus is called the perineum.

Obstetrics is a branch of gynecology that concentrates on all aspects of pregnancy and childbirth, including prenatal care and fetal testing and monitoring. Frequently, many gynecologists are also trained in obstetrics and deliver babies.

OBSTETRICIAN-GYNECOLOGISTS AND OTHER PRACTITIONERS

The various practitioners who offer obstetrical and gynecological care are obstetrician-gynecologists, family practitioners, nurse practitioners, certified nurse-midwives, and lay midwives.

An *obstetrician-gynecologist* is a surgical specialist who has been trained in childbirth procedures as well as in diagnosing and treating gynecologic problems, and has completed approximately four years of ob-gyn residency training after medical school.

In addition, an obstetrician-gynecologist may subspecialize in gynecologic oncology (gynecologic cancers), maternal and fetal medicine (complications of pregnancy), and reproductive endocrinology (hormonal/infertility problems).

The great majority of women choose an ob-gyn for their birth practitioner; in fact, obstetricians deliver four out of every five babies born in this country.

Women may also choose a *family practitioner* (FP) for their obstetrical and gynecological care. A relatively new specialty, family practice, is concerned with the total health of the individual and the family and is not limited to age, sex, organ system, or disease entity. The family practitioner has three years of training following medical school, including a minimum of 3 months of obstetrics and gynecology. Of course, not every FP has obstetrical experience.

A *nurse practitioner* (NP) is a registered nurse who has completed advanced training, in this case most often in gynecologic care, and can offer gynecologic examinations as well as manage gynecologic problems. In a gynecologist's office or a women's health care clinic, a nurse practitioner may do an entire routine gynecological exam—breast exam, pelvic exam, and Pap smear. She can order and interpret routine lab tests, manage minor gynecologic problems such as vaginal infections, and provide care for uncomplicated pregnancies. Nurse practitioners also play an important role in patient education, showing women how to do breast self-exams and use contraceptives such as diaphragms and birth control pills.

A *certified nurse-midwife* (CNM), usually working in conjunction with a physician, has completed graduate training in women's health and obstetrical care. CNMs offer childbirth education, prenatal care, and obstetric care, and can deliver babies and practice privately or in hospitals, birthing centers, or other health centers.

The *lay midwife,* or independent midwife, delivers babies but has no formal obstetrical training, save for the hands-on, practical experience of attending births and delivering babies. Lay midwives deliver babies in a home setting and know, if complications should arise, when to obtain medical assistance.

GYNECOLOGIC EXAMINATION

Gynecologists routinely examine and check the health of female patients. In fact, for a lot of women, gynecologists are their primary care physicians and are doctors to whom they go for preventive care.

See "Women's Health" in section 9, "Family Health and Resources," for a thorough discussion of the typical gynecologic exam, which often is a way for the gynecologist to detect any developing problems.

Another diagnostic test, which is not a regular part of a gynecologic exam but which we mention here because it can be done by the gynecologist, is a D&C (dilation and curettage). The D&C, which can indicate the presence of several disorders or abnormal conditions, dilates the cervix so that the gynecologist can scrape some of the lining of the uterus with a curette. More and more, other procedures such as hysteroscopy or those that use aspiration (use of a suction device to remove uterine tissue contents) are used and are replacing the traditional D&C procedure.

GYNECOLOGIC PROBLEMS AND DISORDERS

Most problems associated with the gynecologic organs are detected by the woman herself (for example, yeast infection and irregular periods) or can be discovered by the gynecologist (fibroids, cancer). Different types of conditions or disorders can occur in and afflict the menstrual cycle, the vulva and vagina, the cervix, the uterus, and the fallopian tubes and ovaries.

Problems of the Menstrual Cycle

Problems of the menstrual cycle can be categorized into problems that cause excessive pain and problems associated with abnormalities in uterine bleeding. These problems can be conditions in themselves or they can be indications of an underlying gynecologic disorder. The experience of excessive pain during periods, termed dysmenorrhea, can also be accompanied by such symptoms as nausea, vomiting, and lower abdominal pain. The pain could be an isolated condition or it could be a sign of various disorders, such as fibroids, endometriosis, or ovarian cysts or tumors.

Diethylstilbestrol (DES)

Diethylstilbestrol (DES), a synthetic estrogen, was used between the years 1941 and 1971 and was given to pregnant women for the purpose of preventing miscarriages. DES primarily affects the reproductive system of the fetus, but may affect other systems as well (immune, cardiovascular). Exposure to DES has been one of the contributing factors to the development of vaginal and cervical cancer (clear cell adenocarcinoma), other gynecologic disorders (menstrual problems, endometriosis), changes in tissues (metaplasia), infertility problems and sterility, cervical as well as vaginal dysplasia, and cervical and uterine deformities (leading to problems and complications in pregnancy).

Some doctors tend to dismiss women's concerns about DES, assuming that DES-related problems are pretty much a thing of the past, and that women age 30 or older are beyond the age when such problems are likely to occur.

Those assumptions can be deadly, says DES Action director Pat Cody. DES-related health problems are still emerging. It's true that the most serious consequence of DES exposure, deadly clear cell adenocarcinoma, is rare. It develops in less than 1 in every 1,000 DES daughters, most often in women aged 15 to 24, with a peak at age 19½. But it's still being diagnosed, in girls as young as 7 and women as old as 38.

And no one knows what possible cancer risks DES daughters face as they grow older, or if they use birth control pills or replacement estrogen. That's one reason DES Action suggests DES daughters and mothers avoid such drugs. It is known that DES mothers have a 44 percent increased risk for breast cancer. So cancer screening is important.

Some doctors also mistakenly believe that a regular Pap smear and pelvic exam can detect DES-related problems. That's just not so. If your gynecologist offers what he or she

---

Abnormal uterine bleeding can describe conditions such as heavy periods (menorrhagia), absence of periods (amenorrhea), infrequent periods (oligomenorrhea), and dysfunctional uterine bleeding (spotting, unpredictable periods). Other disruptions and disturbances of the normal menstrual cycle can be due to abnormalities in the glands or organs that are responsible for hormone production and regulation. Usually, abnormalities or pain in the menstrual cycle can be regulated with hormone therapy (estrogen and progesterone) and analgesics (for pain).

Problems of the Vulva and Vagina

Vulvar and vaginal problems can also occur and affect the health of a woman. Vulvitis, or inflammation of the vulva, produces red itchy skin, swelling, and blisters on the external genitalia and is often caused by vaginitis or herpes. Vulvitis could be the

result of an allergic reaction to a substance or material (detergent, medication) or could be caused by an infection or poor hygiene. Treatment usually includes administration of a cortisone cream (for itching) or antifungal cream (for fungal infections) and a change in personal hygiene. Atrophic vulvar dystrophy, found most often in postmenopausal women, occurs as the vulvar skin becomes red and itchy or papery and white with blisters. This degeneration of vulvar tissue may become malignant and may be caused by a developing cancer.

Cancer of the vulva, a rare condition, produces an itchy lump and ulcers which may bleed. Vulvar cancer, in most cases, is curable with early detection and treatment of the cancer. Treatment includes radiation therapy and a vulvectomy (removal of tumor, cancerous skin, and lymph glands).

Vaginitis, or inflammation of the vagina, can result from a vaginal infection or exposure to a sexually calls a "DES exam," make sure it includes the following:

• A Pap smear not only of the cervix, but four additional smears (called a four-quadrant smear) from the vaginal walls surrounding the cervix. These smears help to determine if a biopsy (tissue sample) needs to be taken to check for clear cell cancer.

• Careful palpation (feeling) of the vaginal walls for any lumps or thickening

• Use of an iodine stain to check the vagina and cervix for adenosis tissue, a glandular tissue not normally found in the vagina that can harbor clear cell cancer. (Regular tissue stains brown; adenosis tissue does not.)

• Some doctors also examine the cervix and vagina with a magnifying instrument called a colposcope. This viewing device helps him or her detect and biopsy areas of tissue abnormality. "Blind," or unguided, biopsies are less accurate than those done with the aid of a colposcope. If an area of abnormal cells is small, a blind biopsy may miss it entirely.

Paradoxically, some DES-related non-cancerous conditions are *overtreated* by ignorant doctors. On a Pap smear, immature adenosis cells can be mistaken for dysplasia (abnormal cells) instead of what they really are, metaplasia (normal, fast-growing cells). That's why it's important that a Pap smear from a DES-exposed woman be labeled as such before it's sent to the laboratory for analysis. If there's any question about the laboratory report, you should request the slide be examined by a pathologist familiar with DES cell changes.

Simple adenosis does not have to be treated; a woman whose doctor suggests this tissue be removed by freezing, burning, or surgery "to prevent cancer" should definitely get a second opinion from a DES specialist.

DES Action offers nationwide referrals to doctors specializing in the treatment of DES-exposed women. The national office of DES Action is at 1615 Broadway, Suite 510, Oakland, CA 94612; telephone 510-465-4011.

---

transmitted disease. The walls of the vagina become irritated and infected by bacteria, which cause vaginal bleeding, itching, irritation, and discomfort, vaginal discharge, and pain in the lower abdomen as well as pain during intercourse.

Common organisms that cause vaginitis include the parasite *Trichomonas vaginalis* (causing trichomoniasis, characterized by a yellow/green foamy discharge); various fungal organisms such as *Candida albicans* (causing yeast infections, characterized by a white, cottage-cheese-like discharge); and organisms such as *Gardnerella vaginalis* (causing bacterial vaginosis, producing a foul-smelling white/gray discharge). Very often these organisms can be transmitted to the body through contact with wet towels, toilet seats, washcloths, and underwear. Treatment of these infections can include the administration of oral antibiotics (such as metronidazole), sulfa drugs, or vaginal suppositories/creams.

Vaginal tumors, rare occurrences in postmenopausal women, cause pain during intercourse or bowel movements, bleeding, and a watery discharge. Most of these tumors are slow-growing squamous cell tumors whose growth can be stopped with surgical removal and with radiation therapy. However, some tumors (called clear cell adenocarcinomas) produce a condition called vaginal adenosis, which may necessitate a complete or partial vaginectomy or a reconstruction of the vagina. The clear cell adenocarcinomas are primarily caused by past exposure to diethylstilbestrol (DES) when the woman was in her mother's womb.

Problems of the Cervix

Cervicitis, or inflammation of the cervix, produces such symptoms as a gray/yellow discharge from the vagina, fever, itching and burning in vulvar area, pain in the lower abdomen, frequent need to urinate, and

Be a DES Detective

What do you need to do to find out if you have been exposed to DES? First, ask your mother:

- Did you take any drugs during the first 5 months of your pregnancy? (DES was given as pills, injections, and suppositories.)

If your mother says yes, ask her why she took the drugs, and if she remembers the brand name. (DES Action, 1615 Broadway, Suite 510, Oakland, CA 94612, has a list of the many brand names under which DES was marketed.) If she's uncertain, ask:

- Did you have any problems during any pregnancy, such as bleeding, miscarriages, premature births, or diabetes?

If your mother did have any of these problems, there's more of a chance she took DES, even if she can't remember.

If your mother's doctor is still practicing, DES Action suggests you ask him in writing for a copy of any records showing prenatal medication. (And send along a self-addressed, stamped envelope.) If the doctor is retired, the practice may have been taken over by another doctor who has the records. Your county medical society may know who has the doctor's records.

The information might also be on your mother's hospital records during the time of your birth. DES Action suggests you write to the medical records department of the hospital. Give the date of birth and mother's name and ask them to let you know what prenatal medicine is listed in the mother's record.

If your mother remembers the pharmacy she used, you can request copies of prescriptions filled for her during her pregnancy. Some pharmacies keep records going back many years; others do not.

If you suspect but are unable to prove that you have been exposed to DES, DES Action recommends you have the DES exam that can detect physical signs of exposure. Besides adenosis tissue, distinct cervical abnormalities (a "collar" or "hood") are common signs. These are most apparent in women under age 30. In women aged 30 or older, the signs may have disappeared.

Clear cell cancer is most likely to be found on the initial DES exam; women who show no signs of cancer during their first exam are less likely to develop it later, although that does sometimes happen.

Women who know they have been exposed to DES are advised to continue to have DES exams throughout their lives. Women who suspect but cannot determine if they have been exposed should have one DES exam. If the exam shows no signs of exposure, most doctors agree they can go back to normal Pap smears. Women with signs of DES exposure are advised to continue with DES exams.

pain and bleeding during or after intercourse. The infection that causes cervicitis may stem from IUD use, an abortion, or childbirth. Cervicitis may also be the result of a vaginal infection or a sexually transmitted disease (STD), or other gynecologic disorder. Treatment of cervicitis can include the administration of oral or injected antibiotics, sulfa drugs, or, in severe cases, the cauterization of the cervix with heat or cryosurgery.

Cervical dysplasia, or cervical intraepithelial neoplasia (CIN), is a condition linked to STD exposure in which cervical cells grow abnormally and may eventually develop into cancer. Even though CIN may produce no symptoms, abnormalities in cervical cells can usually be detected by a Pap smear. Mild forms of dysplasia may disappear by themselves or may be treated by cauterization or laser surgery. However, if any abnormal cervical cells are indicated by a Pap smear and CIN is diagnosed, further diagnostic procedures (such as a colposcopy or a tissue biopsy) are usually recommended.

The abnormal cells can be treated and destroyed with cryosurgery, by laser, or by the loop electrosurgical excision procedure (LEEP) (low-voltage radio waves transmitted by a looplike wire that excises tissue). If cancerous cells do develop, usually in squamous cells, and the cancer is localized (in situ—CIS), a cone biopsy (or conization, in which a cone-shaped piece of tissue is removed) is performed. Cervical cancer produces symptoms such as irregular bleeding from the vagina, general poor health, and aches. If the cancer is invasive (it has spread to other organs), a radical hysterectomy is performed or external and internal radiation therapy can be given.

Problems of the Uterus

Endometriosis is a condition where pieces of the lining of the uterus (endometrium) become detached and grow on other pelvic organs. Monthly, the growths build up tissue as if they were still in the uterine lining. However, because now they are on other organs, the growths may cause internal bleeding, scar tissue, and cysts, and may bind pelvic organs together. Endometriosis generally afflicts women aged 25 to 40 and can produce fatigue, painful intercourse and menstruation, lower-back pain, gastrointestinal discomfort, irregular vaginal bleeding, diarrhea or constipation, and infertility.

The cause of endometriosis is not known, though it is thought that the menstrual flow backs up in the fallopian tubes, creating a spillage of the tissue onto the other pelvic organs (retrograde menstruation theory). A woman can be at risk for endometriosis if there is a history of the condition in her family, if she is prone to yeast infections or immune system diseases, and if she has had a history of dysmenorrhea. The condition is detected by a procedure called a laparoscopy (a small abdominal incision is made and a thin metal scope is used to view the uterus).

Although doctors have recommended pregnancy as a treatment method or cure of endometriosis, for some women this treatment method is not desirable, nor does it entirely guarantee the eradication of the condition. (Further, endometriosis-related scars and adhesions on the ovaries or fallopian tubes can prevent pregnancy.) Other treatment methods such as hormonal treatments (using such drugs as gonadotropin-releasing hormone analogs, synthetic progesteronelike drugs, and oral contraceptives) and cauterization of the growths have been used. If the endometriosis cannot be treated with these methods and if the pain is severe, a hysterectomy is performed.

Fibroids—also called leiomyomas, myomas, and fibromyomas—are benign growths of tissue that form as tumors in the interior of the uterine lining. Small fibroids are usually harmless in nature; however, large fibroids may cause the woman severe abdominal or back pain, irregular or heavy vaginal bleeding, or problems with pregnancy. Often the treatment recommended for removal of numerous, painful, or large fibroids has been a hysterectomy. However, in many cases, there are other, less severe treatment options, such as myomectomies (removal of the fibroids) and hysteroscopic resections (fibroids are shaved off).

Pelvic inflammatory disease (PID) is a bacterial infection of the pelvic organs caused by organisms acquired though sexually transmitted diseases, during childbirth or abortion, or from surgical procedures or IUD insertion. Infection of the uterus (endometritis), the fallopian tubes (salpingitis), and the ovaries (oophoritis) causes many different symptoms in a woman—including pain in the lower abdomen, irregular periods or excessive vaginal bleeding, pain or bleeding during or after intercourse, foul vaginal or urethral discharge, fever, frequent urination or difficulty in urination, and general fatigue.

PID can be detected by a pelvic exam, ultrasound, and laparoscopy and is not serious if it is promptly treated with antibiotics. However, if PID is left untreated, it may develop into chronic PID or peritonitis, cause abscesses to form and produce damage to the fallopian tubes and ovaries, spread to other parts of the body, or cause infertility or even death. Usually, the treatment for severe and uncontrollable PID is a hysterectomy.

Uterine cancer, a common gynecologic cancer, begins in the endometrium of the uterus. In postmenopausal women, uterine cancer produces vaginal bleeding, and in premenopausal women, uterine cancer causes irregular or heavy periods. Women who are considered to be at risk are those who are obese; have never had children; have high blood pressure, a problem with diabetes, or an imbalance in hormones; or have had excessive estrogen replacement therapy. To detect abnormal uterine cells, a D&C or an endometrial biopsy can be performed. Uterine cancer treatment could include surgery, radiation therapy and chemotherapy, or a radical hysterectomy with radiation therapy.

Uterine prolapse occurs as the supportive muscles in the pelvic floor weaken, causing the uterus to descend into the vagina. Uterine prolapse often originates from the relaxation of the pelvic muscles. Pelvic relaxation may manifest itself as the tendency to leak urine when the woman coughs or laughs, a feeling of fullness or discomfort, or a problem in excreting and defecating. Exercises to strengthen the pelvic muscles, called Kegel exercises, are helpful in cases of mild pelvic relaxation. However, in cases of severe uterine prolapse, the uterus can be surgically reattached in its correct position or a pessary can be inserted and fitted around the cervix to support the uterus in place.

Problems of the Ovaries

Ovarian cysts (fluid-filled sacs) or tumors (solid lumps of tissue) may grow on the ovaries. Most of these growths are noncancerous and disappear by themselves. However, when the growths distort, twist, or rupture the ovaries, severe pain or infection may follow. Ovarian cysts and tumors may also put the woman at risk for ovarian cancer.

Because they may produce no symptoms, usually ovarian cysts and tumors are detected by a combination of a pelvic exam, ultrasound, and a laparoscopy. However, ovarian cysts and tumors may cause the woman to experience aching in the lower abdomen, irregular periods, abdominal swelling, and pain during intercourse. If the cysts and tumors persist, grow too large, or produce

severe pain and discomfort, they can be drained or surgically removed. Ovarian cancer, affecting postmenopausal women and women who have never been pregnant, likewise produces few early symptoms and is usually detected during a pelvic exam or through other diagnostic procedures. As the cancer progresses, the woman may experience vaginal bleeding, frequent urination, nausea, abdominal swelling, fatigue, pain in the lower abdomen, or indigestion. The treatment of ovarian cancer may include surgical removal of one or both ovaries (oophorectomy) and its accompanying fallopian tube, radiation therapy, and chemotherapy.

HYSTERECTOMIES

A hysterectomy, or removal of the uterus, is often an elective surgical procedure whose implementation may be lifesaving for some conditions, controversial in some instances, unnecessary in other cases, but normally involves considerable risks and complications. See "Women's Health" in section 9, "Family Health and Resources," for more information.

OBSTETRIC CARE

Obstetric care, care concerned with all aspects of pregnancy and childbirth, can be obtained from a variety of practitioners, as discussed earlier. In addition to choosing the type of practitioner for her prenatal care, a woman can choose the kind of childbirth setting she wants—hospital, birthing center, or home—and the types of fetal tests she wishes to have performed.

PRENATAL CARE AND FETAL TESTING

Prenatal care is the personal health care that a woman takes when she is pregnant. This care involves maintaining a healthful diet and eating habits, avoiding harmful substances such as alcohol and nicotine, exercising, and visiting a practitioner monthly. The first visit to a practitioner, made during the woman's first trimester of pregnancy, will involve a discussion of the woman's personal and family medical history and a physical and gynecologic examination. During the second and third trimesters of pregnancy, a variety of tests can be performed to determine the condition of the fetus. Succeeding visits to the obstetrician will occur monthly (visits become more frequent in the

Emergency Childbirth

It has been calculated that more than 90 percent of births can occur naturally and without any interference. In a childbirth situation away from medical assistance, though, it is a good idea to know a little of what procedures to follow and to be prepared to adequately accommodate the mother and baby. If it appears as if one must deliver the baby without medical assistance, an emergency medical service or a physician should be summoned for advice. If it is possible, prepare some emergency childbirth supplies in advance. If this is not feasible, make use of what supplies are available. Supplies should include a rubber or plastic sheet to place on the flat surface; clean towels, sheets, or fresh newspapers to place under the mother; clean towels or sanitary napkins to control bleeding; clean towels to wrap the baby and keep it warm; sterile rubber gloves; clean, thick string and sterile scissors for tying and cutting the umbilical cord; and a container for the placenta (for later medical examination). Also prepare a flat, clean area, such as a bed, for the woman to deliver her baby.

The woman should be made as comfortable as possible: Pillows can support and prop her up. She can deliver the baby on her back with her legs spread apart, on her side, or in a fashion where she feels comfortable. The childbirth process should not be impeded in any way—the primary job is to guide the baby out, to calm the woman, and to keep the birthing area and anything that touches the baby as clean as possible. One should also make sure one's hands are clean (wash them with soap and water—do not use any antiseptic or chemicals near the mother and baby) or use sterile rubber gloves.

Support the baby's head as it appears, making sure that the umbilical cord is not wrapped around the baby's neck. As the rest of the body follows, continue to support the baby's head and shoulders. When the baby is delivered, allow the fluids to be drained off and breathing to occur by keeping the head lower than the feet. One can gently tap the soles of the feet or rub the baby's back to encourage the baby to breathe. Wrap the baby (taking care not to wipe off the protective coating of the baby) and place the baby on the mother's stomach, keeping the umbilical cord slack.

It is not necessary to cut the umbilical cord if medical assistance is not far away. If it becomes necessary to cut the umbilical cord, two pieces of thick string, one 4 inches away from the baby and another one 8 inches away, should be tied tightly and very securely. The umbilical cord can then be cut in between the two ties with sterile scissors or a fresh razor blade. One should keep the cut end of the umbilical cord wrapped in a sterile dressing.

After the placenta is delivered, put it in a plastic bag for later analysis. To control excess bleeding, use towels or sanitary napkins and gently massage the mother's lower abdomen (where the uterus is) until it is firm. Finally, clean the mother, keep the mother and baby warm, and seek medical assistance.

eighth and ninth months) so that the physician can monitor the health of the mother and the baby.

Women have the option to have certain fetal tests performed in order to check the health of the baby or to warn the mother of the existence of any possible complications concerning the baby. Even though some of these tests might carry health risks for the mother and child, sometimes it is necessary for these tests to be done.

The three most common fetal testing/monitoring procedures are ultrasound, amniocentesis, and alpha-feto protein (AFP) screening. Ultrasound, using sound waves transmitted through an abdominal or vaginal transducer (probe), permits the practitioner to see a picture of the baby's internal organs and position in the womb. Amniocentesis involves extracting a sample of fluid from the amniotic sac (sac that surrounds the fetus) with a long thin needle. Amniocentesis gives the practitioner a sample of the fetus's cells so that various chromosomal and other biochemical disorders can be found. AFP screening tests for neural tube disorders such as spina bifida and anencephaly. Neural tube disorders are associated with the development of the structure that forms the brain and spine.

Other fetal tests include chorionic villus sampling (CVS) and percutaneous umbilical blood sampling test (PUBS). CVS, a newer though somewhat riskier test than amniocentesis, takes a sample of the chorion, the tissue of the amniotic sac. The sample, taken from a needle inserted in the abdomen or through a catheter inserted in the vagina, can detect hereditary and chromosomal disorders. PUBS takes a fetal blood sample from the umbilical vein by way of a needle inserted in the abdomen. PUBS provides the practitioner with an analysis that indicates the existence of any chromosomal disorders more quickly than amniocentesis.

OBSTETRICAL PROCEDURES

In a hospital childbirth setting, there are certain standard obstetrical procedures taken during the last stages of labor and during childbirth itself. The woman may or may not be given an enema, have her pubic area shaved, and be made to lie down and assume the lithotomy position (on her back, her feet in stirrups) before actually delivering the baby. Other so-called interventions that may help or hinder (depending upon the individual case) the natural pro-

gression of labor and childbirth include: the administration of an intravenous solution (for hydration purposes or for giving the mother drugs, such as oxytocin or pitocin, to induce labor); an amniotomy (manual rupture of the amniotic sac to accelerate labor); an episiotomy (perineal incision made to enlarge the baby's passage); vacuum extraction or the use of forceps (to aid the mother in delivering the baby by means of a suction cup or metal tongs); and cesarean section (surgical incision made to deliver the baby abdominally rather than vaginally, used when complications arise during childbirth).

Further, during labor and delivery the heartbeat of the fetus, as well as the contractions of the mother, can be measured and monitored internally or externally by machines. To electrically record data, electrodes can be placed either on the mother's abdomen or on the baby's scalp. At the time of the actual birth, the mother may be given anesthesia injected in the vulva (pudendal block), in the cervix (paracervical block), in the base of the back (caudal anesthesia), or in the middle of the back with the use of a catheter placed around the base of the spinal cord (epidural anesthesia). Or a spinal anesthesia can be given to numb the entire birth area, which stops labor entirely. Many experts question the actual worth of using anesthetics during childbirth, for the perineum naturally becomes numb during childbirth and any drug that the mother has in her system may affect the baby.

RESOURCES FOR OBSTETRICS/ GYNECOLOGY

American Board of Obstetrics and Gynecology
4225 Roosevelt Way N.E., Suite 305
Seattle, WA 98105
206-547-4884

American College of Obstetricians and Gynecologists
409 12th Street S.W.
Washington, DC 20024-2188
202-638-5577

DES Action
1615 Broadway, #510
Oakland, CA 94612
415-465-4011

HERS Foundation (Hysterectomy Educational Resources and Services)
422 Bryn Mawr Avenue
Bala Cynwyd, PA 19004
215-667-7757

International Childbirth Education Association
P.O. Box 20048
Minneapolis, MN 55420
612-854-8660

La Leche League International
9616 Minneapolis Avenue
P.O. Box 1209
Franklin Park, IL 60131-8209
708-455-7730

Sports Medicine

Sports medicine encompasses the prevention and treatment of injuries to athletes, fitness training for nonathletes, the effect of exercise on body functions, the use of exercise for recovery from nonsports injuries, drug use by athletes, and nutrition for athletes and fitness buffs.

SPORTS MEDICINE SPECIALISTS

While you won't find too many medical school graduates who have completed courses in sports medicine, or too many M.D.'s with the phrase "board certified in sports medicine" after their names, you'll certainly find plenty of doctors, chiropractors, physical therapists, exercise trainers, nurses, and nutritionists who will add the title "sports medicine specialist" to their shingles. While sports medicine may be somewhat costly and its methods quite controversial, it has captured the public eye like nothing else in recent memory.

What have doctors done to improve the standards of training in sports medicine? They've decided to go the conventional route—develop a board certification program. In October of 1991, the first sports medicine board exam was administered to twenty-nine physicians. Peter Tyler, M.D., executive director of the American Board of Sports Medicine, explained that the field needed a "recognized standard" of medical competency.

Sports medicine, however, has not yet been recognized by the American Board of Medical Specialties. This board, which stamps the official brand of respectability on any medical discipline, currently recognizes twenty-four mainstream medical specialties.

When we think of sports medicine, we usually think of athletes. But in fact, full-time, competitive athletes constitute only a small percentage of the people who seek out the services of sports medicine doctors. The field caters to people engaging in all levels of fitness and activity. Thus, in broad terms, sports medicine treats all injuries, muscular or otherwise, caused by or related to some kind of motion—most commonly, but not exclusively, athletics. Occasionally, you will find sports medicine centers being used to treat someone who is in need of rehabilitative therapy because of a non-sport-related injury—a car accident victim or an older person who has had a bad fall.

TYPES OF SPORTS INJURIES

Athletes generally sustain two types of injuries: acute trauma and overuse syndrome. Acute trauma is a sudden, violent injury, such as a broken bone or torn ligament, that requires the immediate attention of a doctor. Overuse syndrome results from the repeated stress of an abnormal use of a part of the body and can be treated without professional care.

Athletes and nonathletes who exercise regularly need to learn to recognize the symptoms of developing injuries, to prevent injuries, to treat them, and to identify conditions that require professional care.

As with most of medicine, the equipment and techniques used to treat athletic injuries have become greatly sophisticated in just the last five years. But the best treatment for most sports injuries is prevention. Athletes should know that injured muscles tighten when they heal, and that stretching exercises can reduce some injuries, particularly those to calf and hamstring muscles, by up to 80 percent. Athletes should learn to identify opposing muscles, such as the quadriceps and hamstrings of the leg, and try to ensure that one does not become much stronger than the other, which heightens the risk of injury.

Following is a list of the most common types of sports injuries, along with methods of prevention and treatment.

Foot Injuries

Containing twenty-six bones and acting as interface between body and earth, the foot is vulnerable to many injuries, especially from jogging and basketball, field hockey, tennis, and other sports that require running. Injuries include the following.

Athlete's foot is a fungal skin infection occurring between the toes and on the soles of the foot. It can be prevented with proper bathing and drying of the foot and treated, except in severe cases, with topical ointments.

Black toenails, common among runners and hikers, occur when a blood clot or blister forms beneath the toenail. Resulting from injury or chronic irritation, black toenails can be avoided by wearing socks that are ½ inch longer than the longest toe and shoes that contain a finger's width of extra space at the end of the toe. Nails should be clipped to their natural shape and allowed to extend to the end of the toe. Blood should be drained from an acutely injured toenail; this can be done by applying heat to the top of the nail. If a nail is torn, or if infection or swelling occurs, a doctor should be consulted.

Blisters, one of the most common foot injuries, are collections of fluid between the outer layers of skin, caused by friction or pressure, that can result from starting a new activity or wearing a new pair of shoes. Blisters can be prevented by wearing dry shoes and thicker socks, slowing the level of pressure increase in an activity, or applying petroleum jelly to irritated areas. Treatment requires the blister to be drained without removing the roof, or covering skin. An antibiotic ointment and sterile gauze pad should be applied.

Ingrown toenails result from trauma and from narrow shoes, as well as heredity and foot deformities. Prevention and treatment include the wearing of wide shoes. At home, a small portion of the protruding nail may be removed with a sterilized pair of clippers. The foot should be soaked and a disinfectant applied to the toe. If the problem persists, a doctor should be consulted.

Stress fractures, also called march fractures because they often affect soldiers, are incomplete cracks in a bone caused by repeated stresses of running or jumping. Prevention includes wearing cushioned shoes and avoiding hard surfaces and rapid increases in speed or distance. Treatment includes cessation of the activity that caused the fractures, especially running, while switching to a new activity such as swimming or bicycling to remain fit. Protective padding, heel cups, and, in a few cases, casts can be worn. The athlete should not resume the offending activity for 4 to 8 weeks.

Ankle Injuries
A hinge joint composed of three bones bound together by ligaments, tendons, and connective fibers, the ankle can be pushed suddenly or gradually beyond its limits of flexibility by the forces of propulsion. Injuries include the following.

Achilles tendon injuries, also called tendinitis, affect the tendon extending from the lower calf to the heel, especially in flat-footed athletes or those with high arches. Inflammation of the blood vessels near the tendon can cause a burning sensation; inflammation of the tendon causes shooting pain during activity. An overstressed tendon may pop or rupture. Prevention includes stretching exercises. Treatment for mild or moderate symptoms includes stretching, ice application, heel lifts, avoidance of running on hills, and wearing supportive shoes. Immobility and rehabilitation with physical therapy can be required in severe cases.

Ankle sprains, graded as mild, moderate, or severe, are acute injuries occurring usually when the foot turns under the leg, stretching or tearing the ligaments. Proper treatment is necessary to avoid a chronically unstable ankle. Mild sprains can be treated with RICE (rest, ice, compression, and elevation) of the ankle; activity may be resumed in several days. Moderate and severe sprains should be treated by a doctor; they require immobilization, casts, crutches, and even surgery to repair ligaments. A rehabilitation program is necessary to regain strength and range of motion.

Lower-Leg Injuries
Injuries to the portion of the leg between the ankle and knee often result from repeated stresses and from relying on the leg to absorb too much stress. Injuries include the following.

Leg length discrepancy, or short limb syndrome, results from the body's attempt to compensate for a difference as small as ¼ inch between the lengths of the two legs. The condition can be caused by a fracture during childhood, polio, congenital abnormalities, or a greater flattening in the arch of one foot. Treatment includes shoe lifts and orthotic devices to realign the position and structure of the limb and level the pelvis.

Muscle pulls and tears occur when muscle fibers overstretch, tear, or even rupture, causing pain, swelling, bruising, and loss of function. Muscles prone to pulls and tears include the hamstrings (in the back of the thigh) in sprinters, the groin (inner thigh) in basketball players and others who must change direction quickly, the calf (lower leg) in jumpers, and the shoulder muscles in swimmers. Inadequate warm-up, overdevelopment of some muscles (muscle imbalance), overly ambitious exercise programs, accidents and injuries cause pulls and tears. Minor pulls can be treated by applying heat before activity and ice afterward. A moderate tear requires RICE (rest, ice, compression, and elevation) for 20 minutes three or four times a day for 2 to 3 days, after which heat treatments should replace ice and range-of-motion exercises may be begun. Surgical treatment and extensive rehabilitation may be required for severe tears and ruptures.

Shin splints are tiny tears in the muscles attached to the tibia bone. Pain may be felt in the front or rear portion of the leg. Shin splints may be caused by an imbalance between the stronger posterior leg muscles and the weaker anterior muscles. Other causes include running on the toes, flattening of the arches, tight anterior muscles, and insufficient shock absorption. Prevention includes strengthening and stretch exercises. Treatment includes aspirin to counter inflammation, ice massages after activity, avoiding hills and hard running surfaces, reducing activity by 50 percent, and wearing athletic shoes to overcome arch flattening.

Knee Injuries
The body's largest joint, the knee is a hinge composed of the femur, tibia, and fibula bones and the patella, or kneecap. The knee is vulnerable to acute trauma when perpendicular force is applied. Injuries include the following.

Chondromalacia patella, or runner's knee, occurs when repeated stress causes inflammation and softening of the cartilage under the kneecap. Causes include a flattened or pronated foot, which, when running, causes the lower leg to rotate inward and the kneecap to slide from side to side and rub against the groove of the femur. Prolonged sitting, weak thigh muscles, trauma, muscle imbalance, and neglected ligament injury can also aggravate the cartilage. A doctor, even a specialist, should be consulted. Activity that causes pain should be decreased or stopped. Rest, ice, and anti-inflammatory drugs are helpful. Exercises can be done to strengthen the thighs. Abnormal foot mechanics can be corrected with orthotic devices and physiotherapy.

Knee sprain is an injury to the ligaments that connect the bones of the knee and provide, along with muscles, tendons, and soft tissues, the knee's stability. Knee sprains are less common in running than in contact sports and skiing, which can subject the hyperextended knee to sideways trauma. Treatment, depending on severity, ranges from rest, ice, and crutches to cast immobilization, followed by rehabilitation, and surgery.

Patellar tendinitis, or jumper's knee, results from overuse of the tendon connecting the kneecap to the lower leg, or tibia. Frequent jumping up and down, in an activity such as basketball or volleyball, can cause pain just below the kneecap. Difficulty kneeling may also be experienced. Treatment includes rest and heat, avoiding stressful activity, and taking anti-inflammatory drugs such as aspirin. Braces may be used. Surgery may be necessary to reattach the tendon to the kneecap. Prevention is more effective. If pain is felt, vigorous kicking and jumping should be reduced, and ice, heat, and anti-inflammatory drugs should be taken.

Thigh and Hip Injuries
Groin pulls, acute tears to the muscles of the inner thigh, are common among athletes who must change directions quickly while running, run in bursts, and stop and start while running straight ahead. Sudden pain accompanies the injury. Bruising from the crotch to the knee may follow, although the injury is confined to the inner thigh. Treatment includes rest, ice, compression, and elevation and a wait of 1 to 6 weeks before resumption of activity. Injured muscles tighten while healing and must be stretched gradually during rehabilitation, which consists of stretching and strength exercises.

Hamstring injuries are common among runners and other athletes, such as basketball players and sprinters, who must propel their legs quickly. The three hamstring muscles extend from the base of the buttock down the back of the leg to the top of the lower leg bones, the tibia and fibula. Tears and ruptures to the hamstrings can be prevented by stretching the head to the toes along a straightened leg from a sitting or standing position before activity. Bicycling strengthens the hamstrings. Treatment of hamstring injuries ranges from rest and ice to anti-inflammatory drugs, wraps, and crutches.

Lower-Back Injuries
The lower back, or lumbar region, provides strength to the hips, thighs, and torso, and also absorbs shocks and stresses that pass through the feet and legs. Overuse or abuse of the back, from bending, twisting, and poor posture, can cause a sore back and also impinge on nerves in the spinal vertebrae.

The back is vulnerable to problems caused by imbalance of muscle use. Overuse of the psoas muscle, which bends the hip, can place stress on the spinal column and increase the curvature of the lower back. Tight hamstring muscles, common among long-distance runners, also contribute to lower-back problems by causing a hesitant heel strike and transmitting more stress to the back.

Good posture helps the body tolerate the repeated sideways and back-and-forth stresses imposed by running. Standing with leg, pelvis, and spine aligned reduces the effort required to support the body's weight. High-heeled shoes should be avoided because they cause an imbalance in alignment and place added stress on the feet, ankles, legs, and back.

Runners, especially those with sedentary jobs, should take care to condition and strengthen those muscles, such as abdominal muscles, that are not greatly exercised during running. This helps avoid an imbalance between overused and underused muscles.

Other Injuries and Conditions

Bursitis, in the shoulders or the hips, occurs when a lubricating sac of fluid called the bursa is inflamed during strenuous or repeated outward motions of the arm. The bursa is located near the rotator cuff, a group of muscles that covers the top of the shoulder and helps stabilize it. Treatment of bursitis requires rest and anti-inflammatory drugs, followed by gentle stretching exercises.

Irregular menstrual periods, or amenorrhea, occur when a woman has periods more frequently than once every 25 days or less frequently than once every 35 days. This condition is experienced by 20 to 60 percent of women who exercise vigorously. The causes are not understood, but a woman who experiences amenorrhea is lacking either the hormone progesterone or both estrogen and progesterone. She should consult her doctor, who will probably prescribe hormones.

Muscle cramps occur when muscle fibers contract, usually during exercise. Cramps can last a few seconds or several hours. Causes include injury, a deficiency in salt and other minerals, especially potassium, slowing of blood supply to the muscle by repeated muscular contractions, and hyperventilation. Treatment includes gently stretching and squeezing the affected muscle and eating fruits and vegetables to replace potassium.

Rotator cuff injuries are common among baseball players, tennis players, and other athletes who engage in throwing sports. The rotator cuff, muscles that cover the shoulder, rotate the humerus (upper arm bone) and stabilize the shoulder. As they do their work, they often rub against a small shoulder bone called the acromion. The tendon can become frayed and weakened; the muscles can tear or rupture. Treatment is rest and anti-inflammatory drugs, followed by physical therapy. Steroids are sometimes injected, but with care, as they can wear away the rotator cuff. Surgery is performed in severe cases, but is not always effective, in part because the blood supply to the shoulder is not always generous.

Prevention, by strengthening exercises and stretching before activity, is more effective than treatment.

Tennis elbow is a tear in the tendons that attach the forearm to the elbow. Pain, which is felt when the wrist straightens or bends against resistance, can occur on the inside (forehand tennis elbow) or outside (backhand tennis elbow) of the wrist. Preventive measures include using two hands for a backhand stroke, using the entire upper arm rather than just the wrist to hit the ball, switching to a lighter racket, reducing the tension of the racket strings, and avoiding playing on grass and cement. Treatment is rest and ice. When healing has begun, bending and straightening the wrist while holding small (1-pound) weights helps strengthen the tendon.

SPORTS AND DRUGS

The first drug death in sports occurred in 1890 when a British cyclist died while racing under the stimulant called ephedrine. Little evidence exists to suggest that taking amphetamines or anabolic steroids improves athletic performance, yet athletes continue to take drugs and die from them.

Many athletes and trainers believe that amphetamines, or "uppers," reduce fatigue and promote weight loss. But the drug masks pain and fatigue, increasing the likelihood of injury. They can be habit-forming and can cause heatstroke and even death. Users often think they are performing better than they actually are, need more time to recover muscle strength after an activity, suffer headaches, stomachaches, and irregular heartbeats, and can become severely depressed after the drug's effect wears off.

Many athletes and some medical experts say that steroids, a type of hormone, help the body heal faster and become stronger. The use of steroids has become rampant among professional weight lifters and male teenage athletes. But side effects include acne, decreased or increased sexual desire, sterility, dizziness, fainting, headache, lethargy, aggression, liver disease, intestinal bleeding, cancer, and death.

The American College of Sports Medicine, in a position statement on the use of anabolic steroids by athletes, said that neither medically approved nor extremely large doses hindered or aided performance. The college said oral testosterone derivatives could result in liver disorders, decreased testicular size and function, and decreased sperm production. Not all of these disorders are reversible.

Sports Injuries

Based upon information collected by the National Electronic Injury Surveillance System and reported to the Consumer Product Safety Commission, the following activities were responsible for the majority of sports injuries in 1991.

Sports Injuries by Activity

Activity	Number of Injuries
Basketball	646,678
Baseball	459,542
Football	453,684
Skating (ice/roller)	153,114
Soccer	150,449
Volleyball	129,839
Swimming	128,706
Fishing	84,115
Horseback Riding	71,490
Weight lifting	61,140
Track/field	58,586
Gymnastics	44,877
Wrestling	43,894
Trampoline jumping	38,823
Golf	38,626
Hockey	32,115
Waterskiing	26,633
Boxing	25,417
Martial arts	24,449
Paddleball/squash/racquetball	19,315
Fencing	11,682
Rugby	7,681
Archery	7,397
Billiards	5,610
Cheerleading	5,536
Toy sports equipment	3,597
Horseshoes	3,372
Surfing	3,356
Badminton	3,109
Tetherball	3,095
Handball	3,070
Table tennis/Ping-Pong	2,339
Scuba diving	1,360

4. Settings

INTRODUCTION

Where you go for health care does make a difference. All hospitals are not the same. Nursing homes differ in function and quality. Outpatient surgical centers, sprouting up quicker than the largest fast-food chain can open branches, have no government agencies monitoring the quality of their care. Home health care, the fastest-growing segment of the health care industry, is essentially a puzzle for most consumers.

The informed health care consumer knows that the quality of the facilities and organizations that provide services is as important as the individual practitioners used. Is the laboratory where your specimens are sent certified by a reputable accrediting organization? What are the dangers of hospital-caused infections? Can you do anything to help lower your risk of having a medication error happen to you while hospitalized?

In this section, everything you need to know about hospitals, nursing homes, and other settings where medical services are delivered is explained. You will learn, among other useful information, how to read and understand a hospital bill, what the leading institutions are for major conditions, and how to file a complaint about a medical facility.

Indeed, where you receive medical treatment does make a difference. Now you will have the facts you need to assist in the selection process.

Hospitals

Where you get your medical care is as important as who provides it. The backdrop not only makes a big difference in how much you pay but also dictates what treatment you get or do not get.

Clearly, hospital-based care is the steepest in cost among all medical settings. The charge for an average 4-day stay in the hospital, which does not include intensive care, is $6,400, or $1,600 a day. The average 1-day charge for room and board is approximately $350, with the remaining $1,250 including ancillary services (laboratory, imaging, such as X rays and ultrasound, pharmacy, and general supplies).

While dollar figures like those are enough to convince most people to reduce the time spent in the hospital, the matter of a person's particular medical condition and the diagnostic procedures and treatment it requires is a very important consideration. Not every hospital setting is appropriate for every medical need. Your community hospital is not the place for the kidney transplant you so desperately need, but if all you require is a routine X ray, you have a wide range of hospitals and other medical settings from which to choose.

Here are the various types of hospitals from which to choose.

SPECIALTY HOSPITALS AND GENERAL HOSPITALS

The two major categories of hospitals in the United States are specialty hospitals and general medical/surgical hospitals.

As its name implies, a specialty hospital takes care of only one kind of medical condition or one type of patient. It might admit only those patients with cancer or orthopedic problems, or only children, for example. The selling point of specialty hospitals is that they concentrate on a single disease or condition or type of patient, day in and day out, and presumably the staff becomes expert in dealing with it. The argument goes something like this: There is no better place for someone in your condition than an institution that works on that condition solely.

True, studies do show that hospitals get better at procedures they perform often, and the results are usually better too. But a high rate of successful cesarean births or hysterectomies does not mean that you should enter without concern. The number of successes may be meaningless if these procedures are being performed more often than necessary.

Study after study has documented the fact that some facilities perform far more of one procedure than a hospital only a few miles away with the same number of persons entering with the same conditions. We may not know exactly why, but convenience, habit, the hospital's policies and aims, and even greed have been prominently mentioned.

General medical and surgical hospitals are not necessarily better in terms of efficiency or proficiency than specialty hospitals, but they are equipped to handle a larger variety of medical eventualities. These facilities are what most people envision when they hear the word "hospital." They are, in effect, a conglomeration of little specialty hospitals under one roof. Still, a general hospital occasionally sends a patient to a specialty hospital for better, more focused, and more knowledgeable care.

COMMUNITY HOSPITALS AND MEDICAL CENTERS

Community hospitals, as the name implies, commonly dot the landscape of residential areas; indeed, they are the most common type of hospital in the United States. Such hospitals may have as few as 50 beds or as many as several hundred. A good-size community hospital has around 250 beds, and has virtually every kind of expensive technology that might be required for the best of what hospitals have to offer. The selling point of such places is that they are large enough to give you big-time medicine, yet small enough to provide personal attention.

Traditionally, these hospitals were run as nonprofit corporations, with a board of trustees comprised of lay- and businesspeople and a constant, crying need for government and community support. Nowadays, it is not uncommon for such hospitals to be run as for-profit entities by investor-owned corporations. (We have more to say about for-profit hospitals on the next page.)

The selling point medical centers stress, on the other hand, is that they are big institutions, and because of this they see many different kinds of patients and are able to treat rare conditions that might stump most community hospitals. These medical centers are usually affiliated with universities, an affiliation the medical center considers a plus because it implies that all the newest ideas, machines, techniques, and drugs are available to the practitioners. Many experts, world-famous in their fields, are on the staffs of these hospitals.

But that is only half the story. Certainly, a big hospital is good for providing doctors with lots of patients to see, work on, and learn from. But for a patient hoping for a relaxed and easy recuperation or personalized care, a medical center or other large hospital may not be the place.

While medical centers have just about everything that could possibly be called on to take care of your condition, your condition might just be simply too routine to involve the top staff. Experts and eager young doctors come to these hospitals to pioneer the new medical frontier, to be in the eye of the healing hurricane, which they see as modern medicine. Consequently, they may find a gallbladder operation a chore. You might find yourself feeling like a second-class citizen, relegated to the still highly skilled but second-string medical/surgical team, because you have nothing drastically wrong with you. And you'll be paying a lot of money all the while.

If you do decide on a medical center, don't go there simply because some world-famous authority is on the staff. You might never see her, or she you, while you are there. This physician/researcher/scientist/personality may be too busy with her work or her next grant proposal to see patients.

A hospital's size is not always a reliable clue to the kind of treatment you can expect there. You might have a warm and caring experience at a 750-bed leviathan of a medical center, and you might be treated impersonally at a 100-bed community hospital. Obviously, you need to know more about a hospital than merely its size.

TEACHING AND NONTEACHING HOSPITALS

A teaching hospital is one where there are students in training—both under- and postgraduate medical students. Such hospitals range in size from a few hundred to possibly as high as a few thousand beds, and nearly all teaching hospitals have major medical school ties.

The arguments for going to a teaching hospital are just about the same as the ones for going to a medical center: expertise, newest technology, up-to-the-minute knowledge. Many of the best and best-known teaching hospitals are university medical centers. These hospitals exist as much for the education of the medical students at the university as they do for the care of the patients. As a matter of fact, by virtue of their being admitted, patients have given their implicit permission to be used as teaching examples, because the medical students, interns, and residents need patients to work on and learn from. For all the good they accomplish, teaching hospitals do use patients as teaching tools.

Like medical centers and university-related hospitals, some community hospitals and specialty facilities also have good teaching programs, attracting top students as well as excellent specialists from around the world. These community hospitals are considered the most sophisticated, best-equipped, most desirable places in that category. The fresh, young, eager students are more than happy to attend to you and show off what they know. One thing you'll never be in a

To Profit or Not to Profit

Along with the family farm, the independent community hospital is fast becoming a lone ranger. All sorts of people and organizations own hospitals: religious orders, universities, governments, doctors. Sometimes an owner or ownership group might buy and run a few hospitals in a fairly small and limited region. Not uncommon, such privately owned, for-profit (proprietary) hospitals are growing in number.

But that's not all. What is also happening in the for-profit hospital business is the rise and monumental growth of corporate chain ownership. Whereas privately owned hospitals split the profits among the various owners, the corporately owned, national chain hospitals distribute the wealth to shareholders, who expect solid returns on their investment. The corporations run their hospitals as they would any other business—for maximum profits and earnings. According to the Federation of American Health Systems, a trade association representing proprietary hospitals, 1 in 5 hospitals was investor-owned in 1992.

Today the top three for-profit medical corporations alone—Hospital Corporation of America, Humana, and National Medical Enterprises respectively—either own or manage nearly 42,000 beds in 188 hospitals nationwide. Their total revenues in 1991 exceeded $12.8 billion, with the three giants sharing more than $789 million in profits. The entire proprietary hospital industry generated revenues of $21.5 billion during this same time period.

Critics of medical chains have accused them of promoting overutilization of technology, overtesting of patients, and overpricing of dispensed goods, all in an effort to improve the bottom line.

Of course, for-profit chains in many cases have brought important and valuable services to the medical system. In many instances they have brought hospitals to places that never had them. They have also helped to keep hospital care in some communities by purchasing or contracting to manage a failing local institution, refurbishing it, and putting it back in profit-making operation.

But the fact is that corporate-owned hospitals actually end up costing the consumer more—23 percent more, according to one survey—than a not-for-profit establishment. Paul Starr, in his Pulitzer Prize–winning *The Social Transformation of American Medicine*, states that "national data also indicate that, for every bed-size category, for-profit hospitals have higher costs than the overall average for community hospitals." According to a recent study, reported in *Modern Healthcare*, for-profit hospital charges were 11 percent higher than tax-exempt not-for-profit hospitals. Much of the difference in pricing structure can be attributed to the advantage the not-for-profits enjoy when it comes to taxation and the cost of financing expansion and new services.

What it comes down to is this: The wise consumer, before he or she is admitted to a certain hospital, will find out who owns it and how that ownership might affect his or her care and its cost. The second most important thing a wise consumer can do is to make sure the hospital will accept his or her insurance company's reimbursement as payment in full for services provided. Reaching agreement on this item will avoid misunderstandings and unexpected large out-of-pocket expenses.

teaching hospital is lonely. This form of medicine—with its teaching rounds when students, interns, and residents converge around patients' beds—is just not for everybody.

There is also the matter of cost. Teaching hospitals have greater expenses than nonteaching hospitals. They usually pay a decent salary to postgraduates in training and pay what it takes to attract topflight experts. The research that doesn't earn any money directly for the institution must be underwritten. Enormous sums must be paid for new technological marvels. No wonder the average cost of care in a teaching hospital can be as much as twice that in a nonteaching hospital.

A further explanation for higher cost, in the opinion of some medical experts, is the tendency for the new, inexperienced doctors to order too many tests and unnecessary procedures. They are understandably anxious about what they need to do to pin down a diagnosis, stabilize a condition, or lay down a paper trail for good defensive medicine. So they tend to do a lot. They are, after all, just learning. But bear in mind that they are learning on the patients themselves.

For the consumer trying to decide between a teaching or nonteaching hospital, the person's medical condition and personality, the role high-powered technology can play in treating a particular ailment, and the person's financial situation—these are factors to consider in making the decision.

OSTEOPATHIC HOSPITALS

The osteopathic hospital (staffed with doctors of osteopathy, or D.O.'s) differs little these days from the allopathic hospital (staffed with medical doctors, or M.D.'s). Despite legal and public relations wars, both types of hospitals provide well-rounded doctors and primary care physicians, as well as surgeons and specialists. In fact, some hospitals offer privileges to both D.O.'s and M.D.'s.

There are far fewer osteopathic hospitals than allopathic ones. Osteopaths and their hospitals tend to serve smaller, more rural communities than do M.D.'s and their hospitals.

VETERANS ADMINISTRATION HOSPITALS

Veterans Administration (VA) hospitals and the entire military care system have been under fire for several years, the result of reports that question the quality of military medicine. The VA inspector general's office found cases, it said, in which doctors employed by the VA or performing treatments for the agency were practicing while their medical credentials in one or more states were revoked, suspended, placed on probation, limited, or impaired in some way. A few years later, a General Accounting Office study identified another problem area: the failure to investigate patient injuries and unexpected deaths.

The problems cited were by no means unique to the VA health care system. Civilian hospitals have also fallen prey to physicians who failed to reveal past disciplinary problems or loss of hospital privileges. At the time these problems were discovered, there was no way, short of a costly background investigation, for the VA or private hospitals to quickly check on a physician's disciplinary record. The National Health Care Practitioner Data Bank has corrected this shortcoming and is now available to assist all civilian and VA hospitals in doing physician background checks.

As a result of these studies, corrective action was quickly taken. Together, the VA and the Joint Commission on the Accreditation of Healthcare Organizations (JCAHO) undertook a review of all 172 hospitals in the VA system. While no VA hospital lost its accreditation, it was discovered that VA hospitals had higher levels of noncompliance with JCAHO standards. Fully 70 percent of VA hospitals were not in compliance with Joint Commission standards relative to surgical case review. And in the all-important area of medical staff monitoring and evaluation, 69 percent of hospitals were not in compliance.

Since these shortcomings have been revealed, the VA has established a series of instructional teleconferences designed to help its employees meet Joint Commission standards. In another move to improve quality, medical case review will be done by non-VA physicians. In addition, increased funding of $1 billion, including $26 million for a peer review program, will enable the VA system to improve overall performance.

Another positive development was noted when the VA's assistant inspector general revealed that care delivered by VA hospitals was not only cheaper than in private hospitals, but resulted in similar outcomes. For a system that had taken its share of bumps and bruises, this was indeed an encouraging development.

The VA is also going ahead with plans to form agreements with private providers to automate a number of functions, including prescription drug dispensing. With an improved budgeting system, additional health care workers, and a new emphasis on its mission, the VA has taken major steps toward restoring public confidence in its ability to provide high-quality health care. It should also be remembered that VA hospitals provide medical care to many people who otherwise could not afford it.

State Hospital Licensing Offices

These agencies are responsible for inspecting and licensing hospitals. They conduct surveys to determine that hospitals conform to life-safety codes, infection control programs, sanitation codes, and other construction requirements. Specific complaints about hospitals should be directed to these offices.

Alabama
Hospital Licensure
Alabama Department of Public Health
Environmental Health Service Standards Division
Bureau of Licensing and Certification
State Office Building
434 Monroe Street
Montgomery, AL 36130-1701
205-242-2883

Alaska
Hospital Licensure
Alaska Department of Health and Social Services
Division of Medical Assistance
Health Facilities Licensing and Certification
4433 Business Park Boulevard, Building M
Anchorage, AK 99503
907-561-2171

Arizona
Hospital Licensure
Department of Health Services
Division of Emergency Medical Services and
Health Care Facilities
701 E. Jefferson
Phoenix, AZ 85304
602-255-1177

Arkansas
Hospital Licensure
Arkansas Department of Health
Bureau of Health Resources
Division of Health Facility Services
4815 W. Markham Street
Little Rock, AR 72205-3867
501-661-2201

California
Hospital Licensure
California Health and Welfare Agency
Department of Health Services
Division of Licensing and Certification
714 P Street
Sacramento, CA 95814-2070
916-445-3045

Colorado
Hospital Licensure
Colorado Department of Health
Office of Health Care and Prevention
Division of Health Facilities Regulation
4210 E. 11th Avenue
Denver, CO 80220
303-331-6690

Connecticut
Hospital Licensure
Connecticut Department of Health Services
Hospital and Health Care Division
Licensure and Certification
1049 Asylum Avenue
Hartford, CT 06106-2435
203-566-3880

Delaware
Hospital Licensure
Delaware Department of Health and Social Services
Office of Health Facilities Licensing and Certification
3000 Newport Gap Pike, Building C
Wilmington, DE 19808
302-995-6674

District of Columbia
Hospital Licensure
District of Columbia Department of Consumer and Regulatory Affairs
Service Facility Regulation Administration
Health Facility Division
614 H Street N.W.
Washington, DC 20001
202-727-7194

Florida
Hospital Licensure
Florida Department of Health and Rehabilitative Services
Office of Regulation and Health Facilities
1317 Winewood Boulevard
Tallahassee, FL 32399-0700
904-487-2513

Georgia
Hospital Licensure
Georgia Department of Human Resources
Office of Regulatory Services
Standards and Licensure Section
47 Trinity Avenue S.W.
Atlanta, GA 30334
404-894-5144

Hawaii
Hospital Licensure
Hawaii Department of Health
Hospital and Medical Facilities Branch
P.O. Box 3378
Honolulu, HI 96801
808-548-5935

Idaho
Hospital Licensure
Idaho Health Facilities Authority
1655 Fairview Avenue, Suite 206
Boise, ID 83702
208-342-8772

Illinois
Hospital Licensure
Illinois Department of Public Health
Office of Health Regulation
Health Facilities Standards Division
Hospital Licensing Section
525 W. Jefferson Street
Springfield, IL 62761
217-782-4977

Indiana
Hospital Licensure
Indiana State Board of Health
Division of Acute Care Services
1330 W. Michigan Street, Box 1964
Indianapolis, IN 46206
317-633-8472

Iowa
Hospital Licensure
Iowa Department of Inspections and Appeals
Division of Health Facilities
Lucas State Office Building
Des Moines, IA 50319
515-281-4233

Kansas
Hospital Licensure
Kansas Department of Health and Environment
Division of Health
Bureau of Adult and Child Care Facilities
Hospital Program
Landon State Office Building
900 S.W. Jackson
Topeka, KS 66612
913-296-1240

Kentucky
Hospital Licensure
Kentucky Human Resources Cabinet
Office of Inspector General
Division of Licensing and Regulation
275 E. Main Street
Frankfort, KY 40601
502-564-2800

Louisiana
Hospital Licensure
Louisiana Department of Health and Hospitals
Health Standards Section
Division of Licensing and Certification
1201 Capitol Access Road
P.O. Box 3767
Baton Rouge, LA 70821
504-342-0138

Maine
Hospital Licensure
Maine Department of Human Services
Bureau of Medical Services
Division of Licensing and Certification
Statehouse Station 11
Augusta, ME 04333
207-289-2606

Maryland
Hospital Licensure
Maryland Department of Health and Mental Hygiene
Licensing and Certification Division
4201 Patterson Avenue
Baltimore, MD 21215
410-764-2750

Massachusetts
Hospital Licensure
Massachusetts Executive Office of Human Services
Department of Public Health
Bureau of Health Care Systems
Division of Health Care Quality
150 Tremont Street, 2nd Floor
Boston, MA 02111
617-727-5860

Michigan

Hospital Licensure
Michigan Department of Public Health
Health Facilities Bureau
Division of Health Facilities, Licensing and Certification
3423 N. Logan
P.O. Box 30195
Lansing, MI 48909
517-335-8505

Minnesota

Hospital Licensure
Minnesota Department of Health
Health Resources Bureau
717 Delaware Street S.E., Box 9441
Minneapolis, MN 55440
612-643-2171

Mississippi

Hospital Licensure
Mississippi Department of Health
Division of Licensure and Certification
2688 Insurance Center Drive
Jackson, MS 39216
601-981-6880

Missouri

Hospital Licensure
Missouri Department of Health
Health Resources Division
Bureau of Hospital Licensing and Certification
P.O. Box 570
Jefferson City, MO 65102
314-751-6302

Montana

Hospital Licensure
**Montana Department of Health and
Environmental Sciences**
Division of Health Services
Licensing, Certification and Construction Bureau
Cogswell Building, Room C214
Helena, MT 59620
406-444-2037

Nebraska

Hospital Licensure
Nebraska Department of Health
Health Facilities Standards Bureau
301 Centennial Mall S.
P.O. Box 95007
Lincoln, NE 68509
402-471-2946

Nevada

Hospital Licensure
Nevada Department of Human Resources
Division of Health
Bureau of Regulatory Health Services
505 E. King Street, Room 600
Carson City, NV 89710
702-687-4475

New Hampshire

Hospital Licensure
**New Hampshire Department of Health and
Human Services**
Division of Public Health Services
Bureau of Health Facilities Administration
6 Hazen Drive
Concord, NH 03301
603-271-4592

New Jersey

Hospital Licensure
New Jersey Department of Health
Health Facilities Evaluation and Licensing Division
300 Whitehead Road, CN-367
Trenton, NJ 08625
609-588-7725

New Mexico

Hospital Licensure
New Mexico Department of Health and Environment
Division of Public Health
Licensing and Certification Bureau
1190 St. Francis Drive
Santa Fe, NM 87501
505-827-2409

New York

Hospital Licensure
New York State Department of Health
Office of Health Systems Management
Bureau of Health Standards and Surveillance
Corning Tower, Empire State Plaza
Albany, NY 12237-0001
518-473-3517

North Carolina

Hospital Licensure
North Carolina Department of Human Resources
Division of Facility Services
Council Building
701 Barbour Drive
Raleigh, NC 27603
919-733-2342

North Dakota

Hospital Licensure
North Dakota Department of Health and
Consolidated Laboratories
Health Resources Section
Health Facilities Division
600 E. Boulevard
Bismarck, ND 58505
701-224-2352

Ohio

Hospital Licensure
Ohio Department of Health
Bureau of Medical Services
Division of Licensure and Certification
246 N. High Street
P.O. Box 118
Columbus, OH 43266-0588
614-466-7857

Oklahoma

Hospital Licensure
Oklahoma Department of Health
Medical Facilities Services
1000 N.E. 10th Street
P.O. Box 53551
Oklahoma City, OK 73152
405-271-6868

Oregon

Hospital Licensure
Oregon Department of Human Resources
Division of Health
Office of Environment and Health Systems
Health Facilities Section
State Office Building, Room 608
P.O. Box 231
Portland, OR 97207
503-229-5686

Pennsylvania

Hospital Licensure
Pennsylvania Department of Health
Office of Planning and Quality Assurance
Bureau of Quality Assurance
Division of Hospitals
532 Health and Welfare Building
Harrisburg, PA 17108
717-783-8980

Rhode Island

Hospital Licensure
Rhode Island Department of Health
Family Health Services
Division of Facilities Regulation
3 Capitol Hill
Providence, RI 02908
401-277-2827

South Carolina

Hospital Licensure
South Carolina Department of Health and
Environmental Control
Division of Health Regulation
Health Facilities Regulation Bureau
2600 Bull Street
Columbia, SC 29201
803-734-4842

South Dakota

Hospital Licensure
South Dakota Department of Health
Licensure and Certification Program
Foss Building
523 E. Capitol
Pierre, SD 57501
605-773-3364

Tennessee

Hospital Licensure
Tennessee Department of Health and Environment
Manpower and Facilities Bureau
Division of Health Care Facilities
344 Cordell Hull Building
Nashville, TN 37247-0101
615-367-6303

Texas

Hospital Licensure
Texas Department of Health
Health Facility Licensure and Certification Division
1100 W. 49th Street
Austin, TX 78756
512-458-7245

Utah

Hospital Licensure
Utah Department of Health
Community Health Services Division
Health Facilities Licensing Bureau
288 North 1460 West
Salt Lake City, UT 84116
801-538-6152

Vermont

Hospital Licensure
Vermont Agency of Human Services
Department of Aging and Disabilities
Licensing and Protection Division
19 Commerce Street
P.O. Box 536
Williston, VT 05495
802-863-7250

Virginia

Hospital Licensure
Virginia Department of Health
Office of Planning and Regulatory Services
Division of Licensure and Certification
3600 W. Broad Street, Suite 216
Richmond, VA 23230
804-367-2102

Washington

Hospital Licensure
Washington Department of Social and Health Services
Health and Rehabilitative Services
Health Services Division
Health Facilities Survey Section
Mail Stop OB-44
Olympia, WA 98504
206-753-5851

West Virginia

Hospital Licensure
West Virginia Department of Health and Human Resources
Administration and Finance Bureau
Health Facilities Licensure and Certification Section
Building 3, Room 265
State Capitol Complex
Charleston, WV 25305
304-558-0050

Wisconsin

Hospital Licensure
Wisconsin Department of Health and Social Services
Division of Health
Bureau of Quality Compliance
One West Wilson Street
P.O. Box 7850
Madison, WI 53707
608-267-7185

Wyoming

Hospital Licensure
Wyoming Department of Health
Division of Health and Medical Services
Medical Facilities
Hathaway Building
Cheyenne, WY 82002
307-777-7123

Glossary of Hospital Health Professionals

Anyone who has been in the hospital knows that you encounter a huge variety of non-M.D. and non-D.O. staff members whose presence is more frequent than your own doctor's. Since it's hard to tell the players without a scorecard, the following roll call of medical personnel will help identify the professionals you may meet in the course of your hospital stay or on an outpatient basis.

Adult nurse practitioner—a registered nurse with advanced, specialized training in the primary care of adults.

Anesthetist—a person who administers anesthetics for surgery and diagnostic procedures. May be a nurse-anesthetist or an anesthesia technician.

Certified nurse-midwife (CNM)—a registered nurse who has additional advanced training in childbirth and the care of pregnant women and who has passed a nurse-midwifery certification examination.

Dietitian—a person with special training and skills in menu planning and food preparation.

Family nurse practitioner—a registered nurse with advanced, specialized training in the primary care of adults and family members.

Gerontological nurse—a nurse who cares for older patients.

House staff—doctors in training in a hospital, plus hospital-based physicians, who are the primary physicians for patients who do not have personal physicians and assist in the care of those who do.

Inhalation therapist—a person with training in the area of natural and assisted breathing, including the administration and monitoring of breathing gases, ventilator-assisted breathing, and the teaching of breathing techniques.

Intern—a doctor in the first year of postgraduate training in a hospital. The term is being replaced by "first-year resident."

Licensed practical nurse (LPN) or *licensed vocational nurse (LVN)*—a person who has undergone training in a vocational technical setting, hospital program, or community college and has been granted a license to provide general care to the sick. Considered less well trained than a registered nurse, but functions may overlap considerably, depending on state laws. Often reports to registered nurses.

Maternal-gynecological-neonatal nurse—a nurse who cares for mothers and newborn infants.

Medical-surgical nurse—a nurse who cares for adults with chronic illnesses and for presurgical and post-surgical patients.

Medical technician—a person with training that allows him or her to carry out some of the functions of holders of the M.D. or D.O. degrees, especially in emergency and life-support situations outside of hospitals and during transport to hospitals. May be more highly trained in their limited areas of expertise than nurse practitioners or physician assistants.

Nurse practitioner (NP)—a registered nurse who has taken additional training and is certified to handle some of the functions of a holder of the M.D. or D.O. degree.

Nurse's aide—a person who assists trained nurses in a hospital by performing unspecialized tasks.

Nutritionist—a person who teaches people about nutrition and helps people plan meals tailored to their particular health and diet needs.

Occupational therapist—a person who uses creative activity as a therapy for helping patients recover or rehabilitate from illness, injury, or disability. May have completed an accredited program in occupational therapy and passed a professional examination.

Orderly—a person who does the hospital's routine or heavy work, such as cleaning, moving supplies, and moving patients.

Paramedic—a technician trained and skilled in the delivery of medical care in emergency situations.

Patients' representative—a person employed by the hospital to mediate between patients and hospital staff. Ideally, this person acts as a patient rights activist, dispensing information to patients and getting complaints resolved.

Pediatric nurse practitioner—a registered nurse who has advanced, specialized training in the nursing care of children.

Pharmacist—a person who has graduated from an accredited school of pharmacy and passed a state board examination. Assures safety, efficacy, and efficiency in obtaining, storing, prescribing, dispensing, delivering, administering, and using drugs and related articles. Often maintains medication profiles on patients receiving prescriptions to reduce adverse reactions, allergies, and contraindicated use of drugs.

Physical therapist—a person who has been trained and licensed in physical therapy, primarily to help people rehabilitate from injuries or diseases affecting muscles, joints, nerves, and bones. Works under the direction of a physician.

Physician assistant—a person trained to carry out some of the functions of holders of the M.D. or D.O. degree. May have more training than a nurse practitioner or a medical technician. Works under physicians' supervision.

Physician extender—a term that refers to people who have been trained to do part of what a holder of the M.D. or D.O. degree can do. Physician extenders include nurse practitioners, physician assistants, and medical technicians. They are used heavily in health maintenance organizations.

Private duty nurse—a nurse who is hired to care for one patient exclusively in a hospital or nursing home and is paid directly by the patient or his or her family.

Psychiatric and mental health nurse—a person who cares for patients with mental and emotional disorders.

Radiotherapist—a person who treats cancer and other diseases using X rays and radioactive substances.

Registered dietitian (RD)—a person with education in nutrition who has passed a national registration exam and who plans and directs food service programs in medical care facilities such as hospitals.

Registered nurse (RN)—generally, a highly trained nurse, one licensed by a state to provide general nursing services after passing a qualifying examination. Three types of nursing education lead to registered-nurse licenses: two-year community college programs, three-year hospital-affiliated diploma programs, and four-year baccalaureate degree programs.

Resident—a doctor taking postgraduate training in a hospital, often working toward certification in a specialty area.

Social worker—a person, usually with a master's of social work (M.S.W.) and sometimes with certification, who works with people who are ill, disabled, aged, or handicapped to help them adjust to disabilities or cope with long-term illness.

NOSOCOMIAL INFECTIONS: HAZARDS OF HOSPITALIZATION

While in the hospital, you are at risk of acquiring a condition you did not have when you went in—called iatrogenic disease (from the Greek meaning "doctor-caused" or "doctor-produced"). Iatrogenesis, especially one of its manifestations—nosocomial (pronounced *nohs-oh-KOH-me-ul*) infection—is why it is often said that a hospital is no place for a sick person.

Acquired during hospitalization, nosocomial infections are produced by microorganisms that dwell within hospitals. Nosocomial infections aren't present in patients on admission. In other words, you don't have it when you check in, you get it while you are there. Most of these infections develop at least 72 hours after admission, which means that some may not manifest themselves until after discharge.

It is estimated that the recovery time necessary to combat a nosocomial infection is about 4 extra days of stay at an average additional cost of $1,000 per day (factoring in both room and ancillary charges). That's $4,000 per infection. Nationally, it is estimated that nosocomial infections contribute between $5 and $10 billion to America's medical bill. Robert Haley, M.D., director of the Division of Epidemiology and Preventive Medicine at the University of Texas Southwestern Medical School, states flatly that nosocomial infections are adding "an unnecessary $4 billion a year to our national medical bill." Other experts say the true figure is double that, especially since about one-fourth of all infections acquired in the hospital don't show up until after the patient is discharged. Then work-related expenses and costly readmission to the hospital have to be factored in.

Expensive that it is, a nosocomial infection can also be deadly: Some estimates of infection-related deaths run as high as 100,000 (some even higher, 300,000 or so) a year. Annually, 5 to 10 percent of hospitalized patients (about 2 million people) acquire hospital infections, and in approximately 3 percent of those cases, the infection is the cause of death.

Nosocomial infection rates are highest in large teaching hospitals and lowest in nonteaching hospitals. Obviously, the large teaching facilities attract the sickest patients, but this fact also points out the difficulties large facilities have in maintaining necessary sanitary discipline.

Here are some more disturbing infection-related facts:

- Annually, more than 100,000 hospital patients in the United States acquire nosocomial bacteremia—the presence of bacteria in the blood. Richard E. Dixon, M.D., says the mortality rates "range from 20 percent for patients who do not develop shock, to greater than 80 percent for those who do."

- Infection is the most frequent cause of death in cancer patients.
- Pneumonia, now reported as the most common hospital-acquired infection leading to death, occurs in .5 to 5 percent of all in-hospital patients and in 12 to 15 percent of patients ill enough to require intensive care, and may be responsible for 15 percent of all hospital-associated deaths. It may be introduced into the lungs by way of contaminated respiratory therapy equipment or simply by breathing the air filled with droplets of infection from other patients or coughing medical personnel, especially in the close quarters of intensive care units.

Why is nosocomial infection so widespread, so lethal a problem in modern hospitals? For one thing, as we mentioned before, hospitals are where sick people are. Those who are weak when hospitalized and those weakened in the hospital are highly susceptible to infection. These infections come from the microorganisms and pathogens that thrive in the hospital setting or arrive with new patients from the community at large.

Add to that the increase in invasive procedures and major surgeries. Consider the increased use of drugs that reduce the body's rejection of implants, but at the same time, suppress the body's immune system, leaving the door wide open for infections that can kill—for example, nosocomial pneumonia. Nosocomial infections frequently attack the urinary tract—most usually because of the use of urinary catheters, the cause of approximately 40 percent of all nosocomial infections—surgical wounds (about 25 percent), and the lower respiratory tract (approximately 15 percent).

Another cause of patient susceptibility to hospital infections is, ironically, antibiotics. Typically, when there is a rash of infections, hospitals use additional antibiotics to fight the microorganisms that the antibiotics themselves have nurtured. And it may work for a while—until the aftereffects set in. Not only do patients have bad reactions to the drugs, but there is a rapid development of strains of bacteria resistant to the antibiotics that were once effective against these organisms. The amount of penicillin required to treat an infection today is fifty times greater than it was thirty years ago.

The ways nosocomial infections are spread are numerous. Organisms can be transmitted in food and water, in transfused blood and intravenous fluids, in

How Do You Protect Yourself?

What can be done to protect yourself from nosocomial infections? There is no surefire defense for you if the rest of the hospital is a vast and bubbling breeding ground. So the first step in infection protection is to try to gain admission to a hospital that has a good nosocomial record. Ask your doctor about it. Contact your local department of health. Ask the hospital directly, but be on your guard if the hospital says its infection rate is low while never supplying you with a specific percentage. That may mean that the staff is not properly surveying the facility's infection rate, or not surveying at all.

An active infection control committee is a good sign that the hospital is concerned about infections and is trying to monitor and control them. Ask if that is the case. Another good sign is if someone on the staff is a member of the infection watchdog organization, the Association for Practitioners in Infection Control. Hospitals with a greater than average concern for the nosocomial infection danger will have at least one nurse/epidemiologist on staff to maintain surveillance. Find out if there's one in your hospital.

Little has changed in the nearly three decades since two prominent researchers, H. N. Beaty and R. G. Petersdorf, wrote in the October 1966 *Annals of Internal Medicine* about the most important preventive of iatrogenic disease: "Administer drugs only when they are needed, and . . . perform diagnostic procedures only when they are likely to yield meaningful information."

What Else Can You Do?

While it is true that one-third of all infections treated in hospitals are nosocomial infections, it is also estimated that as many as half of all such infections are preventable. With luck, information, and diligence you might be able to prevent your own. Some things you can do personally and actively while in the hospital are:

- Try to make sure that all hospital personnel who come in contact with you have washed their hands. If you so desire, ask them to do so, in your room, in your presence. You can greatly lower your chances of catching an infection—and paying for its treatment.

- If your roommate becomes infected, or if you are concerned that what he/she has could possibly be transmitted to you via the air or through the use of a common bathroom, ask your doctor or the staff nurse/epidemiologist about your risks. Change your room at once if there is any chance that you might become infected, because once you are infected it is too late. You may have to be put in isolation along with your roommate.

- If you are undergoing surgery or a procedure that requires the removal of hair, refuse to be shaved the night before surgery. One study indicates that among people shaved the day prior to their operations, the nosocomial infection rate was 5.6 percent. Chemical depilatories reduce the rate to just .6 percent. Using barber clippers to remove hair the morning of surgery yields a low infection rate, too.

  Of course, there is a good question you might ask: Is shaving or clipping or any other form of hair removal necessary at all? Maybe not—and especially when it comes to obstetrics/gynecology situations. Removing hair before vaginal delivery or surgery in that area is probably uncalled-for, because the old idea that hair creates a climate for infection is unsubstantiated by clinical studies.

• Have nurses regularly check the drainage of urinary catheters to help you maintain cleanliness.

pharmaceuticals, through the air, by direct human contact, on towels and sheets, and via the housekeeping crew, to name but a few.

Certain places in the hospital must be diligently monitored, for they can be especially hazardous for patients and hospital personnel as well. These include the hemodialysis unit (the equipment can be a source of hepatitis B, a virulent and difficult-to-destroy organism), intensive care units (occupied by patients who are extremely weak and thus susceptible to infection and operated under emergency measures that often have to forsake pristine sanitary procedures in order to save a life), the infant nursery, and the operating room.

To these potential sources of infection add plain old carelessness, if not callousness. The Institute for Child Health reports that many hospital workers who come in direct contact with patients don't take the time to, or are not concerned enough to, take the simplest and best known of precautionary measures: *washing their hands properly.* And doctors are among the worst offenders. No wonder: "Most medical schools don't teach practical prevention, stressing things like washing," explains Timothy R. Franson, M.D., hospital epidemiologist at the Medical College of Wisconsin. Case in point: In two intensive care units studied, hands were washed after patient contact less than half the time. Unwashed hands are prime culprits in the spread of many nosocomial infections.

Equally critical is the antimicrobial chemical used in handwashing. A study reported in the *New England Journal of Medicine* found that a hand-disinfection system using an antimicrobial agent more effectively reduces the rate of nosocomial infections than a system that uses alcohol and soap.

Nosocomial infections can also pass to patients via the procedural chain of the food services department, due to any one or more of the following (nearly all of them with their roots in human error, and any one of them preventable): lack of handwashing; poor per-

sonal hygiene; faulty patient care technique; inadequate refrigeration (the culprit in nearly half of all nosocomial salmonellosis outbreaks); inadequate cooking; inadequate reheating; holding food in warming devices at bacteria-incubating temperatures; using contaminated raw ingredients in uncooked foods; and improper cleaning of equipment.

A myriad of studies also points to other work areas in the hospital that, because of persistently poor and unprofessional hygiene practices, are breeding grounds for nosocomial infections: central service department, the unit responsible for processing, storing, and dispensing hospital supplies; pharmacy; laundry; laboratory (where, more than one story goes, workers have to be admonished not to keep their lunches in the same refrigerators as the ones that contain serum or other specimens)—and the list goes on.

IATROGENIC DISEASE

Iatrogenic disease (literally, doctor-caused) may be considered a nosocomial problem in a general sense because it takes place most often in a hospital. Its origin, though, is with the doctor.

Iatrogenic disease is no small problem. In one major study conducted at a teaching hospital, researchers from Boston University Medical Center found that of 815 consecutive admissions, 36 percent were there because of an iatrogenic problem, and in 2 percent of the patients, iatrogenesis was a contributing factor in the patients' deaths. If one were able to generalize from this study, one would arrive at the conclusion that iatrogenic mishaps kill nearly 500,000 people a year and add at least $1 billion to America's medical bill.

Iatrogenesis comes in all sizes and types. There is the iatrogenesis that occurs when a doctor performs a procedure that has greater risks than benefits, and the gamble is lost. There is the iatrogenesis that occurs when the doctor hasn't prepared himself/herself for the unexpected complication, although it was always a possibility. There is the iatrogenesis that occurs when a doctor makes a mistake, in judgment or handiwork. He/she might go ahead and do something without having adequate knowledge of or skills for the procedure.

High-Risk Areas for Iatrogenesis

There are several areas of medical practice in which iatrogenesis is most prevalent. To avoid becoming a victim of iatrogenesis, you need to know the dangers that could lie in these areas.

Diagnosis

Diagnosing disease is the keystone of medicine, its very foundation. Without an accurate diagnosis, medical practice has no purpose, and patients are treated in ways that are ineffective and expensive or worse—a lot worse. What's the problem? The studies point the finger at too great a reliance on technology and statistics and lab results, and not enough use of human skills, common sense, and brain work. You could say the medical profession has come a long way from the words of Sir William Osler: "Learn to see, learn to hear, learn to feel, learn to smell, and know that by practice alone can you become expert. Medicine is learned by the bedside and not in the classroom."

Doctors may believe the machines and mistrust their own eyes. And the fact of the matter is that, aside from the added costs of high-tech testing, *a person can become ill because of those very tests*. Some very good studies in important journals have made it clear that faulty diagnosis is a major iatrogenic problem. For example, a study by researchers from Baptist Memorial Hospital and the University of Tennessee College of Medicine in Memphis revealed that heart attacks were misdiagnosed 47 percent of the time. From Baylor College of Medicine in Houston came the report that medical residents made diagnostic errors—incorrect findings and oversights—13.1 percent of the time, interns 15.6 percent of the time, and that at least one error occurred during the examination of two-thirds of all patients seen. Both studies appeared in the *Journal of the American Medical Association*.

The *New England Journal of Medicine* reported a Harvard hospital study showing that 10 percent of all patients who had died *might have lived* if they had received the correct diagnosis. In some cate-

gories of disease, the misdiagnosis figures were as high as 24 percent.

Surgery

Unnecessary surgery is an iatrogenic problem. How prevalent is it? Some claim unnecessary surgery comprises somewhere between 10 and 20 percent of all surgery. Heart specialist Robert G. Schneider, M.D., in *When to Say No to Surgery* (Englewood Cliffs, N.J.: Prentice-Hall, 1982) put the unnecessary surgery figure at 15 to 25 percent as an average, multiplies it by the number of operations performed each year, and comes up with a total of somewhere between 3 million and 6.25 million annual unnecessary operations, leading to a ballpark figure of 40,000 to 80,000 unnecessary surgery deaths in America every year—a figure undisputed by most experts today.

In fact, one of the most common vascular operations in this country, carotid endarterectomy—the removal of blockages from arteries carrying blood to the brain—is often done unnecessarily, according to many reports. A Canadian study published in the *New England Journal of Medicine* said that half of the more than 100,000 such operations done in this country every year are performed on patients without symptoms of carotid disease. And there is a 10 percent risk of suffering a stroke or dying from the surgery—roughly five times greater than the condition it's supposed to correct. A five-year Rand Corporation study of 5,000 Medicare patients found carotid endarterectomy to be a common unnecessary surgery, with 65 percent of them done for inappropriate or questionable reasons. Of the people studied, 10 percent died or had a stroke as a direct result of the surgery.

The same Rand study also found that death occurs in roughly 5 percent of heart bypass surgeries (to help or replace constricted or blocked arteries), and even the successful ones can have problems: The new vessel may close within eight years and thus require more surgery.

Other operations most often mentioned as probably unnecessary are many that are elective, many that are female-oriented (mastectomies, hysterectomies, cesarean sections), tonsillectomies, knee operations, and back operations. Indeed, a Blue Cross and Blue Shield Association study in 1991 found that, of the procedures studied, those most often performed inappropriately include tonsillectomies (27 percent of the time), hysterectomies (21.5 percent of the time), and tonsillectomies combined with adenoidectomies (17.6 percent of the time). Further, a 1993 Rand study found that 41 percent of hysterectomies in seven large HMOs are unneeded or questionable.

Because enough evidence exists to charge ample numbers of physicians with performing inappropriate or unnecessary surgery on Medicare patients, the Office of Management and Budget has suggested a reduction in payments to physicians for these procedures:

Arthroscopic, or fiberoptic tube, examinations of knee joints, lungs, esophagus, stomach, and duodenum

Carpal tunnel surgery for hand pain

Lens implant after cataract removal, or lens implant without cataract removal

Coronary bypass surgery

Dilation and curettage of the uterus to diagnose disease

Hip or knee replacement

Heart pacemaker implant

Prostate surgery

Both critics and surgeons agree on one fact: Statistics show that the number of operations each year increases, not in proportion to the rise in population, but rather in proportion to the rise in the number of surgeons. And various Rand Corporation studies point to unnecessary, inappropriate, and overpriced surgeries as substantial causes behind the ever-mounting costs of health care.

Drugs

As an area of iatrogenic abuse, drugs are probably in the lead. Doctors just aren't as well educated in dosages and side effects as they might be. Many doctors learn about the adverse effects of drugs from pharmaceutical company representatives, who are eager to have doctors prescribe their products, and may not always disclose the full extent of adverse effects. Added to this is a great deal of overprescribing, and also unwise, uncertain, or sometimes unethical prescribing.

Michael Cohen, a pharmacist and cofounder of the Institute for Safe Medication Practices, estimates that 2 to 10 percent of all hospital drug doses are administered incorrectly. He cites instances where doctors write orders for the wrong medication, medications are mislabeled, or the wrong patient receives the wrong drug.

Protecting Yourself Against Iatrogenesis

How can you protect yourself against doctor-produced problems, against iatrogenic mishaps? So long as medical care is provided by humans, there will be error and greed and iatrogenesis. That is why you must maintain an attitude of wariness.

If you are not yet in a hospital, be wary of going into one. A hospital ought to be the place your doctor sends you when all else fails, when there is no other choice and no better place to continue your care. If you find yourself in a hospital, be wary of everything scheduled to be done to you. Get as much information as you can about what is to be done to you, what drug is being prescribed for you. Learn the names of the drugs you need to take, their doses and sizes, and even their colors, so that you will be able to spot a mistake or question a change. Before you give the green light to anything, be sure the benefits outweigh the risks. Don't be talked into "fad" operations. Get second opinions and third opinions. When in doubt—and especially if that doubt has to do with elective surgery—don't. Take nothing for granted. And, we'll say it again, question, question, question.

Ask certain specific questions of each surgeon you visit: At what hospital do you operate? What is the nosocomial infection rate there? How often is the operation performed at that hospital? How often do you perform this operation? What's been the result? What are the risks? What will or may the consequences be if you do not perform this surgery?

Numerous studies have demonstrated that the more times a hospital performs certain operations, the lower the death and/or complication rates for people undergoing the procedures. Some of the most recent research on the subject (published in the July 28, 1989, *Journal of the American Medical Association*) found that death rates for four common operations are higher when done by surgeons with less experience. The four procedures studied were: removal of part of the stomach for ulcers; removal of all or part of the colon for cancer; coronary artery bypass grafts for arteriosclerotic heart disease; and repair of the main abdominal artery weakened or torn by an aneurysm. Death rates for these four, plus a fifth operation—gallbladder re-

Medication Errors

Reactions, drug dependency, and allergies may occur even with proper usage of the correct drug, but there is also the possibility that harm to the body (ranging from serious health complications to death) can result due to medication errors committed by a physician, a nurse, a pharmacist, or even the patient.

What are medication errors?

Medication errors are any mistakes, negligence, or miscalculations committed in the process of prescribing and administering a drug to a patient or in monitoring the effects of a drug. Medication errors can involve the type of drug or its dosage, the prescription, the method of dispensing, or the lack of communication between health professionals.

How do medication errors occur?

According to Charles E. Myers, of the American Society of Hospital Pharmacists (ASHP), an organization that has developed a series of guidelines designed to reduce this problem, medication errors commonly arise when there is a breakdown in the communications between various parties who administer and prescribe medication. Myers adds, "In hospitals, the use of medications is a multidisciplinary process involving physicians, pharmacists, nurses, and others. Because it involves multiple parties, errors often can be traced to flaws or lapses in the system where the parties interact."

What can be done to prevent medication errors?

Neil Davis, Pharm.D., a cofounder of the Institute for Safe Medication Practices and a participant in the formulation of the ASHP guidelines, said these guidelines can help reduce the number of hospital medication errors in very practical ways. The ASHP has listed dozens of categories of medication errors and the reasons behind these mistakes.

What can consumers do?

The ASHP hasn't forgotten the important role consumers play in reducing medication errors. Their recommendations are:

1. Inform all your health care providers (physicians, nurses, pharmacists) of your known allergies, sensitivities, and current medications.
2. Ask questions about any recommended procedures or treatments.
3. Learn the names of all the drug products that are prescribed and administered to you.
4. Keep medication logs: Record all drug therapy, including prescribed drugs, nonprescription drugs, home remedies, and medical foods (special diets high in nutrients).
5. Be assertive if something seems incorrect or different from the norm.
6. Take prescription medication as directed.

But these guidelines don't cover everything you can do to prevent a medication error from happening to you. From his own experience with consumer medication errors, Davis has observed other areas where errors can occur. Here's some further advice for medication-error-wary consumers:

1. **Speak up before your treatment.** All too often in hospitals, says Davis, a nurse will give a patient a pill. The patient will swallow it. And then and only then will the patient think to say, "That's funny; an hour ago my pill was red."

2. **Request unit-dose medication.** According to Davis, this is the safest way to administer medication: Each individual dose and strength of medication is individually wrapped; thus, your chances of getting the wrong dose of a drug are more remote.

3. **Take your time at discharge.** When patients are discharged from hospitals, the natural tendency for patients is to hurry this process as much as possible. Before you make your escape, Davis recommends that you take time to verify and understand all of your prescriptions.

4. **Pick out one pharmacy, and get to know the pharmacists.** In the hospital, each new encounter with a doctor brings an added possibility of a new prescription. According to Davis, a good safety check to ensure that you're not being prescribed the same medication twice is to use the same pharmacist and pharmacy.

5. **Write down any new medication allergies you uncover.** Davis recommends that, if you have an allergic reaction, get down in writing the name of this drug and any others in the same drug family that you might be allergic to.

6. **Bring your medications to the hospital.** Again, this simple step can save you a lot of pain and grief. Discuss this with your doctor and have him or her make the arrangements with the nursing station.

moval—were also found to be higher at hospitals that performed them less often.

HOSPITAL BILLS: READING AND UNDERSTANDING THEM

Since most of the money spent on health care in this country is spent in hospitals, it makes obvious sense that the greatest potential for savings is in hospitals. Unless you're one of the lucky few with a spectacular health insurance plan that pays down to the last penny of your hospital costs, chances are you'll be responsible for 10 to 20 percent of the bill when you check out.

What specifically can you do to save money in the hospital? Charges for hospital services are very high, so, obviously, if you are able to manage without some routine services (such as routine admission tests or unnecessary repetition of other tests), you can save considerable sums of money.

Important, too, is your hospital bill. What can you do about it? you ask, since the deed or deeds are done. Just as you would a sizable restaurant tab or an itemized home repair bill, you should review your hospital bill with some care to pick out any inaccuracies, overcharges, and mysterious charges. One might say that's easier said than done. Some hospital bills are long and often hard to read and difficult to understand. That's because most hospital bills are full of abbreviations and shorthand entries, and charges for items and services are often crammed into a catchall category, such as "Miscellaneous."

Sometimes compiling the charges is so tedious and time-consuming that the bill won't be ready for you to examine on the day of your discharge. It will be sent to you instead. Whether you get the bill at the hospital or at home, be certain to get a fully itemized version. While an itemized bill is more detailed and full of charges and services than a summary bill, it is

Sample Hospital Bill

Numbers Correspond to Circled Numbers on Next Page

1. Does the patient identification line or box contain the correct name and account number? (Some hospitals use your Social Security number as an account number, so check it closely—is it accurate?)

2. Are the admission and discharge dates correct? (You don't want to be billed for services if you were discharged before the next billing day.)

3. Is the name of the insurance company entered on the correct line or box?

4. Is the insurance group number correct? (A faulty number here could put you in the wrong group and delay your claim.)

5. Is the insurance policy number correct? (The wrong number here could lead to a rejection of your claim.)

6. Does the "bill to" line or box contain the correct name and address of the person who is responsible for paying the bill? (This line may contain the name of the patient or the patient's spouse. Hospitals want this information even though an insurance company may be paying the bill. They claim that their agreement to provide services is with the patient and not with an insurance company.)

7. Does the hospital bill contain a description of services and a summary of charges for each department?

8. Do any of the individual department charges appear to be higher than they ought to be? (If the hospital billing clerk hits the wrong key, that $37 patient tray kit could end up costing $370.)

9. Do any preadmission testing charges appear on the bill? (Preadmission testing is billed separately and should not be listed on your hospital bill.)

10. Do any of the items listed in the "summary of charges" column appear more than once? (If you only had one chest X ray during your stay, you don't want to be billed for three chest X rays.)

11. Are the dates of the services clearly indicated on the billing statement? (You'll need to have this information if there's a dispute over the bill with either the hospital or your insurance company.)

12. Does the billing statement contain a charge for admission or discharge processing? (Ideally, you should check with your doctor before you're admitted to determine what you will be receiving for these extra charges. The question here is really whether you get *anything* for your money. Very often these charges are little more than the hospital's paper processing fees. You can, however, request that these charges be taken off, but it is best to negotiate all this ahead of time rather than haggle afterward.)

13. Does the amount shown in the "estimated insurance payment" column match the payment schedule as shown on your insurance policy's schedule of benefits? (Many hospitals can tell you how much your insurance company will pay for the care you receive. The estimate is based on the contract the hospital has with your insurance company and your particular plan's coverage.)

14. Is the "patient amount due" column clearly labeled? (Some statements have multiple columns showing various balances due and insurance payments expected, and unless the patient portion of the bill is clearly labeled you might accidentally pay for something that is covered by insurance.)

15. Does the hospital bill contain instructions on how to obtain an itemized bill, inquire about specific charges, or request an audit?

Sample Hospital Bill

PATIENT ACCOUNT STATEMENT

GENERAL INFORMATION

PATIENT'S NAME	ACCOUNT NO.	BIRTH DATE	ADMISSION DATE	DISCHARGE DATE	STATEMENT DATE
JOHN R. DOE (1)	123456	3-5-55	12-29-89 (2)	1-20-90	1-27-90

PRIMARY INSURANCE CO.	GROUP NO.	POLICY NUMBER
HEALTH AMERICA/MAXICARE (3)	584003 (4)	185329253 (5)

BILL TO	MAKE CHECK PAYABLE TO	AMOUNT OF YOUR PAYMENT
MARY ANN DOE (6) 987 10TH STREET TOPEKA, KS 66217	JEFFERSON HOSPITAL PO BOX 1990 J TOPEKA, KS 66201	$3526.80 (14)

IMPORTANT: TO ENSURE PROPER CREDIT, PLEASE DETACH AND RETURN THE TOP PORTION OF THIS STATEMENT WITH YOUR PAYMENT

GENERAL INFORMATION

PATIENT'S NAME	ACCOUNT NO.	STATEMENT DATE	ADMISSION DATE	DISCHARGE DATE	PAGE NO.
JOHN R. DOE	123456	1-27-90	12-29-89	1-20-90 (15)	1

IF YOU HAVE ANY QUESTIONS ABOUT THIS STATEMENT CALL:

BETTY BILLER   PHONE 464-1234   MONDAY THROUGH FRIDAY 8:30 - 4:30

SERVICE DATE		DESCRIPTION	TOTAL AMOUNT	INSURANCE PORTION	PATIENT PORTION
		SUMMARY OF CHARGES (7)			
12-29-89	120	ROOM & DAILY CARE 23 DAYS @$320/day 12-29-89 to 1-20-90	7360.00		
12-29-89	115	PATIENT TRAY-TOWELS, PILLOW, SLIPPERS	370.00		
1-2-90	250	PHARMACY	427.00		
1-4-90	258	IV SOLUTIONS	1052.00		
1-4-90	260	IV THERAPY	632.50		
1-4-90	270	MEDICAL-SURGICAL SUPPLIES	9.50		
1-2-90	300	LABORATORY	214.50		
1-5-90	301	LABORATORY/CHEMISTRY	63.00		
1-9-90	302	LABORATORY/IMMUNOLOGY	583.00		
1-11-90	305	LABORATORY/HEMATOLOGY	189.00		
1-15-90	306	LABORATORY/BACTERIOLOGY-MICROBIOLOGY	308.00		
1-17-90	307	LABORATORY/UROLOGY	154.50		
12-27-89	309	LABORATORY/PREADMISSION TESTING	480.00		
1-2-90	320	DIAGNOSTIC X-RAY	27.00		
1-2-90	320	DIAGNOSTIC X-RAY	27.00		
1-3-90	324	DIAGNOSTIC X-RAY/CHEST	213.50		
1-4-90	360	OPERATING ROOM SERVICES	90.00		
1-4-90	370	ANESTHESIA	452.00		
12-30-89	390	BLOOD/STORAGE PROCEDURES	20.00		
1-5-90	410	RESPIRATORY SERVICES	376.50		
1-8-90	420	PHYSICAL THERAPY	73.00		
1-4-90	710	RECOVERY ROOM	59.00		
1-3-90	730	ELECTROCARDIOGRAM	147.00		
1-20-90	999	ADMISSION/DISCHARGE PROCESSING	160.00		
		TOTAL CHARGES (12)	$13488.00		
		AMOUNT BILLED TO INSURANCE		$9961.20	
		PAY THIS AMOUNT			$3526.80 (14)

THANK YOU FOR CHOOSING JEFFERSON HEALTH SERVICES FOR YOUR MEDICAL CARE.

FINAL DIAGNOSIS	PLEASE READ REVERSE SIDE OF THIS STATEMENT
ACUTE ENDOCARDITIS	

Circled annotation numbers: (8) (9) (10) (11) (13)

preferable because without it you can never determine whether you were billed accurately and fairly. If the itemized bill comes in full of undecipherable computer codes, ask for a bill you can understand.

There's no getting around it: If you want to avoid paying for what you did not get, you have to go over the hospital bill item by item, no matter how long it takes. A daily log and other records, kept during a hospital stay, can serve as guides and evidence.

The sample hospital bill provided marks and explains areas of pertinent information and potential inaccuracy.

How good are your chances of finding errors? Equifax Services, an Atlanta firm that audits around 40,000 hospital bills annually for insurers, found in one audit of selected bills that more than 97 percent of hospital bills contain errors! And, according to the firm's calculations, hospital overcharges exceed undercharges by three to one. You can spot these errors only if you receive an itemized bill, and nine times out of ten a hospital will not give you an itemized bill unless you ask for it.

The way most hospital billing systems operate is to charge patients for treatments, services, and supplies *before* they are actually received—in fact, usually when they are ordered by the physician. If the treatments or services are never rendered or the supplies not received, because of a change in the doctor's orders or an early discharge from the hospital, the charges may still remain on the bill. Many errors also occur when surgery is involved, because surgery is a high-dollar item with a myriad of accompanying services and charges. An error here can be significant. Then there's the problem of clerical or simple typographical errors: a charge of $30 for an aspirin tablet instead of $.30, or a bill for twelve blood tests instead of one umbrella test that analyzes twelve components.

In reviewing your own hospital bill, put a check mark next to the items that seem unclear or odd. Before you pay, you should clarify any portions of the bill that you believe are wrong or questionable. If the bill is riddled with inaccuracies, errors, and overcharges, to the point where you question the entire bill, *don't pay it.*

To clarify and rectify any errors, first approach the hospital: Talk to the head of the billing office or even a hospital administrator. If there are major problems that nobody at the hospital seems able to resolve, or if they refuse to clear an error or explain a muddled entry, you have other avenues open to you.

Call your attorney if you need help or guidance. If your bill is going to be paid by your insurer, be sure to inform your insurer directly, and in writing, of any inaccuracies in the bill. Everyone saves money by making sure that insurers do not overpay hospitals, and gone are the days when nobody cared enough to scrutinize a hospital bill—including the insurance company paying it. In fact, some employers and insurance companies now offer rewards to people who spot overcharges and other errors on their hospital bills. But even if yours doesn't, you can save money by giving any bill a checkup.

Explain the situation to your insurance company—the fact that the bill is wrong and you are trying to correct the errors—and instruct them not to pay your bill when the hospital submits it. Your employer, or any other group or association who may be paying a good chunk of your insurance, should be informed about what you are doing, why you are refusing to accept or pay the bill.

When you contact your insurance company, you are requesting an audit of your account. This audit is called a utilization review. And, of course, any documentation (the daily log, record of tests and medications administered, and so on) you have will be valuable in pleading your case. If you suspect fraud, contact your state attorney general's office.

Always remember that you have the right to refuse to pay a bill that is questionable. Bear in mind, though, that the hospital has a right to send collection agencies after you or sue for your actions, if you and the hospital don't come to an agreement. Even here you have recourse: If the hospital threatens you with legal action or has a collection agency after you, contact your state's consumer protection office.

HOSPITAL EMERGENCY DEPARTMENTS

Hospital emergency departments (EDs), at one time called emergency rooms, are designed primarily for treating patients with severe, life-threatening conditions. These conditions may be the result of illnesses (such as a heart attack or stroke), accidents (auto, recreation- or work-related), or violence (muggings, stabbings, shootings) and other traumas. Some hospital emergency departments offering highly specialized emergency care are designated area-wide trauma centers. Most EDs are open 24 hours a day, 7 days a week, and are required by law to provide care to any-

Hospital Bill Errors:
17 Surefire Questions to Ask

American Claims Evaluation, Inc., a firm in the business of auditing hospital bills, recommends you ask yourself the following questions to help identify possible errors on a bill:

1. Was I billed for the right kind of room (semiprivate, private, etc.)?
2. Was I billed for the correct number of days I occupied the hospital room?
3. Was I billed correctly for any time spent in specialized units (intensive care unit, coronary care unit, etc.)?
4. If I left before "checkout time," was I billed for an extra day even though I'd already gone?
5. Was I billed only for those X rays and tests that I actually received?
6. If I had preadmission testing, did the hospital bill me for the "standard admission test battery" even though I never had it?
7. Was I charged only for supplies, medications, therapy, dressings, injections, etc., that I received? Were the quantities correct?
8. Were medications that my doctor prescribed billed over the entire stay even though I took them only once or twice?
9. Were drugs prescribed for me to take home actually received?
10. Was I billed for bedpans, humidifiers, admission kits, thermometers, etc., that I never received and/or was not allowed to take home?
11. If I received a blood transfusion, was I charged for blood that a donor, blood bank, Red Cross family, or community assurance program replaced?
12. If admitted to a maternity unit, was I billed for a labor room that may not have been used because of a swift delivery?
13. If I was able to keep my newborn in my room, was I charged for excess nursery care?
14. Was I charged for personal items not received or not allowed to take home?
15. Was I billed for daily hospital visits by my doctor or surgeon that did not occur?
16. Was I billed for consultations with specialists to whom I was referred but that did not take place?
17. Was I charged for the correct type of treatment and number of hours of treatment by physical, radiation, inhalation, speech, and/or occupational therapists?

one entering the department. A requirement of hospital licensure is that hospitals treat all patients who present themselves for care.

Hospital EDs, however, are not generic, not all the same. Emergency departments in small rural hospitals are primarily designed to treat and care for small emergencies and to stabilize more seriously ill or injured patients, then transfer them to a larger facility. Emergency departments in medium-size hospitals are equipped to treat a broad range of problems, includ-

ing heart attacks, strokes, and trauma. These emergency departments may also stabilize severely ill patients before transferring them to a larger tertiary, or specialty care, hospital.

Emergency departments in large, well-equipped hospitals are able to handle the more seriously ill or injured patients, many of whom are transferred from small and medium-size hospitals. These hospitals are designated as major trauma centers and, as such, have a staff of highly trained trauma nurses and doctors always ready to provide care. In addition, a full range of specialists is either present or on standby should the severely ill or injured patient require such services. Air ambulance support enables them to transport ("medevac") patients from an accident site directly to the hospital. These air ambulances are also used to pick up and transport trauma patients who have been stabilized at other EDs.

Recognized Levels of Emergency Departments

Standards for EDs have been developed by the Joint Commission on the Accreditation of Healthcare Organizations (JCAHO). While JCAHO recognizes four levels of service, most hospital EDs fall into one of three distinct groups:

Level I is the most sophisticated level of service, with comprehensive emergency care 24 hours a day. Such an ED is staffed full-time by physicians specializing in emergency care, with additional coverage by hospital staff physicians in other specialties. In some cases other specialists must be available for consultation within 30 minutes.

Level II EDs also provide comprehensive emergency care and are staffed by at least one physician with a specialty in emergency medicine. Other specialists, if not physically present in the hospital, must be available within 30 minutes for consultation or to provide care.

Level III EDs are available to provide emergency care 24 hours a day; however, a physician is not necessarily physically present in the emergency department. In these situations, a physician must be available within 30 minutes of the need for emergency care. Level III EDs usually stabilize patients before transferring them to other hospitals.

Level IV EDs are not much more than aid stations that can determine if an emergency exists, render first aid, and arrange for transfer of a patient to a larger facility.

Personnel

Staffing an ED 24 hours a day is no easy task, as doctors, nurses, technicians, and other support staff must be available if services are to be provided when needed. Ideally, EDs should be under the direction of a doctor with a specialty in emergency medicine, although this may not always be the case, especially in rural areas and even some urban areas. (However, this does not mean that doctors who lack emergency medicine backgrounds are not qualified to treat emergencies.) Staffing of EDs has always

been difficult, and it was not unusual to have doctors with non-emergency medicine specialties "moonlighting" in the ED just to pick up some extra income.

With the passage of the Emergency Medical Services Act of 1973, however, emergency medicine began to receive the type of attention it required. Another leap forward was the development of the emergency medicine specialist and the recognition of this specialty by mainstream medicine. The American Board of Emergency Medicine is recognized by the American Board of Medical Specialties and grants certificates to those doctors who meet the criteria and pass the examination for board certification.

According to the American Board of Medical Specialties, an emergency medicine specialist is:

> a doctor who focuses on the immediate medical needs of the patient, and takes all action necessary to prevent further injury or death. This means that the emergency doctor immediately evaluates the patient as to his or her medical condition, selects the proper care, and determines the proper disposition of the patient. In some cases, this includes discharge to home, admission to the hospital or transfer to another facility for further treatment and recovery.

Emergency department doctors may also be board-certified in the subspecialty of pediatric emergency medicine.

In addition to doctors, nurses also play a very important role in the services provided by EDs. These specially trained nurses perform a function known as triage, which means separation of the patients according to the need for service. The triage nurse performs a medical assessment of each patient to ensure that those most in need of lifesaving or life-supporting care receive it on a priority basis. This priority selection process enables a severely injured accident victim to receive treatment ahead of someone, for instance, with a fishhook in the finger.

Emergency departments also require support staff such as reception and registration personnel, and X-ray, laboratory, and pharmacy technicians. Hospitals with air ambulances also have helicopter pilots, flight surgeons, and flight nurses on staff.

Hospital EDs are also responsible for directing pre-hospital care provided by ambulance and rescue squads. Emergency medical personnel, using sophisticated communications equipment (called telemetry), relay vital patient information to doctors and nurses at the hospital ED. Using this information, they advise the emergency personnel attending the patient on the proper course of treatment until the patient and medical team arrive at the ED.

Equipment

Obviously, a great amount of medical equipment and supplies is needed to outfit today's modern emergency department. Even Level III EDs have the ability to stabilize seriously ill or injured patients before they are transferred to larger facilities.

The EDs of today resemble a large open room with treatment areas extending from the walls, separated by movable curtains. Each area contains a gurney (movable treatment table) for the patient, and access to oxygen, anesthesia gases, suction and telemetry (monitoring) equipment. One or two of these areas are fully equipped to become an emergency operating room if the patient requires emergency surgery.

Portable X-ray equipment, laboratory supplies, medications, sutures, bandages, surgical instruments, and hypodermic needles are all part of the supplies necessary to provide emergency care.

Going to the Emergency Department

What should you expect when you arrive at an ED?

Upon arriving at the ED, whether under your own power or by emergency vehicle, you'll need to complete some paperwork before being seen by a doctor. (This protocol would not apply if you were obviously bleeding or experiencing other signs of distress.) Your first stop is the reception or registration desk, where your name, address, telephone number, insurance carrier, and name of personal physician are taken, along with your complaint or reason for the visit.

This information then goes to the triage nurse, who takes your vital signs (blood pressure, pulse, temperature) and asks you a few more questions. For example: Are you allergic to any medications? Are you presently taking any medications? If so, what are they? When did you last have a tetanus shot?

Depending upon the determination of the triage nurse, you may be seen next or you may await your turn with the other sore throats, bruised fingers, and twisted ankles.

It's important to add here that the function of performing triage is not taken lightly. In it there is no intent to demean what you may consider a medical emergency, which in reality is a medical urgency. You must remember that a medical urgency is *not* the same as a true medical emergency.

If your condition is serious, such as loss of blood from an open wound or loss of consciousness, severe burns, or obvious broken bones, you will be seen ahead of patients with less serious conditions.

Once in the treatment area, the doctor will review the notes made by the triage nurse and ask you a few more questions about your complaint. If your condition is something obvious, such as a gash on your forehead as a result of falling from a ladder, the physician attends to your wound with a bandage or stitches.

Should your condition be much more serious, very likely the physician will want to take X rays of suspected broken bones or to look for internal damage. There may also be a need for laboratory tests, in which case a technician would be summoned to draw blood and get the specimen to the lab "stat" (medical talk for "quickly"). Depending upon what is learned from the X rays and lab work, you may be treated and released, or admitted to the hospital for further study and observation.

When a person in a full-fledged cardiac emergency arrives at the ED, the entire area shifts into high gear with a flurry of activity. A "crash cart"—a special cart containing cardiac emergency supplies such as stimulants, anticlotting medications, blood pressure monitor, electrical defibrillator (those paddlelike devices you see on TV medical shows), oxygen, and a cardiac monitor—is wheeled to the treatment area.

Once the patient is stabilized and out of danger, he or she is transferred to the hospital's cardiac care unit or to another facility.

Leading Medical Centers

Finding the best medical center for your particular condition should not require the skills of Ellery Queen, Miss Marple, or Sherlock Holmes. Your personal physician should be able to direct you to the top medical centers and some of the top-name specialists in your region or the nation who cover the suspected disorder. From time to time major city and national magazines, such as *New York* magazine, *Philadelphia* magazine, *Washingtonian*, *Prevention* magazine, and

U.S. News & World Report, run listings of top medical centers and specialists.

We asked specialists and medical experts around the United States to recommend the leading hospitals for a variety of specialties in serious diseases and complex conditions. The results appear below. This list is by no means all-inclusive, but it can provide a good lead to some of the best care in the nation.

The hospitals listed under each condition or specialty are those that were mentioned most often by the medical experts. They are listed in alphabetical order, not in order of expertise or quality within a given heading. The fact that many hospitals appear more than once is a reflection of the reputation many of them have developed among medical professionals.

AIDS

Beth Israel Medical Center
First Avenue at 16th Street
New York, NY 10003

Jackson Memorial Hospital
1611 N.W. 12th Avenue
Miami, FL 33136-1096

Johns Hopkins University Hospital
600 N. Wolfe Street
Baltimore, MD 21205

Massachusetts General Hospital
32 Fruit Street
Boston, MA 02114-2698

Memorial Sloan-Kettering Cancer Center
1275 York Avenue
New York, NY 10016

St. Luke's–Roosevelt Medical Center
Amsterdam Avenue and 114th Street
New York, NY 10023-7409

St. Vincent's Hospital and Medical Center
153 W. 11th Street
New York, NY 10011-8397

San Francisco General Hospital
1001 Potrero Avenue
San Francisco, CA 94110-3594

University of California at San Francisco Medical Center
505 Parnassus Avenue
San Francisco, CA 94143

Cancer

Dana-Farber Cancer Institute
44 Binney Street
Boston, MA 02115-6084

Fred Hutchinson Cancer Research Center
1124 Columbia Street
Seattle, WA 98104

Georgetown University Medical Center
Vince Lombardi Cancer Research Center
3800 Reservoir Road N.W.
Washington, DC 20007

Johns Hopkins University Hospital
600 N. Wolfe Street
Baltimore, MD 21205

Mayo Clinic
200 First Street S.W.
Rochester, MN 55905

Memorial Sloan-Kettering Cancer Center
1275 York Avenue
New York, NY 10016

Presbyterian University Hospital
DeSoto at O'Hara Street
Pittsburgh, PA 15213-2525

University of Texas M. D. Anderson Cancer Center
1515 Holcombe Boulevard
Houston, TX 77030

Cardiology

Barnes Hospital
One Barnes Hospital Plaza
St. Louis, MO 63110

Baylor University Medical Center
3500 Gaston Avenue
Dallas, TX 75246-2088

Brigham and Women's Hospital
75 Francis Street
Boston, MA 02115

Cedar's Sinai Hospital UCLA
8700 Beverly Boulevard
Los Angeles, CA 90048-0750

Cleveland Clinic
9500 Euclid Avenue
Cleveland, OH 44195

Columbia-Presbyterian Medical Center
622 W. 168th Street
New York, NY 10032-3784

Duke University Hospital
P.O. Box 3708
Durham, NC 27704

Emory University Hospital
1364 Clifton Road
Atlanta, GA 30322

Massachusetts General Hospital
32 Fruit Street
Boston, MA 02114-2698

Mayo Clinic
200 First Street S.W.
Rochester, MN 55905

Mid-America Heart Institute
St. Luke's Hospital of Kansas City
Kansas City, MO 64111-3238

Stanford University Hospital
300 Pasteur Drive
Stanford, CA 94305

Texas Heart Institute
St. Luke's Episcopal Hospital
1101 Bates Street
Houston, TX 77030

Yale–New Haven Medical Center
333 Cedar Street
New Haven, CT 06510

Endocrinology

Cleveland Clinic
9500 Euclid Avenue
Cleveland, OH 44195

Jackson Memorial Hospital
1611 N.W. 12th Avenue
Miami, FL 33136-1096

Jewish Hospital, St. Louis
216 S. Kings Highway
St. Louis, MO 63110

Massachusetts General Hospital
32 Fruit Street
Boston, MA 02114-2698

Mayo Clinic
200 First Street S.W.
Rochester, MN 55905

Stanford University Hospital
300 Pasteur Drive
Stanford, CA 94305

UCLA Medical Center
10833 LeConte Avenue
Los Angeles, CA 90024

Gastroenterology

Johns Hopkins University Hospital
600 N. Wolfe Street
Baltimore, MD 21205

Massachusetts General Hospital
32 Fruit Street
Boston, MA 02114-2698

Mayo Clinic
200 First Street S.W.
Rochester, MN 55905

Mt. Sinai Hospital
One Gustave L. Levy Place
New York, NY 10029

Presbyterian University Hospital
DeSoto at O'Hara Street
Pittsburgh, PA 15213-2525

University of Chicago Hospitals
5841 S. Maryland Avenue
Chicago, IL 60637-1470

Neurology

Hospital of the University of Pennsylvania
3400 Spruce Street
Philadelphia, PA 19104-4228

Johns Hopkins University Hospital
600 N. Wolfe Street
Baltimore, MD 21205

Massachusetts General Hospital
32 Fruit Street
Boston, MA 02114-2698

Mayo Clinic
200 First Street S.W.
Rochester, MN 55905

Tufts New England Medical Center
750 Washington Street
Boston, MA 02111-1526

UCLA Medical Center
10833 LeConte Avenue
Los Angeles, CA 90024

University of California at San Francisco Medical Center
505 Parnassus Avenue
San Francisco, CA 94143

Obstetrics/Gynecology

Georgetown University Medical Center
3800 Reservoir Road N.W.
Washington, DC 20007

Irvine Medical Center
16200 Sand Canyon Avenue
Irvine, CA 92718-3701

Jones Institute for Reproductive Medicine
601 Colley Avenue
Norfolk, VA 23507

Northwestern Memorial Hospital
250 E. Superior Avenue
Chicago, IL 60611-3095

Ohio State University Hospital
410 W. 10th Avenue
Columbus, OH 43210-1236

St. Barnabas Medical Center
94 Old Short Hills Road
Livingston, NJ 07039-5668

University of California at San Diego Medical Center
225 Dickinson Street
San Diego, CA 92103-6999

University of Kansas Medical Center
2105 Independence Avenue
Kansas City, MO 64124-2395

University of Southern California Medical Center
1441 Eastlake Avenue
Los Angeles, CA 90033-1085

Psychiatry

C. F. Menninger Memorial Hospital
P.O. Box 829
Topeka, KS 66601-0829

Columbia-Presbyterian Medical Center
622 W. 168th Street
New York, NY 10032-3796

Dartmouth Hitchcock Medical Center
2 Maynard Street
Hanover, NH 03756

Duke University Medical Center
Erwin Road
Durham, NC 27710

Johns Hopkins Hospital
600 N. Wolfe Street
Baltimore, MD 21205-2182

Massachusetts General Hospital
32 Fruit Street
Boston, MA 02114-2698

Mayo Clinic
200 First Street S.W.
Rochester, MN 55905

McLean Hospital
115 Mill Street
Belmont, MA 02178-1048

New York Hospital–Cornell Medical Center
525 E. 68th Street
New York, NY 10021-4885

North Carolina Memorial Hospital
Manning Drive
Chapel Hill, NC 27514-4216

Payne Whitney Psychiatric Clinic
525 E. 68th Street
New York, NY 10021-4873

Sheppard and Enoch Pratt Hospital
6501 N. Charles Street
Towson, MD 21204-6899

Southwestern Medical Center
233 W. 10th Street
Dallas, TX 75208-4592

The Institute of Living
400 Washington Street
Hartford, CT 06106-3392

University of California at Los Angeles Medical Center
10833 LeConte Avenue
Los Angeles, CA 90024-6972

University of Washington Medical Center
1959 N.E. Pacific Street
Seattle, WA 98195

Yale–New Haven Hospital
20 York Street
New Haven, CT 06510-3202

Leading Psychiatric Treatment Centers

The following list of the leading psychiatric treatment centers was compiled by *U.S. News & World Report* in its annual ranking of America's best hospitals. A survey was conducted among some 2,400 physicians, representing sixteen specialties, who were asked to rank the hospitals based upon a list of service indicators such as mortality rate, RNs-to-bed ratio, board-certified physicians, and the facility's reputation. The list of psychiatric hospitals was based solely on reputational scores achieved in previous surveys conducted for *U.S. News & World Report* in 1991, 1992, and 1993.

McLean Hospital
115 Mill Street
Belmont, MA 02178-1048

C. F. Menninger Memorial Hospital
P.O. Box 829
Topeka, KS 66601-0829

New York Hospital–Cornell Medical Center
525 E. 68th Street
New York, NY 10021-4885

Massachusetts General Hospital
32 Fruit Street
Boston, MA 02114-2698

Johns Hopkins University Hospital
600 N. Wolfe Street
Baltimore, MD 21205-2182

Sheppard and Enoch Pratt Hospital
6501 N. Charles Street
Towson, MD 21204-6899

The Institute of Living
400 Washington Street
Hartford, CT 06106-3392

Mayo Clinic
200 First Street S.W.
Rochester, MN 55905

University of California at Los Angeles Medical Center
10833 LeConte Avenue
Los Angeles, CA 90024-6972

Columbia-Presbyterian Medical Center
622 W. 168th Street
New York, NY 10032-3796

Yale–New Haven Hospital
20 York Street
New Haven, CT 06510-3202

Duke University Medical Center
Erwin Road
Durham, NC 27710

© *U.S. News & World Report*, July 12, 1993. Used with permission.

Burn Care Centers

Burn care centers are capable of providing the specialized treatment services that burn victims require, such as skin grafting and extensive rehabilitation therapy. The following hospitals operate dedicated burn care units or offer a burn care program. Shriners hospitals and dedicated children's hospitals limit their admissions to pediatric cases.

Hospital-Based Burn Care Centers

Alabama

Children's Hospital
1600 7th Avenue S.
Birmingham, AL 35233
205-939-9100

University of Alabama Hospitals
619 S. 19th Street
Birmingham, AL 35233
205-934-3411

University of Southern Alabama Medical Center Hospital
2451 Fillingim Street
Mobile, AL 36617
205-471-7000

Alaska

Providence Hospital
3200 Providence Drive
Anchorage, AK 99504
907-562-2211

Arizona

Maricopa Medical Center
2601 E. Roosevelt Street
Phoenix, AZ 85008
602-267-5700

St. Mary's Hospital
1601 W. St. Mary's Road
Tucson, AZ 85745
602-662-5833

Arkansas

Arkansas Children's Hospital
804 Wolfe Street
Little Rock, AR 72202
501-370-1323

University Hospital
University of Arkansas Medical Science Campus
4301 W. Markham Street
Little Rock, AR 72205
501-661-5000

California

Alta Bates Hospital
3001 Colby Street at Ashby
Berkeley, CA 94705
510-204-1573

Valley Medical Center of Fresno
445 S. Cedar Avenue
Fresno, CA 93702
209-453-4220

Los Angeles County/University of Southern California Medical Center
1200 N. State Street
Los Angeles, CA 90033
213-226-7991

Children's Hospital of Oakland
747 52nd Street
Oakland, CA 94609
510-428-2876

University of California at Irvine Medical Center
101 The City Drive
Orange, CA 92668
714-634-5304

University of California at Davis Medical Center
2315 Stockton Boulevard
Sacramento, CA 95817
916-453-3636

University Hospital/University of California Medical Center
225 Dickinson Street
San Diego, CA 92103
619-294-6502

St. Francis Memorial Hospital
900 Hyde Street
San Francisco, CA 94120
415-775-4321

Santa Clara Valley Medical Center
751 S. Bascom Avenue
San Jose, CA 95128
408-279-5242

Brookside Hospital
2000 Vale Road
San Pablo, CA 94806
510-235-7000

Sherman Oaks Community Hospital
4929 Van Nuys Boulevard
Sherman Oaks, CA 91403
818-907-4580

Dameron Hospital
525 W. Acacia Street
Stockton, CA 95203
209-944-5550

Torrance Memorial Hospital Medical Center
3330 Lomita Boulevard
Torrance, CA 90505
310-517-4622

Colorado
Children's Hospital
1056 E. 19th Avenue
Denver, CO 80218
303-861-8888

University Medical Center
4200 E. 9th Avenue
Denver, CO 80262
303-394-8052

Northern Colorado Medical Center
1801 16th Street
Greeley, CO 80631
303-352-4121

Connecticut
Bridgeport Hospital
267 Grant Street
P.O. Box 5000
Bridgeport, CT 06610
203-384-3728

Yale–New Haven Hospital
20 York Street
New Haven, CT 06504
203-785-2573

District of Columbia
Washington Hospital Center
110 Irving Street N.W.
Washington, DC 20010
202-541-7241
202-541-6662

Florida
Shands Hospital
University of Florida
Gainesville, FL 32610
904-392-3054
904-392-3055

James M. Jackson Memorial Hospital
1611 N.W. 12th Avenue
Miami, FL 33136
305-325-7085

Orlando Regional Medical Center
1414 S. Kuhl Avenue
Orlando, FL 32806
305-841-5176

Tampa General Hospital
Davis Islands
Tampa, FL 33606
813-253-0711

Georgia
Grady Memorial Hospital
80 Butler Street S.E.
Atlanta, GA 30335
404-588-4307

Humana Hospital
3651 Wheeler Road
Augusta, GA 30910
404-863-3232

Hawaii
Straub Clinic and Hospital
888 S. King Street
Honolulu, HI 96813
808-523-2311

Illinois
Cook County Hospital
1825 W. Harrison Street
Chicago, IL 60612
312-633-6564
312-633-6570

University of Chicago Hospitals
950 E. 59th Street
Chicago, IL 60637
312-962-6736

Foster G. McGraw Hospital
Loyola University of Chicago
2160 S. First Avenue
Maywood, IL 60153
312-531-3988

Trinity Medical Center
2701 17th Street
Rock Island, IL 61201
309-793-3173

Memorial Medical Center
800 N. Rutledge Street
Springfield, IL 62781
217-788-3325

Indiana
St. Joseph's Hospital
700 Broadway
Fort Wayne, IN 46802
219-425-3431

J. W. Riley Hospital
1100 W. Michigan Street
Indianapolis, IN 46223
317-264-3927

W. N. Wishard Memorial Hospital
1001 W. 10th Street
Indianapolis, IN 46202
317-630-6471

Iowa
University of Iowa Hospitals and Clinics
650 Newton Road
Iowa City, IA 52242
319-356-2496

Iowa Methodist Hospital
1200 Pleasant Street
Des Moines, IA 50309
515-241-5042

St. Luke's Regional Medical Center
2720 Stone Park Boulevard
Sioux City, IA 51104
712-279-3440

Kansas
University of Kansas Medical Center
39th Street and Rainbow Boulevard
Kansas City, KS 66103
913-588-6540

St. Francis Regional Medical Center
929 N. St. Francis Avenue
Wichita, KS 67201
316-268-5388

Kentucky
University Hospital
800 Rose Street
Lexington, KY 40536
606-233-5260

Humana Hospital University
530 S. Jackson
Louisville, KY 40217
502-562-3000

Kosair-Children's Hospital
200 E. Chestnut
Louisville, KY 40202
502-562-6300

Louisiana
Baton Rouge General Hospital
3600 Florida Street
P.O. Box 2511
Baton Rouge, LA 70821
504-387-7716

Louisiana State University Medical Center Hospital
1541 Kings Highway
P.O. Box 33932
Shreveport, LA 71130
318-674-6133

Maine
Maine Medical Center
22 Bramhall Street
Portland, ME 04102
207-871-2991

Maryland
Johns Hopkins Bayview Hospital
4940 Eastern Avenue
Baltimore, MD 21224
301-955-0886

Massachusetts
Brigham and Women's Hospital
75 Francis Street
Boston, MA 02115
617-732-7712

Massachusetts General Hospital
32 Fruit Street
Boston, MA 02114
617-726-3354

Shriners Burns Institute
51 Blossom Street
Boston, MA 02114
617-722-3000

Baystate Medical Center
759 Chestnut
Springfield, MA 01199
413-784-4800

University of Massachusettes Medical Center
55 Lake Avenue, N.
Worcester, MA 01655
508-856-5129

Michigan
University of Michigan Medical Center
1500 E. Medical Center Drive
Ann Arbor, MI 48109
313-936-9666

Children's Hospital of Michigan
3901 Beaubien Boulevard
Detroit, MI 48201
313-494-5678

Detroit Receiving Hospital and University Health Center
4201 St. Antoine
Detroit, MI 48201
313-745-3078

Hurley Medical Center
One Hurley Plaza
Flint, MI 48502
313-257-9188

Blodgett Memorial Medical Center
1840 Wealthy Street S.E.
Grand Rapids, MI 49506
616-774-7670

Bronson Methodist Hospital
252 E. Lovell Street
Kalamazoo, MI 49007
616-383-6485
800-632-3430

Edward R. Sparrow Hospital
1215 E. Michigan Avenue
Lansing, MI 48909
517-483-2677

St. Mary's Hospital
830 S. Jefferson Avenue
Saginaw, MI 48601
517-790-5055

Minnesota

Miller-Dwan Hospital and Medical Center
502 E. 2nd Street
Duluth, MN 55805
218-727-8762

Hennepin County Medical Center
701 Park Avenue
Minneapolis, MN 55415
612-347-2915

St. Paul–Ramsey Medical Center
640 Jackson Street
St. Paul, MN 55101
612-221-3351

Mississippi

Delta Medical Center
1400 E. Union Street
P.O. Box 5247
Greenville, MS 38701
601-378-3783

Missouri

University of Missouri Health Sciences Center
One Hospital Drive
Columbia, MO 65212
314-882-7994

Children's Mercy Hospital
24th at Gillham Road
Kansas City, MO 64108
816-234-3520

St. John's Regional Health Center
1235 E. Cherokee Street
Springfield, MO 65802
417-885-2876

Barnes Hospital
Barnes Hospital Plaza
St. Louis, MO 63110
314-362-4060

St. John's Mercy Medical Center
615 S. New Ballas Road
St. Louis, MO 63141
314-569-6055

Montana

St. Vincent Hospital
1233 N. 30th Street
Billings, MT 59101
406-657-7067

Nebraska

St. Elizabeth Community Health Center
555 S. 70th Street
Lincoln, NE 68510
402-489-7181

Nevada

University Medical Center
1800 W. Charleston Boulevard
Las Vegas, NV 89102
702-383-2268

New Jersey

St. Barnabas Medical Center
Old Short Hills Road
Livingston, NJ 07039
201-533-5920

New Mexico

University of New Mexico Hospital
2211 Lomas Boulevard N.E.
Albuquerque, NM 87106
505-843-2111

New York

Bronx Municipal Health Center
Pelham Parkway S. and Eastchester Road
Bronx, NY 10461
212-430-8065

Eric County Medical Center
462 Grider Street
Buffalo, NY 14215
716-898-5231

Nassau County Medical Center
2201 Hempstead Turnpike
East Meadow, NY 11554
516-542-3207

St. Joseph's Hospital
555 E. Market Street
Elmira, NY 14902
607-733-6541

New York Hospital–Cornell Medical Center
525 E. 68th Street
New York, NY 10021
212-472-5132

Strong Memorial Hospital
601 Elmwood Avenue
Rochester, NY 14642
716-275-5475

University Hospital
Stony Brook, NY 11794
516-444-2701

Upstate Medical Center
750 E. Adams Street
Syracuse, NY 13210
315-473-6083

Westchester County Medical Center
Grasslands Reservation
Valhalla, NY 10595
914-347-4909

Good Samaritan Hospital
1000 Montauk Highway
West Islip, NY 11795
516-957-4000

North Carolina

North Carolina Jaycee Burn Center
Hospitals of the University of North Carolina
Chapel Hill, NC 27514
919-966-3571

Duke University Hospital
Duke University
Durham, NC 27710
919-681-2404

North Carolina Baptist Hospital
300 S. Hawthorne Road
Winston-Salem, NC 27103
919-748-7766

Ohio

**Children's Hospital Medical Center—Akron
Regional Burn Center**
281 Locust Street
Akron, OH 44308
216-379-8224

Shriners Burns Institute
202 Goodman Street
Cincinnati, OH 45219
513-751-3900

University of Cincinnati Hospital
234 Goodman Street
Cincinnati, OH 45267
513-872-3100

MetroHealth Medical Center
2500 MetroHealth Drive
Cleveland, OH 44109
216-459-5643

Children's Hospital
700 Children's Drive
Columbus, OH 43205
614-461-2000

Ohio State University Hospital
410 W. 10th Avenue
Columbus, OH 43210
614-421-8744

Children's Medical Center
One Children's Plaza
Dayton, OH 45404
513-226-8300

Miami Valley Hospital
One Wyoming Street
Dayton, OH 45409
513-223-6192

St. Vincent's Medical Center
2213 Cherry Street
Toledo, OH 43608
419-259-4734

Oklahoma

Baptist Medical Center
3300 N.W. Expressway
Oklahoma City, OK 73112
405-949-3345

Oklahoma Children's Memorial Hospital
940 N.E. 13th Street
Oklahoma City, OK 73104
405-271-4733

Hillcrest Medical Center
1120 S. Utica Avenue
Tulsa, OK 74104
918-584-1351

Oregon

Oregon Burn Center at Emanuel Hospital
2801 N. Gantenbein Avenue
Portland, OR 97227
503-280-4233

Pennsylvania

Lehigh Valley Hospital Center
1200 S. Cedar Crest Boulevard
P.O. Box 689
Allentown, PA 18105
610-776-8734

Crozer-Chester Medical Center
15th Street and Upland Avenue
Chester, PA 19013
610-876-0356

Hamot Medical Center
201 State Street
Erie, PA 16550
814-459-0344

Saint Agnes Medical Center
1900 S. Broad Street
Philadelphia, PA 19145
215-339-4339

St. Christopher's Hospital for Children
5th Street and Lehigh Avenue
Philadelphia, PA 19133
215-427-5000

Mercy Hospital
1400 Locust Street
Pittsburgh, PA 15219
412-232-8225

Western Pennsylvania Hospital
4800 Friendship Avenue
Pittsburgh, PA 15224
412-363-2876

South Carolina

Medical University Hospital
171 Ashley Avenue
Charleston, SC 29425
803-792-3681

South Dakota

McKennan Hospital Burn Unit
800 E. 21st Street
Sioux Falls, SD 57101
605-333-8425

Tennessee

Baroness Erlanger Hospital
975 E. 3rd Street
Chattanooga, TN 37403
615-778-7881

Regional Medical Center
842 Jefferson Avenue
Memphis, TN 38103
901-528-5500

Vanderbilt University Hospital
1161 21st Avenue
Nashville, TN 37232
615-322-7311

Texas

Parkland Memorial Hospital
5201 Harry Hines Boulevard
Dallas, TX 75235
214-637-8546

Sun Towers Hospital
1801 N. Oregon Street
El Paso, TX 79902
915-532-6281

Brooke Army Medical Center
Fort Sam Houston, TX 78234
512-221-4604

John Peter Smith Hospital
1500 S. Main Street
Fort Worth, TX 76104
817-921-3431

Shriners Burns Institute
610 Texas Avenue
Galveston, TX 77550
409-761-2516

University of Texas Medical Branch Hospitals
8th and Mechanic Street
Galveston, TX 77550
713-761-2023

Hermann Hospital
1203 Ross Sterling Avenue
Houston, TX 77030
713-797-4350

University Medical Center
P.O. Box 5980
Lubbock, TX 79417
800-345-9911

St. Luke's Lutheran Hospital
7930 Floyd Curl Drive
San Antonio, TX 78229
210-517-7000

Utah

University of Utah Hospital
50 N. Medical Drive
Salt Lake City, UT 84132
801-581-2700

Vermont

Medical Center Hospital of Vermont
Colchester Avenue
Burlington, VT 05404
802-656-2434

Virginia

University of Virginia Medical Center
Lee Street
Charlottesville, VA 22908
804-924-2876

Norfolk General Hospital
600 Gresham Drive
Norfolk, VA 23507
804-628-3117

Medical College of Virginia Hospital
1200 E. Broad Street
Box 510, MCV Station
Richmond, VA 23298
804-786-9240

Washington
St. Joseph's Hospital
3201 Ellis Street
Bellingham, WA 98225
206-734-5400 ext. 2501

Harborview Medical Center
325 9th Avenue
Seattle, WA 98104
206-223-3127

Sacred Heart Medical Center
W. 101 8th Avenue
Spokane, WA 99220
509-455-3344

St. Joseph's Hospital
1718 S. I Street
Tacoma, WA 98401
206-591-6677

West Virginia
Cabell-Huntington Hospital
1340 Hal Greer Boulevard
Huntington, WV 25701
304-526-2390

Wisconsin
University of Wisconsin Hospital and Clinics
600 Highland Avenue
Madison, WI 53792
608-263-1490

St. Mary's Hospital
2323 N. Lake Drive
Box 503
Milwaukee, WI 53211
414-225-8000

Source: Burn Foundation, 1128 Walnut Street,
Suite 301, Philadelphia, PA 19107.

Freestanding Children's Hospitals in the United States (Short- and Long-Term Care)

The following is a listing of freestanding children's hospitals, which are physically separate from any other hospital but which may be a part of a larger hospital system.

Alabama
Children's Hospital of Alabama
1600 7th Avenue S.
Birmingham, AL 35233
205-939-9100

Arizona
Phoenix Children's Hospital
1111 E. McDowell Road
Phoenix, AZ 85006
602-239-2400

Westbridge
1830 E. Roosevelt
P.O. Box 5750
Phoenix, AZ 85010
602-254-0884

Westbridge Center for Children
720 E. Montebello
Phoenix, AZ 85014
602-277-5437

Desert Hills
5245 N. Camino de Oeste
Tucson, AZ 85745
602-622-5437

Arkansas
Rivendell Psychiatric Center
100 Rivendell Drive
Benton, AR 72015
501-794-1255

Arkansas Children's Hospital
800 Marshall Street
Little Rock, AR 72202
501-320-1100

California
Rancho Park Hospital
109 E. Chase Avenue
El Cajon, CA 92020
619-579-1666

Valley Children's Hospital
3151 N. Millbrook
Fresno, CA 93703
209-225-3000

Children's Hospital of Los Angeles
4650 Sunset Boulevard
P.O. Box 54700
Los Angeles, CA 90027
213-660-2450

Crossroads Hospital
6323 Woodman Avenue
Los Angeles, CA 91401
818-782-2470

Shriners Hospital for Crippled Children
3160 Geneva Street
Los Angeles, CA 90020
213-388-3151

Newport Harbor, An Adolescent Hospital
1501 E. 16th Street
Newport Beach, CA 92663
714-650-9752

Children's Hospital Oakland
747 52nd Street
Oakland, CA 94609
510-428-3000

Children's Hospital of Orange County
455 S. Main Street
Orange, CA 92668
714-997-3000

Lucile Salter Packard Children's Hospital at Stanford
725 Welch Road
Palo Alto, CA 94304
415-497-8000

Children's Hospital and Health Center
8001 Frost Street
San Diego, CA 92123
619-576-1700

Shriners Hospital for Crippled Children
1701 19th Avenue
San Francisco, CA 94122
415-665-1100

Colorado

Cleo Wallace Center Hospital
8405 W. 100th
Box 345
Broomfield, CO 80038
303-466-7391

The Children's Hospital
1056 E. 19th Avenue
Box 020
Denver, CO 80218
303-861-8888

Connecticut

Henry D. Altobello Children and Youth Center
P.O. Box 902
Meriden, CT 06450
203-238-6054

Riverview Hospital for Children
River Road
Box 621
Middletown, CT 06457
203-344-2700

Newington Children's Hospital
181 E. Cedar Street
Newington, CT 06111
203-667-5437

Housatonic Adolescent Hospital
Box W
Newtown, CT 06470
203-270-2700

Delaware

Meadow Wood Hospital
575 S. DuPont Highway
New Castle, DE 19720
302-328-3330

Alfred I. DuPont Institute
1600 Rockland Road
P.O. Box 269
Wilmington, DE 19899
302-651-4000

District of Columbia

Children's National Medical Center
111 Michigan Avenue N.W.
Washington, DC 20010
202-745-5000

The Hospital for Sick Children
1731 Bunker Hill Road N.E.
Washington, DC 20017
202-832-4400

Florida

HCA Grant Center Hospital of North Florida
U.S. Highway 301
P.O. Box 100
Citra, FL 32113
904-595-3500

Florida Camelot
P.O. Box 1101
Land o' Lakes, FL 33549
813-949-7491

Devereux Hospital and Children's Center of Florida
8000 Devereux Drive
Melbourne, FL 32940
407-242-9100

HCA Grant Center Hospital
20601 S.W. 157th Avenue
Miami, FL 33197
305-521-0710

Miami Children's Hospital
6125 S.W. 31st Street
Miami, FL 33155
305-666-6511

All Children's Hospital, Inc.
801 6th Street S.
St. Petersburg, FL 33701
813-898-7451

Shriners Hospital for Crippled Children, Tampa Unit
12502 N. Pine Drive
Tampa, FL 33612
813-972-2250

Georgia

Charter Brook Hospital
3913 N. Peachtree Road
Atlanta, GA 30341
404-457-8315

Egleston Children's Hospital at Emory University
1405 Clifton Road N.E.
Atlanta, GA 30322
404-325-6000

Hillside Hospital
690 Courtney Drive N.E.
Atlanta, GA 30306
404-875-4551

Scottish Rite Children's Medical Center
1001 Johnson Ferry Road N.E.
Atlanta, GA 30363-3101
404-256-5252

Inner Harbour Hospitals
4685 Dorsett Shoals
Douglasville, GA 30135
404-942-2391

Devereux Center—Georgia
1980 Stanley Road
Kennesaw, GA 30144
404-427-0147

Hawaii

Shriners Hospital for Crippled Children
1310 Punahou Street
Honolulu, HI 96826
808-941-4466

Illinois

LaRabida Children's Hospital and Research Center
E. 65th Street at Lake Michigan
Chicago, IL 60649
312-363-6700

Shriners Hospital for Crippled Children
2211 N. Oak Park Avenue
Chicago, IL 60635
312-622-5400

The Children's Memorial Hospital
2300 Children's Plaza
Chicago, IL 60614
312-880-4000

Indiana

Lifelines Children's Rehabilitation Hospital
1707 W. 86th Street
P.O. Box 40407
Indianapolis, IN 46240-0407
317-872-0555

Kansas

St. Francis at Ellsworth
P.O. Box 127
Ellsworth, KS 67439
913-472-4453

St. Francis at Salina
5097 Cloud Street
Salina, KS 67401
913-825-0563

Children's Division of Menninger Clinic
P.O. Box 829
Topeka, KS 66601
913-273-7500

Kentucky

Children's Psychiatric Hospital of Northern Kentucky
502 Farrell Drive
Box 2680
Covington, KY 41012
606-331-1900

Shriners Hospital for Crippled Children, Lexington Unit
1900 Richmond Road
Lexington, KY 40502
606-266-2101

Valley Institute of Psychiatry
1000 Industrial Drive
P.O. Box 4010
Owensboro, KY 42302
502-686-8477

Louisiana

Greenwell Springs Hospital
Greenwell Springs Road
Greenwell Springs, LA 70739
504-261-2730

Children's Hospital
200 Henry Clay Avenue
New Orleans, LA 70118
504-899-9511

Shriners Hospital for Crippled Children, Shreveport Unit
3100 Samfort Avenue
Shreveport, LA 71103
318-222-5704

Maryland

Mt. Washington Pediatric Hospital, Inc.
1708 W. Rogers Avenue
Baltimore, MD 21209-4597
410-578-8600

The Kennedy Institute
707 N. Broadway
Baltimore, MD 21205
410-550-9000

Massachusetts

Children's Hospital
300 Longwood Avenue
Boston, MA 02115
617-735-6000

Franciscan Children's Hospital and Rehabilitation Center
30 Warren Street
Boston, MA 02135
617-254-3800

Shriners Hospital for Crippled Children, Boston Unit
51 Blossom Street
Boston, MA 02114
617-722-3000

Massachusetts Hospital School
3 Randolph Street
Canton, MA 02021
617-828-2440

Shriners Hospital for Crippled Children, Springfield Unit
516 Carew Street
Springfield, MA 01104
413-787-2000

Michigan

Children's Hospital of Michigan
3901 Beaubien Boulevard
Detroit, MI 48201
313-745-5437

Hawthorn Center
18471 Haggerty Road
Northville, MI 48167
313-349-3000

Minnesota

Wilson Center for Adolescent Psychiatry
Box 917
Faribault, MN 55021
507-334-5561

Minneapolis Children's Medical Center
2525 Chicago Avenue S.
Minneapolis, MN 55404
612-863-6100

Shriners Hospital for Crippled Children, Twin Cities Unit
2025 E. River Road
Minneapolis, MN 55414
612-335-5300

Gillette Children's Hospital
200 E. University Avenue
St. Paul, MN 55101
612-291-2848

The Children's Hospital
345 N. Smith Avenue
St. Paul, MN 55102
612-220-6110

Missouri

Crittenton Center
10918 Elm Avenue
Kansas City, MO 64134
816-765-6600

The Children's Mercy Hospital
2401 Gillham Road
Kansas City, MO 64108
816-234-3000

Cardinal Glennon Children's Hospital
1465 S. Grand Boulevard
St. Louis, MO 63104
314-577-5600

SSM Rehabilitation Institute
555 N. New Ballas Road, Suite 150
St. Louis, MO 63141
314-994-0157

Shriners Hospital for Crippled Children
2001 S. Lindbergh Avenue
St. Louis, MO 63131
314-432-3600

St. Louis Children's Hospital
400 S. Kingshighway
St. Louis, MO 63110
314-454-6000

Montana

Shodair Crippled Children's Hospital
840 Helena Avenue
Box 5539
Helena, MT 59604
406-444-7500

Nebraska

Boys Town National Research Hospital
555 N. 30th Street
Omaha, NE 68106
402-498-6511

Children's Hospital
8301 Dodge Street
Omaha, NE 68114
402-390-5400

New Hampshire
Spofford Hall Hospital
Route 9A, Box 225
Spofford, NH 03462
603-363-4545

New Jersey
Children's Specialized Hospital
New Providence Road
Mountainside, NJ 07091
908-233-3720

Matheny School
Main Street
Peapack, NJ 07977
908-234-0011

Voorhees Pediatric Facility
1304 Laurel Oak Road
Voorhees, NJ 08043
609-346-3300

New Mexico
Carrie Tingley Hospital
1127 University N.E.
Albuquerque, NM 87102
505-272-5200

**University of New Mexico Children's
Psychiatric Hospital**
1001 Yale Boulevard N.E.
Albuquerque, NM 87131
505-843-2945

New York
St. Mary's Hospital for Children, Inc.
29-01 216th Street
Bayside, NY 11360
718-990-8800

Queens Children's Psychiatric Center
74-03 Commonwealth Boulevard
Bellerose, NY 11426
212-264-2900

Bronx Children's Psychiatric Center
1000 Waters Place
Bronx, NY 10461
212-892-0808

The Children's Hospital of Buffalo
219 Bryant Street
Buffalo, NY 14222
716-878-7000

Sagamore Children's Psychiatric Center
197 Half Hollow Road
Dix Hills, NY 11747
516-673-7700

Rockland Children's Psychiatric Center
Convent Road
Orangeburg, NY 10962
914-359-7400

Blythedale Children's Hospital
Bradhurst Avenue
Valhalla, NY 10595
914-592-7555

Western New York Child's Psychiatric Center
1010 East and West Road
West Seneca, NY 14224
716-674-9730

North Carolina
Amos Cottage Rehabilitation Hospital
3325 Silas Creek Parkway
Winston-Salem, NC 27103
919-765-9916

Ohio
Children's Hospital Medical Center of Akron
281 Locust Street
Akron, OH 44308
216-379-8200

Children's Hospital Medical Center
Elland and Bethesda Avenues
Cincinnati, OH 45229-2899
513-559-4200

**Shriners Hospital for Crippled Children—Burn
Institute**
202 Goodman Street
Cincinnati, OH 45219
513-751-3900

Health Hill Hospital for Children
2801 Martin Luther King Jr. Drive
Cleveland, OH 44104
216-721-5400

Children's Hospital
700 Children's Drive
Columbus, OH 43205
614-461-2000

The Children's Medical Center
One Children's Plaza
Dayton, OH 45404
513-226-8300

Sagamore Hills Children's Psychiatric Hospital
11910 Dunham Road
Northfield, OH 44067
216-467-7955

Belmont Pines Hospital
615 Churchill Hubbard Road
Youngstown, OH 44505
216-759-2700

Oklahoma
Willow Crest Hospital
130 A Street S.W.
Miami, OK 74354
918-542-1836

Children's Medical Center
5300 E. Skelly Drive
P.O. Box 35648
Tulsa, OK 74153-0648
918-664-6600

Shadow Mountain Institute
6262 S. Sheridan
Tulsa, OK 74133
918-492-8200

Oregon

Shriners Hospital for Crippled Children
3101 S.W. Sam Jackson Park Road
Portland, OR 97201
503-241-5090

Pennsylvania

The Devereux Foundation
119 Old Lancaster Road
P.O. Box 400
Devon, PA 19333
610-964-3000

Shriners Hospital for Crippled Children
1645 W. 8th Street
Erie, PA 16505
814-452-4164

The Devereux Foundation—The Mapleton Psychiatric Institute—Earl D. Bond Center
655 Sugartown Road
P.O. Box 400
Malvern, PA 19355
610-296-6923

Children's Rehabilitation Hospital
Ford Road at Fairmont Park
Philadelphia, PA 19131
215-581-3100

Children's Seashore House
Philadelphia Center for Health Care Sciences
3405 Civic Center Boulevard
Philadelphia, PA 19104
215-895-3600

Shriners Hospital for Crippled Children, Philadelphia Unit
8400 Roosevelt Boulevard
Philadelphia, PA 19152
215-332-4500

St. Christopher's Hospital for Children
Erie Avenue at Front Street
Philadelphia, PA 19134-1095
215-427-5000

The Children's Hospital of Philadelphia
34th Street and Civic Center Boulevard
Philadelphia, PA 19104
215-590-1000

Children's Hospital of Pittsburgh
One Children's Place
3705 5th Avenue at DeSoto Street
Pittsburgh, PA 15213-2583
412-692-5325

Southwood Psychiatric Hospital
2575 Boyce Plaza Road
Pittsburgh, PA 15241
412-257-2290

The Children's Home of Pittsburgh
5618 Kentucky Avenue
Pittsburgh, PA 15232-2696
412-441-4884

Eastern State School and Hospital
3740 Lincoln Highway
Trevose, PA 19047
215-671-3141

Rhode Island

Emma Pendleton Bradley Hospital
1011 Veterans Memorial Parkway
Riverside, RI 02915
401-434-3400

South Carolina

Shriners Hospital for Crippled Children, Greenville Unit
950 W. Faris Road
Greenville, SC 29605
803-271-3444

South Dakota

Crippled Children's Hospital and School
2501 W. 26th Street
Sioux Falls, SD 57105
605-336-1840

Tennessee

East Tennessee Children's Hospital
2018 W. Clinch Avenue
P.O. Box 15010
Knoxville, TN 37916
615-546-7711

Le Bonheur Children's Medical Center, Inc.
One Children's Plaza
848 Adams Avenue
Memphis, TN 38103
901-522-3000

St. Jude's Children's Research Hospital
332 N. Lauderdale Street
Box 318
Memphis, TN 38101
901-522-0300

Vanderbilt Child and Adolescent Psychiatric Hospital
1601 23rd Avenue S.
Nashville, TN 37212
615-320-7770

Texas

Willow Creek Hospital
7000 Highway 287 S.
Arlington, TX 76017
817-572-3355

Ada Wilson Children Center for Rehabilitation
3511 S. Alameda Street
Corpus Christi, TX 78411
512-853-9977

Driscoll Children's Hospital
3533 S. Alameda Street
Corpus Christi, TX 78411
512-850-5000

Children's Medical Center of Dallas
1935 Motor Street
Dallas, TX 75235
214-920-2000

Texas Scottish Rite Hospital for Children
2222 Welborn
P.O. Box 19567
Dallas, TX 75219
214-521-3168

Cook–Fort Worth Children's Medical Center
801 7th Avenue
Fort Worth, TX 76104
817-885-4000

Shriners Hospital for Crippled Children—Burns Institute
610 Texas Avenue
Galveston, TX 77550
409-770-6600

Shriners Hospital for Crippled Children, Houston Unit
1402 N. MacGregor Drive
Houston, TX 77030
713-797-1616

Texas Children's Hospital
6621 Fannin Street
Houston, TX 77030
713-798-1000

Southwest Neuropsychiatric Institute—Woodlawn
2939 W. Woodlawn
San Antonio, TX 78228
512-736-4273

Devereux Foundation—Texas Center
120 David Wade Drive
Victoria, TX 77902
512-575-8271

Methodist Home Children's Guidance Center
1111 Herring Avenue
Waco, TX 76708
817-753-0181

Utah

Primary Children's Medical Center
100 N. Medical Drive
Salt Lake City, UT 84113
801-588-2000

Shriners Hospital for Crippled Children, Intermountain Unit
Fairfax Avenue and Virginia Street
Salt Lake City, UT 84103
801-532-5307

Rivendell Psychiatric Center
5899 W. Rivendell Drive
West Jordan, UT 84084
801-561-3377

Virginia

Graydon Manor
301 Children's Center Road
Leesburg, VA 22075
703-777-3485

Cumberland Hospital for Children
Route 637
P.O. Box 150
New Kent, VA 23124
804-966-2242

Children's Hospital of the King's Daughters, Inc.
800 W. Olney Road
Norfolk, VA 23507
804-628-7000

Children's Hospital
2924 Brook Road
Richmond, VA 23220
804-321-7474

Psychiatric Institute of Richmond
3001 5th Avenue
Richmond, VA 23222
804-329-3400

De Jarnette Center
Richmond Road, Drawer 2309
P.O. Box 2309
Staunton, VA 24401
703-332-8800

Washington

Children's Hospital and Medical Center
4800 Sand Point Way N.E.
P.O. Box C-5371
Seattle, WA 98105
206-526-2000

Shriners Hospital for Crippled Children
911 W. 5th Avenue
Spokane, WA 99204
509-455-7844

Wisconsin

Children's Hospital of Wisconsin
9000 W. Wisconsin Avenue
P.O. Box 1997
Milwaukee, WI 53201
414-266-2000

Source: The National Association of Children's Hospitals and Related Institutions, Inc., Nov. 1991.

Nonfreestanding Children's Hospitals in the United States

The following is a listing of nonfreestanding children's hospitals. In order to be designated a nonfreestanding children's hospital, a facility must be part of a larger medical center; must have a separate board of directors, independent of the larger facility; and must have its own medical director and medical staff.

Arizona

Children's Health Center
St. Joseph's Hospital
350 W. Thomas Road
Phoenix, AZ 85013
602-285-3160

University Medical Center
Children's Hospital
1501 N. Campbell Avenue
Tucson, AZ 85724
602-694-0111

California

Memorial Miller Children's Hospital
2801 Atlantic Avenue
P.O. Box 1428
Long Beach, CA 90801-1428
213-595-2000

Children's Hospital Foundation
15405 Los Gatos Boulevard, Suite 103
Los Gatos, CA 95032
408-358-1665

University Children's Hospital
University of California at Davis Medical Center
2315 Stockton Boulevard
Sacramento, CA 95817
916-734-2011

Florida

Memorial Hospital Children's Center
3501 Johnson Street
Hollywood, FL 33021
305-987-2000

Jacksonville Wolfson Children's Hospital at Baptist Medical Center
800 Prudential Drive
Jacksonville, FL 32207
904-393-2000

Arnold Palmer Hospital for Children and Women
Orlando Regional Medical Center
1414 Kuhl Avenue
Orlando, FL 32806
407-649-9111

Children's Hospital at Sacred Heart Hospital
5151 N. 9th Avenue
Pensacola, FL 32504
904-474-7000

Georgia

Children's Medical Center
Medical College of Georgia
1120 15th Street
Augusta, GA 30912-6001
404-721-0211

The Children's Hospital at the Medical Center of Central Georgia
777 Hemlock Street
P.O. Box 6000
Macon, GA 31201
912-744-1104

Illinois

Sylvain and Arma Wyler Children's Hospital
University of Chicago Hospitals
5841 S. Maryland, Hospital Box 426
Chicago, IL 60637
312-702-6239

United Medical Center
501 10th Avenue
Moline, IL 61265
309-757-2968

Lutheran General Children's Medical Center
1775 Dempster Street
Park Ridge, IL 60068
708-696-2210

Children's Hospital of Illinois at St. Francis Medical Center
530 N.E. Glen Oak Avenue
Peoria, IL 61637
309-655-7171

Rockford Memorial Hospital—Children's Center
2400 N. Rockton Avenue
Rockford, IL 61103
815-968-6861

Indiana

James Whitcomb Riley Hospital for Children
Indiana University Hospital
1100 W. Michigan Street
Indianapolis, IN 46202
317-274-5000

Kentucky

Kosair Children's Hospital
Alliant Health System
200 E. Chestnut
P.O. Box 35070
Louisville, KY 40232-5070
502-629-6000

Maryland

Johns Hopkins Children's Center
600 N. Wolfe Street
CMSC 2-111
Baltimore, MD 21205
410-955-5000

Massachusetts

Floating Hospital for Infants and Children
New England Medical Center
750 Washington Street
Boston, MA 02111
617-956-5000

Minnesota

Variety Club Children's Hospital at the University of Minnesota Hospital and Clinic
Harvard Street at East River Parkway
Box 604 UMHC
Minneapolis, MN 55455
612-626-3330

Nebraska

University of Nebraska Medical Center
600 S. 42nd
Omaha, NE 68198
402-559-4281

Nevada

Humana Children's Hospital—Las Vegas
3186 Maryland Parkway
P.O. Box 98530
Las Vegas, NV 89193
702-731-8000

New Jersey

Children's Hospital of New Jersey
United Hospital Medical Center
15 S. 9th Street
Newark, NJ 07107
201-268-8760

New York

Schneider Children's Hospital
Long Island Jewish Medical Center
269-01 76th Avenue
New Hyde Park, NY 11042
718-470-3000

North Carolina

North Carolina Children's Hospital
University of North Carolina Hospitals
101 Manning Drive
Chapel Hill, NC 27514
919-966-4131

Carolinas Medical Center
1000 Blythe Boulevard
P.O. Box 32861
Charlotte, NC 28232-2861
704-355-2000

Cape Fear Valley Medical Center
Cumberland County Hospital System
1638 Owen Drive
P.O. Box 2000
Fayetteville, NC 28302
919-323-6151

North Dakota

Children's Hospital—Meritcare
720 4th Street N.
Fargo, ND 58122
701-234-6000

Ohio

Cleveland Clinic Children's Hospital
9500 Euclid Avenue
Cleveland, OH 44195-5045
216-444-6479

Rainbow Babies and Children's Hospital
2074 Abington Road
Cleveland, OH 44106
216-844-3762

Oklahoma

Children's Hospital of Oklahoma
Oklahoma Medical Center
940 N.E. 13th Street
P.O. Box 26307
Oklahoma City, OK 73126
405-271-6165

The Children's Center
St. Francis Hospital
6161 S. Yale
Tulsa, OK 74136
918-494-2200

Oregon

Children's Healthcare Center at Emanuel Hospital and Health Center
2801 N. Gantebein Avenue
Portland, OR 97227
503-280-3500

Pennsylvania

Geisinger Children's Hospital Center
Geisinger Medical Center
N. Academy Avenue
Danville, PA 17822
717-271-5200

The Rehabilitation Institute of Pittsburgh
6301 Northumberland Street
Pittsburgh, PA 15217
412-521-9000

Rhode Island

Department of Pediatrics
Rhode Island Hospital
593 Eddy Street
Providence, RI 02903
401-277-4000

South Carolina

Children's Hospital
University of South Carolina
171 Ashley Avenue
Charleston, SC 29425
803-792-3131

Tennessee

Children's Hospital of Vanderbilt University
1211 22nd Avenue S.
Nashville, TN 37232
615-322-3377

Texas

Hermann Children's Hospital
6411 Fannin
Houston, TX 77030-1501
713-797-2170

Santa Rosa Children's Hospital
Santa Rosa Health Care Corporation
519 W. Houston Street
San Antonio, TX 78207-3108
512-228-2011

Washington

Mary Bridge Children's Hospital and Health Center
317 S. K Street
P.O. Box 5299
Tacoma, WA 98405-0987
206-594-1000

West Virginia

Children's Hospital of West Virginia
University Hospitals
Medical Center Drive
Morgantown, WV 26506-8111
304-293-7086

Source: The National Association of Children's Hospitals and Related Institutions, Inc., Nov. 1991.

Ambulatory Care

The medical market is a free-for-all, with private practice doctors being hurt and the traditional role of hospitals challenged in every possible scenario. This phenomenon is never more evident than in a relatively new development on the health care scene in America: ambulatory medical care.

Borrowing a page from the fast-food industry, entrepreneurs in the early 1980s began moving in droves to provide people with a more convenient and less costly medical setting. And the novel approach to medical care has met with speedy success. Just since 1984 the number of freestanding (that is, not in a doctor's office or hospital) ambulatory care centers has more than doubled, from nearly 1,800 to more than 4,600 in 1993, according to the SMG Marketing Group as reported in *Modern Healthcare*.

TYPES OF AMBULATORY CARE CENTERS

Ambulatory care centers, offering essentially walk-in/walk-out care, first sprang up in order to attract business away from the hospital emergency room, where an estimated 80 percent of visits are not considered true emergencies. Today these facilities emphasize primary rather than emergency care and offer a broad range of services. Generally, ambulatory centers fall into two categories:

Primary/Emergency/Urgent Care

The mission here is to treat minor injuries or short-term illnesses and provide immediate treatment for routine problems—for example, cuts, sprains, dislocated or broken bones, sore throats, earaches, and so on. Because they are alternatives to the hospital emergency room or doctor's office, they have been labeled everything from emergicenter, urgicenter, and medi-center to the less flattering "doc-in-a-box." To the savvy consumer they offer many advantages, primarily convenience and, depending upon the individual case, less expensive care.

Typically, they are open 10 to 16 hours a day, and some around-the-clock. Even with the extended office hours many doctors have launched in response, the competition from ambulatory centers is still fierce because many are open 6 to 7 days a week. Located where traffic is brisk—in shopping malls or along commercial avenues—they usually operate on a no-appointment, walk-in basis (although it is becoming more common for centers to see people by appointment as well), and you are promised only a short wait (in the neighborhood of 15 to 20 minutes), unless your injury requires even quicker attention. Most offer ancillary services such as X rays and simple laboratory tests (urine and blood tests and the like) on site, with some facilities even adding sophisticated diagnostic equipment and specialists' services ranging from physical therapy to psychological counseling.

The thorny side of this rosy picture? Generally, little attention is paid to comprehensive or follow-up care. That doesn't mean the nurse or another staff member will not phone you the next day to ask how that dog bite is healing, but it does mean that most of these centers downplay the taking of extensive medical history. In short, they don't expect you to become a regular visitor. But perhaps that is not your wish anyway.

As for costs—treatment at an emergency or urgent care clinic is usually less expensive than a hospital visit. However, depending on how the clinic operates and how sick or hurt you are, it may cost more than a physician's office visit.

Surgery

Ambulatory surgery is a natural outgrowth of the shift, for cost-cutting purposes, to outpatient surgery (surgery that avoids an overnight hospital stay). Outpatient surgery is performed in three kinds of settings: doctors' offices; freestanding (apart from a hospital or doctor's office) surgery centers; and hospital outpatient facilities (which currently account for most of such surgery done in this country). As to cost differences—costs are generally higher at hospitals' outpatient departments than at freestanding centers, which are somewhat higher than at doctors' offices.

Most freestanding surgery centers, 60.7 percent, are independently owned; corporate ownership accounts for 28.3 percent of facilities; hospitals account for only 11 percent of ownership. According to industry analysts, large multiunit corporations are expected to emerge as the predominant owners of freestanding facilities by the end of this decade. California and Texas have the most surgery centers, followed by Florida, Arizona, Tennessee, Washington, and Ohio, according to the Federated Ambulatory Surgery Association of Alexandria, Virginia.

More than anything else, advances in medical and surgical technology, especially anesthesia administra-

tion, have been responsible for the surge in popularity of freestanding centers, also called surgicenters. With today's sophisticated equipment and delicate instruments such as lasers, surgicenters can perform minor surgical procedures—cataract surgery, oral surgery, tubal ligation, arthroscopic procedures, and the like—and send patients home a few hours after the operation.

CONSUMER CRITERIA FOR AN AMBULATORY CARE FACILITY

Ambulatory care may be convenient, accessible, and less costly, and have the bright future that predictions describe, but as the consumer you have to make sure your future after such care is bright—or that you have a future at all. When choosing any ambulatory care facility—for whatever service, be it routine medical care, urgent or emergency care, or surgery—you must face one essential question: *whether quicker and less expensive medical care means a lowering of the quality of that care and less concern for safety.*

When shopping around for the right setting for your needs, bear in mind that competition is fierce and multipronged: walk-in medical clinics, hospital emergency rooms, private practice physicians, group medical practices, hospital outpatient surgery departments, and freestanding surgical centers—all vying for your dollar. So you don't have to settle on less than the best. But you do have to snoop around first. Why waste your money and time on a clinic that's not for you? Here are some pointers:

- Schedule a get-acquainted visit.
- Find out whether the center is licensed and/or accredited, the only two means by which you can ascertain whether the facility has met certain objective standards for medical care. A possible roadblock here is that not every state licenses (and, in turn, regulates) ambulatory care facilities or has comprehensive standards, and the accreditation process is voluntary. But there's another avenue open to you. Insurance companies and Medicare/Medicaid do certify facilities that participate in their programs. While their inspection teams may be checking for compliance with standards more along the lines of staffing, equipment, plant, and record keeping, this is better than no certification and no standards at all.
- Verify the above information in any of these ways: Contact your state health department, who

Taking Care of Business

With business in "same day" surgery booming, surgicenters continue to carve out a bigger niche than ever before. According to a Chicago-based marketing firm, by the end of 1992 there were 1,696 surgery centers performing more than 2.8 million procedures annually. By 1996 surgicenters will account for nearly 4 million outpatient procedures (*Modern Healthcare*, June 28, 1993).

Not to be outdone in the race for business, doctor's office surgery is supposed to match the volume growth of these freestanding centers, and account for around 3 million procedures in 1996, says the same marketing firm.

With so much trade in outpatient surgery, is it any wonder that the number of freestanding ambulatory surgery centers is increasing? Another factor fueling the growth in outpatient surgery is Medicare and the need to provide more cost-effective care to beneficiaries. In 1986 Medicare approved some 1,500 formerly inpatient procedures for reimbursement on an outpatient basis. The success of this program and the real cost savings convinced Medicare to increase the number of procedures approved for outpatient reimbursement.

The most common types of surgical procedures these centers perform are, in descending order of volume: ophthalmologic (31 percent of all freestanding centers offer only cataract surgery), gynecologic, gastroenterologic, otolaryngologic (ear, nose, and throat), orthopedic, general surgery, plastic surgery, urologic, podiatric, and neurologic.

will tell you whether the facility is licensed. Call the facility's business manager and ask whether the clinic is certified by Medicare/Medicaid and any private insurance companies. Contact the two major accrediting organizations (but be prepared—only a handful of centers have gone through a voluntary review for accreditation):

Accreditation Association for Ambulatory Health Care
9933 Lawler Avenue
Skokie, IL 60077-5702
708-676-9610

Joint Commission on the Accreditation of Healthcare Organizations
One Renaissance Boulevard
Oakbrook Terrace, IL 60181
708-916-5635

• Find out how the center functions, including its hours of operation and holiday schedule, whether appointments are necessary or recommended, and what medical problems it is prepared to treat.

What does it *not* treat? Ask how the center works with local hospitals and emergency ambulance services. Should the need arise, can the center arrange rapid transportation to a hospital?
• Ask how the center maintains its records and whether you will be given copies of your medical record. If not, what provisions does it make for follow-up care elsewhere? Will the center send a copy to your regular physician?
• Find out how the center handles follow-up care such as having a cast removed or having additional lab tests done. Is there a onetime charge or must you pay again for a follow-up visit?
• Ask about the ancillary services available: Does the center have X-ray equipment? When was it last inspected/calibrated? Is there a laboratory on the premises? If so, what are the credentials of the lab staff? Is there an orthopedic room for treating broken bones and dislocations? A suture room?
• Find out what life-support equipment is available on site—a critical issue if the center offers emergency and/or surgical care. A cardiac defibrillator? A properly supplied "crash cart"? Are the

medical personnel trained in life-support techniques, especially cardiopulmonary resuscitation? Does the facility have the necessary equipment to handle a heart attack?

- Find out who the staff are and their credentials. Call your state's medical licensing board (see listing in section 3, "Healing Arts") and make sure all the doctors who work there are licensed. Whether the doctors, especially in the ambulatory surgery centers, are board-certified in their specialties is extremely important too. For that information you must check the particular medical specialty board (see section 3, "Healing Arts"). At what hospitals do the doctors have admitting privileges? In the case of a surgery center, is there an anesthesiologist on staff? Will he/she be present during the procedure?

- Ask what the typical charges are. Must you pay at the time of treatment? Credit card or cash only, or can a payment schedule be arranged? What health insurance coverage does the center accept? You will want to check your insurance policy to find out what constitutes "emergency care" and under what conditions outpatient care and surgery will be covered. There is a chance that, if you are treated at a less expensive facility than a hospital, your plan will pay full costs and waive the usual deductible and copayment or perhaps just adjust the copayment. It's worth asking.

- Find out what volume of surgeries the surgicenter performs a year. More and more studies are corroborating what many people already suspected regarding quality of surgical care: Practice makes perfect. One report's estimate of the optimum number is 1,200 to 1,500. Also ask the surgeon how many times a year he/she performs the procedure you are about to undergo.

Emergency Care

Emergency care is defined as care for patients with severe, life-threatening, or potentially disabling conditions that require intervention within minutes or hours.

Most people are familiar with the image of emergency medical personnel rushing to the aid of accident and heart attack victims, rendering care and then whisking them off to the hospital. In the strictest sense of the definition, this is true emergency care.

However, there are other situations that might not be life-threatening, but are nonetheless medical emergencies, such as sprained ankles and broken bones. While these may not require the services of an ambulance squad, there are several other ways of obtaining emergency care when these situations occur.

The simplest and most basic emergency care is first aid, which you might be able to do for yourself or receive from someone else. Anyone who has participated in scouting can probably recall the course on first aid. You learned what to do to remove a splinter, stop the bleeding, or treat an insect bite. In addition, many people have completed Red Cross first-aid classes, especially in cardiopulmonary resuscitation (CPR).

Organized emergency care is best provided through a system of emergency personnel, well coordinated to ensure that proper care is rendered in an efficient and timely manner.

THE EMERGENCY MEDICAL SERVICES SYSTEM

The Emergency Medical Services Systems Act of 1973 provided for the development of an integrated emergency medical system that would serve a designated geographical area. The goal then was to improve all segments of the system, including the training of personnel, establishment of a 911 telephone system, improvements in communication, and categorization of hospital emergency departments.

As a result of this legislation, the position of emergency medical technician (EMT) was introduced and training programs standardized. Classes on emergency medical procedures are offered by hospitals, and EMT candidates are required to pass a comprehensive examination on proper emergency care procedures. This was done to ensure that only qualified people serve on ambulance and rescue squads.

The next step in the development of an emergency medical system was to improve the communications system between the ambulance squads and the hospitals. Up until the enactment of the law, there had been many instances in which vital communication between hospitals and ambulances was impossible because of incompatible radios. Very often an ambulance squad would arrive at a hospital emergency department with a severely injured or ill patient only to discover that the hospital was unprepared to receive the patient. Funds made available through the

First Aid

First aid is immediate health care given to a person who is injured due to a sudden illness, an accident, or a life-threatening situation. First aid is given by individuals who tend to a victim's injuries before proper medical services have been summoned to the scene. The primary goals of first aid are to call for medical assistance, to tend to the victim's injuries, to comfort and reassure the victim, to protect the victim from further harm, and to avoid worsening the victim's condition.

An individual who gives first aid must quickly and calmly assess the situation of the victim and the nature of the accident: whether or not it is safe to approach the victim, whether or not the victim's life is in danger and should be moved, and the extent of injuries involved. When assessing the victim's condition, the rescuer should check and monitor important bodily functions, such as breathing and heart functions. The rescuer must keep the victim's airway open and check on the victim's *breathing* and *circulatory functions*—a process easily remembered as ABC. Regardless of the injury, a victim should not be moved unless his/her life is threatened and, then, should not be moved without proper assistance. If a spinal or neck injury is suspected, a rescuer should move the victim only if his/her life is in danger.

After having gathered initial information about the condition of the victim, the rescuer can effectively respond to the victim's immediate needs (whether the victim is unconscious, has no pulse, is bleeding severely, has broken bones, is going into shock, etc.). The rescuer should call the local EMS (Emergency Medical Services System) number in order to obtain proper medical attention for the victim. Persons giving first aid should be prepared to tell EMS the essential information surrounding the injury or accident: the victim's name, age, address, present condition, location, and what first-aid procedures have already been taken. With medical help on the way, the rescuer can continue to administer first aid, to monitor the victim's vital signs, and to comfort the victim.

Any individual may administer first aid, be it in the form of performing rescue breathing or simply comforting a victim, but must first procure the consent of the victim. If the victim is unconscious or is unable to answer for himself or herself, the consent is implied. In the event that any liability in giving first aid is leveled at the rescuer, he or she can be protected by Good Samaritan laws, which are found in most states. To give first aid effectively, it is wise for the rescuer to be trained properly (by taking a first-aid course), to be knowledgeable of the different types of emergency procedures, and to know the extent of his or her own capabilities in aiding another person.

legislation provided for the upgrading of all communications equipment.

Hospital emergency departments capable of handling true emergencies are categorized according to the level of care they are able to provide. (See "Hospital Emergency Departments" earlier in this section for more information.)

Categorizing hospitals also enables the ambulance squad to take the patient to the hospital with the most appropriate level of care. Once on the scene, the EMTs perform a medical assessment of the patient and communicate this information to doctors at the hospital. Depending upon the extent of the illness or injury, the ED doctor may direct the EMTs to take the patient to the nearest hospital or divert to a hospital with special treatment programs.

State, county, and municipal governments are responsible for developing and implementing a universal 911 emergency telephone system. This system enables callers to contact an emergency communications center and request ambulance assistance when seconds may literally mean the difference between life and death.

WHO PROVIDES EMERGENCY CARE?

Emergency care may be provided by individuals, first responders (fire and police), EMTs, paramedics, and other health professionals (doctors and nurses). Any individual who has satisfactorily completed a first-aid course may provide emergency care. However, even people who have not completed a formal course in first aid may render assistance, even if it's just comforting the person, until trained emergency personnel arrive.

First responders are police and fire personnel who arrive at an accident or injury scene before medical personnel. They are trained to make a quick assessment of the situation and provide comfort and assistance until the EMTs arrive. The primary responsibilities of a first responder are to prevent further injury or exposure to risk and to comfort the person. It may involve performing CPR, removing people from an accident scene, or assisting in the emergency birth of a baby.

Emergency medical technicians must complete an approved course of study comprising some 126 hours of instruction in various emergency situations and procedures. The course is a combination of classroom instruction and hands-on experience in assisting with emergency calls. EMTs must be ready for everything from major trauma and serious illness to emergencies involving mental health problems. Depending upon the victim's particular state, EMTs may even defibrillate cardiac arrest patients and intubate (insert a breathing tube in the airway of) patients who have stopped breathing.

The course of instruction includes topics in anatomy, physiology, patient assessment, cardiac arrest, bleeding and shock, emergency childbirth, burns and hazardous materials, and the lifting and moving of patients.

Paramedics complete a longer course of instruction and are trained in advanced life-support systems. In addition, they are qualified to administer medications, especially intravenous lines. Paramedics use radios and telemetry equipment to stay in contact with doctors at the hospital ED, who monitor and direct the on-the-scene care. Paramedics may not be available in every locale or city.

Doctors and nurses are the mainstays of the hospital ED; however, when they are part of an air ambulance crew, they provide emergency care along with the EMTs and paramedics.

Emergency care is also available at urgicare centers, although such facilities should not be used for life-threatening emergencies, unless no other assistance is available. These centers are ideal for treating sunburns, elbow scrapes, sprained ankles and wrists, splinters in the foot or hand, and so forth. Often located in suburbs or even shopping malls, urgicare centers tend to be easily accessible and may be open anywhere from 12 to 24 hours a day. They are an excellent choice when a person needs more than mere first aid, but are not appropriate substitutes for the high-tech care of a hospital emergency department.

FIRST AID BOOKS

General First Aid Books

AMA Staff. *AMA Handbook of First Aid and Emergency Care.* rev. ed. 352p. 1990. pap. $9.95 (0-679-72959-3) Random House, Inc.

Amalfitano, Andrew M. *First Aid in Schools: A Thorough, Easy-to-Use Reference for All School Personnel.* LC 91-72716. (Illus.). 112p. 1991. pap. text ed. $19.95 (1-880036-10-X) Emergency Training of Colorado.

American Red Cross Staff and Handal, Kathleen A. *The American Red Cross First Aid and Safety Handbook.* 1992. $29.95 (0-316-73645-7); pap. $14.95 (0-316-73646-5) Little, Brown & Co.

Auerbach, Paul S. *Medicine for the Outdoors: A Guide to Emergency Medical Procedures and First Aid.* rev. ed. 1991. $27.95 (0-316-05932-3) Little, Brown & Co.

Baldwin, Shirley. *First Aid for the Office and Workplace.* (Illus.). 192p. 1991. $15.00 (0-87527-258-4) Warren H. Green, Inc.

Baughman, Henry, and Niva, George. *First Aid for Injury and Illness.* 256p. 1990. $28.95 (0-8403-6081-9) Kendall/Hunt Publishing Co.

Bergeron, Dave. *First Responder: Self-Instructional Workbook.* (Illus.). 166p. 1982. $10.95 (0-89303-227-1) Prentice Hall.

Blate, Michael. *First-Aid Using Simple Remedies.* (Illus.). 196p. 1983. pap. $12.95 (0-916878-17-1) G-Jo Institute/Falkynor Bks.

Bowman, Warren. *Outdoor Emergency Care: Comprehensive First Aid for Non-Urban Settings.* (Illus.). 488p. 1988. pap. text ed. $23.50 (0-929752-00-7) National Ski Patrol System, Inc.

Brennan, William T., and Crowe, James W. *Guide to Problems and Practices in First Aid and Emergency Care.* 4th ed. 196p. 1981. (0-697-07390-4) Brown & Benchmark.

Brown, Andrew J., ed. *First Aid: Principles and Practices.* 2nd ed. (Illus.). 320p. 1987. pap. text ed. (0-02-327150-7) Macmillan Publishing Co., Inc.

Cain, Harvey D. *Flint's Emergency Treatment and Management.* 7th ed. (Illus.). 842p. 1985. text ed. $38.40 (0-7216-2313-1) W. B. Saunders Co.

Clayman, Charles B., ed. *Accidents and Emergencies.* LC 91-45392. (The American Medical Association Home Medical Library) (Illus.). 144p. 1992. $16.98 (0-89577-423-2) Reader's Digest Assn., Inc.

Consumer Guide Editors and Mosher, Charles. *Emergency First Aid.* 96p. 1980. pap. $2.50 (0-449-90023-1) Fawcett Bk Group.

Cooper, Martin J. *First Aid for Kids: An Emergency Guide Book for Parents.* 1991. pap. $5.95 (1-55874-093-7) Health Communications, Inc.

Do Carmo, Pamela B., and Patterson, Angelo T. *First Aid Principles and Procedures.* (Illus.). 256p. 1976. pap. text ed. $30.00 (0-13-317933-8) Prentice Hall.

Dranov, Paula. *Random House Personal Medical Handbook: First Aid Away from Home.* 1990. pap. $8.95 (0-679-72930-5) Random House, Inc.

Dworkin, Gerald M. *CPR for Infants and Children: A Guide to Cardiopulmonary Resuscitation.* (Illus.). 79p. 1989. pap. $13.95 (0-87868-272-4) Child Welfare League of America, Inc.

Eastman, Peter F. *Advanced First Aid for All Outdoors.* LC 87-44658. (Illus.). 175p. 1976. pap. $6.00 (0-87033-233-6) Cornell Maritime Press, Inc.

Feller, Irving, and Jones, Claudella A. *Teaching Basic Burn Care.* LC 75-15373. (Illus.). 1975. $120.00 (0-917478-27-4) National Institute for Burn Medicine, Ann Arbor, MI.

First Aid Book. rev. ed. (Illus.). 247p. 1990. pap. $6.50 (0-16-024145-6) U.S. Government Printing Office.

First Aid Book. (Illus.). 240p. 1991. $5.99 (0-517-46668-6) Outlet Bk Co., Inc.

Fleischer, Gary. *First Aid for Kids.* (Illus.). 20p. 1987. $9.95 (0-8210-5814-3) Barron's Educational Services, Inc.

Forgey, William W. *First Aid for the Outdoors: The Basic Essentials.* LC 88-32997 (Illus.). 72p. 1988. pap. $4.95 (0-934802-43-2) ICS Bks, Inc.

Gardner, Ward. *New Advanced First Aid.* 3rd ed. (Illus.). 288p. 1984. pap. $14.95 (0-7236-0803-2) Butterworth-Heinemann.

Gosselin, James, and Smith, Paul W. *Mosby's First Responder Workbook.* (Illus.). 352p. 1988. pap. $9.95 (0-8016-1932-7) Mosby-Year Bk, Inc.

Hafen, Brent Q. *First Aid for Health Emergencies.* 4th ed. 598p. 1988. pap. text ed. $34.25 (0-314-65674-X) West Publishing Co.

Hafen, Brent Q., et al., eds. *First Aid: Contemporary Practices and Principles.* LC 72-82623. pap. $42.60 (0-8357-9049-5) Bks on Demand.

Henderson, John. *Emergency Medical Guide.* 4th ed. 1978. pap. text ed. $9.95 (0-07-028169-6) McGraw-Hill Publishing Co.

Hewett, Peter R. *Beyond First Aid.* (Illus.). 256p. 1992. pap. text ed. (0-443-04579-8) Churchill Livingstone, Inc.

Home Medical Dictionary. rev. ed. 256p. 1991. pap. $2.49 (0-517-67043-7) Outlet Bk Co., Inc.

James, Gay, and Heath, P. J. *First Aid: A Programmed Study Guide.* 176p. 1988. pap. text ed. $14.95 (0-912855-87-8) Eddie Bowers Publishing, Inc.

Judd-Gosselin. *First Responder, Pkg. 2.* 1988. $26.95 (0-8016-3353-2) Mosby-Year Bk, Inc.

Koester, Robert J. *Outdoor First-Aid: A Field Guide Recognition and Treatment of Outdoor Injuries and Illnesses.* LC 91-72633 (Illus.). 104p. 1992. $22.95 (1-879471-13-2) DBS Productions.

Lavalla, Patrick. *Handbook: Living Life's Emergencies.* (Illus.). 72p. 1981. pap. $4.00 (0-913724-25-4) Emergency Response Institute, Inc.

Malstrom, Stan. *Natural First Aid.* 19p. pap. $3.95 (0-913923-38-9) Woodland Health Bks.

National Safety Council First Aid and CPR, Level 1. 96p. 1991. pap. $7.00 (0-86720-154-1) Jones & Bartlett Publishers, Inc.

——, *Level 2.* 192p. 1991. pap. $12.00 (0-86720-155-X) Jones & Bartlett Publishers, Inc.

——, *Level 3.* 288p. 1991. pap. $22.50 (0-86720-156-8) Jones & Bartlett Publishers, Inc.

Parcel, Guy S. *Emergency Care*. 4th ed. (Illus.). 368p. 1989. pap. $17.95 (0-8016-4267-1) Mosby-Year Bk, Inc.

Rogers, James H., et al. *First Aid and Emergency Medical Care*. 128p. 1980. $19.95 (0-8403-2242-9) Kendall/Hunt Publishing Co.

Sevelius, Gunnar. *First Aid—You Are It!* (Illus.). 80p. 1988. pap. $2.00 (0-933435-11-8) Health & Safety Publications.

Thygerson, Alton. *Teaching First Aid and Emergency Care Resource Book*. 96p. 1988. pap. text ed. $37.50 (0-86720-096-0) Jones & Barlett Publishers, Inc.

———. *First Aid and Emergency Care Workbook*. 352p. 1987. pap. $27.50 (0-86720-071-5) Jones & Bartlett Publishers, Inc.

———. *The First Aid Book*. 2nd ed. (Illus.). 352p. 1986. pap. text ed. $26.00 (0-13-318015-8) Prentice Hall.

———. *First Aid Essentials*. 224p. 1989. pap. $12.00 (0-86720-116-9) Jones & Bartlett Publishers, Inc.

Vasu, C. Mark. *Vital Response: A First Responder Training Manual*. (Illus.). 240p. 1991. pap. text ed. $22.95 (0-9629479-4-6) Cordith & Assocs.

Vogel, Stephen N., and Manhoff, David H. *Emergency Medical Treatment: Children*. (Illus.). 28p. 1984. pap. $7.95 (0-916363-00-7) E.M.T., Inc.

Whiddon, Thomas R., et al. *A Laboratory Guide to First Aid and Emergency Care*. 2nd ed. rev. and updated. LC 85-25707. (Illus.). 145p. 1986. pap. $16.00 (0-942280-20-2) Publishing Horizons, Inc.

Wood, J. A. *Theory of Advanced First Aid*. 1986. $35.00 (0-82500-892-9) Kluwer Academic Publishers.

Zucker, Elana. *The Homemaker—Home Health Aide Pocket Guide*. 256p. 1989. pap. text ed. $12.00 (0-89303-691-9) Prentice Hall.

First-Aid Books for Children

Berger, Melvin. *Ouch! A Book About Cuts, Scratches, and Scrapes*. (Illus.). 32p. (gr. k-3). 1991. $12.95 (0-525-67323-7) Dutton Children's Bks.

Boelts, Maribeth, and Boelts, Darwin. *Kids to the Rescue! First-Aid Techniques for Kids*. LC 91-5066 (Illus.). 80p. (gr. ps-6). 1992. PLB $17.95 (0-943990-83-1); pap. $7.95 (0-943990-82-3) Parenting Press.

Boy Scouts of America. *Emergency Preparedness*. (Illus.). 64p. (gr. 6-12). 1972. pap. $1.85 (0-8395-3366-7) Boy Scouts of America.

———. *First Aid*. (Illus.). 96p. (gr. 6-12). 1988. pap. $1.85 (0-8395-3276-8) Boy Scouts of America.

Greeley, Sheila. *Star-Junior First Aid*. LC 89-51922. (Illus.). 72p. 1989. pap. $7.95 (0-936029-19-6) Western Bk Journal Press.

Justus, Fred. *Basic Skills First Aid Workbook*. 32p. (gr. 5-9). 1983. $1.98 (0-8209-0576-3) ESP, Inc.

———. *First Aid*. 24p. (gr. 5-9). 1980. $5.00 (0-8209-016-4) ESP, Inc.

Kittredge, Mary. *Emergency Medicine*. 112p. (gr. 6-12). 1991. $18.95 (0-7910-0063-X) Chelsea House Publishers.

Ward, Brian R. *First Aid*. (Illus.). 48p. (gr. 4-12). 1987. PLB $12.40 (0-531-10260-2) Franklin Watts, Inc.

Nursing Homes

The term "nursing home" is actually a very general name for several different types of medical care facilities. It has the connotation of being a "last stop" for the elderly, but it actually can be a place for people of all ages to convalesce following an accident or serious illness, or a temporary placement for an elderly person while the family evaluates and arranges for alternative modes of care.

Nursing homes are for people who have difficulty caring for themselves, and as such provide three basic types of services:

- Nursing/medical care—for example, injections of medications, catheterizations, physical therapy, and other forms of rehabilitative services
- Personal care—for example, assistance in eating, dressing, bathing, and getting in and out of bed
- Residential services—for example, providing a clean room, good food, and a pleasant atmosphere with appropriate social activities

Nursing homes can be classified in many different ways, but two common classifications are level of care they provide and type of ownership.

LEVELS OF CARE

Skilled nursing. In a skilled nursing facility, care is delivered by registered and licensed practical nurses on the orders of an attending physician. The person who requires skilled nursing is often bedridden and not able to help him/herself, and may be placed in the facility for a short or an extended period of time, depending on the prognosis. (By the way, skilled nursing facilities are the only type of nursing homes Medicare will reimburse for, and then only a very limited amount of coverage is provided.)

Intermediate care. The immediate care facility provides less intensive care than the skilled facility and usually costs less. Normally not confined to a bed, the resident has a greater degree of mobility. Here, too, care is delivered by registered and licensed practical nurses and an array of therapists. Intermediate care stresses rehabilitation therapy to enable the resident to go home or at least to regain and/or retain as many functions of daily living as possible. For people with chronic conditions, the immediate care facility offers a full range of medical, social, recreational, and support services.

Sheltered, or custodial, care. This level of care is nonmedical in that residents do not require constant attention from nurses or aides, but do need help with such routine activities as getting out of bed, walking, eating, and bathing. The custodial care facility is for people who are capable of independent living but who may require some assistance with personal care and homemaking services.

OWNERSHIP

Aside from the obvious matter of the level of care needed, another key point is ownership. Opinions differ as to which type offers the best quality of care.

Nonprofit. Operated by various religious, fraternal, charitable, or community groups, nonprofit homes use any cash surpluses they may have to improve operations, purchase new equipment, and so forth. So, when well funded and well managed, these homes can be an excellent choice. Because they are subsidized by their parent organizations, care in these homes may sometimes be less expensive.

For-profit. Also called proprietary nursing homes, for-profit homes are operated specifically to earn a profit for their investors, who may be individuals or corporations. Because these homes are often better funded and more responsive to competitive pressures, some people argue that the care is of a higher quality than that in nonprofit homes. In actuality the quality of care varies from facility to facility.

Government/public nonprofit. Some local or state governments operate nursing homes offering various levels of care. These homes are classified as public nonprofit institutions because they are funded through the collection of taxes or the sale of municipal bonds. When they are operated by the city or county, they are generally referred to as the city or county home/hospital, and, as such, admissions are usually restricted to local residents.

CHOOSING A NURSING HOME

An important first step in choosing the right nursing home is to verify any home's licensure status through the state's nursing home licensing office (see later in this section). Important, too, is a close, firsthand inspection. Call the homes under consideration for appointments. Ask to speak to the administrator and plan to tour the home. Set aside several hours for each appointment.

- *Licensing.* Find out if the facility is properly licensed and certified. Issued by governmental authority, usually the state, a license means that the home has been inspected and has met certain standards established by law relating to matters such as fire protection, the physical plant, housekeeping, maintenance, and standards of care. Another related matter is certification, as it applies to Medicare/Medicaid payments. If a home applies for certification under either program, it agrees to certain conditions—for example, the home agrees to set aside a certain number of beds for Medicare/Medicaid residents and accept the prevailing rate paid by these programs, even though it may be less than the normal daily rate.
- *Building and grounds.* Inspect the building and grounds. The physical layout and beauty of the facility should be among the least important considerations, but safety and livability are two of the most important. Regarding safety, things to look for or ask are: Does the building appear to be fireproof? Are the emergency exits well marked? Are there sufficient smoke detectors? Is fire-fighting equipment—fire extinguishers and a sprinkler system—prominent?

Whether or not a building is livable depends upon things such as convenience, appearance, and the quality of life. Is the outside of the building neat and well maintained? Do the sidewalks have wheelchair ramps? Is there an area where residents can sit outside? Are the corridors wide enough for two wheelchairs to pass easily? Is there enough room in general for the residents? These are just some of the questions to ask.

Evaluating and Selecting a Nursing Home

As daunting and difficult as it may seem, it is possible to select a nursing home by yourself. Inadequate or poorly run nursing homes can be avoided if you know what to look for.

It is not necessary to be a trained professional to rate and pick a nursing home. What you need is information. And to get that information you need to know whom to ask, what to ask, what to look for, and how to evaluate that information. Picking a nursing home for a loved one is like buying a home. You need to do a great deal of research to make sure that the facility selected is the one that will meet the needs of the placed person, be acceptable as a place to live, and be affordable and within the means of those who will pay the bill.

Let us assume that you have narrowed down the nursing homes in your area to a manageable number by screening out those that are:

1. Too far away to allow you and other family members to visit the patient frequently
2. Not properly certified/licensed
3. Too expensive for your resources, and
4. Not appropriate in other ways, such as not offering the range of medical services the person needs

Now comes the face-to-facility encounter! There is absolutely no substitute for your own close, firsthand inspection. What you must now do is call for appointments at those homes still under consideration. Make it clear that you not only want to talk to the home's administrator but also plan to make an extensive tour of all the home's facilities.

What follows is a checklist of questions that you actually take with you to the nursing homes you decide to visit.

You don't necessarily have to answer every single question on the checklist, but you should try very hard to answer the ones that are important to you.

Evaluating a Nursing Home: Questions to Ask

The Building and Grounds

Outside:

1. Is the building neat and well maintained?
2. Does it appear fireproof? (Wood-framed buildings can be dangerous.)
3. Are the sidewalks clean and well maintained?
4. Do the sidewalks have wheelchair ramps?
5. Does the entrance have handrails and wheelchair ramps?
6. Is the home located within easy walking distance of public transportation?
7. Are the grounds spacious?
8. Are they well maintained?
9. Is there an area where patients can sit?
10. Do they sit outside (weather permitting) or otherwise use the outside area?

continued on next page

Inside:

11. Is the lobby clean and well furnished?
12. Do residents use the lobby?
13. Are the corridors well lighted? Are they wide enough for two wheelchairs to pass easily?
14. Does there seem to be enough room in general for the residents?
15. Are emergency exits well marked?
16. Is there an emergency lighting system?
17. Is there an actively functioning safety committee?
18. Is fire-fighting equipment (such as fire extinguishers) prominent?
19. Are there sufficient smoke detectors?

The Rooms

1. Are the rooms neat and clean?
2. Is there sufficient light?
3. Are there curtains on the windows?
4. Do all the rooms open on a hallway?
5. Do residents hang their own pictures?
6. Is there sufficient closet space?
7. Does each resident have a sink and mirror?
8. Is there counter space for personal objects?
9. Is the room nicely furnished?
10. Is the room air-conditioned?
11. Do the rooms have individual thermostats?
12. Is there an adjoining bathroom?
13. Are the bathrooms shared by no more than four residents?
14. Do residents have a choice between single and shared rooms?
15. In general, do residents have enough personal space?
16. Are procedures for changing roommates liberal and clearly spelled out?
17. If the rooms have TV sets, are they equipped with earphones?
18. Do the beds have bedspreads?
19. Are there grab bars on the toilet and bathtub?
20. Do the tubs have nonslip surfaces?
21. Do bathrooms and toilet areas have sufficient privacy?
22. Do the rooms have private telephones?

The Personnel

1. Does the home's administrator have a current license?
2. Was the administrator or his/her representative courteous to you?
3. Did he/she see you promptly?

4. Were the home's administrative policies well explained?

5. Was the administrator open to your questions?

6. Does the home employ:

   a. a physical therapist

   b. an occupational therapist

   c. a speech pathologist

   d. a dietitian

   e. a nurse practitioner

7. Is the nursing supervisor an RN?

8. Are all the head nurses RNs?

9. Do there seem to be enough nurses, nurse's aides, and orderlies on duty?

10. Was the staff generally friendly toward you?

11. Were they neatly dressed?

12. Did the residents seem at ease with the staff?

13. Did the staff speak to the residents in respectful, noncondescending terms?

14. Did the staff seem to like the residents?

15. Did the staff generally have pleasant expressions on their faces?

The Medical/Nursing Care

1. Is a physician on the premises for a fixed period of time each day?

2. Is a physician on call in case of emergency?

3. Is a registered nurse on duty during the day, 7 days a week?

4. Is at least one RN or one LPN on duty day and night?

5. Are dental services provided in the home itself?

6. Are there facilities outside of the residents' rooms for physical examinations?

7. May the resident select his/her own physician?

8. May the resident select his/her own hospital?

9. Does the home have a contract with an ambulance service?

10. Does the home have access to a pharmacist who maintains records on each resident and reviews them when new medications are ordered?

11. Is the family allowed to make alternative arrangements for purchasing prescription drugs?

12. Are arrangements made for patients who wish to use alternative professional services, such as podiatrists or chiropractors?

13. Does the home make arrangements for private duty nurses when the family thinks one is required?

14. Does the home have policies that severely restrict the use of physical restraints?

15. Are the majority of the residents free of physical restraints?

16. Are the rooms and halls free of any smell of human excrement?

17. Do they smell of heavy perfume?

continued on next page

18. Does each resident have a call button within easy reach?

19. Can it be turned off only at the patient's bed?

20. Are there call buttons in the bathrooms and bathing areas?

21. Does each resident have a water container and clean glass in his/her room?

22. Are the more inactive residents' fingernails trimmed; are the men cleanly shaved?

23. Does the home keep its own medical records?

24. Does the resident (or resident's family) have access to them?

The Recreational/Social Arrangements

1. Does the home employ a full-time social director?

2. Are residents permitted to entertain visitors in their rooms?

3. Are visiting hours liberal?

4. Are residents given reasonable leeway in establishing when they go to bed?

5. Are members of the opposite sex permitted to visit one another in their rooms with the doors closed?

6. Is alcohol permitted in the home?

7. Are there no limitations on outgoing or incoming telephone calls?

8. Do the published rules and regulations seem reasonable to you?

9. Are children permitted to visit?

10. Is there a quiet, private place where residents can entertain visitors?

11. Does there seem to be a wide range of recreational activities?

12. Are residents included in this planning in some formal way?

13. Is there an actively functioning patient council?

14. Is there sufficient room for the residents to engage in recreational/social events?

15. Are calendars of such events posted in convenient places?

16. Did you observe a substantial number of patients engaging in the recreational/social events?

17. Is there a newsletter for families of residents?

18. Are religious services held on the premises?

19. Are arrangements made to allow patients to attend outside religious services if they wish?

20. Is there a library with recent magazine issues and a good selection of books?

21. Does the home sponsor frequent outings for those residents who are able to go?

22. Is there a canteen?

23. Do patients appear to socialize with one another?

24. Does the home have any special programs with area schools to bring young people in to interact with the residents?

25. Does the home subscribe to (and provide you with a copy of) a liberal Patient Bill of Rights?

26. Is there a formal health education program for residents?

27. Does the home provide frequent continuing-education courses for its staff?

The Food

1. Are fresh fruits and vegetables served in season?
2. Does the home prepare meals from scratch rather than use frozen or prepackaged meals?
3. Do the residents have a choice in the selection of meals?
4. Are provisions for special diets made?
5. Is help available for residents requiring feeding assistance?
6. Is this help available both in the resident's room and in the dining area?
7. Are residents served in their rooms if they prefer?
8. Is there a reasonable amount of flexibility as to when residents can eat?
9. Are dining hours for the convenience of the residents rather than the staff?
10. Are residents given sufficient time to eat their meals?
11. Does the food appear appetizing to you?
12. Can the kitchen accommodate special, nonmedically prescribed diets (e.g., for religious reasons)?
13. Is the kitchen basically clean by your standards?
14. Does the kitchen staff appear neat and clean?
15. Is the menu cycle adequately varied?
16. Does the meal being served match the one on the menu?
17. Are the food carts closed for sanitation purposes?
18. Does the kitchen have a dishwashing machine?
19. Are snacks available between meals and at bedtime?
20. Do residents have access to a refrigerator to store their snacks?
21. Is the dining area clean and attractive?
22. Are the tables convenient for wheelchair use?

• *The rooms*. Inspect some of the rooms and observe the comfort they provide, the atmosphere they permit, and their safety. Here important factors include the amount of light, closet space, and spaciousness in general; whether residents have a choice between single and jointly occupied rooms; the placement of bathrooms and thermostats; whether the beds have screens or curtains for privacy; whether the toilet and bathtub have grab bars; whether the tubs have nonslip surfaces. Whether all rooms open to a hallway is an important safety consideration in case of fire or the need for prompt nursing/medical attention.

• *The personnel*. Ask who the staff are, what their credentials are, and how available key personnel are. Does the home's administrator have a current license? Are all the head nurses RNs? Is a physician on the premises for a fixed time each day? On-call 24 hours a day? Is a registered nurse on duty during the day, 7 days a week? Go around to as many sections of the home as possible and observe the staff's demeanor to the residents. Are the staff friendly? Do the residents seem at ease with the staff?

• *The recreational/social arrangements*. Determine if the home has a well-run recreational/social program. Both formal programs—such as social events, religious services on premises, outings, an on-site library and canteen—and atmosphere-related issues along the lines of visiting hours and designated nonsmoking areas can add to the quality of the residents' lives.

• *The food.* Assess the sanitation with which the food is prepared and the aesthetic appeal and nutritional value of the final product. Although it may seem like a minor consideration to some people, an elderly person's meals are a crucial part of his/her life. This is especially true of an institutionalized person. Surveys have identified food as the most frequently voiced complaint.

An extensive list of questions to ask in evaluating a nursing home appears on pages 273–77.

ALTERNATIVES TO NURSING HOMES

Long a concern among policymakers, the nation's overemphasis on nursing home-based institutionalization rather than home or other community-based care is a growing problem. The fact is that nursing home placement is not, and should not be, the sole solution to the plight of an elderly person who is debilitated by ill health and who has increasing difficulty taking care of him- or herself. Nothing mandates nursing home placement if there is someone available to administer the needed care in the home and/or coordinate delivery of alternative services. Humane and relatively inexpensive alternatives are out there if you know what they are and where to look.

First thing to do is take stock of the person's needs and attempt to match those needs with the alternative forms of care available in your area. Good sources of information on what your community has to offer are the local telephone directory, Office on Aging, welfare office, Visiting Nurses Association, United Way office, senior citizen organizations, veteran and fraternal organizations, home health agencies, and Red Cross.

While there is no way to list all the creative solutions that families have discovered, the following alternatives to nursing home care are the most common and widely used. We have placed them under three broad categories.

Alternatives for People Requiring Constant Care or Monitoring

Most of these services can be combined with each other as well as with those in the second category.

Adult day care. An adult day care center lets an elderly person enjoy a full range of activities—including arts and crafts, games, and just plain old conversation—on a daily basis in a supervised setting. Nursing care is not provided. Many centers are operated by church groups and senior citizen organizations, and often funded by United Way.

Ambulatory services. With more and more medical procedures being performed on an outpatient basis, thus saving the costs—and hazards—of an in-hospital stay, outpatient clinics may be viable options for people who need frequent medical care or monitoring that is difficult to provide in the home.

Home health care. This program provides nursing services—from the very basic, such as giving medication, to providing extensive physical or speech therapies—right in the person's home. Home health care, provided on the orders of a doctor or purchased individually, may be covered under Medicare, as long as certain conditions are met and the agency administering the services is certified. The Visiting Nurses Association is noted for its work in home care.

Family education. Some agencies—for example, the Visiting Nurses Association and Red Cross—and church groups give instruction to the family members who will be caring for the person in need. The skills taught include monitoring vital signs, providing nutritional meals, preventing bedsores, and changing bandages.

Respite care. More for the family or caregiver than the person needing care, respite care simply provides a break for the person who is providing the care and who needs to get out of the house once in a while. Under such a program, someone from the respite agency will come to the home and spend a fixed number of hours there. Some hospitals and nursing homes are getting into this business. They board the person needing care for a specific amount of time and provide round-the-clock care.

Alternatives for More Independent People

A number of excellent programs for elderly people who do not require constant supervision or that much nursing care may actually delay their need for nursing homes for many years.

Homemaker service. The primary purpose of homemaker services is to provide nonmedical support to a homebound person, the ideal candidate being an ambulatory person who maintains a relatively independent lifestyle but who may require some assistance in the preparation of meals or with housework. Such services are often contracted for by a home health agency, and not covered under Medicare or Medicaid, so other sources of reimbursement must be explored.

Home sharing. Persons who can still get around and take care of themselves may consider home sharing if they are tired of living alone and no longer want to be totally responsible for home maintenance. A typical home-sharing experience finds five to six older people renting a house together and sharing the expenses. The arrangement usually includes a resident manager who attends to day-to-day matters, leaving the residents free for other pursuits. A relatively expensive setup, home sharing is not for everyone.

Meals on Wheels. An excellent program designed to provide hot, nutritious meals to homebound people, Meals on Wheels is usually operated by a social service agency or community group. The service delivers one hot meal a day directly to the person's residence, and the price of such a service is nominal, often based on ability to pay.

Telephone reassurance. For an elderly person living alone, telephone reassurance can take some of the worry out of being alone and can help the person maintain an independent lifestyle without risking total isolation.

Shopping services. Tailored to the homebound elderly or convalescing person, this program entails having groceries and other needed items delivered. Some senior citizen centers and church groups offer this service.

Special transportation. Special transportation services, with vehicles equipped to handle wheelchairs and other devices, are valuable to people with limited mobility. Check in your telephone directory under county government or under "Transportation," or call the Red Cross or other local groups working with handicapped citizens.

Special health aids or devices. Special devices such as walkers, mechanical feeding devices, geriatric chairs, artificial limbs, and orthopedic shoes can facilitate personal independence or make it more feasible for a family member to assist.

Institutional Alternatives

Nursing homes are not the only institutional arrangements for people who cannot or do not wish to be cared for at home. Three of the most common alternatives are:

Adult foster care. This permits a person 60 years of age or older to be placed in a home setting with another person or family, and there have all the care required. This can be a very useful program for people who do not require intensive nursing care.

Hospice. Hospices are for people who are terminally ill, and the program's hallmarks are control of pain and relief from suffering, as well as preparation for death and support for survivors. The mission of hospices is to inspirit death with dignity and allow the family to maintain close contact with the patient, free from the intrusive high technology of the hospital. Hospice services can be delivered in the home or in a separate facility with a homelike atmosphere. Medicare covers hospice care.

Life care communities. A relatively new concept, these communities provide residential care in an apartmentlike setting, along with skilled and intermediate nursing care. As residents require nursing care, they are transferred to the nursing home section of the community, and once they recover return to their apartments. The life care community covers all costs of hospitalization, so the services do not come cheap. This option often requires a substantial, nonrefundable down payment as well as monthly fees. An excellent source of information on life care communities is available from the American Association of Homes for the Aging, 1129 20th Street N.W., Washington, DC 20036. You can call them at 202-296-5960. Two other groups who may help are:

American Health Care Association
1200 15th Street N.W.
Washington, DC 20005
202-833-2050

National Consumers League
1522 K Street N.W., Suite 406
Washington, DC 20005
202-797-7600

State Nursing Home Ombudsman Offices

These offices investigate complaints about care provided in nursing homes, regardless of the type or level of care provided.

Alabama
Alabama Commission on Aging
136 Cotoma Street
Montgomery, AL 36130
205-261-5743

Alaska
Alaska Older Alaskans Commission
Department of Administration
2600 Denali Street, Suite 403
Anchorage, AK 99503
907-279-2232

Arizona
Arizona Aging and Adult Services
Department of Economic Security
P.O. Box 6123-950A
Phoenix, AZ 85007
602-255-4446

Arkansas
Arkansas Division of Aging and Adult Services
Department of Human Services
Donaghey Building
7th and Main Streets
Little Rock, AR 72201
501-682-2441

California
California Department of Aging
Office of the Long-Term Care Ombudsman
1600 K Street
Sacramento, CA 95814
800-231-4024

Colorado
Colorado State Care Ombudsman Program
455 Sherman Street, Suite 130
Denver, CO 80218
303-772-0300
800-582-7410

Connecticut
Connecticut Department of Aging
175 Main Street
Hartford, CT 06106
203-566-7770

Delaware
Delaware (Northern) Division on Aging
Delaware State Hospital
1901 N. DuPont Highway
New Castle, DE 19720
302-421-6791

Delaware (Southern) Division of Aging
Milford State Services Center
11-13 Church Street
Milford, DE 19963
302-422-1386

District of Columbia
District of Columbia Office on Aging
1424 K Street N.W., 2nd Floor
Washington, DC 20005
202-724-5622

Florida
Florida State Long-Term Care Ombudsman Council
1317 Winewood Boulevard
Building 1, Room 308
Tallahassee, FL 32399-0700
904-488-6190

Georgia
Georgia Office of Aging
Department of Human Resources
878 Peachtree Street N.E., Room 642
Atlanta, GA 30309
404-894-5336

Hawaii
Hawaii Executive Office on Aging
Office of the Governor
335 Merchant Street, Room 241
Honolulu, HI 96813
808-548-2593

Idaho
Idaho Office on Aging
Statehouse, Room 114
Boise, ID 83720
208-334-3833

Illinois
Illinois Department on Aging
421 E. Capitol Avenue
Springfield, IL 62701
217-785-3140

Indiana
Indiana Department of Human Services
251 N. Illinois
P.O. Box 7083
Indianapolis, IN 46207-7083
317-232-1223
800-622-4484 in Indiana only

Iowa

Iowa Department of Elder Affairs
914 Grand
236 Jewett Building
Des Moines, IA 50319
515-281-5187

Kansas

Kansas Department on Aging
Docking State Office Building
915 S.W. Harrison, Room 122-S
Topeka, KS 66612-1500
913-296-4986

Kentucky

Kentucky Department of Social Services
Division of Aging Services
CHR Building, 6 West
275 E. Main Street
Frankfort, KY 40621
502-564-6930

Louisiana

Louisiana Governor's Office of Elderly Affairs
P.O. Box 80374
Baton Rouge, LA 70898-0374
504-925-1700

Maine

Maine Long-Term Care Ombudsman Program
Maine Committee on Aging
Statehouse Station 127
Augusta, ME 04333
207-289-3658
800-452-1912

Maryland

Maryland Office on Aging
301 W. Preston Street, Room 104
Baltimore, MD 21201
410-225-1083

Massachusetts

Massachusetts Executive Offices—Elder Affairs
38 Chauncy Street
Boston, MA 02111
617-727-7750

Michigan

Michigan Citizens for Better Care
David Whitney Building
1553 Woodward, Suite 525
Detroit, MI 48226
313-962-5968

Minnesota

Minnesota Board on Aging
Human Services Building
444 Lafayette Road
St. Paul, MN 55155-3843
612-296-2770

Mississippi

Mississippi Council on Aging
421 W. Pascagoula Street
Jackson, MS 39203-3524
601-949-2029

Missouri

Missouri Division of Aging
Department of Social Services
2701 W. Main Street
Jefferson City, MO 65102
314-751-3082

Montana

Montana Seniors Office—Legal and Ombudsman Services
P.O. Box 232, Capitol Station
Helena, MT 59620
406-444-4676

Nebraska

Nebraska Department on Aging
P.O. Box 95044
Lincoln, NE 68509
402-471-2307

Nevada

Nevada Division for Aging Services
Kinkead Building, Room 101
505 E. King Street
Carson City, NV 89710
702-885-4210

New Hampshire

New Hampshire Long-Term Care Ombudsman Program
Department of Elderly and Adult Services
6 Hazen Drive, 3rd Floor East
Concord, NH 03301-6508
603-271-4375

New Jersey

New Jersey Ombudsman for the Institutionalized Elderly
28 W. State Street, Room 305
Trenton, NJ 08625
609-292-8016
800-624-4262

New Mexico

New Mexico State Agency on Aging
224 E. Palace Avenue, 4th Floor
Santa Fe, NM 87501
505-827-7640
800-432-2080

New York

New York State Office for Aging
Agency Building Number 2, 2nd Floor
Empire State Plaza
Albany, NY 12223
518-474-7329

North Carolina

North Carolina Division of Aging
1985 Umstead Drive
Raleigh, NC 27603
919-733-3983

North Dakota

North Dakota Long-Term Care Ombudsman
Aging Services Division
State Capitol
Bismarck, ND 58505-0250
701-224-2577

Ohio

Ohio Department on Aging
State Ombudsman
50 W. Broad Street, 9th Floor
Columbus, OH 43266-0501
614-466-1220
800-282-1206

Oklahoma

Oklahoma Department of Human Services
Office of Client Advocacy
Long-Term Care Ombudsman
P.O. Box 25352
Oklahoma City, OK 73125
405-521-2281

Oregon

Oregon Long-Term Care Ombudsman's Office
2475 Lancaster Drive N.E.
Building B, Suite 9
Salem, OR 97305
503-378-6533
800-522-2602

Pennsylvania

Pennsylvania Department of Aging
Bureau of Advocacy
231 State Street
Harrisburg, PA 17101
717-783-7247

Puerto Rico

Puerto Rico Office of the Ombudsman
San Juan Bank Building
1205 Ponce de León Avenue
Santurce, PR 00908
809-725-1886

Rhode Island

Rhode Island Department of Elderly Affairs
160 Pine Street
Providence, RI 02903
401-277-2894

South Carolina

South Carolina Governor's Office
Ombudsman Division
Edgar A. Brown Building
1205 Pendleton Street
Columbia, SC 29201
803-734-0457

South Dakota

South Dakota Office of Adult Services and Aging
State Ombudsman
700 Governor's Drive
Pierre, SD 57501-2291
605-773-3656

Tennessee

Tennessee Commission on Aging
706 Church Street
Nashville, TN 37219
615-741-2056

Texas

Texas Department on Aging
P.O. Box 12786
Austin, TX 78711
512-444-2727

Utah

Utah State Division of Aging and Adult Services
Long-Term Care Ombudsman
120 North 200 West, 4th Floor
Salt Lake City, UT 84103
801-538-3929

Vermont

Vermont Office on Aging
Long-Term Care Ombudsman Program
103 S. Main Street
Waterbury, VT 05676
802-241-2400
800-642-5119

Virginia

Virginia Department for the Aging
700 E. Franklin Street
700 Center, 10th Floor
Richmond, VA 23219-2327
804-225-2271
800-552-3402

Washington

Washington State Long-Term Care Ombudsman
Legislative and Constituent Services
Mail Stop OB-44Y
Olympia, WA 98504
206-838-6810

West Virginia

West Virginia Commission on Aging
State Capitol Complex
Charleston, WV 25305
304-558-3317

Wisconsin

Wisconsin Governor's Ombudsman Program for the Aging and Disabled
819 N. 6th, Room 619
Milwaukee, WI 53203
414-227-4386

Wyoming

Wyoming Nursing Home Ombudsman
P.O. Box 94
Wheatlyn, WY 82201
307-322-5553

State Nursing Home Licensing Offices

These state agencies inspect nursing homes and issue licenses, based on state criteria in areas such as life-safety codes, staffing, food preparation, and quality of care.

Alabama

Alabama Nursing Home Licensure Office
Division of Licensure and Certification
Alabama Department of Health
434 Monroe Street
Montgomery, AL 36103-1701
205-261-5113

Alaska

Alaska Nursing Home Licensure Office
Department of Health and Social Services
Health Facilities Certification and Licensing
4433 Business Park Boulevard, Building M
Anchorage, AK 99503
907-561-2171

Arizona

Arizona Department of Health Services
Office of Health Care Licensure
701 E. Jefferson Street, Suite 300
Phoenix, AZ 85034
602-255-1177

Arkansas

Arkansas Department of Health
Certification and Licensure Section
Office of Long-Term Care
P.O. Box 8059
Little Rock, AR 72203-8059
501-682-8430

California

California Nursing Home Licensure Office
Licensure and Certification Division
Facilities Licensing Section
714 P Street, Room 823
Sacramento, CA 95814
916-445-3281

Colorado

Colorado Nursing Home Licensure Office
Colorado Department of Health
Health Facilities Division
Evaluation and Licensure Section
4210 E. 11th Avenue, Room 254
Denver, CO 80220
303-331-4930

Connecticut

Connecticut Nursing Home Licensure Office
Connecticut State Department of Health
Division of Hospital and Medical Care
150 Washington Street
Hartford, CT 06106
203-566-5758

Delaware

Delaware Office of Health Facility Licensing and Certification
Nursing Home Division
Division of Public Health
3000 Newport Gap Pike
Wilmington, DE 19808
302-571-3499

District of Columbia

District of Columbia Office of Licensing and Certification
Nursing Home Division
Department of Human Services
614 H Street N.W., Suite 1014
Washington, DC 20001
202-727-7190

Florida

Florida Nursing Home Licensure Office
Licensure and Certification Branch
Division of Health
Department of Rehabilitation Services
2727 Mahan Drive
Tallahassee, FL 32308
904-487-3513

Georgia

Georgia Nursing Home Licensure Office
Standards and Licensure Unit
Office of Regulatory Services
878 Peachtree Street N.E., Suite 803
Atlanta, GA 30309
404-894-5137

Hawaii

Hawaii Nursing Home Licensure Office
Hospital and Medical Facility Branch
Hawaii State Department of Health
P.O. Box 3378
Honolulu, HI 96801
808-548-5935

Idaho

Idaho Nursing Home Licensure Office
Facilities Standards and Development
Idaho Department of Health and Welfare
450 W. Washington Street, 2nd Floor
Boise, ID 83720
208-334-6626

Illinois

Illinois Nursing Home Licensure Office
Illinois Department of Public Health
Health Facilities and Quality of Care
525 W. Jefferson, 4th Floor
Springfield, IL 62721
217-782-5180

Indiana

Indiana Nursing Home Licensure Office
Division of Health Facilities
Indiana State Board of Health
1330 W. Michigan Street
P.O. Box 1964
Indianapolis, IN 46206-1964
317-633-8442

Iowa

Iowa Nursing Home Licensure Office
State Department of Health
Division of Health Facilities
Lucas State Office Building
Des Moines, IA 50319
515-281-4115
800-523-3213

Kansas

Kansas Department of Health and Environment
Bureau of Adult and Child Homes
Landon State Office Building, 10th Floor
Topeka, KS 66602-1290
913-296-1240

Kentucky

Kentucky Nursing Home Licensure Office
Division for Licensing and Regulation
Office of the Inspector General
CHR Building, 4th Floor East
275 E. Main Street
Frankfort, KY 40621
502-564-2800

Louisiana

Louisiana Nursing Home Licensure Office
Department of Health and Human Resources
Division of Licensure and Certifcation
P.O. Box 3767
Baton Rouge, LA 70821-3767
504-342-5774

Maine

Maine Nursing Home Licensure Office
Division of Licensure and Certification
249 Western Avenue
Statehouse Station 11
Augusta, ME 04333
207-289-2606

Maryland

Maryland Nursing Home Licensure Office
Office of Licensing and Certification Program
Department of Health and Mental Hygiene
4201 Patterson Avenue
Baltimore, MD 21215
410-764-2770

Massachusetts

Massachusetts Nursing Home Licensure Office
Long-Term Care Facilities Program
Department of Public Health
80 Boylston Street, 11th Floor
Boston, MA 02116
617-727-5864

Michigan

Michigan Nursing Home Licensure Office
Bureau of Health Care Administration
Department of Public Health
3423 N. Logan Street
Lansing, MI 48909
517-335-8505

Minnesota

Minnesota Nursing Home Licensure Office
Minnesota Department of Health
Survey and Compliance Section
393 N. Dunlop Street
P.O. Box 64900
Minneapolis, MN 55440-0900
612-643-2102

Mississippi

Mississippi Nursing Home Licensure Office
Health Facilities Certification and Licensure
Mississippi State Board of Health
P.O. Box 1700
Jackson, MS 39215
601-960-7769

Missouri

Missouri Department of Social Services
Division of Aging
1440 Aaron Court
P.O. Box 1337
Jefferson City, MO 65102
314-751-2712

Montana

**Montana Department of Health and
Environmental Sciences**
Bureau of Licensing and Certification
Cogswell Building
Helena, MT 59620
406-444-2037

Nebraska

Nebraska Division of Licensure and Standards
Nursing Home Division
Department of Health
301 Centennial Mall S.
P.O. Box 95007
Lincoln, NE 68509
402-471-2946

Nevada

Nevada Nursing Home Licensure Office
Bureau of Regulatory Health Services
505 E. King Street
Carson City, NV 89710
702-885-4475

New Hampshire

**New Hampshire Department of
Health and Human Services**
Division of Public Health
Bureau of Health Facilities Administration
6 Hazen Drive
Concord, NH 03301
603-271-4592

New Jersey

New Jersey Nursing Home Licensure Office
New Jersey State Department of Health
Licensing, Certification and Standards
CN-367
Trenton, NJ 08625-0367
609-588-7726

New Mexico

New Mexico Nursing Home Licensure Office
Health and Social Service Department
Public Health Division
Harold Runnels Building
1190 St. Francis Drive
Santa Fe, NM 87503
505-827-2434

New York

New York Bureau of Long-Term Care Services
Corning, Second Tower
Empire State Plaza, Room 1882
Albany, NY 12237
518-473-1564

North Carolina

North Carolina Nursing Home Licensure Office
Licensure and Certification Section
Health Care Facilities Branch
701 Barbour Drive
Raleigh, NC 27603
919-733-2786

North Dakota

North Dakota Division of Health Facilities
State Department of Health
Nursing Home Division
State Capitol
600 East Boulevard
Bismarck, ND 58505-0200
701-224-2352

Ohio

Ohio Nursing Home Licensure Office
Medical Services
Licensing and Certification Division
Ohio Department of Health
246 N. High Street, 8th Floor
Columbus, OH 43216-0118
614-466-2070

Oklahoma

Oklahoma Nursing Home Licensure Office
Licensure and Certification Division
Oklahoma State Department of Health
P.O. Box 53551
Oklahoma City, OK 73152
405-271-6868

Oregon

Oregon Senior Services Division
Long-Term Care Licensing
Licensing and Certification
313 Public Service Building
Salem, OR 97310
503-378-3751

Pennsylvania

Pennsylvania Nursing Home Licensure Office
Commonwealth of Pennsylvania
Division of Long-Term Care
Health and Welfare Building, Room 526
Harrisburg, PA 17120
717-787-1816

Rhode Island

Rhode Island Nursing Home Licensure Office
Rhode Island Department of Health
Division of Facilities Regulation
3 Capitol Hill
Providence, RI 02908
401-277-2566

South Carolina

South Carolina Nursing Home Licensure Office
Division of Health Facilities and Services
Department of Health Licensing
2600 Bull Street
Columbia, SC 29101
803-734-4680

South Dakota

South Dakota Department of Health
Division of Licensure and Certification
523 E. Capitol Street
Pierre, SD 57501
605-773-3364

Tennessee

Tennessee Department of Health and Environment
Board of Licensing Health Care Facilities
283 Plus Park Boulevard
Nashville, TN 37219-5407
615-367-6303

Texas

Texas Nursing Home Licensure Office
Texas Department of Health
Quality Standards Division
1100 W. 49th Street, Room T201
Austin, TX 78756-3188
512-458-7490

Utah

Utah Nursing Home Licensure Office
Utah Department of Health
Bureau of Health Facilities Licensing
P.O. Box 16660
Salt Lake City, UT 84116-0660
801-538-6152

Vermont

Vermont Nursing Home Licensure Office
Vermont Department of Health
Medical Regulation
60 Main Street
P.O. Box 70
Burlington, VT 05402
802-863-7250

Virginia

Virginia Nursing Home Licensure Office
Division of Licensure and Certification
1013 Madison Building
109 Governor Street
Richmond, VA 23219
804-786-2081

Washington

Washington Nursing Home Licensure Office
DSHS-Health Services Division
Aging and Adult Services Administration
623 8th Avenue S.E.
Mail Stop HB-11
Olympia, WA 98504-0095
206-753-5840

West Virginia

West Virginia Nursing Home Licensure Office
Health Facilities and Licensure Certification Section
1900 Kanawha Boulevard
Building 3, Room 535
Charleston, WV 25305
304-558-0050

Wisconsin

Wisconsin Department of Health and Social Services
Division of Health
Bureau of Quality Compliance
One W. Wilson Street, Room 150
P.O. Box 309
Madison, WI 53701
608-266-3024

Wyoming

Wyoming Department of Health and Social Services
Division of Health and Medical Services
Medical Facilities
Hathaway Building, 4th Floor
Cheyenne, WY 82002-0717
307-777-7121

Home Health Care and Homemaker Services

Home health care, as the name implies, is care delivered to an individual in the home setting. It may be medical or nonmedical in nature, depending upon the particular needs of the person. Care that is medical in nature is called home health care, while nonmedical care is referred to as homemaker services.

The market for home care services is growing rapidly as many people who were once kept in the hospital for a few extra days are now being discharged to return to their home environment and continue their recuperation and recovery. Not only do these people generally recover more quickly at home, but there is also the added benefit of lower costs to the individual and the entire health care system. The following examination of charges for services in the home versus the hospital clearly demonstrates cost savings.

Comparison of Selected Monthly
Home and Hospital Costs

Condition	Hospital Cost	Home Cost	Savings
Infant w/breathing, feeding problems	$60,970	$20,209	$40,761
Neurological disorder w/respiratory problems	$17,783	$196*	$17,587
Ventilator-dependent patient care	$22,569	$1,766	$20,803
Nutrition infusions	$23,670	$9,000	$14,670
Antibiotic infusions	$7,290	$2,070	$5,220
Patient requiring respiratory support	$24,715	$9,267	$15,448
Quadriplegic w/ spinal cord injury	$23,862	$13,931	$9,931
Cerebral palsy patient	$8,425	$4,867†	$3,558

* After initial cost of equipment.
† In extended care unit of hospital.

Most home health care services are covered under Medicare, Medicaid, county health programs, or private insurance companies. In order for home health services to be reimbursed by Medicare, the patient's physician must write an order for home care; a written treatment plan must also be included.

HOME HEALTH CARE A GROWTH INDUSTRY

Expenditures for home health care are increasing rapidly and are projected to exceed $18 billion in 1993. This is quite an increase from 1980, when expenditures for home care services were just over $1 billion.

In 1992 Medicare spent $8.2 billion, or 6.1 percent of its total budget, on home health care. The agency paid for 138.5 million home health visits, and 2.87 million Medicare beneficiaries received home health care that year.

As of February 1993, Medicare had certified 6,497 home health agencies, or more than two and one-half times the agencies certified in 1977. In addition, the National Association for Home Care (NAHC) in 1993 estimated that there were 5,714 non-Medicare home health care agencies, 1,223 Medicare-certified hospices, and 477 non-Medicare hospices, bringing the total number of agencies in the U.S. to 13,911.

According to NAHC, the home health care industry is growing at about 10 percent per year. That estimate is based in part on Bureau of Labor statistics showing that home health care enjoyed a 19.2 percent jump in new job growth in 1990, almost three times the rate for the entire health care industry. Professions most in demand include homemaker health aides, physical therapists, respiratory therapists, occupational therapists, X-ray technicians, physician's assistants, medical secretaries, and support personnel.

HOME HEALTH CARE SERVICES

Home health care services must be ordered by a physician and delivered by a certified home health care provider, especially if insurance coverage is involved.

The services may be provided by a Visiting Nurses Association (VNA), home health agency, hospital, county or municipal government, or other organized community group.

Home health care services generally include:

• Diet and nutritional counseling
• Health assessment (determining the health status of the person)
• Hospice care for the terminally ill
• Nursing services
• Social services

Other home health services may be quite specialized, such as intensive nursing care, respiratory therapy, intravenous antibiotics, and occupational, physical, or speech therapy. Providers may include physicians, nurses, county or city health department workers, family, and friends.

Intravenous (IV) antibiotic therapy is poised to become one of the fastest-growing services provided in the home, as technological improvements enable doctors to prescribe it for patients with certain types of conditions. Patients with urinary tract infections, osteomyelitis, endocarditis, infected wounds, septic arthritis, and other infections that respond to IV therapy are treated at home under the following conditions.

- Their condition is stable and they can monitor their own therapy.
- They understand the responsibilities and potential problems of home IV therapy.
- Their home is equipped with a phone for emergency communications and a refrigerator to store antibiotics.
- The prescribed antibiotic has low toxicity, a long half-life, and a broad spectrum of activity.

Homemaker Services

The primary purpose of homemaker services is to provide nonmedical support to a homebound individual who does not otherwise require nursing home care. The ideal candidate for such services is an ambulatory individual who maintains a relatively independent lifestyle, but who may require some assistance in the preparation of meals or with housework.

Homemaker services are very often available from home health agencies; however, these nonmedical services are not covered by Medicare or Medicaid. While these two government insurance plans do not cover homemaker services, some commercial insurance companies may. (The schedule of benefits received with the plan would indicate if this is the case.)

Homemaker services (such as nutrition care) and home chores are covered under the federal Older Americans Act. For more information on eligibility and coverage, contact the Agency on Aging in your state (see listing of state aging offices in section 9, "Family Health and Resources").

Who Provides Home Care Services?

There are five types of home care providers:

Visiting Nurses Associations (VNA) are voluntary and nonprofit, governed by a board of directors, and financed by tax-deductible contributions and earnings.

Public agencies are operated by a state, county, city, or other local government. Their major responsibilities are disease prevention and community health education.

Proprietary agencies are for-profit home care agencies that provide nursing care and other services to homebound individuals. Many of these agencies are certified and eligible to participate in the Medicare and Medicaid programs.

Private not-for-profit (PNP) agencies are privately owned and governed home health agencies. They provide a full range of nursing and therapy services and may contract for homemaker services with other agencies. Many of these home health agencies are eligible to participate in both Medicare and Medicaid.

Hospital-based agencies are operating units or departments of a hospital. Many of these agencies are outgrowths of the social services department and are closely linked to the discharge planning office. Coordination between the home care department and discharge planning enables the patient to receive the proper type of aftercare. Properly certified hospital-based home care departments are eligible to participate in both Medicare and Medicaid.

Home Health Care Agencies Funded Through Medicare

Agencies	Number	Percent
VNA	604	9.9
Public	1,149	18.7
Proprietary	1,953	31.9
PNP	594	9.7
Hospital	1,688	27.5

Medical Laboratories

The modern clinical laboratory is a high-tech marvel, with its automatic analyzers that can perform anywhere from twenty to forty different tests from a single sample of blood. It's possible to monitor the functioning of various body systems from one blood sample. Tests may be designed, for example, to look for certain levels of enzymes secreted by the liver or

Blood Tests and Urinalysis

Blood tests and urinalyses can tell your doctor a great deal about your state of health.

Blood Tests

A complete blood count (CBC), a commonly performed test, provides information on the three types of blood cells—red and white blood cells and platelets.

If your doctor suspects anemia, he or she may order a CBC to determine if the values of your different cells are within the acceptable range. The blood is checked for:

Red blood cell count. Determines the number of red blood cells in 1 cubic millimeter of blood. Normal values for men are 4.6 to 6.2 million per cubic millimeter, women 4.2 to 5.4 million, and children 4.6 to 4.8 million. A low red cell count might indicate anemia; too many cells may result in clotting in smaller blood vessels.

White blood cell count. These cells form part of the immune system and have the ability to recognize and attack invading organisms. The normal range of white blood cells is 4,500 to 11,000; however, if an invading agent is present, their numbers rapidly increase. Very high levels of white blood cells may indicate leukemia, a lower than normal count may indicate aplastic anemia (a blood defect in which the bone marrow no longer makes blood cells) or pernicious anemia (a form of anemia affecting mainly older persons).

Platelet count. Platelets are tiny, cell-like structures that are very important to blood clotting, and are produced in the bone marrow. Normal values are between 150,000 to 400,000 per cubic millimeter of blood. Elevated levels of platelets may be found when certain types of cancer, leukemia, or inflammatory disease are present. Lower levels may indicate a bone marrow disease, or decreased production as a result of medications.

Urinalysis

A urinalysis is a chemical, microscopic, or physical examination of urine. Urine may be analyzed for chemicals such as blood, ketones, protein, and sugar, or may be analyzed microscopically for bacteria, blood cells, crystals, or pus. Physically, urine is examined for acidity, color, and specific gravity.

Normal values for urine would be: slightly acidic, amber color, and a specific gravity varying from 1.005 to 1.030. Abnormal material found in urine include blood, fat, glucose, hemoglobin, ketones, proteins, and pus. The presence of any of these materials could indicate a disease-causing pathogen.

the level of minerals present in the bloodstream. Hormonal levels may also be determined by blood analysis.

Laboratories make extensive use of microscopes to examine tissue and cell samples and look for disease-causing agents or changes in cellular structures. Bacteria cultures are grown in temperature-and-climate-controlled incubators, robotic arms automatically place specimens in test tubes, and other mechanized equipment performs hundreds of dipstick tests quickly and accurately.

Laboratory medicine is big business, with expenditures topping some $33 billion a year (this figure does not include the expenditures for diagnostic pro-

Clinical Laboratory Improvement Act (CLIA) of 1988

In an effort to improve the overall quality of laboratories, the federal government, through CLIA, will inspect all levels of laboratories every two years. This means that previously exempt labs in physicians' offices now come under the scrutiny of CLIA inspectors, along with hospital and commercial labs.

CLIA divides labs into three categories: waived (performs simple tests); Level I (performs moderately complex tests); and Level II (performs highly complex tests). Provisions in CLIA require over time that laboratories hire better-trained and -qualified personnel.

Assisting the federal government in this effort is the Commission on Office Laboratory Accreditation. This organization, which already does voluntary inspections, will become part of the overall CLIA effort. When an inspector pays a visit to a laboratory, certain items are checked. For example, lab records and personnel records are checked, and proficiency testing (to determine if the equipment is functioning properly) is done. The inspector may also observe tests in progress.

Following the review, an inspector makes a verbal report to the laboratory supervisor noting deficiencies and suggesting remedies. Later, a written report follows with more specific information concerning problem areas and the corrective actions that need to be taken.

cedures such as imaging and endoscopic examinations) for approximately 10 billion tests performed in more than 120,000 laboratories nationwide. Most laboratories are found in doctors' offices, with some 5,000 located in hospitals and another 5,000 in independently owned commercial labs.

A major problem for all laboratories is accuracy, which led to the passage of the Clinical Laboratory Improvement Act of 1966, ushering in the first clinical quality standards. This first effort, aimed primarily at labs performing tests for Medicaid and Medicare patients, did not quite do the job; therefore, Congress passed the Clinical Laboratory Improvement Act of 1988. This time Congress responded to complaints from consumers and passed a measure that sets forth credentials for laboratory personnel, and requires all labs to be inspected, including those located in doctors' offices.

LABORATORY PERSONNEL

Medical laboratories are under the supervision of a pathologist (a doctor with a specialty in pathology). According to the American Board of Medical Spe-

cialties, pathology "is that specialty of the practice of medicine dealing with the cause and nature of disease. It contributes to diagnosis, prognosis, and treatment through knowledge gained by the laboratory application of the biologic, chemical, and physical sciences to humans."

What this means is that pathologists examine the various types of specimens that are collected from body tissues, cells, and fluids (blood, urine) in order to determine if the sample is normal or a disease-causing agent is present. Laboratory tests may be used to establish the presence of disease, rule out a disease, monitor a condition, or identify tissue removed from the body during a biopsy or surgery.

There are three groups of laboratory personnel recognized by the American Society of Clinical Pathologists (ASCP), an organization that promotes standards in education, training, and certification. The categories are technicians, technologists, and specialists.

The differences in these positions is related to the duties they perform and the educational requirements for certification. Medical laboratory technicians are required to have an associate degree or a combination

Physician In-Office Laboratories

Diagnostic testing has moved out of the medical laboratory and into the doctor's office, where, according to an American Public Health Association study, about half of the lab tests in this country are now performed. Doctors in great numbers (some estimates go as high as 200,000) do in-office testing—especially since it has become another source of revenue.

For an investment as low as $1,000, a physician can buy an analyzer, and with a little training a person can operate this scaled-down version of its commercial counterpart. These machines are compact enough to fit into any office and deliver almost instantaneous readings on blood chemistries, hemoglobins, electrolytes, therapeutic drug levels, and more.

However, along with these conveniences come some serious questions. Are tests being ordered because they are needed or just because the equipment is there? Are the results of these tests accurate? What type of quality-control mechanism is in place? And are more sophisticated tests being bypassed in favor of easy-to-perform in-office tests?

Obviously, the answers to many of these questions will depend upon the individual practitioner, but red flags have been raised over this issue. Critics of office-based testing point to problems with accuracy, quality and quality control, the lack of adequately trained laboratory staff and staff turnover—and the incentive to increase revenues through overtesting. Study after study shows that small in-office laboratories tend to have a greater variability in test results than do large, regulated labs.

The passage of the Clinical Laboratory Improvement Act of 1988 means that office-based labs are now subject to regulation. The Department of Health and Human Services is responsible for developing uniform certification, inspection, and licensure for all labs, including those in doctors' offices.

of courses in the medical sciences and laboratory work experience. Medical technologists are required to have a baccalaureate degree and a combination of work-related experience. Specialists may be required to be registered nurses, and hold baccalaureate, master's, or doctorate degrees.

Medical laboratory technicians collect specimens and prepare them for examination or perform certain procedures on them. A common example is the blood test. For it, a medical technician "sticks" you to collect the blood. The test tube with your blood sample is marked with your name and sent to the laboratory. When it arrives, depending upon the particular test ordered, laboratory technicians prepare the specimen for viewing under the microscope or load it into the automatic chemical analyzer.

Medical technologists perform many of the actual tests on the specimens that are collected. When tissue samples are collected through biopsy or surgery, the specimens are labeled and sent to the laboratory for analysis. These tissue samples are analyzed using sophisticated chemical tests or are examined under the microscope. Technologists are also responsible for writing their preliminary findings and reporting these results to the pathologist.

Specialists, as the name implies, have expertise in specific areas, such as blood banking, chemistry, cytology (the study of cells), hematology (blood), immunology, and microbiology. They are responsible for conducting some of the most sophisticated laboratory work done, such as identifying biologically matched donors in the case of bone marrow transplants. With their expertise at the tissue and cellular levels, they are involved in identifying disease-causing agents and looking for the effects of these agents on tissue and cells.

There's more, however, to medical testing than just collecting a sample of blood, urine, sputum, or stool. The specimen must first be collected properly to ensure that it is not contaminated in any way. Failure to collect a specimen properly can easily lead to inaccurate and incorrect results. For this reason, it's very important that laboratory personnel be properly trained and certified for the very important work they do.

QUALITY AND CERTIFICATION OF LABORATORIES

Laboratory tests are subject to two fatal flaws, the "false-positive" and "false-negative" results.

A false-positive result indicates that an abnormality exists or a disease is present when in reality none is present. A false-negative result means that an abnormality or disease-causing agent is indeed present but the test fails to detect it. If a medical decision is made on the results of one test, then a patient may undergo treatment he or she does not require or may not receive adequate care for a condition that is present.

Organizations such as the American Society of Clinical Pathologists and the National Accrediting Agency for Clinical Laboratory Sciences work to improve the educational requirements for medical laboratory personnel. They establish standards, conduct examinations, and accredit those who meet their requirements.

RESOURCES FOR LABORATORY QUALITY PROGRAMS

American Society of Clinical Pathologists
2100 W. Harrison Street
Chicago, IL 60612
312-738-1336

College of American Pathologists
325 Waukegan Road
Northfield, IL 60093-2750
708-446-8800

Commission on Office Laboratory Accreditation
8701 Georgia Avenue, Suite 610
Silver Spring, MD 20910
301-588-5882

5. Procedures

INTRODUCTION

Medical tests and procedures have become as commonplace as a physician's office visit. In fact, most encounters with a physician, or other health care practitioner, usually involve at least one test and quite likely a treatment. While some tests and treatments are benign, the vast majority have risks associated with them. In some cases, the risks are significant and the decision to proceed may rest on your judgment of whether the benefit outweighs the risk.

Each year there are more than 30 million major operations performed in American hospitals. An equal number of operations, many of them quite serious, are performed in outpatient facilities or physicians' offices. As the technology of medicine improves and expands, the ability of practitioners to do more complicated procedures grows. But so do the risks for the uninformed consumer. Therefore, the more you know about the benefits and risks of procedures, the more likely you are to choose the most appropriate one.

In this section, you will learn the important facts about the 100 most commonly performed hospital operations. You will find out which operations have the highest risk, the most commonly performed outpatient procedures, and much more. New technologies are described and discussed too.

Medical studies show that consumers who are knowledgeable about the treatments they receive and who participate in the decision-making process tend to have better medical outcomes.

100 Most Commonly Performed Operations

On the following pages, we present 100 of the most commonly performed operations in the U.S., complete with their nonmedicalese name (when there is one) and a brief description of the procedure. The number found in parentheses following the name of the operation is the ranking—calculated from highest in volume to lowest, in terms of operations performed annually—of this particular procedure within the list of 100. Some procedures are diagnostic in nature and performed to determine a disease or problem. Others are surgical treatments, performed to solve or alleviate a medical problem. And some, like balloon angioplasty, are used both diagnostically and therapeutically.

The 100 procedures reviewed were selected in two ways. The majority are those procedures most frequently performed in U.S. hospitals, either on an inpatient or on an outpatient basis. Others, like lens implantation and circumcision, are not necessarily performed in hospitals, but are still major procedures in terms of volume and/or the controversial issues surrounding various aspects of the procedure. (It is because they are often not performed in hospitals that these two common operations are not given a numerical rank here.)

The shift from hospital-based surgery to outpatient surgery represents a major trend now occurring in American medicine: Because of improved practice techniques and advanced technology, operations like lens implantation are done in a matter of minutes, with little risk to the patient, and therefore do not require overnight or prolonged hospitalization.

Determining the 100 most frequently performed procedures is not as easy as you might think. Doctors and hospitals are not required to report each operation they perform to some central data bank. Even the federal government does not track fully 100 of the most common procedures. So a great deal of research went into finding out just what were the most often performed operations.

Our data came from two sources. The major one was Healthcare Knowledge Resources of Ann Arbor, Michigan, which produces such a list by keeping a data base of 16 percent of all hospital discharges in the U.S. Healthcare Knowledge Resources then extrapolates those figures to find the national number. Our other source of information was the federal government, which does gather and publish selected data concerning procedures. We combined the data from these two sources to arrive at the 100 procedures covered here.

It is also important to have a perspective of the actual volume for each procedure in a given year. For example, cesarean sections, which top the list, were performed 962,622 times in 1989. There were 267,868 appendectomies (the eighth most frequently performed procedure) and 149,444 ureteral catheterizations (number 100 on our list). But these numbers may be less than the actual number performed for certain procedures.

100 Most Commonly Performed Operations (in rank order)

- Circumcision*
- Cataract removal with intraocular lens implant*
1. Cervical cesarean section
2. Total cholecystectomy
3. Total abdominal hysterectomy
4. Left cardiac catheterization
5. Repair of obstetric laceration
6. Transurethral resection of the prostate
7. Intervertebral disk excision
8. Appendectomy
9. Low-forceps delivery with episiotomy
10. Aortocoronary bypass—2-, 3-, and 4-vessel procedure combined
11. Tonsillectomy and adenoidectomy
12. Percutaneous transluminal coronary angioplasty
13. Intercostal catheter insertion
14. Esophagogastroduodenoscopy with closed biopsy
15. Transurethral destruction of bladder lesion
16. Open reduction and internal fixation of fracture of the femur
17. Combined right and left cardiac catheterization
18. Cystoscopy
19. Vacuum extraction delivery with episiotomy
20. Wound debridement and excision
21. Vaginal hysterectomy
22. Open reduction and internal fixation of fracture of the tibia and fibula
23. Placement of central venous catheter
24. Total knee replacement
25. Unilateral external simple mastectomy
26. Myelogram with contrast enhancement
27. Hemodialysis
28. Dilation and curettage, postdelivery
29. Fetal monitoring
30. Bone marrow biopsy
31. Vascular shunt and bypass
32. Endoscopic large bowel examination
33. Head and neck endarterectomy
34. Medical induction of labor
35. Peritoneal adhesiolysis
36. Skin suture
37. Total hip replacement
38. Endoscopic biopsy of the bronchus
39. Spinal canal exploration
40. Aortocoronary bypass—3 coronary arteries
41. Skin lesion: subsequent incision and destruction
42. Sigmoidectomy
43. Dilation and curretage (diagnostic)
44. Contrast phlebogram of the leg
45. Surgical repair of indirect inguinal hernia
46. Right hemicolectomy
47. Arterial catheterization
48. Joint replacement revision
49. Contrast cerebral arteriogram
50. Repair of obstetric laceration of the rectum and anus
51. Aortocoronary bypass—2 coronary arteries
52. Tonsillectomy
53. Hemorrhoidectomy
54. Transurethral removal of ureter obstruction
55. Aortocoronary bypass—4 or more coronary arteries
56. Diagnostic laparoscopy

100 Most Commonly Performed Operations
(in rank order)

57. Surgical repair of direct inguinal hernia
58. Exploratory laparotomy
59. Endoscopic lung biopsy
60. Unilateral salpingo-oophorectomy or salpingo-ovariectomy
61. Fetal electrocardiogram
62. Local destruction of ovarian lesion
63. Removal of tube and ectopic pregnancy
64. Abdominal aorta resection and replacement
65. Local destruction of skin lesion
66. Fiber-optic bronchoscopy
67. Partial small bowel resection
68. Dialysis arteriovenostomy
69. Revision of vascular procedure
70. Repair of vessel
71. Left hemicolectomy
72. Open reduction and internal fixation of fracture of the radius and ulna
73. Closed fracture reduction of the tibia and fibula
74. Shoulder arthroplasty
75. Cruciate ligament repair
76. Percutaneous liver biopsy
77. Toe amputation
78. Bilateral tubal division
79. Closed fracture reduction of the radius and ulna
80. Closed reduction and internal fixation of fracture of the femur

81. Incisional hernia repair
82. Aspiration and curettage, postdelivery
83. Nephroureterectomy
84. Surgical repair of unilateral inguinal hernia
85. Above-the-knee amputation
86. Lobectomy of lung
87. Below-the-knee amputation
88. Unilateral thyroid lobectomy
89. Rotator cuff repair
90. Contrast aortogram
91. Bilateral salpingo-oophorectomy or salpingo-ovariectomy
92. Endoscopic colon polypectomy
93. Uterine lesion destruction
94. Free skin graft
95. Temporary pacemaker system insertion
96. Ligation and stripping of varicose veins of the legs
97. Repair of cystocele or rectocele
98. Bilateral tubal destruction
99. Septoplasty
100. Ureteral catheterization

*These two procedures are given no rank order within the top 100, because they are not necessarily performed in hospitals and, indeed, are often *not* performed in hospitals. Nevertheless, these are two very common operations.

Words that are italicized appear in the glossary following the procedures.

DIAGNOSTIC PROCEDURES

Arterial Catheterization (47)
Placement of a *catheter* in an artery to measure intraarterial pressures, administer chemotherapy drugs, or remove *emboli* blocking an artery

Aspiration and Curettage, Postdelivery (82)
Use of a suction *catheter* to remove all of, or samples of, the womb lining for diagnostic or therapeutic purposes following the birth of a baby

Bone Marrow Biopsy (30)
Removal of marrow from the central channel of a bone for study to assist in the treatment of various serious diseases

Combined Right and Left Cardiac Catheterization (17)
X ray of the arteries and chambers of the heart using a *contrast medium* injected via a *catheter* threaded into the heart through an artery in the arm or leg

Contrast Aortogram (90)
X ray of the *aorta* with a *contrast medium* injected into an artery

Contrast Cerebral Arteriogram (49)
X ray of one or more arteries of the head with a *contrast medium* injected into the arteries

Contrast Phlebogram of the Leg (44)
X ray of one or more veins of the leg using a *contrast medium* injected into a vein

Cystoscopy (18)
Examination of the inside of the bladder through a *fiber-optic scope* inserted through the *urethra*

Diagnostic Laparoscopy (56)
Examination of the organs within the abdominal cavity via a *fiber-optic scope* inserted through an incision in or just below the navel

Dilation and Curettage (43)
Widening of the mouth of the womb and removal of samples of the womb lining for diagnostic purposes

Endoscopic Biopsy of the Bronchus (38)
Examination of the inside of the *bronchial tree* of the lungs through a *fiber-optic scope* and the removal of tissue specimens for analysis

Endoscopic Large Bowel Examination (32)
Examination of the large bowel (colon) via a *colonoscope* or *sigmoidoscope*

Endoscopic Lung Biopsy (59)
Examination of the lungs with a flexible *endoscope* and removal of tissue samples for pathological examination

Esophagogastroduodenoscopy (EGDS) with Closed Biopsy (14)
Examination of the *esophagus,* stomach, and *duodenum* with a flexible *fiber-optic scope,* and removal of small pieces of tissue for examination

Exploratory Laparotomy (58)
Opening the abdomen to explore the contents when other diagnostic methods have failed or are not applicable

Fetal Electrocardiogram (61)
Lay title: Fetal EKG
Monitoring of the health status of a fetal heart before and during birth using electrodes attached to the scalp

Fetal Monitoring (29)
Monitoring of the health status of a fetus using one or more instruments, some of which are electronic

Fiber-Optic Bronchoscopy (66)
Examination of the bronchial tubes with a flexible *fiber-optic scope,* which may also be used for treatment

Left Cardiac Catheterization (4)
X ray of the arteries and chambers of the heart using a *contrast medium* injected via a *catheter* threaded into the heart through an arm or leg artery

Myelogram with Contrast Enhancement (26)
Lay title: Myelogram
X ray of the spinal column with *contrast medium* inserted into the spinal canal via spinal tap

Percutaneous Liver Biopsy (76)
Lay title: Needle biopsy of the liver
Obtaining a piece of liver tissue with a needle placed through the skin and into the liver

Spinal Canal Exploration (39)
Surgical exploration of the spinal canal

SURGICAL PROCEDURES

Abdominal Aorta Resection and Replacement (64)
Replacement of the abdominal portion of the *aorta,* with a flexible *graft*

Above-the-knee Amputation (85)
Amputation of the leg at a point above the knee

Aortocoronary Bypass (10, 40, 51, 55)
Lay title: Coronary artery bypass graft (CABG)
Replacement of blocked coronary arteries with transplanted veins or arteries
   Regardless of the number of arteries bypassed, this procedure is essentially the same; therefore, we have combined their ranking in the top 100 procedures.

   Aortocoronary bypass—2 coronary arteries (51)
   Aortocoronary bypass—3 coronary arteries (40)
   Aortocoronary bypass—4 or more coronary arteries (55)
   Aortocoronary bypass— 2-, 3-, and 4-vessel procedures (10)

Appendectomy (8)
Removal of the appendix through a small incision

Below-the-Knee Amputation (87)
Removal of the lower leg below the knee joint

Bilateral Salpingo-Oophorectomy or Salpingo-Ovariectomy (91)
Removal of the ovaries and the *fallopian tubes;* "female castration"

Bilateral Tubal Destruction (98)
Destruction (through nonreversible methods, such as cutting with surgical scissors or using a device to clog and seal the ends) of the *fallopian tubes* to avoid pregnancy

Bilateral Tubal Division (78)
Lay title: Having your tubes tied
Cutting of the *fallopian tubes* for sterility

Cataract Removal with Intraocular Lens Implant
Lay title: Cataract surgery
Surgical removal of a hard opacity of the lens of the eye and implanting an *intraocular* plastic lens

Cervical Cesarean Section (1)
Lay title: C-section
Removal of infant from the womb through an incision in the lower abdomen

Circumcision
Surgical removal of the *prepuce* covering the *glans* of the penis

Closed Fracture Reduction of the Radius and Ulna (79)
Manipulating and splinting or casting of the forearm to fix broken bones in the arm

Closed Fracture Reduction of the Tibia and Fibula (73)
Repair of broken bones of the lower leg by splinting or casting

Closed Reduction and Internal Fixation of Fracture of the Femur (80)
Repair of a fracture of the *femur* with an *internal fixation* device without use of an incision to expose the site of the break

Cruciate Ligament Repair (75)
Repair of the crisscross *ligaments* at the back of the knee

Dialysis Arteriovenostomy (68)
Surgical creation of a direct union of a vein and artery in the wrist, forearm, or thigh as a site for *hemodialysis*

Dilation and Curettage, Postdelivery (28)
Lay title: D&C
Widening of the mouth of the womb and removal of specific areas of the womb lining for therapeutic purposes following the birth of a baby

Endoscopic Colon Polypectomy (92)
Removal of benign or malignant polyps of the colon via a *colonoscope*

Free Skin Graft (94)
Grafting of skin from one location on the body to another to cover wounds where skin is missing, to cover burns, and to aid in the repair of scars

Head And Neck Endarterectomy (33)
Removal of blockages in the arteries of the head and neck

Hemodialysis (27)
Lay title: Kidney dialysis
Use of an artificial kidney machine or of fluid inserted in front of the *peritoneum* to remove waste products and excess minerals from the blood of a person whose kidneys have temporarily or permanently failed

Hemorrhoidectomy (53)
Removal of *prolapsed* veins of the rectum

Incisional Hernia Repair (81)
Repair of a *hernia* that has occurred through a new surgical wound or an old surgical scar

Intercostal Catheter Insertion (13)
Insertion of a small plastic tube between the ribs into the *pleura* for pain relief or under the pleura for relief of *pneumothorax*

Intervertebral Disk Excision (7)
Removal of all or part of the fibrous disk found between the *vertebrae;* may be accompanied by a spinal fusion of two or more vertebrae

Joint Replacement Revision (48)
Revision of the replacement of a natural joint—for example, hip, knee, ankle, shoulder, elbow, or wrist—with a *prosthesis*

Left Hemicolectomy (71)
Removal of the left (descending) half of the *colon*

Ligation and Stripping of Varicose Veins of the Legs (96)
The *ligation* and removal of damaged veins in the legs to avoid clotting, circulatory problems, and ulceration, or to improve cosmetic appearance

Lobectomy of Lung (86)
Removal of one of the three divisions of the lung

Local Destruction of Ovarian Lesion (62)
Destruction of a *lesion* on the ovary without removal of the intact ovary

Local Destruction of Skin Lesion (65)
Destruction of *lesions* of the skin by various methods

Low-Forceps Delivery with Episiotomy (9)
Use of instrument to deliver baby stuck low in the vagina, plus a surgical incision to enlarge the vaginal opening

Medical Induction of Labor (34)
Lay title: Inducing labor
Starting or strengthening labor by the use of chemicals injected and/or applied to the *cervix*

Nephroureterectomy (83)
Removal of a kidney and all or part of a *ureter*

Open Reduction and Internal Fixation of Fracture of the Femur (16)
Repair of a broken leg with an *internal fixation* device

Open Reduction and Internal Fixation of Fracture of the Radius and Ulna (72)
Opening of the forearm to fix broken bones

Open Reduction and Internal Fixation of Fracture of the Tibia and Fibula (22)
Repair of broken bones of the lower leg by the insertion of a device to hold the broken bones together

Partial Small Bowel Resection (67)
Removal of a part of the *small intestine*

Percutaneous Transluminal Coronary Angioplasty (PTCA) (12)
Lay title: Balloon angioplasty
Crushing of *plaque* in an artery with an inflatable balloon inserted into the artery through a *catheter* threaded through the *femoral* or *brachial artery*

Peritoneal Adhesiolysis (35)
Destruction of abnormal tissue connections inside the abdomen that result from inflammatory diseases, injury, or prior surgery

Placement of Central Venous Catheter (23)
Placement of a *catheter* into the *central venous system* of the body, specifically the *superior vena cava* as opposed to the *peripheral venous system*

Removal of Tube and Ectopic Pregnancy (63)
Removal of a *fallopian tube* in which a fertilized egg has implanted itself

Repair of Cystocele or Rectocele (97)
Repair of a *herniation* of the bladder or the rectum into the vaginal vault

Repair of Obstetric Laceration (5)
Repair of tears to the soft tissue of the pelvis following childbirth

Repair of Obstetric Laceration of the Rectum and Anus (50)
Repair of damage to the rectum and anus (anorectal region) occurring during childbirth

Repair of Vessel (70)
Repair of a blood vessel damaged through disease or injury

Revision of Vascular Procedure (69)
Reoperation on a vessel for a repair of other surgery that did not work the first time

Right Hemicolectomy (46)
Removal of the right (ascending) half of the *colon*

Rotator Cuff Repair (89)
Surgical repair of damage to the soft tissues of the shoulder joint

Septoplasty (99)
Repair or revision of the *septum* between the two nostrils

Shoulder Arthroplasty (74)
Resurfacing, repair, or replacement of the shoulder joint

Sigmoidectomy (42)
Removal of the *sigmoid colon*

Skin Lesion: Subsequent Incision and Destruction (41)
Destruction of *lesions* of the skin by various methods after an initial attempt does not produce complete removal

Skin Suture (36)
Lay title: Stitches
Sewing up a wound or incision in the skin

Surgical Repair of Indirect Inguinal Hernia (45)
Surgical Repair of Direct Inguinal Hernia (57)
Surgical Repair of Unilateral Inguinal Hernia (84)
Direct Inguinal Hernia: Surgical repair of a tear in the abdominal wall that allows a loop of intestine to protrude

Indirect Inguinal Hernia: Surgical repair of a tear in the abdominal wall that allows a loop of intestine to slip through the pelvic floor and into the *inguinal canal*

Inguinal hernias are divided into two classes: direct and indirect. The hernia is called direct when a loop of the intestine emerges through a gap or tear in the muscles of the abdominal wall between the deepest-lying artery (the epigastric artery) and the abdominal muscles. The hernia is called indirect when a loop of the intestine slips through a gap or tear in the muscles of the pelvic floor and drops through the inguinal canal and into the scrotum in men or into the analogous area to the left or right of the vagina in women.

The procedure Surgical Repair of Unilateral Inguinal Hernia is just like treatment of direct or indirect hernia, but the term is used for billing purposes when the surgeon fails to specify the hernia as direct or indirect. Its inclusion in the most frequently performed procedures is attributable to a quirk of reimbursement.

Temporary Pacemaker System Insertion (95)
Insertion of wiring and devices for temporary control of heart rate and rhythm

Toe Amputation (77)
Surgical removal of one or more toes (with possible use of the toes to replace fingers lost to trauma)

Tonsillectomy (52)
Removal of lymph nodes at the back of the throat that, when swollen due to repeated infections, can cause various problems such as recurrent infections

Tonsillectomy and Adenoidectomy (11)
Removal of lymph nodes at the back and top of the throat that, when swollen due to repeated infections, can cause various problems such as recurrent infections

Total Abdominal Hysterectomy (3)
Lay title: Hysterectomy
Removal of the uterus through an incision low in the abdomen. This procedure involves removal of the uterus and is to be distinguished from hysterectomy that includes removal of the ovaries and tubes, technically called a hysterectomy and salpingo-oophorectomy.

Total Cholecystectomy (2)
Gallbladder removal

Total Hip Replacement (37)
Replacement of the hip socket and upper portion of the *femur* with metal and plastic prosthetic parts

Total Knee Replacement (24)
Replacement of the knee with an artificial joint

Transurethral Destruction of Bladder Lesion (15)
Examination of the inside of the bladder through a *cystoscope* or resectoscope inserted through the *urethra* and destruction of abnormal tissue by cutting, *electrocautery,* or laser beam

Transurethral Removal of Ureter Obstruction (54)
Insertion of a thin tube into the *ureters* to remove an obstruction

Transurethral Resection of the Prostate (6)
Lay title: TURP
Removal of a portion of the prostate gland by means of a *cystoscope*

Unilateral External Simple Mastectomy (25)
Removal of a single breast without removal of underlying muscle or lymph nodes

Unilateral Salpingo-Oophorectomy or Salpingo-Ovariectomy (60)
Removal of a single ovary and *fallopian tube*

Unilateral Thyroid Lobectomy (88)
Removal of one of the two lobes of the thyroid gland

Ureteral Catheterization (100)
Insertion of a thin tube into the one or both of the *ureters*

Ureteral catheterization is the all-encompassing name for any procedure that consists of inserting a *catheter* through the urethra, into the bladder, and into one or both of the ureters.

Uterine Lesion Destruction (93)
Destruction of a *lesion* in or on the uterus by various means

Vacuum Extraction Delivery with Episiotomy (19)
Use of a suction instrument to deliver a baby stuck low in the vagina, after making a surgical incision to enlarge the vaginal opening

Vaginal Hysterectomy (21)
Removal of the uterus through the vaginal opening without an abdominal incision

Vascular Shunt and Bypass (31)
Rerouting of a blood or fluid flow within the body to relieve circulatory problems, accumulation of fluid, etc.

Virtually any circulatory system disorder, whether *congenital* or acquired, can be corrected by surgically rerouting the vessels causing the problem.

Wound Debridement and Excision (20)
Removal of dead tissue and restructuring of wounds to allow closure, reduce scarring, and lessen the chance of infection

Glossary for "100 Most Commonly Performed Operations"

Aorta—the body's primary artery that receives blood from the heart's left ventricle and distributes it to the body.

Brachial artery—the major artery in the arm.

Bronchial tree—tubes, composed of fibrous, elastic rings, that run off the windpipe and divide in two, with one running to each lung, just above the top of the heart.

Catheter—a thin, flexible plastic tube that can be placed inside some part of the body; for example, a Foley catheter, which is used to drain urine from the bladder.

Central venous system—large veins of the trunk of the body (thorax and abdomen).

Cervix—mouth of the uterus.

Colon—the part of the large intestine that extends to the rectum.

Colonoscope—a flexible fiber-optic instrument inserted through the anus to examine the large intestine from the anus to the cecum (the first part of the large intestine).

Congenital—present at birth.

Contrast medium—a solution of iodine compounds that block X rays; often called a dye or radiopaque dye.

Cystoscope—a rigid instrument with a viewing lens and light source that is used to view the urethra and bladder. Inserted through the urethra, the cystoscope may also be used to obtain urine and tissue samples.

Duodenum—first part of the small intestine just below the stomach.

Electrocautery—the use of electric current to seal blood vessels by heat and, thus, stop bleeding.

Emboli—a solid particle, usually a fragment of clotted blood or a fatty deposit, carried along in the bloodstream.

Endoscope—a rigid or flexible tube that is used to look inside of a body cavity or organ.

Esophagus—the tube from the mouth to the stomach.

Fallopian tubes—paired structures that carry eggs from the ovaries to the uterus.

Femoral artery—the major artery in the thigh.

Femur—the thighbone.

Fiber-optic scope—a thin, flexible tube containing bundles of glass filaments that can transmit light around bends and curves to illuminate the inside of the body. Forceps, scissors, or other tiny instruments can be threaded through channels in some scopes, to facilitate surgical procedures.

Glans—the head of the penis.

Graft—any tissue or organ for implantation or transplantation.

Hemodialysis—the use of a machine to cleanse the blood in a patient whose kidneys have failed.

Hernia—the protrusion of an organ or part of an organ through a muscular wall that usually supports it.

Herniation—the abnormal protrusion of an organ or other body part through a defect or natural opening in a membrane covering muscles or bone.

Inguinal canal—a canal containing two rings of fibrous tissue located in the groin in both men and women; in men, where the spermatic cord passes out of the abdomen into the scrotum, supporting the testicles, vas deferens (tubes that carry sperm from the testicles to the seminal vesicles), and blood vessels; in women, where the round ligament of the uterus leaves the abdomen to connect with the labium majus.

Internal fixation—the use of plate, nails, screws, wires, or some combination thereof in the repair of a broken bone.

Intraocular—within the eye.

Lesion—an abnormal growth or localized condition, such as a tumor, wart, or cyst.

Ligament—strong fibrous tissue that connects a bone to another bone.

Peripheral venous system—veins of the limbs and head of the body.

Peritoneum—the transparent covering of the organs that lies just behind the muscular wall of the abdomen.

Pleura—the membrane surrounding the lungs.

Pneumothorax—air in the chest cavity that can cause lung collapse.

Prepuce—the foreskin of the penis.

Prolapse—the slippage of a body part from its normal position.

Prosthesis—an artificial body part.

Resurfacing—planing off any bone spurs or protrusions to create a very smooth surface for repair or replacement of joints.

Revision—a surgical alteration performed to reverse a previous surgery.

Septum—generally refers to a dividing wall or partition, such as the nasal septum, that separates the nasal cavities.

Sigmoid colon—lower portion of the large intestine just above the rectum; it looks like an angular "S."

Sigmoidoscope—a rigid or flexible tube inserted through the anus to examine the sigmoid colon (the S-shaped portion of the colon just above the rectum). The rigid sigmoidoscope is a lighted tube about 12 inches long and 1 inch in diameter. The flexible sigmoidoscope employs fiber optics and is about 2 feet long.

Small intestine—the part of the digestive tract concerned with the digestion of food and the absorption of food into the bloodstream.

Superior vena cava—a major vein that drains blood from the head, neck, upper extremities, and chest and returns it to the right atrium of the heart.

Ureters—tubes that carry the urine from the kidneys to the bladder.

Urethra—the tube through which urine is excreted from the bladder.

Vertebrae—bones that make up the spinal column.

High-Risk Surgical Procedures

There is probably no word that evokes more fear than "surgery." And the first fearful thought most people have after hearing the word is "Am I going to die?"

Modern medicine has come a long way since the turn of the century when surgical death rates made dying from an operation as likely as surviving one. Today only 1 out of every 75 persons dies as a direct result of all surgery performed. (The exact rate is 1.33 percent.) The percentage of people who die during or as a direct result of an operation is termed the mortality rate. The eighteen surgical procedures, or operations, discussed below have a mortality rate of 1.33 percent or greater.

Yet overall mortality rates are of little significance to you who must deal with one operation. Of importance to you is the mortality rate for the procedure you are contemplating and what factors increase or decrease those percentages.

For each procedure, we discuss the mortality rate and the factors that affect it. We also discuss the morbidity rate (rate of complications)—but more on that later. For now let's concentrate on how to assess your chances of surviving a surgical procedure.

The mortality rates associated with the procedure are calculated on the total number of procedures performed. For example, the procedure Closed Reduction and Internal Fixation of Fracture of the Femur (surgical repair of a broken leg) has a mortality rate of 3.7 percent based on 28,000 procedures studied. That translates into 1,036 deaths resulting from the procedure or 1 death for every 27 procedures performed. The important point to consider is the percentage of deaths, rather than the actual numbers. The percentage gives you a much better perspective on what your survival chances are. Thus, in this case your chance of surviving the operation is 96.3 percent.

As you will find as you review each operation, certain factors may raise the overall mortality rate. Depending on the procedure, age may be a factor. In other instances, other medical conditions that you might have may lower your chances of survival.

Therefore, it is important to not only read this part carefully but also assess (and discuss with your doctor) your overall condition as compared to the points noted in the discussion.

Mortality is not the only hazard facing consumers considering surgery. There is also the prospect of complications—conditions that develop as a result of the procedure—some of which may be life-threatening. The rate at which these complicating factors occurs is called the morbidity rate. It, too, is expressed as a percentage.

While there are standard definitions of what a complication is, there are no standards for what is major, minor, or countable. Thus, a very meticulous study of one set of practitioners that looks at every event that extends the hospital stay or increases the cost of care could report a very high complication rate, while a sloppy study that counts only events that ultimately led to a bad outcome could report a very low one.

It is well understood among medical researchers that wide variations in surgical outcomes and complications associated with specific surgical procedures are fairly routine. Work conducted by Dartmouth Medical School professor Jack Wennberg, M.D., and studies conducted by the Pennsylvania Council on Health Care Cost Containment (both have done extensive studies on variations in mortality and morbidity rates) indicate that there is at least two standard deviations' difference between doctors in the same hospital. Translated into common English: If the mean mortality rate for a particular procedure per doctor is 5 percent and the standard deviation is 5 percent, this would allow for a mortality rate range of zero to 15 percent.

CALCULATING YOUR RISK

With all that said, how do you translate the numbers and percentages you will find in each of the operations covered below? In other words, how do you calculate your risk of death or complications?

It is important that you understand the combined risks of mortality and morbidity. Keep in mind that as the percentage increases, so does your risk. Obviously, your risk is lower as the percentage decreases. As noted earlier, the overall mortality rate for all surgical procedures is calculated to be 1.33 percent. That, as we said before, means that 1 death occurs for every 75 surgical procedures. Nationally, there are some 30 million surgical procedures performed in hospitals each year resulting in 400,000 deaths.

The following table will help you translate the mortality and morbidity percentages associated with procedures described here. The percentages are found in the left-hand column and your risk is listed in the right-hand column.

Percentage	Your Risk
100%	1 out of 1
50	1 out of 2
25	1 out of 4
10	1 out of 10
5	1 out of 20
4	1 out of 25
3	1 out of 33
2	1 out of 50
1	1 out of 100
.75	1 out of 133
.60	1 out of 166
.50	1 out of 200
.40	1 out of 250
.25	1 out of 400
.20	1 out of 500
.15	1 out of 666
.10	1 out of 1,000

To calculate a risk from a percentage not shown:
1. Put the percentage in decimal form (always move the decimal point two places to the left). For example, 1.33 percent becomes .0133.
2. Next, divide the decimal into the number 1. In the case described, it would be 1 divided by .0133. Your answer will be expressed as a whole number. In this case, the answer is 75.

Two final notes to help you better use this presentation: In many of the procedures, we note a risk related to the use of general anesthesia. Because the risk is the same regardless of the procedure, we have included the *anesthesia risk* explanation in the glossary at the end of this part. The glossary also defines terms that are italicized in our discussions.

Finally, be sure to keep risks in perspective. Many people who die as a result of surgery may have been so ill that their likelihood of surviving was minimal to begin with. The same applies to complications.

Remember that your condition and situation are unique; The mortality and morbidity statistics presented here should only be used as a guide. For your own peace of mind, ask your surgeon to discuss his or her individual mortality and morbidity statistics for the procedure you are having.

18 HIGH-RISK SURGICAL PROCEDURES

The following diagnostic and surgical procedures fall into a high-risk category because their mortality rates exceed the national average of 1.33 percent for all operations.

Abdominal Aorta Resection and Replacement
Replacement of the abdominal portion of the *aorta* with a flexible *graft*

Mortality (Death) and Morbidity (Complication) Rates
Mortality rates as low as 2% to 5% are reported regularly, but there is considerable variation in the results depending upon the age of the patient, seriousness of the condition, whether the operation is elective or emergency, and what technique is used. Complication rates as low as zero have been reported.

About one-third of patients whose grafts were examined by *ultrasonography* on several occasions following surgery showed incipient major or minor problems, suggesting a complication rate of about 33%.

A 1989 study of the use of a sutureless, ringed *prosthesis* for the aorta showed that the portion of the operation when blood supply to the lower body was cut off took only 17 minutes and had a mortality rate of 6% (due to heart attacks) and a zero complication rate. A 1990 study with the same device showed a mortality rate of 8%, with a restricted flow time of only 9 minutes. The authors of this study recommend that surgeons use sutureless, ringed grafts, because they can be inserted quickly. In contrast, the careful and minute suturing required for the sutured grafts consumes most of the surgeon's time. Speed is essential because surgery on the aorta requires cutting off the blood supply to the lower body, which can result in kidney or nerve damage.

As with many other operations, the mortality rate is vastly higher for emergency than for elective procedures. An Israeli study showed a 4.6% mortality rate for elective replacements and a 45.2% mortality rate in emergency operations. A German study found 50% mortality for emergency operations.

Replacement of an infected aortic replacement graft has an operative mortality rate of 10% and an additional mortality of 15% within the first year. The 85% of patients who survive the first year have no further problems. The traditional operation for infected aortic grafts requires complete removal of the graft and a bypass operation to establish an alternate flow channel for the arterial blood, rather than graft replacement. This operation results in a high rate of loss of one or both legs due to restricted circulation to the lower body during excessively long operations. The direct replacement operation described above resulted in no leg loss in one study.

Use of a rigid, sutureless graft—made of Dacron woven over metal, either titanium or Vitallium—has an early postoperative mortality rate of 11.25% and a late mortality rate (within an average follow-up of about two years) of 6%. About 40% of patients will require some further suturing of the aorta when this device is used.

Complications and Possible Side Effects
About 7.3% of patients will require replacement of a tube graft within an average follow-up period of about four and a half years.

Obstruction of the *ureter* or ureters where a Dacron tube graft crosses it is a possible but uncommon complication. Whether a patient is at risk for it depends on the patient's anatomy and the positioning of the graft. Only about 3.1% of patients who are at risk for this complication will actually develop it. Whether the Dacron graft is passed over or under the ureter seems to make no difference.

While misdiagnosis is not, strictly speaking, a complication, the discovery of an *aneurysm* of the thoracic aorta, which is the part in the chest above the *diaphragm,* strongly points to the possibility of abdominal aortic disease, and patients who have a tho-

racic aorta problem should have full aorta studies to make sure that there are no problems in the abdomen.

Paralysis of the lower body can occur if the blood supply to the spine is destroyed, but this can be avoided by proper surgical technique. Some surgeons construct a temporary blood supply to the kidneys and use electronic monitoring of electrical activity in the spine to avoid complications; others rely on speed of operation to avoid them. Although the complicated procedure of constructing a temporary blood supply seems logical, this increases operating time, which exposes the patient to greater risk.

As with any procedure in which anesthesia is used, death from reaction to the anesthetic drugs, error on the part of the anesthetist, or machine failure is a remote possibility.

Above-the-Knee Amputation
Amputation of the leg at a point above the knee

Mortality (Death) and Morbidity
(Complication) Rates
As with some other procedures presented in this section, many of the conditions that require the surgery can in themselves be fatal. The mortality rate following amputation for trauma is about 2.3%. Another series of patients without trauma were found to have an operative mortality rate of 15% and two-year postoperative mortality of an additional 26%. Causes of death were *sepsis* in 54%, heart disease in 16%, and stroke in 11%. All of the patients in this series required above-the-knee amputation for various systemic diseases, such as diabetes, that cause vascular problems.

Burn patients who have above-the-knee amputations of both legs as a result of concomitant trauma—albeit a rare occurrence—have a mortality rate of 33%.

Mortality is higher after failed *thromboembolectomy* and for infection that cannot be controlled with antibiotics.

An artificial blood vessel *graft* may be used to repair traumatically damaged vessels as part of an amputation procedure or may be used to increase blood flow in an attempt to avoid amputations. In either case, it can be a source of blood clots that block nearby arteries and veins. A 1976 study using a mathematical model predicted greater success using vein transplants from other parts of the body rather than artificial materials. Current materials—for example, polytetrafluoroethylene and Dacron—have a better record, but 45% still show blockage four years after the operation.

A study in the late 1980s of World War II veterans who had above-the-knee amputations during the war found that 5.8% of them had abdominal aortic *aneurysms,* a condition marked by ballooning of the *aorta,* which can rupture with fatal results, compared with 1.1% of veterans with two good legs. The change in blood flow that accompanies above-the-knee amputation appears to alter the circulatory pattern in a way that causes aneurysms in some people.

Measures of the energy expenditure required to walk with a prosthesis for an above-the-knee amputation indicate that it is much more difficult than walking with a below-the-knee prosthesis or with two good legs. This is one reason for a surgeon to try to save the knee if at all possible. A high level of physical fitness is required to use an above-the-knee prosthesis successfully.

Well-engineered, newer artificial legs can reduce the energy demand required for walking by about 50% with improvements in gait and walking speed. An artificial leg has been developed that is better for jogging than the usual artificial leg, designed primarily for walking. However, it is regarded as needing improvement. Designing the ideal artificial limb continues to present problems because there are many variables to consider, such as the normal gait of the person; the amount of pressure put on the socket as the person shifts weight; and the general condition of the stump relative to blood flow and health of the tissue. Attempts have been made to write computer programs that take these variables into account, so that artificial limbs may be better designed; however, preliminary studies have shown that the use of such computer-aided design and manufacturing techniques did not result in an artificial limb notably superior to conventional manufacturing methods.

Problems have also arisen with "robotized" artificial limbs that use computers and an elaborate system of motors to create the walking motion. Researchers have discovered the difficulty of creating an artificial limb that responds to twitching of the thigh muscle or contraction of the buttocks and produces a normal gait. They also discovered that going from one mode (straight-level walking) to another (going up an incline) can produce problems for the computer system. Further research is needed to determine how best to match patient and computer system.

As with virtually all surgery of the lower body, *pulmonary embolism* is a possibility.

The risk of amputation for patients who have an infected knee prosthesis is about 4%.

Seventy-two percent of patients have "phantom limb" pain, in which pain is felt in the missing part of the limb, or stump pain.

Complications and Possible Side Effects
Unrecognized damage to vessels has been reported. This may lead to further surgery.

A poorly fitted prosthesis can result in a noncancerous skin condition resembling Kaposi's sarcoma.

As with any procedure in which anesthesia is used, death from reaction to the anesthetic drugs, error on the part of the anesthetist, or machine failure is a remote possibility.

Aortocoronary Bypass
Replacement of blocked coronary arteries with transplanted veins or arteries

Mortality (Death) and Morbidity (Complication) Rates
Mortality for this procedure has steadily fallen since its invention, and current (1990–91) literature notes that overall operative mortality of zero to 3% can be achieved with current techniques. Based on a review of some 400 articles from the National Library of Medicine database, this rate of 1% to 3% reflects the results with carefully selected patients in the best centers. Five-year survival following surgery, even in patients over 65, can be as high as 96.9%. As with all surgeries, mortality rises with age, with the number and severity of coexisting diseases, and with the presence of any medical problems that are likely to cause problems with anesthesia. One 1990 study dealing with emergency bypasses found 14.5% *operative mortality* and 35.9% *major morbidity* (for example, the breastbone does not show signs of healing or there is infection of the sac that surrounds the heart); operative mortality was 4% for those taken directly to the operating room from the cardiac catheterization suite and 22.4% for those who had to be taken to the operating room from a general ward or the intensive care unit. Results in other series range between these two extremes. Mortality increased with the number of vessels replaced.

Major complications include problems with sternal (breastbone) wounds, which occurred in 1.1% of patients in a study covering 1985–87. Of those who had sternal wound problems, 14.1% died of multiorgan failure; the presence of bacteria in cultures of the sternal wound was an indication of a stormy course, even if the patient lived. Other problems include various cardiac complications, which can be expected in about 18% of patients both over and under age 70; patients over age 70 can expect noncardiac complications to occur in 31% of cases. One study comparing patients under and over age 70 found *perioperative* heart attacks in 4.1% and 7.9% of patients respectively; a need for prolonged respiratory support in 3.1% and 7.9%; and major neurologic complications in 1.1% and 4%. (Examples of major neurologic complications include stroke resulting from fat clots in the brain and brain damage due to lack of oxygen.)

Complications and Possible Side Effects
In addition to the usual surgical risks, depression following cardiac surgery is somewhat more severe than that following other surgeries, and about 16% to 31% of those operated on display mild to severe psychiatric symptoms. Very extensive pre- and postsurgical testing in one study indicated that about 11% of patients will fail to recover fully from the effects of cardiac surgery on the nervous system. Postoperative depression, especially in the elderly, is a persistent finding; however, it seems to respond well to standard pharmacological treatment for depression.

The cause of cognitive impairments following cardiac surgery is unknown; one theory is that patients suffer "microstrokes" from clots released from the walls of arteries and veins while the cardiac bypass machine is in use. The machine reverses the usual direction of blood flow, and this may create turbulence that releases tiny *emboli* from the vessel walls. Other theories point to alternating sensory deprivation and sensory overload in the cardiac intensive care unit, and the patient's having to face the extreme seriousness of his or her medical situation and the possibility of death. Most patients recover fully, but the full impact of mental health problems following coronary artery bypass grafting is unknown.

Stroke during or immediately following the operation has been rising, from about .57% to 2.4% over the five-year period 1979–83, largely due to the increasing age of patients being operated on. A 1988 study showed a risk of 2.9% for patients who had a prior history of stroke and had general anesthesia for any surgery. In yet another study, for patients with diagnosis of severe *carotid artery* narrowing, the risk of stroke was 9.2% versus 1.9% for those without severe narrowing. Other studies have found stroke rates in the 2.4% range as well, and have found that this probability of stroke correlates very highly with increasing age of those having CABG.

Several risk factors, none of them significantly avoidable or modifiable by either patient or physician, have been identified. *Carotid bruits* raise the risk to 2.9% for having a stroke during or immediately after the surgery, a risk not dramatically greater than the overall risk of 2.4% found in several studies. Depending upon the size of the clot, the region of the brain affected, and the speed and competence of poststroke therapy, the consequences of perioperative stroke can range from trivial to devastating.

Below-the-Knee Amputation
Removal of the lower leg below the knee joint

Mortality (Death) and Morbidity (Complication) Rates
The mortality rate for two different techniques of constructing stumps was 11% and 17% for the two methods in a 1991 controlled trial. Not statistically significant, the difference suggests that mortality rates around 14% are to be expected. About 5% of cases have complications serious enough to require above-the-knee amputation. In patients over age 80, problems with healing of the stump flaps can be expected in about 10% of cases. Seventy-two percent of patients have "phantom limb" pain, in which pain is felt in the missing part of the limb, or stump pain.

Complication rates recently cited for joint replacement surgery are broadly applicable to most lower-limb surgery: 40% to 70% risk of deep venous thrombosis without anticlotting treatment; 2% to 16% risk of nonfatal *pulmonary embolism;* and 1.8% to 3.4% risk of fatal pulmonary embolism. Various courses of treatment with anticlotting drugs can reduce these risks appreciably.

Complications and Possible Side Effects
Injury to the vessels in the region of the knee can occur, and can be serious but unrecognized at the time

of operation. When the injury is discovered, vessel repair operations are possible.

As with any procedure in which anesthesia is used, death from reaction to the anesthetic drugs, error on the part of the anesthetist, or machine failure is a remote possibility.

Bone Marrow Biopsy
Removal of marrow from the central channel of a bone for study to assist in the treatment of various serious diseases

Mortality (Death) and Morbidity (Complication) Rates
Data drawn from the Commission on Professional and Hospital Activities (CPHA), which include a large sample of U.S. hospitals, show a mortality rate of 7.7% for patients having this procedure. This very high figure reflects the fact that serious underlying diseases, most often cancer, lead to the need for the bone marrow biopsy in the first place. Aplastic anemia, for example, has a 38% mortality rate when treated without bone marrow transplant, and the mortality rate for some leukemias is 50% within two years of diagnosis.

A multiyear study of more than 1,000 patients found zero mortality and minor complications in .2% of patients. Failure to obtain adequate specimens that were apparent to the surgeon at the time of operation occurred in 1.6% of the cases, and later discovery by the laboratory that a specimen was unsuitable occurred in 5% of the cases, meaning that 6.6% of procedures had to be repeated.

Complications and Possible Side Effects
Although infections are not a direct risk of bone marrow biopsy (as opposed to the conditions and treatments for which bone marrow biopsy is a diagnostic step), they can be devastating in patients who have had bone marrow transplants. Frequent use of antibiotics and failure to maintain the patients in laminar flow rooms are both associated with increased infections in these patients. (Laminar flow rooms are those in which the airflow is controlled to prevent the entry of airborne bacteria.) The patient's immune system recovers within about a year if the transplant is successful.

As with any procedure in which anesthesia is used, death from reaction to the anesthetic drugs, error on the part of the anesthetist, or machine failure is a remote possibility.

Closed Reduction and Internal Fixation of Fracture of the Femur
Repair of a fracture of the *femur* with an *internal fixation* device without use of an incision to expose the site of the break

Mortality (Death) and Morbidity (Complication) Rates
Closed intermedullary nailing (the use of rods or nails placed in the bone, or wires and screws placed across the bone to assure proper alignment) produces a 6-week mortality rate of 3.7% and an 8-month rate of 10.4%, with a 2.3% shifting of the bones at the fracture site, a complication that necessitates reoperation. In patients over age 65, use of a sliding plate and screws produces a one-year mortality rate of 25% and a one-year reoperation rate of 25%. Later results with another type of intermedullary nail that locks to prevent rotation of the broken ends of the bone resulted in no mortality and roughly a 33% complication rate.

Complications and Possible Side Effects
As with all lower-limb procedures, *pulmonary embolism* can occur in up to 5% of patients. Closed procedures, which do not involve cutting tissues, seem to produce a lower rate of infection than open procedures, but total mortality and total morbidity for the two procedures are similar.

As with any procedure in which anesthesia is used, death from reaction to the anesthetic drugs, error on the part of the anesthetist, or machine failure is a remote possibility.

Exploratory Laparotomy
Opening the abdomen to explore the contents when other diagnostic methods have failed or are not applicable

Mortality (Death) and Morbidity (Complication) Rates
Reported mortality rates range from 2.58% to 16% for trauma patients at first laparotomy, to 40% for trauma patients at repeat laparotomy, to 86% at repeat laparotomy for patients over age 65.

The medical literature clearly indicates that initial and repeat laparotomies are very different entities. Second laparotomies that are attempts to find a focus of infection in patients with *intraabdominal sepsis* and that are not directed by positive clinical findings—second laparotomies that are "fishing expeditions"—have a 93% mortality rate.

Exploratory laparotomy for gunshot wounds of the abdomen has a 2.7% mortality rate if major arteries or veins were not injured, and a 39.2% mortality rate if major vascular structures were injured. An incidental finding was that the heroic effort of emergency resuscitative *thoracotomy* was successful in only 10% of the patients on whom it was attempted. The most common postoperative complication was *abscess* formation, which occurred in 3% of patients. The seriousness of the patients with vascular injuries is perhaps best indicated by the fact that 50% of them required more than eighteen units of blood.

Mortality from exploratory laparoscopy rises with age, primarily because of the increased susceptibility of the elderly to infection and their inability to recover from the surgery as well as younger patients do. Mortality for second laparotomies in patients over age 65 is 86%, versus 21% for those under age 65. For patients who had signs of organ failure prior to second laparotomy, the mean survival following the procedure was 4 days for patients both over and under 65 years.

Repeat exploratory laparotomy to determine the stage of disease and the response to treatment has very low mortality in patients with Hodgkin's disease. Even so, a special analysis indicates that in hospitals with a 1% mortality rate for laparotomies on patients with Hodgkin's, the operation is too risky for 1 in 7 patients—and in institutions with a 3% mortality, too risky for 1 in 3. This means that it is unwise to perform even the safer variations in most hospitals.

Exploratory laparotomy for lymphogranulomatosis has essentially a zero mortality rate and a 13.2% complication rate.

Emergency first laparotomy for cancer patients receiving chemotherapy and *corticosteroids* who develop intestinal perforations has a mortality rate of 53% and a major complication rate of 50%.

Complications and Possible Side Effects
Misdiagnosis can be a devastating "complication." A study of thirty-six patients who were referred for exploratory laparotomy for undiagnosable liver disease showed that 100% of them had been misdiagnosed and that the correct diagnosis could have been made from information recorded in the history and physical in thirty-one of them, and from additional laboratory

testing in the other five. The thirty-six patients had a 31% mortality rate and a 61% complication rate.

Rupture of the abdominal wound occurs in .6% of all laparotomies and has a mortality rate of 34%. Necrotizing fasciitis (a condition in which the fascia, the tough tissue containing the muscles, is destroyed) is a rare but devastating infectious complication that may require reconstruction of the entire abdominal wall if the patient is to live.

As with any procedure in which anesthesia is used, death from reaction to the anesthetic drugs, error on the part of the anesthetist, or machine failure is a remote possibility.

Head and Neck Endarterectomy
Removal of blockages in the arteries of the head and neck

Mortality (Death) and Morbidity (Complication) Rates
As of 1989, mortality for this procedure in community hospitals was 2.8%. The risk of stroke during an endarterectomy is 1.6%.

Nerve damage is apparently much more common than usually thought. One British study found a 25% incidence of vocal cord nerve palsy, or incomplete paralysis, and damage to the transverse cervical nerves of the neck in 69% of patients, although there was some recovery of function over a 6-month follow-up period. The same rate of injury to the vocal nerves was found in another study.

Following this procedure, 48% of patients develop vascular headache syndromes, which are induced by trauma to the veins in the neck, the pain of which can be severe enough to lead patients to attempt suicide during attacks. The fact that 100% of these patients have the pain on the operated side suggests that the procedure causes hidden injury to the vessels on that side of the head.

Complications and Possible Side Effects
Hematomas are a rare but potentially lethal complication of this procedure, because they can produce pressure on the arteries sufficient to cause a stroke. (The rate of hematomas is 1.9%.) They can be treated easily, under a local anesthetic, by evacuation, or drainage, with a small incision.

Massive swelling of the neck has also been reported.

Airway obstruction requiring emergency treatment can develop in up to 40% of patients who have this procedure following radiation treatment for cancers of the head and neck.

As with any procedure in which anesthesia is used, death from reaction to the anesthetic drugs, error on the part of the anesthetist, or machine failure is a remote possibility.

Hemodialysis (Kidney dialysis)

Use of an artificial kidney machine or of fluid inserted in front of the *peritoneum* to remove waste products and excess minerals from the blood of a person whose kidneys have temporarily or permanently failed

Mortality (Death) and Morbidity (Complication) Rates

As with many other surgeries, mortality rates vary widely with age and other health problems. The bad news is that for all patients on any form of dialysis, the annual mortality rate seems to be about 14% per year. The good news is that, for dialysis patients with no problems other than kidney failure, the survival curves (life expectancy measures of the probability of death, adjusted for age) are no worse than for the overall population of the United States as of 1990. The key to age-adjusted tables, in this instance, is that (all things being equal) a person on dialysis with proper medical care statistically could enjoy a life span equal to the general population.

A 1990 study indicates that 90% of dialysis patients without complications survive at least three years of dialysis, for a mortality rate of 10%. In the patients in whom complications develop, the three-year survival rate is 60%—for a three-year mortality rate of 40%. For all patients, the one-year survival rate is 73% to 79%—depending on the condition that produced kidney failure—and the one-year mortality rate is 27% to 21% accordingly. A study of patients using continuous ambulatory peritoneal dialysis found 12-, 24-, 36-, and 43-month survival rates of 90% at 12 months, 80% at 24 months, 70% at 36 months, and 70% at 43 months; mortality appeared to stabilize at 30% after 43 months.

As with many other surgical procedures, mortality rates are lower for younger patients. A study of children on dialysis found survival rates of 100% at 6 months and 95% at five years for hemodialysis; 92% at 6 months and five years for kidney transplants from living related donors; and 88% at 6 months and 85% at five years for kidney transplants from corpses.

Thus, the mortality rates at five years were 5% for hemodialysis, 8% for kidney transplants from living related donors, and 15% for kidney transplants from corpses.

Being on dialysis is associated with a higher than normal surgical mortality rate. For elective procedures (other than dialysis), the mortality and morbidity rates in a group of dialysis patients over a seven-year period were 6% and 12%, and 47% and 62% for emergency procedures. Even so, appropriate surgical correction of problems—for example, repair of a broken leg, removal of a cataract, or removal of a tumor—can lead to longer survival and a better quality of life.

The mortality rate for dialysis patients is likely to increase substantially in the future because of changes in the patient populations accepted for dialysis. Contrary to past practice, it is now customary to start extremely ill patients on dialysis. Indeed, one 1990 study found that almost all of the increase in dialysis mortality seen in recent years was due to acceptance of sicker patients. The overall mortality rate for dialysis is also highly sensitive to the age distribution of the patients: One-year survival is 95.1% for patients aged 15 to 24 but only 52.5% for patients over the age of 85. Diabetics and whites generally have worse survival rates than other classes of patients. Five-year survival on dialysis for all patients is about 41%.

Morbidity of one sort or another is common in patients on dialysis. As a result of distressing complications (discussed below), voluntary withdrawals from treatment accounted for 9% of all deaths of dialysis patients and 12% of deaths in patients aged 65 or over in 1988. There is a high correlation between paper-and-pencil scales of patient functioning and quality of life and probability of death; those who show the lowest quality of life on the paper-and-pencil tests are most likely to die. (A paper-and-pencil test is a questionnaire in order to gain a psychological profile of a person, to determine any psychological and physical limitations under which the person lives.)

Much of the short-term morbidity, which may resolve at the end of treatment or shortly thereafter, is related to the inability of dialysis equipment to respond rapidly enough to changes in the patient's blood composition to prevent large and rapid swings in the concentration of water, *electrolytes,* and other substances in the patient's blood. Even when rapid control over one or two elements is possible, only about 50% of patients fit the simple mathematical models that would allow the equipment to be programmed to respond properly.

Common dialysis-associated problems include cramps, low blood pressure, problems with access sites, and reactions to first use of the dialyzer membrane. Dialysis prescriptions (combination of chemicals in the dialysate, time on the machine, and use of pressure filtration) that reduce the average blood urea nitrogen, or BUN (a measure of waste products in the blood), as low as possible are associated with lower morbidity.

As you might expect, some data suggest that poor nutritional status and low protein intake are associated with higher probability of death while on dialysis. Some doctors prefer to restrict protein intake to control *uremia,* but it appears that this approach can be overdone and actually can contribute to mortality. One study suggests that inadequate protein intake is associated with an 81.8% increase (from 4.4% to 8%) in mortality when dialysis patients were compared with an otherwise similar group who had adequate protein intake and adequate dialysis. For at least some patients on hemodialysis, malnutrition is clearly the chief cause of morbidity and mortality.

A study conducted by the Institute of Medicine, a branch of the National Academy of Sciences, found indications that mortality among dialysis patients has also been increasing as a result of cuts in federal payments for dialysis: The cuts have led to shorter treatment times and thus to a greater buildup of waste products in the blood of dialysis patients. Treatment times shorter than 3.5 hours per session were associated with an increase in mortality. Another study, however, found that reduction in treatment time from an average of 17 hours to 2.7 hours was not associated with any increase in mortality, provided that concentrations of breakdown products in the blood were kept constant and not allowed to rise with shorter treatments. Another study found no increase in mortality when treatment times were shortened to 3 hours.

Complications and Possible Side Effects
Other than kidney disease itself, the major cause of morbidity and mortality among dialysis patients is circulatory problems of one sort or another, usually resulting in atherosclerotic heart disease and stroke. The kidneys have a complicated role in the mainte-

nance of blood pressure and blood chemistry, and it has proven impossible to exert total control over blood pressure in some patients on dialysis. Uncontrolled high blood pressure is associated with a higher rate of heart disease and stroke.

The major cause of morbidity among patients on peritoneal dialysis is infection. *Peritonitis* can be devastating and carries with it a high mortality rate. Careful attention to sterile technique can reduce the incidence of infection to about one episode per 18 months.

In two cases reported in the medical literature, *cerebral edema* occurred after patients with the bacterial infection leptospirosis were put on dialysis. This resulted in death for one patient and partial paralysis for the other.

Accumulation of aluminum in bone, which is found in about 50% of dialysis patients, is strongly associated with increased morbidity and mortality. It is unclear whether this is a result of the kidney condition, a doctor-caused problem associated with dialysis (such as the dialysate not mixed properly to sufficiently filter aluminum, or the use of aluminum-coated tubs for water filtration), or the procedure's failure to exactly duplicate kidney function. Both dialysis and uremia are associated with bone disorders.

Ascites can also occur, with either dialysis method. This can usually be relieved by a form of dialysis called ultrafiltration or by implanting a *shunt* that drains peritoneal fluid into a vein via a one-way valve.

As of 1990, about 42% of patients on dialysis showed evidence of infection with hepatitis, even if they did not develop the full-blown disease. It is unclear to what degree this is related to treatment-acquired infection or transfer of antibodies in the many blood transfusions required by dialysis patients.

Psychiatric complications are common in both transplant and dialysis patients—46% of transplant patients and 48% of dialysis patient were found to have at least some evidence of psychiatric problems. Another study found a 33% rate of psychiatric complications among patients undergoing dialysis. Depression while on dialysis is strongly associated with a higher probability of death.

An associated complication of sorts is the labeling by dialysis-unit staff of some patients as sicker, or more problematic. Indeed, one study suggests that, to some extent, such labeling is a self-fulfilling prophecy, because it may lead to poorer care for patients whose conditions are perceived to be worse, even if this perception is inaccurate.

Left Hemicolectomy
Removal of the left (descending) half of the *colon*

Mortality (Death) and Morbidity (Complication) Rates
This is not a trivial procedure. Mortality is low in patients who are being operated on under ideal conditions. However, the diseases or injuries that require removal of the left colon have often weakened the patient prior to any operation. Consequently, the surgeon may be confronted with the need to operate on a patient in a very bad state of health.

Operative mortality rates of around 6.2% are reported in the literature. Complications with the anastomosis, the point where the intestines are rejoined, range around 4%.

Complications and Possible Side Effects
As with any abdominal procedure, infections, formation of *adhesions,* and postoperative bleeding may occur. The anastomosis may fail to heal in patients whose nutritional status is poor or who have widespread cancer. *Hyperalimentation* may help speed healing, especially in patients with radiation injury to the bowel or Crohn's colitis. There is some evidence that intravenous feeding with solutions of branched-chain amino acids (types of the building blocks of protein that have "Y" shapes in their molecular structure) is helpful in fighting severe infections.

Diarrhea after the operation is a potential problem, but it can be controlled by avoiding foods that produce diarrhea, use of antidiarrheal drugs such as Imodium and Lomotil, and eating more water-soluble fiber or taking over-the-counter drugs containing water-soluble fiber, such as Metamucil, Citrucel, and Fiberall.

As with any procedure in which anesthesia is used, death from reaction to the anesthetic drugs, error on the part of the anesthetist, or machine failure is a remote possibility.

Open Reduction and Internal Fixation of Fracture of the Femur
Repair of a broken leg with an *internal fixation* device

Mortality (Death) and Morbidity (Complication) Rates
In-hospital mortality rates for this procedure in community hospitals in the U.S. were 4.5% for 1989. *Perioperative* mortality rates reported in the medical literature range from zero to 21%. Mortality rates have been steadily improving over the last two decades.

Representative studies of complications found rates of 26% to 46% and 35.6%. Infection is a relatively common problem; rates as high as 28% have been reported, although rates as low as 3% can be achieved.

Complications and Possible Side Effects
The chief complication, which is better described as complete failure of the procedure, is failure of the broken bone ends to join. Rates of nonunion reported in various studies range from zero to 33%. Other complications include rotation of the broken pieces relative to one another around a fixation device. The result of this rotation is that the anatomical position of the lower leg relative to the upper leg is altered, so that the foot turns inward or outward more than it should. The effects of this on the ability of the patient to walk and on the appearance of the limb may be serious enough to require reoperation.

As with any procedure in which anesthesia is used, death from reaction to the anesthetic drugs, error on the part of the anesthetist, or machine failure is a remote possibility.

Partial Small Bowel Resection
Removal of a part of the small intestine

Mortality (Death) and Morbidity (Complication) Rates
Mortality varies greatly with the underlying condition, age of the patient, and the amount of intestine removed. Mortality and complication rates of zero have been reported for removal of small cancers of the small intestine.

On the other hand, massive small intestine resection (defined as average loss of 91% of bowel) required because of bowel infarction had a reported mortality rate of 46% in a group of men whose average age was 64. Mortality rates of 60% have been reported when 89% of the bowel is lost. Long-term follow-up of pediatric patients with massive bowel resection shows a long-term mortality rate of 48%.

Complications and Possible Side Effects

Most resections remove so little of the small intestine that there are few, if any, noticeable changes in digestion. When much of the small bowel is removed, however, the patient is unable to absorb sufficient calories and nutrients. Nearly all nutrient absorption takes place in the small intestine; the large intestine essentially recycles water, minerals, and bile.

Investigations in both humans and animals have shown that, when part of the small bowel is removed, the small intestine compensates rather heroically by increasing the size of its absorptive structures and making other adaptations. There is a limit to the rate at which absorption can be increased, however, so eventually there is some loss of ability to digest food. Many patients who have had large portions of the small bowel removed (more than 75% or so) cannot tolerate any fats. Such patients may suffer from diarrhea and abdominal discomfort, and may be unable to absorb enough food to allow them to perform even light tasks. Also, some drugs may be poorly absorbed, thereby making treatment of the results of the resection even more difficult. Absorption of certain critical amino acids may be reduced. In one study, all patients who had lost two-thirds or more of the small intestine and whose diets were not carefully supplemented were found to be in a state of subclinical malnutrition, which is a form of malnutrition that does not result in symptoms of the disease but can be detected by laboratory tests.

Long-term intravenous feeding called *total parenteral nutrition (TPN)* is not an acceptable solution to the loss of the small bowel for several reasons: The small intestine plays a role in regulation of excretion of calcium by the kidneys, and long-term TPN leads to loss of bone. Liver damage can also occur and be severe enough to require liver transplantation.

Even when oral feeding is resumed, other problems may occur, including kidney stones, gallstones, bone fractures caused by mineral loss, delayed growth, and delayed or absent puberty.

Whether a return to oral feeding is possible depends on the length of the remaining small intestine. The critical breaking point seems to be between 20 and 30 cm of remaining bowel—roughly between 8 and 12 inches. Although adults with less than 20 cm of remaining intestine may return to eating solid foods, children with less than 20 cm remaining can rarely return to oral feeding; those with more than 30 cm nearly always can.

The output of ileostomies—substances and secretions such as gastric juices, stomach acid, bile, and enzymes—is very high and largely liquid, and failure to replace the fluid loss can lead to dehydration, particularly in the elderly.

Pseudo-obstruction of the small intestine can occur after massive intestinal resection for Crohn's disease. Because of pain and vomiting brought about by both the residual Crohn's disease and by continuing partial obstruction, TPN may be required even if adequate bowel is left.

As with any procedure in which anesthesia is used, death from reaction to the anesthetic drugs, error on the part of the anesthetist, or machine failure is a remote possibility.

Percutaneous Transluminal Coronary Angioplasty (PTCA) (Balloon angioplasty)

Crushing of *plaque* in an artery with an inflatable balloon inserted into the artery through a *catheter* threaded through the *femoral* or *brachial artery*

Mortality (Death) and Morbidity (Complication) Rates

Mortality for this procedure has steadily fallen since it was first done, and the current (1984–91) literature reflects operative mortality rates of 5%; .8% to 3.8%; .7% to .9%; 1%; 7.2% (for patients operated on during or after a heart attack, 43% of whom had single-vessel disease); and .2% to 8.5%. One-year survival rates of 95%, and one-year heart attack rates of 3% are typical for patients who undergo PCTA. It is not possible to disentangle results for single-vessel disease in all studies reviewed, but the mortality rate is lower when fewer vessels are treated. One study cites a mortality rate of 1.9% per vessel treated with PCTA.

As for complications, rates of under 2% for *perioperative* heart attack and emergency bypass surgery and 12% for *acute reocclusion* of the vessel are achievable. Significant bleeding can be expected in 2% to 3% of patients. Heart attack during the procedure occurs in about 1% to 5% of patients. A 1984 study from the National Heart, Lung, and Blood Institute cites occurrence of coronary artery dissection (essentially, a tearing apart of the artery) in 3%, vessel *occlusion* in 1%, prolonged chest pain in 1%, and artery spasm in 1%, noting that these rates declined as surgeons gained experience. Cardiac rupture, which involves massive tearing of the wall of the heart and profuse bleeding in the chest, is a rare event.

Remarkably, there is only one study of a group of patients who died following PTCA. Unfortunately, we don't know what percentage of the total number of patients having PTCA these patients—a group of 26—represent. The study findings for the 21 of the 26 patients who died within 3 weeks of operation showed demonstrable cardiac complications in 19 patients; clots formed from platelets in 10 patients (48%); coronary artery disintegration was seen in 17 patients (81%); blood clots that had moved from the site where they formed to other parts of the body were noted in 13 patients (62%); *atheroemboli* were found in 7 patients (33%); and heart attacks occurred in 17 patients (81%). An increased incidence of clots formed from *fibrin* platelets in the heart and coronary vessels was noted when compared with a non-PTCA cardiac autopsy population (5 of 53 patients).

Complications and Possible Side Effects
Groin *hematomas* at the point where the catheter is inserted, and two heart rhythm disturbances—*atrial fibrillation* and *left bundle branch block*—were reported in under 1% of elderly patients in one study. Rates are probably lower in younger patients.

Repair of the artery used for the catheterization, even in experienced hands, is required in 1% to 3% of the cases.

Removal of Tube and Ectopic Pregnancy
Removal of a *fallopian tube* in which a fertilized egg has implanted itself

Mortality (Death) and Morbidity
(Complication) Rates
The mortality rate associated with this procedure is 1% to 2%, even when some quoted morbidity figures (for example, infection) seem high. Zero mortality and a 2% complication rate have been reported for the laparoscopic procedure. Complication rates of zero to 2% have been reported.

The chief concern mentioned in the literature is whether the surgeon can remove the entire pregnancy and maintain the ability of the woman to have a normal pregnancy in the future. For this reason conservative alternatives to the procedure have been developed and are being refined.

Earlier detection of ectopic pregnancy (through *ultrasound* studies or *laparoscopic* examination) has reduced rates of morbidity and mortality. Infection can

occur in up to 22% of women, but may cause no symptoms and be detectable only by bacterial culture.

Bleeding as a major complication has been reported in 2.53% of laparoscopically treated ectopic pregnancies, with a mortality of zero and no hospital stay longer than 24 hours.

In ectopic pregnancies treated with laparoscopy, reoperation required because of failure to remove the entire pregnancy the first time occurs in up to 5.12% of cases. Rates of pregnancy inside the womb (following microsurgery to correct tubal defects) are variable, but have been reported to be as low as 19.4%.

Complications and Possible Side Effects
Depending on the degree of scarring of the fallopian tubes, and the functioning of the other tube if only one was removed, fertility may be impaired. Among women who want to get pregnant again after ectopic pregnancy, success rates (as measured by objective evidence of pregnancy) vary from 61% to 100%. Both the rate of fertilizations and the rate of pregnancies carried to term have been reported to be around 90%, with 10.9% of the pregnancies failing because of a repeat ectopic pregnancy.

Adhesions, which can interfere with the chances of future pregnancy, occur by the eighth day after surgery in more than 50% of women operated on for ectopic pregnancy. They can be repaired by laparoscopy and tend not to recur following such surgery.

While removal of the ovaries is not, strictly speaking, a part of this procedure, ovarian damage in a woman who has only one functioning ovary will make estrogen supplements necessary. If the woman takes the drug assiduously, her survival rate is as good as that for women with intact ovaries. True, hormone replacement therapy is controversial—the use of replacement estrogens is believed to increase the incidence of breast cancer. However, studies of this question have given equivocal results. Current research strongly suggests that the combined effect in reducing bone loss and heart disease (a major and growing problem in women) more than outweighs any risk of breast cancer that might be associated with hormone replacement therapy.

A complication of ectopic pregnancy itself is hemolytic uremic syndrome. This condition is characterized by anemia, bleeding, and kidney failure, and has been reported following the successful removal of an ectopic pregnancy.

Endometriosis is a condition in which tissue from the uterine lining somehow escapes the uterus and becomes implanted on pelvic organs, usually causing pain. There is a small chance following this procedure that this endometrial tissue can become entrapped in scar tissue, but this is relatively rare.

In women treated with the laparoscope, possible complications include a bulging of the navel where the laparoscope was inserted, cardiac arrest, and electrical burns of the abdominal viscera, usually the small intestine.

Puncture of the womb is a rare complication. So is the need to convert a closed operation, as laparoscopy is, to an open procedure, such as laparotomy, to finish it.

The operation, if done through the vagina, is carried out on the stirrup table with the woman in the lithotomy position. If the procedure is lengthy and the woman is not shifted to relieve pressure on various parts of the body, permanent nerve damage can occur.

Ovarian remnant syndrome, which is characterized primarily by pelvic pain, can occur when a surgeon is removing both tubes and ovaries and fails to remove all of an ovary. Because the doctor thinks that the ovaries are gone, the woman's pain is dismissed as psychosomatic, and she is either ignored or referred to a psychiatrist. Although relatively rare, ovarian remnant syndrome may progress to tissue damage requiring bowel and bladder surgery. Necrotizing fasciitis, in which the tough tissue containing the muscles is destroyed, with destruction spreading to the overlying and underlying tissues, is a rare but absolutely devastating complication. In some cases, loss of the full thickness of the abdominal occurs and multiple reconstructive surgeries are required.

Formation of a *fistula* occurs in about 1.9% of women. It is also possible for the tube to recanalize, affording an unbroken route from the ovary to the uterus, which may cause another ectopic pregnancy.

Studies in monkeys indicate that there are no hormonal changes following removal of one or both tubes if the ovaries are left intact.

As with any procedure in which anesthesia is used, death from reaction to the anesthetic drugs, error on the part of the anesthetist, or machine failure is a remote possibility.

Revision of Vascular Procedure

Reoperation on a vessel for a repair or other surgery that did not work the first time

Mortality (Death) and Morbidity (Complication) Rates

A recent Japanese study warns, "Since vascular disease is always progressive and a perfect vascular *prosthesis* has yet to be developed, postoperative complications are almost inevitable." Further, the study indicates that about 8.4% of patients with initially successful repairs will have late graft (replacement blood vessel) failure. Some vascular procedures have a reoperation rate as high as 75%. A Hungarian study of revisions following cardiovascular surgery shows a mortality rate of 12.5% and a failure rate of 17.5%.

Mortality is hard to estimate for this procedure, which is actually a catchall group of procedures. Doctors bill insurers for services under procedure codes. Some procedures that are infrequently performed or are so variable that they defy more detailed classification are lumped together, like this one: It applies to any revision to any prior vascular procedure, if the revision is not clearly described by a separate code.

In vascular repairs and reconstructions, and reoperations for them, death rarely results directly from the repair, but instead results from failure to reestablish adequate blood flow to the organ or limb in question. Universally, in terms of morbidity and mortality, the results for second and later operations are worse than for initial operations, and emergency procedures invariably carry a high mortality.

Take, for instance, a late complication of vascular reconstruction—formation of a pseudoaneurysm, at the suture line. The mortality rate for reoperation for this complication is 2.08% when the procedure is done electively, and 50% for emergency procedures. The authors of the study cited recommend early operation, for obvious reasons.

The need for revision due to bleeding after surgery ranges from 2.8% to 4.2%, depending on the operative site. There are significantly more complications, mainly infections, if the reoperation is done more than 48 hours after the first procedure.

A 1989 study of microsurgical repairs of leg vessels indicated that patency (how open or unobstructed the vessel is) fell steadily during the first 90 days from a high of 86.1% right after surgery to a low of 68.4% after 5.4 months; further, there seemed to be little change in patency after the first 90 days. This suggests that the final failure of patency rate is in the range of 32% of microsurgical repairs attempted, and this figure is probably lower with larger vessels.

The surgical folk wisdom that it is important to suture all layers of the vessel wall to avoid plugging by flaps of the innermost layer has not been proven in animal studies. However, the conventional technique of suturing all layers seemed to produce a higher long-term patency rate.

Complications and Possible Side Effects

In one study bacteria were cultured from 79% of grafts that were removed during the revision procedure. *Subclinical infection* may be a reason for graft failure. The rate of deep infection following vessel reconstruction is about 1.2%.

Vascular procedures are often done in attempts to prevent loss of a leg due to inadequate blood flow. If the first procedure fails, and one or more attempts at reconstructing the blood vessel(s) are required, it can be much harder for the surgeon to perform a successful below-the-knee amputation if it is needed later. This is because an adequate flow of blood to the stump is needed for postoperative healing.

Wound complications occur in up to 62.5% of patients who have had revised vascular procedures in the groin area. In the attempt to repair or replace the vessel that preceded the revision procedure, use of the sartorius muscle, located in the groin/hip region, to cover the graft reduces later complications significantly.

As with any procedure in which anesthesia is used, death from reaction to the anesthetic drugs, error on the part of the anesthetist, or machine failure is a remote possibility.

Right Hemicolectomy

Removal of the right (ascending) half of the *colon*

Mortality (Death) and Morbidity (Complication) Rates

This is not a trivial procedure. Mortality is low in patients who are being operated on under ideal conditions, but the diseases or injuries that require removal of the right colon frequently leave such people in poor health.

Operative mortality rates from 5.7% to 12.5% in cancer patients have been reported. Mortality and complication rates of 7% have been reported in another study. Complications with the *anastomosis* range around 4%. Mortality in patients being treated for radiation injury to the colon can be as high as 14%. For patients receiving emergency right hemicolectomies for trauma, the mortality rate has been reported as high as 29% and the complication rate 11%.

Complications and Possible Side Effects

As with any abdominal procedure, infections, formation of *adhesions*, and postoperative bleeding may occur. The anastomosis may fail to heal in patients whose nutritional status is poor or who have widespread cancer. *Hyperalimentation* may help speed healing, especially in patients with radiation injury to the bowel or Crohn's disease. There is some evidence that intravenous feeding with solutions of branched-chain amino acids (types of the building blocks of protein that have "Y" shapes in their molecular structure) is helpful in fighting severe infections.

As with any procedure in which anesthesia is used, death from reaction to the anesthetic drugs, error on the part of the anesthetist, or machine failure is a remote possibility.

Spinal Canal Exploration

Surgical exploration of the spinal canal

Mortality (Death) and Morbidity (Complication) Rates

Most studies of patients having this procedure were small, so mortality and morbidity figures may be exaggerated. Mortality rates of up to 14% have been reported, the immediate cause of death being tuberculosis infection of the spine. Spinal canal exploration can be expected to cause permanent nerve damage in varying degrees of severity, depending on the study, in about 1.36% to 14% of patients.

Complications and Possible Side Effects

As with any procedure in which anesthesia is used, death from reaction to the anesthetic drugs, error on the part of the anesthetist, or machine failure is a remote possibility.

Vascular Shunt and Bypass

Rerouting of a blood or fluid flow within the body to relieve circulatory problems, accumulation of fluid, etc. Virtually any circulatory system disorder, whether *congenital* or acquired, can be corrected by surgically rerouting the vessels causing the problem.

Mortality (Death) and Morbidity (Complication) Rates

When a peritoneovenous shunt, which routes fluid from the abdominal cavity into the venous circulation for disposal by the kidneys, is inserted, operative mortality ranges from 10% to 25%, depending on how sick the patient is when the operation begins. Drainage of the *ascitic fluid* before the shunt is opened, so that the venous circulation is not hit with a massive amount of ascitic fluid, lessens the mortality. Around 81% of patients survive the first year with the shunt in place.

Bleeding from *esophageal varices* occurs in 7.9% of patients, as does late infection after placement of the shunt. Of the patients studied, 30.5% had a recurrence of *ascites;* most were attributed to obstructions of the shunt. Dr. LeVeen, who invented the shunt, achieved a mortality rate of under 1% in patients who were not jaundiced and did not have fluid accumulation in the chest cavity.

In patients in whom the cause of the accumulation of ascitic fluid is cancer, the major complication rate is 4% and the rate of *embolization of tumor* through the shunt is 5%. The outcome of tumor embolization can range from no symptoms to death, depending on the size of the tumor *emboli* and the veins or arteries that are ultimately blocked by them.

Other studies indicate that infection occurs in up to 21% of cases and usually requires removal of the shunt to clear up the infection. The shunt can be an occasional source of a fatal air embolism (the presence of air in the blood that blocks the flow of blood through a vessel); the surgeon can avoid this during repair procedures by clamping off the shunt before opening the *peritoneum.*

LeVeen shunts can also trigger a fatal condition called adult respiratory distress syndrome (ARDS), which is an inability to adequately oxygenate the blood through breathing. ARDS can result from a wide variety of conditions that affect the way the alveoli (the small sacs in the lungs) exchange air with the blood. It is unknown precisely why LeVeen shunts can trigger this condition, but they probably cause a disturbance in the circulation of blood in the lungs. For the shunt to function effectively, the venous end must lie within the *superior vena cava.* Shunts can occasionally move out of position; this can be detected on X rays if the shunt has a radiopaque line on it. (A radiopaque line on a shunt allows detection of the otherwise invisible shunt on an X ray.)

Complications and Possible Side Effects

For LeVeen shunts, subclinical disorders of blood clotting develop in about 75% of patients (subclinical disorders are those that are detectable on lab tests but do not produce symptoms). Few develop clotting problems or bleeding, although both have been noted.

Blockage of a LeVeen shunt occurs in about 12% of cases. It must be treated with some delicacy, usually by detection of the blocked portion followed by surgical replacement, because flushing obstructions out of the tube into the venous circulation under pressure can be fatal. Even if the LeVeen shunt controls the ascites, patients can die at a later time of the underlying liver disease (infectious and alcoholic *cirrhosis,* mainly) that causes the ascites. Patients should be aware that placement of the shunt can be fatal if system-wide clotting occurs when the ascitic fluid enters the bloodstream.

Some patients develop fluid in the lungs due to circulatory changes induced by the placement of the shunt; most respond to *diuretics,* but in a few, removal of the shunt may be required to avoid fluid accumulation in the lungs.

A LeVeen shunt may occasionally cause *perforation* of the *colon* if the abdominal end migrates out of position.

As with any procedure in which anesthesia is used, death from reaction to the anesthetic drugs, error on the part of the anesthetist, or machine failure is a remote possibility.

Glossary for "18 High-Risk Surgical Procedures"

Abscess—a collection of pus that forms as the result of infection.

Acute reocclusion—a sudden reclogging of a vessel.

Adhesion—a band of scar tissue that forms between cut surfaces of organs; an abnormal union of body surfaces caused by fibrous scars.

Anastomosis—the joint formed by the sewing together of small and large intestines.

Anesthesia risk—the rate of death due to anesthesia of all types was estimated to be between .001% and .004% in the 1970s and early 1980s. The most recent figures available from several Western nations suggest a death rate in the range of .0004% to .0007%, roughly a tenfold reduction. This is further supported by a close study of closed malpractice cases in Massachusetts. If an anesthesia complication is serious enough to warrant admission to an intensive care unit, the mortality is about 17%.

Aneurysm—a bulging and ballooning of the wall of an artery due to the pressure of blood flowing through a weakened area.

Aorta—the body's primary artery that receives blood from the heart's left ventricle and distributes it to the body.

Ascites—an accumulation of fluid in the abdomen.

Ascitic fluid—fluid in the abdomen as a result of the condition ascites.

Atheroemboli—clots composed of plaque.

Atrial fibrillation—a heart rhythm disturbance marked by rapid, unsystematic contractions of the upper heart chambers.

Brachial artery—the major artery in the arm.

Carotid artery—any of the four principal arteries of the neck and head.

Carotid bruits—sounds in the carotid arteries attributable to narrowing of the arteries.

Catheter—a thin, flexible plastic tube that can be placed inside some part of the body—for example, a Foley catheter, which is used to drain urine from the bladder.

Cerebral edema—retention of water in the tissues of the brain.

Cirrhosis—the formation of fibrous scar tissue in place of healthy cells, obstructing the flow of blood through the liver. As a result, the various functions of the liver deteriorate.

Colon—the part of the large intestine that extends to the rectum.

Congenital—present at birth.

Corticosteroids—a group of drugs used principally as anti-inflammatories.

Diaphragm—muscle that separates the abdomen from the chest.

Diuretic—a drug that increases the output of urine and thus drains fluid from the body.

Electrolytes—mineral salts that are involved in nerve signal transmission and muscle contractions.

Emboli—solid particles, usually fragments of clotted blood or fatty deposits, carried along in the bloodstream.

Embolization of tumor—the plugging of a blood vessel due to tumor fragments, especially from stomach cancer.

Esophageal varices—varicose veins of the esophagus, which have lost the support of the surrounding tissue and are bulging into the channel of the esophagus, and are irritated by the passage of food. They are almost always due to changes in the liver circulation caused by cirrhosis, which in turn is generally due to alcoholism. Although rare, a few cases are due to congenital weakness of the esophageal tissue.

Fallopian tubes—paired structures that carry eggs from the ovaries to the uterus.

Femoral artery—the major artery in the thigh.

Femur—the thighbone.

Fibrin—a protein in the blood that is the major component of blood clots.

Fistula—a passage or tunnel formed in the body by disease, injury, congenital abnormalities, or, occasionally, surgery.

Graft—any tissue or organ for implantation or transplantation.

Hematoma—a collection of blood and clots usually in an organ, a cavity, or tissue.

Hyperalimentation—feeding a complete protein/carbohydrate/fat/vitamin/mineral solution through a central venous catheter placed in the neck or the chest.

Internal fixation—the use of plate, nails, screws, wires, or some combination thereof in the repair of a broken bone.

Intraabdominal sepsis—infection within the abdomen.

Laparoscopic—pertaining to the laparoscope, a thin, lighted instrument that is inserted through a small incision in the abdomen, usually near the naval, to examine the liver, spleen, intestines, and in women the uterus, ovaries, and fallopian tubes.

Left bundle branch block—a heart rhythm disturbance.

Major morbidity—any complication that extends the length of stay in the hospital beyond the expected discharge date.

Occlusion—blockage of any passage, canal, vessel, or opening in the body.

Operative mortality—death that occurs during a surgical procedure; depending upon other factors, could also include death that occurs in the process of recovery.

Perforation—tearing or boring through a vessel, duct, intestine, or organ.

Perioperative—the time period from admission to the hospital for surgery to discharge from the hospital.

Peritoneum—the transparent covering of the organs that lies just behind the muscular wall of the abdomen.

Peritonitis—an inflammation of the transparent membrane that covers most of the abdomen beneath the muscle layer.

Plaque—a deposit of fatty buildup in the inner lining of the artery wall.

Prosthesis—an artificial body part.

Pulmonary embolism—a blood clot that lodges in the pulmonary artery or in another vessel in a lung.

Sepsis—presence of disease-causing microorganisms in the bloodstream.

Shunt—a tube, with or without a one-way valve, that carries some fluid from one place to another place; a passage between two natural channels, especially between blood vessels.

Subclinical infection—an infection with no detectable symptoms or signs (such as pain, fever, redness, or swelling) but that nonetheless destroys tissue or prevents healing after surgery.

Superior vena cava—a major vein that drains blood from the head, neck, upper extremities, and chest and returns it to the right atrium of the heart.

Thoracotomy—surgical incision of the chest wall.

Thromboembolectomy—removal of a blood clot blocking a vein or artery.

Total parenteral nutrition (TPN)—a type of extremely nutritious long-term intravenous feeding that bypasses the stomach and contains all of the necessary fats, proteins, and carbohydrates (and nutrients in general) that the body requires.

Ultrasonography—the process of imaging deep structures of the body by recording the reflection of high-frequency sound waves for diagnostic purposes.

Ultrasound—use of sound waves at very high frequency for diagnostic purposes. The resulting echoes are translated into pictures on a TV monitor; the image itself is called a sonogram.

Uremia—accumulation of waste products in the blood.

Ureters—tubes that carry the urine from the kidneys to the bladder.

Source: From *Good Operations—Bad Operations: The People's Medical Society's Guide to Surgery,* by Charles B. Inlander and the staff of the People's Medical Society. New York: Viking, 1993.

Most Frequently Performed Outpatient Procedures

Not all diagnostic tests or surgical procedures require an overnight stay at a hospital. An increasing number of procedures are done on an outpatient, or ambulatory, basis, which means that the patient comes in the day of the procedure, checks out on the same day, and recuperates at home. The following tables list the most frequently performed hospital-based outpatient nonsurgical procedures and the ten most frequently performed hospital-based outpatient surgical procedures.

To help you better understand these procedures, we have included short definitions of equipment or medical terms where appropriate.

10 Most Frequently Performed Hospital-Based, Outpatient Nonsurgical Procedures

1. Transabdominal endoscopy and colonoscopy (inserting a tubelike lighted instrument through the abdominal wall to examine abdominal organs, such as the liver, spleen, and small intestine, or the reproductive organs of women; or examining the colon [the large intestine] with a tubelike lighted instrument)

2. Transabdominal and other endoscopy (inserting a tubelike lighted instrument through the abdominal wall to examine abdominal organs, such as the liver, spleen, and small intestine, or the reproductive organs of women; using a tubelike lighted instrument called an endoscope

to examine parts of the body—lungs, bladder, or stomach, for example—or bone joints, such as the hip, shoulder, or knee)

3. Soft tissue X ray of thorax (chest)
4. Diagnostic ultrasound (using sound waves to examine body cavities or parts)
5. Cystoscopy and urethroscopy (examination of the tube leading from the bladder and the bladder itself with a tubelike lighted instrument)
6. Computerized axial tomography (also called CAT or CT scan; a noninvasive diagnostic procedure that takes a series of cross-sectional X rays, then uses a computer to construct highly detailed pictures of internal body parts)
7. Endoscopy and flexible sigmoidoscopy (examination of the S-shaped portion of the colon [the large intestine] with a flexible tubelike lighted instrument)
8. Transfusion of blood and blood components
9. Physical therapy and/or therapeutic procedures
10. Other diagnostic and therapeutic procedures

10 Most Frequently Performed Hospital-Based, Outpatient Surgical Procedures

1. Suture of skin and subcutaneous tissue (stitches)
2. Local excision or destruction of intestinal lesion (removal of an abnormal growth of tissue in the intestines by cutting, burning, or freezing)
3. Extracapsular extraction of lens, by fragmentation and aspiration technique (using sound waves to liquefy the lens of the eye and removing the material with a needle-shaped vacuum device)
4. Local excision and/or destruction of lesion of breast (removal of an abnormal growth of tissue in the breast by cutting, burning, or freezing)
5. Immobilization, pressure, and attention to wound (preventing movement of the wound site, control of bleeding, and application of bandage)
6. Diagnostic and therapeutic procedures on nervous system
7. Other extracapsular extraction of lens (removing the outer covering of the lens of the eye by cutting with a scalpel)
8. Local excision and/or destruction of lesion or tissue of skin (removal of a growth, such as a wart or mole, by cutting, burning, or freezing)

9. Unilateral repair of inguinal hernia (repair of a hernia on only one side of the groin)
10. Other cataract extraction (removal of a cataract by removing the entire lens of the eye)

Source: Healthcare Research Systems, Inc., 1992. Used with permission. The Lake Forest, Illinois, company used data from about 12 million UB-82 claim forms (standardized forms used by insurance companies to pay claims based on diagnoses and treatments) submitted during 1991 by 305 hospitals that participate in the electronic claims system of CIS Technologies, Tulsa, Oklahoma, according to Robert Simmons, Jr., vice-president of sales and marketing. The researchers then extrapolated those results to all U.S. community hospitals. For additional information, telephone 800-826-2477.

Cosmetic Surgery

Cosmetic surgery is the permanent alteration of a part of the body that is done not because of medical necessity, but in order to approve the appearance of the patient. The fifteen most common types of cosmetic surgery are given here.

FACIAL

Facelift. Sagging skin and underlying facial muscles are lifted and repositioned. Excess skin and fat removed. Incisions usually begin in temple hair above and in front of ear, extend down in front of ear, around earlobe, up behind ear, and backward into hair of the scalp. Possible complications: hematoma, or excessive bleeding into the site of the incision; hair loss around incision; heavy scarring; paralysis of part of face; skin slough (interference with blood supply to surgical site).

Rhinoplasty (nose surgery). Nose made smaller by removing excess bone and cartilage. Incisions usually hidden just inside rim of the nostrils. Ideal age for procedure: 15 for girls, 18 for boys. Possible complications: nasal bleeding; whites of eyes can turn red due to leaking blood.

Otoplasty (protruding ears). Incision made in back of ear, in the crease where ear joins the back of head. Small amount of skin and cartilage is removed. Ideal age for procedure: 5 to 6 years. Possible complications: hematoma; formation of new deformity.

Blepharoplasty (eyelid lift). Removes excess skin from upper eyelid or protruding fatty tissue from lower eyelid. Excess skin in upper lid removed through incision in natural crease above the eye. Fatty tissue in lower lid removed through incision just below lower eyelid. Possible complications: dry-eye syndrome; epiphora (excessive tear production); corneal injury; telangiectasia (increase in small blood vessels); enophthalmous (sunken eye); hematoma.

Augmentation mentoplasty (chin implant). Small incision inside the mouth, between the lower lip and gum, or in small crease under the chin. Implant made from semisolid, spongelike, or mesh synthetic materials.

Reduction mentoplasty. Incision made beneath the chin, and instrument like a dental drill is used to shave off excess bony tissue of the chin.

Malar augmentation (cheek implants). Provides cheekbones, adding definition to face. Incision usually made between upper gums and cheek. Soft cheek tissue is elevated and pocket created over cheekbone. Implant is slid through the incision. Implants come in a variety of sizes and shapes and are made of medical-grade plastic.

Forehead lift. Improves droopy or heavy eyebrows and permanently furrowed brow. Incision made across hairline. Forehead and brows lifted and redraped upward, resulting excess skin removed.

Eyebrow lift. Recommended for men in place of forehead lift, since incision in hairline could become visible with balding. Incision made above eyebrows, often in a natural forehead wrinkle.

OTHER TYPES OF PLASTIC SURGERY

Reduction mammoplasty (breast reduction). Both horizontal and vertical incisions are made that follow the contour of the breast in an inverted "T" shape from the nipple area down to and within the crease below the breast. Excess tissue, fat, and skin from both sides of breast removed. Possible complications: hematoma; infection; poor healing of scars; diminished sensation in the nipple.

Mastopexy (lifting of sagging breasts). Incisions following natural contour of breast and around the areola. Excess skin removed from lower section of breast. Nipple, areola, and underlying breast tissue moved up. Possible complications: hematoma; infection; lessened sensitivity in the breast.

Augmentation mammoplasty (breast augmentation). Removable silicone implant inserted through an

Controversy Surrounding Silicone Breast Implants

The issue of silicone gel-filled implants for breast enlargement became a medical controversy in the 1990s after many women who had augmentation surgery began complaining of flulike symptoms. The only thing these women shared in common were breast implants.

Effective April 1992, the Food and Drug Administration (FDA) announced that it would allow silicone gel-filled implants to be available but only through clinical scientific studies. At the present time, silicone gel-filled implants are only available to women who need breast reconstruction surgery (see pg. 321). They are not available for purely cosmetic reasons.

However, women can still have their breasts enlarged with saline-filled implants, which are made with salt water contained in a silicone envelope. Although saline-filled implants are still on the market for reconstruction and augmentation as of 1993, they will be allowed to remain so only if the FDA decides that information submitted by manufacturers shows that they are safe and effective.

Although the safety of saline-filled implants has not been proven, leakage or rupture of these implants results in release of salt water, which is not foreign to and does not remain in the body. But because saline-filled implants use a silicone envelope, whose long-term safety has not been demonstrated, the saline-filled implants may not be entirely without risk.

If a saline-filled implant leaks or ruptures, it deflates and usually must be replaced.

History of Breast Implants

Breast implants have been available in the United States since the 1960s. As of 1992 approximately 1.5 million women had chosen breast implants, either for reconstruction or for augmentation.

About 20 percent of these implants have been used for reconstruction of breasts after mastectomy—the surgical removal of the breast due to cancer or injury—or to correct other deformities. The rest have been used for augmentation—to increase the size or improve the shape of the woman's natural breast(s).

In recent years, the Food and Drug Administration has received information regarding possible serious health risks of breast implants. This information, and a need for more research on their long-term safety, have led the FDA to require manufacturers to conduct additional scientific studies on the risks. Studies are also continuing on their benefits.

incision beneath the breast, beneath either the breast tissue or the muscle. Possible complications: hematoma; infection, which requires removal of implant; diminished sensation in nipple; formation of scar tissue, causing breast to become hard; and rupture, in which the gel filling is released into surrounding tissue. If the problems are severe, the implants may have to be removed permanently.

Breast reconstruction. Surgery to restore normal breast contour as much as possible, most often following removal of cancerous breast. Existing scar is opened and mammary implant is inserted beneath the muscle. Technique similar to breast augmentation. Nipple can be reconstructed at same time. Possible complications: hematoma; if blood supply compromised by radiation treatments, skin loss may result and implant may need to be removed; extensive scarring.

Because of FDA's concerns about the possible risks of silicone gel-filled implants, these devices are only available to women who are enrolled in a clinical study sponsored by the implant manufacturer and approved by the FDA. This includes women who have had breast cancer surgery or a severe injury to the breast, or who have a medical condition causing severe breast abnormality. Women who need to have an existing implant replaced are also eligible for the program.

Abdominoplasty (tummy tuck). Incision made in shape of "W" running from side to side and across the lower part of the abdomen. Excess fat and skin removed. Possible complications: bleeding and hematoma.

Lipolysis (body contouring). Fat deposits are sucked out of the body through plastic tubing into collection bottles. Incisions very tiny. Method used for removing fat from thigh, buttock, hip, abdomen, upper arm, and chin. Possible complications: rippling, dimpling, or sagging skin.

Medical Testing

Medical tests are one way your doctor has of obtaining the accurate and reliable information needed to give you the best medical care possible. After your doctor gathers your medical history and conducts a physical exam, chances are he or she will recommend medical tests to fill in the picture.

Medical tests can be divided into four categories:

Screening is usually a simple test to determine if a particular problem is present in a patient who appears healthy and has no complaints.

Diagnostic tests confirm or deny a doctor's impressions.

Prognostic tests are conducted after a diagnosis has been made to gather additional information.

Monitoring is done to evaluate medical treatment given to a patient.

Medical tests can also be divided into two classifications—invasive and noninvasive. A test that involves penetration of the body is an invasive test. Such tests normally pose greater risks than a test that does not penetrate the body. The prudent patient will ask, whenever an invasive test is ordered, if a noninvasive test is available that would be just as efficient.

You can increase the accuracy of tests your doctor has ordered by making sure your doctor knows the name of every medicine or drug that you've taken recently—even over-the-counter medications. Be certain to follow all the directions given to you for the test, and be certain that the technician performing the test knows your name and that the right test is being done.

Always ask your doctor the reason for a particular test. And if you change doctors, be sure your new physician knows what tests you've had in the past to avoid unnecessary repetition.

We've broadly defined the diagnostic tests and procedures most requested by medical practitioners today.

Amniocentesis—a sampling of the amniotic fluid that surrounds the fetus; used to detect certain birth defects and brain and blood disorders.

Angiogram—an X-ray picture of a blood vessel made after injecting an opaque substance or dye through a thin tube (catheter) into blood vessels to make them visible on X-ray film. An angiogram of the arteries is called arteriogram; of the veins, venogram or phlebogram; of the lymph vessels, lymphangiogram; of the heart's arteries, coronary angiogram.

Arteriogram—an X-ray picture used to locate blockages in the arteries. See *Angiogram*.

Arthrogram—an X-ray picture of a joint; used to detect injury or damage.

Arthroscopy—an examination of a joint by means of a long, flexible viewing tube inserted into the joint; used to detect injury or damage.

Barium enema—X-ray pictures of the large intestine (colon) made after injecting barium sulfate into the rectum; used to locate abnormalities in the colon. Often called a lower GI (gastrointestinal) series.

Barium meal—X-ray pictures of the esophagus, stomach, and duodenum (first part of the small intestine) made after the patient swallows barium sulfate on an empty stomach. Used to locate problems or abnormalities. Often called an upper GI (gastrointestinal) series.

Biopsy—the removal of a small portion of body tissue for microscopic analysis; often used to check growths that might be cancerous.

Bronchoscopy—an examination of the bronchi (air passages) of the lungs with a flexible, fiber-optic viewing tube that has been inserted down the throat.

Cardiac catheterization—the insertion of a thin, flexible tube (a catheter) through a vein or artery into the heart. Used to collect information about the heart's structure and performance and to inject an opaque substance (dye) so that an X ray can be made.

Carotid or cerebral arteriogram—an X-ray picture of the blood vessels of the brain; used in diagnosing stroke. See *Angiogram*.

Cholesterol test—a sampling of the blood to determine the amount of cholesterol in the blood.

Colonoscopy—an examination of the colon with a flexible, fiber-optic viewing tube.

Complete blood cell count (CBC)—an examination of blood samples to get a count of the number of red cells, white cells, and hemoglobin in the blood and to determine the percentage of red cells in the blood. Used to check for infection or screen for blood disorders.

Computerized axial tomography (CAT) scan—a highly detailed picture of internal body parts constructed by a computer from hundreds of X rays; frequently used to locate disease, tumors, or abnormalities in the selected part of the body.

Coronary angiogram—an X-ray picture of the heart's arteries. Coronary angiography is a form of cardiac catheterization.

Cystogram—an X ray of the bladder made by inserting a thin tube through the urethra into the bladder.

Dilation and curettage (D&C)—the removal of a layer of tissue from the wall of the uterus; as a diagnostic test, it is used to diagnose the cause of excessive bleeding or other problems.

Echocardiogram—an ultrasound recording of the heart's internal structures; used to locate heart valve problems or heart deformities.

Electrocardiogram (ECG or EKG)—a recording of the heart muscle's activity that is collected by electrodes placed on the body. Used to detect heart damage, as after a heart attack, and to monitor the effect of certain drugs.

Electroencephalogram (EEG)—a recording of the brain's electrical impulses and brain patterns that is collected by electrodes placed on the scalp. Often used to detect brain damage, diagnose epilepsy, or confirm brain death.

Electromyogram (EMG)—a recording of the electrical activity of resting and contracting muscles that is collected by an electrode and a thin needle attached to the skin. Used to detect weakness, paralysis, or other problems in the muscle.

Endoscopy—the use of a hollow tube that contains a light source and a viewing lens to examine interior parts of the body. Some of the tubes are rigid for direct viewing, while others are flexible and can be "snaked" through various parts of the body. The newer flexible scopes owe their success in large part to the development and application of fiber optics technology. Fiber-optic devices are thin, flexible tubes containing bundles of glass filaments that can transmit light around bends and curves to illuminate the inside of the body. Utilizing a sort of light-at-the-end-of-the-tunnel approach, scopes are viewing instruments, but some offer more than just a look. In some cases forceps, scissors, or other tiny instruments can be threaded through channels in the scope to facilitate surgical procedures. In addition, the pictures taken by the lens of the scope can be fed to a television monitor for better viewing.

Here are some of the more common endoscopes:

Arthroscope. A fiber-optic instrument used to examine the interior of a joint such as a knee or shoulder. The arthroscope is inserted through a small incision made above the joint.

Bronchoscope. An instrument inserted through the mouth to examine the lungs and bronchial tree. The rigid bronchoscope is a straight, hollow tube that permits direct viewing of the airway passages. The flexible bronchoscope uses a fiber-optic system that permits the doctor to perform an inspection of the full bronchial system.

Colonoscope. A flexible fiber-optic instrument inserted through the anus to examine the large intestine from the anus to the cecum (the first part of the large intestine).

Coloposcope. A thin, lighted instrument that is inserted into the vagina to permit examination of the cervix and to obtain tissue samples for biopsy.

Culdoscope. A thin, lighted instrument that is inserted through an incision made in the vagina to view the uterus, fallopian tubes, and rectal wall.

Cystoscope. A rigid instrument with a viewing lens and light source that is used to view the urethra and bladder. Inserted through the urethra, the cystoscope may also be used to obtain urine and tissue samples.

Gastroscope. A flexible fiber-optic instrument that is inserted through the mouth or the nose and used to examine the upper portion of the digestive tract—esophagus, stomach, and duodenum.

Hysteroscope. A short, rigid instrument with a light source that is inserted through the vagina and cervix to examine the uterus.

Laparoscope. A thin, lighted instrument that is inserted through a small incision in the abdomen, usually near the navel, and is used to examine the liver, spleen, intestines, and in women the uterus, ovaries, and fallopian tubes.

Laryngoscope. A thin fiber-optic instrument that is inserted through a nostril in order to view the base of the tongue, epiglottis, larynx, and vocal cords.

Proctoscope. A short (about 5 or 6 inches), rigid or flexible tube that is inserted through the anus to examine the rectum.

Sigmoidoscope. A rigid or flexible tube inserted through the anus to examine the sigmoid colon (the S-shaped portion of the colon just above the rectum). The rigid sigmoidoscope is a lighted tube about 12 inches long and 1 inch in diameter. The flexible sigmoidoscope employs fiber optics and is about 2 feet long.

Hysterosalpingogram—an X-ray picture of the uterus and fallopian tubes.

Lower gastrointestinal (GI) series—See *Barium enema.*

Magnetic resonance imaging (MRI)—the use of a magnetic field (instead of radiation) to produce detailed, computer-generated pictures of the body.

Mammogram—an X-ray picture of the breast; used to diagnose certain conditions, including breast cancer.

15 Common Medical Tests and Any Risks Associated with Them

Allergy Skin Tests

Prick. Up to thirty to thirty-five possible allergens (substances you might be allergic to) can be tested for at once. The front of the arm or the back is chosen as a test site and cleansed with alcohol. A drop of solution from each allergen is placed on the skin, then pricked with a needlelike object. Reactions are charted. If you are sensitive to a certain substance, slight swelling and itching will occur. Medication is given if reactions are severe. Antihistamines need to be discontinued for 1 to 2 days before test. Swelling and itching are likely.

Scratch. Similar to the prick test. A small scratch is made on the skin of the arm with a very fine needle before a drop of solution is placed on it.

Intradermal. Testing solutions are injected under your skin rather than placed on it. This technique is used when the doctor suspects a sensitivity is present despite negative results from a prick or scratch test. But this can result in a larger number of false-positive results and more serious reaction than swelling and itching.

Patch. This test is used to discover if a rash is caused by skin contact with a substance such as metal nickel, which is used in jewelry. Patches containing possible offensive materials are taped onto the back and results are noted 2 days later. Cream is prescribed for scaly, itchy reactions.

The major risk in skin testing is anaphylactic reaction, an extreme allergic response. This occurs in less than 1 in 2,000 cases and is treated with Adrenalin.

Electrocardiogram (EKG)

Resting. Patient lies on table and electrodes are attached to the wrists and ankles. A paste that conducts electricity is applied between the electrode and the skin to pick up the heart's electrical activity. A fifth wire attached to a suction cup is placed on the chest. Results appear on graph. EKGs can detect arrhythmias (abnormal cardiac rhythms), myocardial infarction (heart attack), hypertrophy (enlarged heart), rheumatic fever, and pulmonary embolus.

No risk is associated with this test. Errors in recording and interpreting can occur, so EKG results should always be interpreted in light of symptoms, history, physical exam, and other test results. EKGs are accurate in discovering a problem approximately 80 percent of the time. Accuracy rises to 90 percent if an isotope is injected into a vein.

Exercise (stress test). This test determines if the heart's demand for blood can be met during monitored exercise. Similar to resting EKG, but only chest monitors are used. Stress tests are sometimes performed several weeks following a heart attack as an indicator of how much exercise can be tolerated by a recovering patient. The test can also diagnose angina pectoris (periodic chest pain caused by insufficient oxygen supply to the heart).

Exercise testing is generally safe, with death occurring in less than 1 in 10,000 patients.

MRI (Magnetic Resonance Imaging)

This is the most high-tech of all medical tests. Images of internal body parts are made

15 Common Medical Tests and Any Risks Associated with Them (cont.)

possible by the use of magnetic fields and radio frequency pulses. The major benefit is that the patient is not exposed to radiation. Many patients are bothered by the noisiness of the procedure. Claustrophobia is not a problem with the newer models.

The powerful magnet that is used may affect pacemakers, artificial limbs, and other implanted or prosthetic medical devices that contain metal.

Ultrasound Imaging

Sound waves are used to provide images of internal body parts. Like the MRI, the major benefit is that the patient is not exposed to radiation. Lubricant is applied to the skin over the area to be examined. A transducer, an instrument that records the sound waves, is passed over the lubricated area and an image appears on a monitor or TV screen. This test is routinely used in pregnancy to determine the age and health of the fetus and detect congenital anomalies.

It should be mentioned that the findings of the largest-ever study on prenatal ultrasound screening—a study reported in the September 16, 1993, *New England Journal of Medicine*—indicate that the routine use of ultrasound does not improve the outcome of pregnancies for low-risk women. As to the issue of safety of ultrasonography in general, exposure to the sound waves used in ultrasound has not been shown to cause ill effects. However, this does not mean that it has been proven safe.

X Rays

Rays with a shorter wavelength than those of visible light are routinely used to diagnose broken bones and dental cavities. X rays can damage the body in three ways. They can damage individual cells; rarely this can lead to cancer. They can injure a developing fetus, resulting in birth defects. And they can injure the sperm or egg cells in the testes or ovaries.

Endoscopy

The direct visualization of a body cavity by a special optical instrument. This is usually performed if X rays are not definitive or if tissue is required for analysis because something was found. Gastrointestinal endoscopy includes a look at the esophagus, stomach, and duodenum. Sigmoidoscopy is the visual examination of the sigmoid colon, rectum, and anus; it is usually the first test done to evaluate unexplained rectal bleeding.

Endoscopy is generally very safe, with a complication rate of less than 1 in 1,000.

Biopsy

The single most important test to see if cancer is present. Biopsies may be done during surgery, endoscopy or as a separate procedure. The three types of biopsy are:

Excisional—when the entire lump, node, or suspicious area and some of the surrounding tissue are removed

Incisional—when only a slice or wedge of the suspicious area is removed

Needle—when a long, thin needle is inserted into the suspect tissue and a core of tissue is removed

Risks vary as to the type and location of the biopsy to be performed.

15 Common Medical Tests and Any Risks Associated with Them *(cont.)*

Mammography

X-ray examination of the breast. This is the most sensitive detector of early breast disease. It is generally recommended that women undergo a baseline mammogram between the ages of 35 and 39, and then every one to two years between the ages of 40 to 49, and yearly thereafter.

Newer X-ray techniques have dramatically reduced the radiation exposure in mammograms.

Pap Smear

A type of biopsy known as scraping. This is the most frequently performed screening study for the detection of cancer of the uterine cervix. Cells are scraped from the surface of the cervix during a pelvic examination and then rubbed onto a slide, where the smear is examined. Little or no risk is involved. About 10 percent of cancers are not detected with this test. Even if a report says cancer cells were seen, there is about a 20 percent chance no cancer is present.

Spinal Tap

This test examines the spinal fluid that bathes the brain and spinal cord. In various diseases and injuries, the spinal fluid may contain red or white blood cells, increased amounts of protein, and elevated or lowered levels of sugar. In addition, many diseases will cause the pressure of the spinal fluid to be higher than normal. A needle is inserted into the lower spine to draw the fluid for testing. Spinal taps can help determine brain tumors, meningitis, brain cancer, and multiple sclero-

sis. Procedure is moderately painful and headaches are not uncommon.

About 1 in 1,000 people having this test suffer some nerve injury, which usually heals on its own with time. A slight risk of infection is present.

Glaucoma Screening

A battery of tests to detect the buildup of pressure in the fluid inside the eye. Glaucoma is most prevalent in those over 40, in African-Americans, and in diabetics. Tests include:

Visual acuity examination—reading an eye chart

Refraction—reading eye chart with one eye covered and using various lenses

Pupillary reflex response—testing the pupil with a penlike flashlight

Visual field measurement—measuring how well objects are seen above, below, and on either side of a direct line of sight

Slit-lamp examination—eyedrops given to dilate the pupil and allow visual examination of the eye as far back as the retina

Intraocular pressure determination—also known as tonometry, the procedure that tests for eye pressure

Retinal examination—visual examination of retina using an ophthalmoscope, which looks like a fat flashlight with a disk at its end. Risks include a slight chance that cornea may be scratched or that infection will occur.

Audiogram

Measurement of your hearing in one ear and in both ears together. The test is performed inside a booth where patient wears earphones and identifies various sounds when heard. No risks involved.

15 Common Medical Tests and Any Risks Associated with Them *(cont.)*

Pulmonary Function Tests

Lung disease tests. Patient performs a series of different breathing maneuvers into a tube as requested by the tester. Results are recorded on a graph. The tests measure vital capacity (how much air is forcibly exhaled after inhaling as deeply as possible), residual volume (how much air remains in the lungs after a forcible exhalation), tidal volume (how much air is expired with each normal breath), and compliance (how well the lungs stretch with each breath in and how well they collapse with each breath out).

Little risk is involved except if a severe or unstable heart or lung condition is present.

Blood Tests

About fifty different tests can be performed on blood. These tests can be divided into two types—those that are concerned with the blood itself and those that are concerned with the various substances carried by the blood. Blood can be drawn to test for substances such as sugar, cholesterol, digitalis, and alcohol; for harmful bacteria; and for antibodies from previous diseases.

Blood is drawn in three ways: Venipuncture draws blood from a vein, usually from the inside of an elbow or from the back of a hand. Artery puncture draws blood from an artery; not many tests require blood from this source, but artery puncture is used to measure the amount of oxygen or carbon dioxide in the blood. In finger sticks, blood is drawn from the tip of a finger using a lance (sharp needle).

The risks include a slight chance of fainting. If bleeding or swelling occurs at the site of an artery puncture, see your doctor.

Urine Tests

About 100 different tests can be performed on urine. Depending on the type of test ordered, the time of day and method of collecting the urine can vary. Following exact collection orders improves the accuracy of these tests. No risks are involved.

Myelogram—an X-ray picture of the fluid-filled space around the spinal cord; used to locate tumors, nerve injuries, and slipped disks.

Pap test—a sampling of the tissue of the cervix; used to detect abnormal cells and cancer. Also called a cervical smear.

Positron emission tomography (PET)—a technique for making computer-generated images of the brain or other body organs by means of radioactive isotopes injected into the body; used to locate abnormal tissue.

Spinal tap—a sampling of cerebrospinal fluid removed from the spinal canal by means of a long needle; used to diagnose diseases of and injuries to the brain and spinal cord, especially in suspected cases of meningitis and stroke.

Thermogram—a photograph of the surfaces of the body made by a camera with heat-sensitive film; often used to detect varicose veins and breast tumors.

Ultrasound scan—a picture of organs and structures deep inside the body that has been made with high-frequency sound waves. Used to gather information about some part of the body; also used on pregnant women to gain information about the health or development of the fetus.

Upper gastrointestinal (GI) series—See *Barium meal*.

Venogram—an X-ray picture of the interior of a vein. See *Angiogram*.

X ray—a picture of the body's internal structures made with electromagnetic rays with a short wavelength.

SCREENINGS AND TESTS FOR COMMON FAMILIAL CONDITIONS

Suppose you have found that leukemia runs in your family. So you want to keep an eye out for symptoms of the disease in you and your family—among them, fatigue and other symptoms of anemia, pressure under the left side of your ribs resulting from an enlarged spleen, swollen lymph nodes, and weight loss. A good medical guide can provide essential data on symptoms.

But sometimes there are no overt symptoms, so more scientific methods may be worth pursuing.

The simplest screen for leukemia is a blood test, including a complete blood count. Indeed, leukemia is often discovered in routine blood testing for other problems before symptoms of this blood cancer present themselves. If chronic myelogenous leukemia (CML) is part of your family tree, you should have your genes screened for the so-called Philadelphia chromosome, which is found in 90 percent of people with CML.

Regular blood testing may be advisable for your young children if your family has a history of acute lymphocytic leukemia (ALL). When detected early in younger children, ALL is successfully treated 70 percent of the time; for older children and adults, the survival rate is only 20 percent.

Other kinds of screening are appropriate for different afflictions—digital rectal exams for prostate cancer; blood pressure and cholesterol tests for heart disease and stroke; mammograms for breast cancer.

If a certain disease or condition runs in your family, you may want to consider the associated screening tests listed below. They can help detect the disease as early as possible.

NIPPING FAMILY DISEASES IN THE BUD
Family Affliction Associated Screening Test

Cancers

Breast cancer	Mammograms at least every other year beginning at age 35. Self-examination for lumps. CEA and CA 15-3 blood tests
Cervical and vaginal cancers	Annual Pap smear and pelvic exam commencing at age 20
Colon cancer	Test annually for blood in the stool, starting at age 30. (The fecal occult [hidden] blood test has come into question because of the high number of false-positive results it produces. This means the test indicates blood is present in the stool when in actuality it's not. When blood is present, a colonoscopy is recommended.) CEA blood test for carcinoembryonic antigen. Periodic colonoscopy. Annual proctosigmoidoscopy beginning at age 45. Rigid proctoscopy
Leukemia	Complete blood count, chromosome analysis, bone marrow biopsy
Lung cancer	Annual chest X ray and sputum exam beginning at age 50. NSE blood test
Oral cancer	Annual dental examination. Biopsy
Ovarian cancer, cysts, and tumors	Annual pelvic exam. Ultrasonography. CA 125 blood test
Pancreatic cancer	CA 19-9 blood test
Prostate cancer	Digital rectal exam annually after age 40. Prostate-specific antigen (PSA) blood test that picks up presence of protein secreted by cancerous glands
Stomach cancer	Periodic endoscopic examination, particularly if Barrett's syndrome is present
Testicular cancer	AFP blood test for alpha-fetoprotein. Regular self-examination. Ultrasound
Cancer of the uterus	Endometrial biopsy

Other Diseases

Cystic fibrosis	Regular tests of lung function, stool, and perspiration salinity of infants and young children who may be at risk from this inherited disorder diagnosed at, or shortly after, birth
Diabetes	Regular blood sugar tests in persons of any age who have a family history of diabetes. Urinalysis
Glaucoma	Glaucoma exam at age 40
Heart attack, heart disease, atherosclerosis, stroke	Regular blood pressure, serum cholesterol, and triglyceride tests. Electrocardiogram. Exercise-tolerance test
Mood disorders	Psychiatric evaluation when symptoms—chronic depression, major mood swings—first present themselves
Osteoporosis	Bone density assessment before menopause
Polycystic kidney disease, kidney tumors	Urinalysis, ultrasound, CAT scan
Schizophrenia	Psychiatric evaluation when symptoms—delusions, hallucinations, incoherence—first present themselves

A Caveat on Screening

Screening tests—from Pap smears to cholesterol counts—can help add years to your life. But beware: They can also cut your life short and drain your wallet if a test is inaccurate. All screening tests, especially the newest ones, are prone to error—both positive and negative results that are ultimately proven false (known as false positive and false negative).

The new PSA blood test, which plumbs the blood for prostate-specific antigens related to prostate cancer, comes up false positive or false negative 36 percent of the time; but the Pap smear produces a false result 35 percent of the time it's positive, too. Even a basic blood pressure reading can be thrown off if the person administering the test is inexperienced or the cuff is not the right size for the dimensions of a particular arm. A recently developed test is likely to be more prone to error just because the test giver's body of experience with the test is short-lived and not extensive.

How can testing kill? In most cases a test itself doesn't do that, but an erroneously recommended procedure might. For example, medical experts estimate that 15 to 25 percent of all surgery is unnecessary. Misdiagnosis and/or poor testing creates the justification and demand for that unnecessary surgery. All major surgery involves approximately a 1.3 percent risk of death through complications. A bad test result could send you needlessly into the operating room and on to your grave.

Relatively less dramatic damage can be caused by inaccurate test results: unnecessary removal of an organ, unnecessary chemotherapy or radiation treatment, nonfatal complications, pain or discomfort from a recommended procedure.

So whenever you are screened, use *all* test results the way the Pentagon uses the Distant Early Warning anti-nuclear-attack system. When a worrisome blip shows up on their screens, they don't automatically press the button and launch Armageddon; the blip could have been a flock of geese, not incoming nuclear warheads. So, too, when health screens indicate potential trouble for you, don't assume Judgment Day has arrived. Always request reconnaissance—additional or repeat testing, second opinions—to get more evidence to substantiate the early warning.

Because testing can be expensive, consult with your physician to get a professional and gut-level opinion about the need for further testing, factor in cost when choosing tests, and use your own common sense. If three successive tests have found no evidence of the suspected disease but your doctor suggests an $800 magnetic resonance imaging to "eliminate the last .01 percent chance," you may want to call off the diagnostic hounds and bet with the odds that are already in your favor.

Abortion

Abortion is expulsion or extraction of the embryo or fetus from the uterus before it is viable. Spontaneous abortion, or miscarriage, can be caused by the death of the fetus from abnormality or disease or from trauma to the expectant mother.

Therapeutic and elective abortions are intensely personal and controversial issues in the United States today. With the Supreme Court ruling in 1973 in the landmark *Roe v. Wade* decision, abortions have been legal up to the twenty-fourth week. In the majority of states, the decision is the woman's until the twelfth week of pregnancy. A few states have passed laws affecting that decision after the twelfth week.

Not only performed as a matter of choice, however, abortions also are performed for medical reasons, specifically the woman's physical and/or mental health.

When it comes to abortion, there's something of a paradox among gynecologists. A survey by the American College of Obstetricians and Gynecologists (ACOG) shows that 84 percent of its members favor the availability of legal abortions. But only 34 percent perform abortions, and less than 2 percent do more than twenty-five abortions a month.

Fear of harassment or losing patients may stop some doctors. Others may have more personal reasons. The Alan Guttmacher Institute in New York reported, in a 1989 survey, that 86 percent of abortions are performed in freestanding outpatient medical facilities, such as family planning clinics or women's health centers. Ten percent are performed in hospitals or hospital outpatient centers. The remaining 4 percent are performed in physicians' offices. In all states but Vermont, law requires an abortion be performed by a medical doctor, such as a gynecologist, family practitioner, or osteopath. In Vermont, abortions may be performed by a trained nurse practitioner.

If safety records are an indication, this setup works well. As with any kind of surgical procedure, practice means perfect. It means the doctor or nurse practitioner is performing the operation often enough to remain proficient, and the support staff know what to do when a problem arises. "Doing abortions at a clinic means you can schedule them sooner and perform them more efficiently and more safely than you would in a doctor's office," says Morton Lebow, a spokesman for the ACOG. Their statistics show that most doctors who perform abortions in their offices do four or fewer a month. At a clinic, a doctor could easily do that many in an hour.

There's no doubt that the safety record for abortion has improved since 1973, when abortion first became legal in the United States. (Illegal abortions are defined as those done by a woman herself or by an untrained person.) Better-trained doctors, improved techniques, earlier abortions, and better management of complications such as infection have all helped make abortion safe.

Statistics show that a legal abortion, early in pregnancy, is seven times safer than carrying a pregnancy to term, and nearly twice as safe as a penicillin injection. According to the Centers for Disease Control and Prevention, the overall risk of dying from a legal abortion has dropped from 4.1 deaths per 100,000 abortions in 1972 to .4 per 100,000 in 1987—more than a ninefold decrease. The few deaths that do occur are often a fatal reaction to the use of general anesthesia, which may be used at some facilities at the woman's request for midterm or even early abortions. (Most abortions are done with a local anesthetic injected in the cervix, and sometimes, with intravenous sedation. General anesthesia is never used for a late abortion.)

Women experience complications that require hospitalization in less than .05 percent of abortions. The most common complications are a perforated uterus, infection, or an incomplete abortion.

There's no doubt that the earlier an abortion is done, the safer it is.

METHODS

Up to 14 weeks of pregnancy, most abortions are done by a procedure called suction curettage or vacuum aspiration. The woman lies on her back, legs in stirrups, on an examining table, just as she would for a gynecological exam. Her cervix is swabbed with a disinfectant, and, often, a local anesthetic is injected around the cervix. The cervix is slowly dilated, then a suction tube about the diameter of a pencil is inserted. The tube is used to suck out the contents of the uterus, including the fetus and placenta. The entire procedure takes about 10 minutes. Some women experience cramping during the procedure and for up to an hour afterward.

Between approximately 14 and 24 weeks of pregnancy, a technique known as *dilation and evacuation (D&E)* or *dilation and curettage (D&C)* is more often

An Analysis of State Laws Mandating Parental Involvement or Counseling for Abortion for Minors

Snapshot—Laws by State

State	Status	Year Enacted*	Type of Involvement	Number of Parents or Other Adult	Judicial or Other Bypass	Waiting Period
Alabama	enforced	1987	consent	one	yes	
Alaska	not enforced	1970	consent	one	no	
Arizona	enjoined	1989	consent	one	yes	
Arkansas	enforced	1989	notice	two	yes	48 hr
California	enjoined	1987	consent	one	yes	
Colorado	enjoined	1967	consent	one	no	
Connecticut	enforced	1990	counseling			
Delaware	not enforced	1970	consent	two	no	
District of Columbia	no law					
Florida	no law					
Georgia	enforced	1988	notice	one	yes	24 hr
Hawaii	no law					
Idaho	enforced	1983	notice "if possible"	two	no	24 hr
Illinois*	enjoined	1983	notice	two	yes	24 hr
Indiana	enforced	1984	consent	one	yes	
Iowa	no law					
Kansas	enforced	1992	notice	one	yes	
Kentucky	enjoined	1986	consent	two	yes	
Louisiana*	enjoined	1991	consent	one	yes	
Maine†	enforced	1989	counseling	one or adult relative	yes	
Maryland	enforced	1991	notice	one	physician bypass	
Massachusetts	enforced	1980	consent	two	yes	
Michigan	enforced	1990	consent	one	yes	
Minnesota	enforced	1981	notice	two	yes	48 hr
Mississippi	enforced	1986	consent	two	yes	
Missouri	enforced	1979	consent	one	yes	
Montana	not enforced	1974	notice	one	no	
Nebraska	enforced	1991	notice	one	yes	48 hr
Nevada	enjoined	1985	notice	one	yes	
New Hampshire	no law					
New Jersey	no law					
New Mexico	not enforced	1969	consent	one	no	

Snapshot—Laws by State *(cont.)*

State	Status	Year Enacted*	Type of Involvement	Number of Parents or Other Adult	Judicial or Other Bypass	Waiting Period
New York	no law					
North Carolina	no law	1967 repealed				
North Dakota	enforced	1981	consent	two	yes	
Ohio	enforced	1985	notice	one	yes	24 hr
Oklahoma	no law					
Oregon	no law	1969 repealed				
Pennsylvania	enforced	1989	consent	one	yes	24 hr
Rhode Island	enforced	1982	consent	one	yes	
South Carolina	enforced	1990	consent	one or grandparent	yes	
South Dakota	enjoined	1993	notice	one	no	
Tennessee	enforced	1988	notice	two	yes	
Texas	no law					
Utah	enforced	1974	notice "if possible"	two	no	
Vermont	no law					
Virginia	no law	1970 repealed				
Washington	no law	1970 repealed				
West Virginia	enforced	1984	notice	one	yes or physician bypass	24 hr
Wisconsin	enforced	1992	consent	one or adult relative	yes or clergy bypass	
Wyoming	enforced	1989	consent	one	yes	48 hr
Totals	25 enforced (24 with parent; 1 [Conn.] no parent) 9 enjoined 4 not enforced 13 + District of Columbia no law			20 consent 15 notice 1 consent *or* counseling† 1 counseling		

* Where a state has more than one law, only the most recent has been included.

† "Counseling" laws include those that require intensive counseling or encourage minors to involve their parents.

Source: National Abortion Rights Action League, Feb. 1994.

used. The cervix is dilated and the lining of the uterus is scraped with a sharp, spoonlike instrument, a curette. Suction is used to remove the contents, and forceps may be used to remove fetal parts too big to pass through the suction tube. This procedure can take up to 30 minutes, and is more likely to require sedation or general anesthesia.

After the twenty-fourth week of pregnancy, most abortions are done by the *induction,* or *instillation, method.* Less than 3 percent of all abortions in the U.S. are done this way. A prostaglandin or urea solution or a combination of both is injected through the abdomen into the fluid around the fetus. Uterine contractions soon start, and hours later the fetus and placenta are expelled. This method of abortion involves a hospital stay of a day or two.

Menstrual extraction is a technique for removing an embryo from uterus in very early pregnancy or suspected pregnancy a few days after the first missed menstrual period. In the 1970s self-help groups in some cities nationwide developed this technique, in which the woman—or a woman performing it on another—uses a small flexible plastic instrument (cannula) to remove the uterine lining at around the time that her period is due or a few days after.

Not only is the procedure potentially unnecessary—when the pregnancy has not been definitely established—but it carries some risk of infection, since a foreign body is inserted into the uterus. Further, a pelvic examination and repeat pregnancy test is usually recommended a few weeks after the procedure, in order to determine whether fragments of fetal and placental tissue are retained.

RU-486 (developed in France by Dr. Etienne Baulier and the Roussel Uclaf company and commonly called the abortion pill) is a substance that can induce abortion of an early known pregnancy, or it can be used as a contraceptive (if taken monthly around the time of an expected menstrual period). In its capacity as an abortifacient, it breaks the fertilized egg's bond to the uterine wall, resulting in miscarriage. When used in the first 2 months of a pregnancy, it causes abortion a reported 85 percent of the time, and tends to be more effective when administered along with prostaglandins.

RU-486 is not currently approved for use in the United States and Canada. However, clinical trials are set to begin with final FDA approval expected by 1996.

Given the ever-changing national and state political climate regarding the issue of abortion, your best source for your state's current statutes is the National Abortion Rights Action League.

ABORTION RESOURCES

NARAL—National Abortion Rights Action League
1156 15th Street N.W., Suite 700
Washington, DC 20005
202-973-3000

Planned Parenthood Federation of America, Inc.
810 7th Avenue
New York, NY 10019
212-541-7800

American Victims of Abortion
Olivia Gans, Director
419 7th Street N.W., Suite 402
Washington, DC 20004
202-626-8800

WEBA—Women Exploited by Abortion
24823 Nogal Street
Morena Valley, CA 92388
714-247-1278

End Stage Renal Dialysis

End stage renal dialysis is a procedure that treats a condition in which kidney function has decreased to 5 to 10 percent of its normal ability to function or has ceased altogether. End stage kidney disease does not occur suddenly but instead over a long period of time. Usually, a chronic renal condition or other kidney disease has preceded the end stage disease. Inevitably, because the proper functioning of the kidneys is vital to sustain life, end stage renal disease is fatal.

The kidneys belong to the urinary system, whose other members include the ureters, a urinary bladder, and a urethra. The kidneys are responsible for removing wastes (water and solutes in the form of urine) from the blood, regulating the composition and volume of the blood, participating in red blood cell production and vitamin D activation, and regulating blood pressure. Kidney failure can occur due to severe injury to the kidneys, infection, exposure to toxins, and kidney diseases. When the kidneys fail to function, as in end stage renal disease, kidney transplantation and kidney dialysis are the only available options for the patient.

CHRONIC KIDNEY FAILURE

Chronic kidney failure, usually a precursor to end stage renal disease, is a slow, progressive condition that destroys the kidneys over a period of years. Diseases that cause chronic kidney failure include glomerulonephritis (marked by blood and proteins in the urine, decreased urine, and swelling), diabetes mellitus (the most common disease to cause end stage renal disease), hypertension (high blood pressure), polycystic kidney disease (in which the kidneys have become too big and have many cysts, or lumps), pyelonephritis (a pus-forming infection of the kidney), and vesicoureteral reflux (an abnormal backflow of urine from the bladder to the ureter, resulting from a defect at birth or infection of the lower urinary tract).

Symptoms of chronic kidney failure—although they do not often appear in its early stages—include hypertension, vomiting, weight loss, headache, gastrointestinal bleeding, decreased urine output, fatigue, muscle cramps, and decreased mental activity. A urinalysis (a test on urine to check the function of the kidneys) may also indicate the presence of infections and of developing problems associated with the kidneys. Chronic renal failure damage is not limited to the urinary system itself: It cripples, affects, and impedes the normal functioning of the skeletal system, digestive system, cardiovascular system, and central nervous system. Chronic kidney failure may be treated by identifying and treating the underlying disease that initiated the kidney trouble and by following a low-protein, low-salt diet.

END STAGE RENAL DISEASE

End stage renal disease occurs when the kidneys fail to function and are no longer capable of sustaining life. Symptoms of end stage renal disease include uremia (a condition in which toxic levels of urea exist in the blood), urinary infection, intractable nausea and vomiting, hypertension, bone disease, gastrointestinal difficulties, congestive heart failure, anemia, and dementia. As mentioned earlier, end stage renal disease can be treated only by kidney transplantation or by dialysis. Transplantation is considered for those patients who are young or who are relatively healthy otherwise. Dialysis is an option for individuals who have complex medical problems or infections.

DIALYSIS: HEMODIALYSIS AND PERITONEAL DIALYSIS

Dialysis is the process by which the blood is filtered using artificial means. There are two basic types of dialysis: hemodialysis and peritoneal dialysis.

Hemodialysis, the most common form of dialysis, uses a kidney machine in order to remove impurities from the blood. In dialysis, the blood is diffused across a semipermeable membrane in order to separate large and small particles. Blood is pumped from the patient through access devices, called arteriovenous fistulas or arteriovenous shunts, located on either the lower leg or the forearm. Fistulas and shunts allow blood from the patient's radial artery to exit, enter the kidney machine, and then return back into the patient's cephalic vein. The blood travels through tubes to one side of the semipermeable membrane (made of cellophane sheets) in the kidney machine. On the other side of the membrane, a solution (dialysate) of water and a concentrated solution of sodium, chloride, potassium, acetate, calcium, and magnesium regulates the filtered substances as they move across the membrane. The blood that passes through the artificial kidney—approximately 500 ml of blood is in the machine at a time—is then treated with an anticoagulant substance before it enters the patient's body.

Each session of dialysis treatment lasts 3 to 4 hours and occurs about three times a week. Hemodialysis can be done in a hospital dialysis unit, at an outpatient center, in an intensive care unit, or at home. Even though a partner is usually required to help in home hemodialysis, it offers the patient a more independent lifestyle and is less expensive. Dialysis treatments, however, are not without complications. These may include seizures, infection, stroke, hypotension (abnormally low blood pressure), hemorrhage, heart attack, air embolism, hypokalemia (a deficiency of potassium in the blood), obesity, hernia, hemolytic anemia (the escape of hemoglobin outside the red blood cell), peritonitis (a swelling of the peritoneum), and even dementia.

Peritoneal dialysis utilizes the patient's own peritoneum as the dialyzing semipermeable membrane needed to filter and clean the blood. The peritoneum, the large membrane that lines the abdominal cavity, used in conjunction with a dialysate can function as an artificial kidney. The composition of the dialysate utilized in peritoneal dialysis is similar to the dialysate used in hemodialysis and is comparable to the composition of the body's interstitial fluid. The dialysate is made up of glucose, sodium, chloride, acetate, calcium, and magnesium.

In peritoneal dialysis, a catheter (hollow, flexible tube) is placed in the peritoneal cavity, the dialysate is passed through the catheter to the small blood vessels in the cavity, and the waste products along with the dialysate are drained from the cavity. Sessions of peritoneal dialysis in which the peritoneal cavity is irrigated with blood and dialysate can last between 24 and 72 hours.

The more convenient and less time-consuming type of peritoneal dialysis is continuous ambulatory peritoneal dialysis (CAPD), which can be performed at home. The sessions last 4 to 8 hours and are done throughout the duration of the day, 7 days a week. Side effects particular to CAPD include weight gain, backaches, and peritonitis. Complications of peritoneal dialysis may include bleeding (in the abdominal cavity at the puncture site of the catheter), peritonitis, hypotension, loss of proteins, and atelectasis (collapsed lung).

SPECIFIC PROBLEMS OF DIALYSIS PATIENTS

The diets and psychological states of dialysis patients must be monitored. A dialysis patient must follow a special diet consisting of restricted amounts of protein, sodium, potassium, fluids, and phosphorus. Medications such as vitamin B complex and vitamin C, calcium carbonate, folic acid, anabolic steroids, ferrous sulfate, propranolol, and hydralazine (for hypertension) are prescribed to supplement dietary needs or to control other health problems that may exist. A dialysis patient is also affected mentally by his condition.

As for the importance of monitoring the dialysis patient's psychological state, it should be noted that the person is dependent upon a machine to sustain his life and knows he must endure continuous dialysis treatments the rest of his life. In effect, the patient's life is permanently disrupted. He may not be able to maintain a regular job or follow his customary schedule because his daily activities are planned around dialysis treatments. At home, the dialysis patient's role in the family may change—from an active member to a passive one—and, if the dialysis is actually done at home, the treatments themselves could place additional strains on family members. The dialysis patient may be hostile, deny his condition, feel guilty about the high costs of his treatment, or be ambivalent to his condition. Because the constant threat of dying and his deteriorating physical condition are so prevalent in the dialysis patient's mind, he may become depressed or may become completely dependent upon others, having no interest in his own life. Even though dialysis treatment does place a physical and mental strain on the patient, it is still possible to cope with the condition and to achieve some kind of independence: with home dialysis treatments, self-care dialysis, and through a modified lifestyle.

Hormone Replacement Therapy

One of the most mind-boggling health decisions a menopausal woman faces is whether or not to take supplemental hormones to replace those no longer being produced by her aging ovaries.

Hormone replacement therapy (HRT) includes estrogen, a major female hormone that has many functions, including thickening the uterine lining. It often includes progesterone (usually a synthetic mix of progestins), a hormone that counterbalances estrogen, making the uterine lining shed each month as menstrual bleeding. And HRT occasionally includes androgen, male hormones that women, too, naturally produce in small amounts, and which are thought to influence sex drive, energy levels, and mood.

Why is the decision so confusing?

- Because even among well-done studies published in prestigious medical journals, results are sometimes contradictory or hard to interpret, especially when it comes to hormone replacement therapy and heart disease or breast cancer.
- Because many questions about HRT remain unanswered, especially questions about the benefits and risks of long-term use of estrogen-progestin combinations.
- Because even doctors have trouble separating hype from fact, especially when it comes to estrogen's alleged ability to preserve youthful good looks and ensure a sense of well-being. As the National Women's Health Network points out in

What Is Known About the Cancer Risks of HRT?

Doctors say that women who decline to take replacement hormones often do so because of a fear of cancer. The unknown possible risks, perhaps, scare women most.

It's clear that estrogen, taken alone, in any form, increases a woman's risk of developing cancer of the endometrium (uterine lining) from four to fifteen times. Estrogen causes the uterine lining to grow and thicken, which eventually can lead to abnormal cell growth that can become cancerous.

That's why progestins are added during therapy. Progestin allows the uterine lining to break down and be shed as menstrual fluid. The monthly shedding prevents cancer from developing. Women who take progestins run less risk of endometrial cancer than women who take no replacement hormones.

Problems with both cyclic estrogen-progestin therapy (given in staged doses during a month, resulting in monthly menstrual periods) and estrogen alone are leading an increasing number of doctors to experiment with a combination of continual estrogen-progestin therapy (given in the same dosage throughout the month). This may provide the benefits of both estrogen and progestins without monthly periods. The problem with this therapy, according to Wulf Utian, M.D., director of obstetrics and gynecology at University McDonald Women's Hospital in Cleveland, is that no one knows whether it creates a risk for endometrial cancer. "Most of us think the excess risk is eliminated, but that has not yet been proven," he says.

The risks for breast cancer from HRT are much less clear. Most researchers agree that, theoretically, both estrogen and progestins could cause breast cancer, because they stimulate the growth of cells in the breast (and breast cancer can be induced by estrogen in laboratory animals). But most researchers think this effect is weak in older women, whose breast tissue cells are fairly inactive.

Most of the few studies done show no connection between hormone replacement therapy (mostly estrogen) and breast cancer.

But a study by Swedish researchers, published in the August 3, 1989, *New England Journal of Medicine,* did show a connection. Women who took replacement hormones had a 10 percent greater risk of developing breast cancer than women who had not taken hormones. That's a very slight risk.

Several higher-risk groups stood out: women who took estrogen for six years or more, and women who took more potent forms of estrogen not generally used in the United States.

More important to U.S. women, those who took estrogen-progesterone combinations for more than six years appeared to have 4.4 times the average risk of developing breast cancer. A major problem with this part of the study was that there were only ten women in this group, a number much too small to provide a statistically reliable result, according to experts reviewing the study for the *Harvard Medical School Newsletter.* Their consensus: The Swedish study highlights the need for more research, especially in the area of long-term estrogen/progestin therapy.

its booklet *Taking Hormones and Women's Health,* some doctors continue to claim estrogen relieves depression and keeps skin "young-looking" even after a National Institutes of Health Conference in 1979 found no evidence of those effects. (For a copy of the booklet, send $5 to: National Women's Health Network, 1325 G Street N.W., Washington, DC 20005.)

And drug companies are constantly marketing their various hormone replacement products—and funding research in this area—because the potential for profits is great.

Despite this confusion, most gynecologists apparently think hormone replacement benefits outweigh the risks, especially for women who have had their ovaries removed. And some 4-million-plus women do choose to take hormones. They either simply follow their doctor's recommendation, or, wisely, they get more information and decide that, for them, the benefits of HRT outweigh the risks, including, they hope, those risks that are still unknown.

So how can you decide if HRT is for you? Well, you can start by asking your gynecologist or family physician a few questions. Start with "Why do you think I should have HRT?"

If you are bothered by hot flashes (upper body flushing usually followed by heavy sweating) or vaginal atrophy (thinning and dryness, which can cause painful intercourse), HRT definitely can help.

Estrogen *is* FDA-approved to treat both these very uncomfortable symptoms of menopause. It controls hot flashes in about 2 weeks of use, provided the dose is adequate. Vaginal atrophy is more slowly resolved, depending on the severity of the condition. Without hormone treatment, hot flashes usually eventually lessen, but vaginal atrophy only gets worse. (If it is a woman's only menopausal symptom, vaginal atrophy is often treated with an estrogen-containing topical cream for as long as a woman remains sexually active.)

Although anecdotal evidence, and some studies, suggest estrogen therapy can help such other symptoms as urinary incontinence, vaginal infections, muscle and joint pains, mood swings and insomnia, it is *not* FDA-approved to treat these symptoms. "But women whose hot flashes disturb their sleep do sometimes find that estrogen helps relieve symptoms of anxiety or depression," says Isaac Schiff, M.D., chief

of Vincent Memorial Gynecology Service at Massachusetts General Hospital.

You may decide to try HRT to see if it helps relieve any of these symptoms, but keep in mind that you may need other, or additional, treatment.

Even if you aren't bothered by hot flashes, vaginal atrophy, or other symptoms, your physician may recommend HRT. Her reasons? To help prevent osteoporosis (porous, fragile bones) and heart disease, the number-one killer of women after they reach the age of menopause.

Admittedly, these both seem like good reasons to take HRT, but is the evidence of benefits strong enough to subject yourself to the possible risks of prolonged hormone treatment? That's something you'll have to decide for yourself.

Pap Smears

For most women, the benefit of routine Pap smears seems obvious. The test offers the chance to detect cervical cancer early enough to treat it successfully. Many organizations, including the American Cancer Society and the National Cancer Institute, recommend periodic or annual Pap smears. Women who follow those recommendations probably believe they are doing the best thing they can to prevent cervical cancer. And, indeed, they may be.

But the fact is, like many other medical screening tests, the results of a Pap smear are best evaluated with caution. Even though it's one of the most common cancer-screening tests, it's also one of the most inaccurate. The test as done today fails to detect 20 to 40 percent of cases of cancer or precursor cell abnormalities.

And even when the Pap smear *is* accurate, the results can create confusion. A woman may end up being treated for a condition that would have disappeared on its own, or at least, never developed into cancer during her lifetime. She might even be told she has cancer, or a precancerous condition, not knowing that doctors sometimes disagree on exactly what cervical cell abnormalities fit those categories. All in all, there are lots of good reasons for a woman to question her doctor closely about any abnormal Pap smear, and to beware of any treatment recommended on the basis of a Pap smear alone. It's also important for her to check out any symptoms of abnormal bleeding even though she may recently have had a normal Pap smear.

What Is a Pap Smear?

A Pap smear is a scraping of cells from the cervix, the part of the uterus that extends into the vagina. The cells are collected from the mouth of the cervical canal, a narrow opening into the uterus where cell changes that can lead to cervical cancer are most likely to begin.

The cells are smeared onto a glass slide, sprayed with a fixative to preserve them, and sent to a laboratory to be examined under a microscope for abnormalities. Each smear is classified (see below) and a report of any abnormalities is sent back to the doctor.

Why is the Pap smear so inaccurate? Doctors' failure to take an adequate cell sample accounts for about half the errors, says the American College of Obstetricians and Gynecologists. Some doctors may be poorly trained; others, simply in a hurry.

What can you do? Ask your gynecologist if the laboratory he or she uses sends back inadequate smears, rather than simply reporting them as normal. That's an important way for your doctor to get feedback on how well he or she is performing Pap smears. If your doctor uses a cone-shaped "cyto" brush rather than a wooden stick or cotton swab to scrap the cervix, he or she is also more likely to get a good sampling of cells.

Misreading Pap smears at the laboratory also accounts for about half of the errors.

In 1987 the *Wall Street Journal* investigated the Pap-screening industry. They found high-volume cut-rate laboratories with overworked, undersupervised technicians, many paid on a piecework basis that encouraged them to rush the analysis. They also found that the few laws regulating the industry were often ignored.

Since that time, federal regulations have put a ceiling on the number of Pap smears a lab technician can do per week at labs receiving federal funds or doing interstate business. They have also established proficiency testing and standards to check a lab's error rate. It's too soon to tell whether these laws will improve the quality of Pap smear testing. So it's important to ask your gynecologist these questions:

Where will my Pap smear be sent?

Is the laboratory certified by the College of American Pathologists or the American Society of Cytology? Experts say either of these certifications is most likely to indicate reliability.

If the lab does testing for Medicare or Medicaid-funded patients, chances are it is accredited and has passed an on-site inspection. But that doesn't necessarily give the kind of quality assurance as does accreditation by either of the above professional organizations, because, apparently, Medicare inspectors don't always know what to look for when they visit a lab. A survey sponsored by the Health Care Financing Administration in 1989 showed that routine Medicare inspections failed to detect potentially serious discrepancies in slide interpretation at 8 out of 17 labs. So don't count on Medicare inspection alone as assurance of a lab's reliability.

Is the lab near here? Your doctor is likely to communicate more often with a lab that's close. If it's far away, that may mean it's a high-volume, cut-rate lab that's prone to errors. Find out.

How Are Pap Smears Classified?

The results of a Pap smear are classified according to how much of the surface tissue of the cervix is affected and the degree of cell changes that exist.

Right now, many laboratories are in the process of updating and improving how they classify and describe Pap smears. (They are switching from the old Papanicolaou class 1-5 system to the new Bethesda method.) In the meantime, doctors have to sift through a hodgepodge of terminology.

It's important that your gynecologist use a lab that provides a full descriptive report, that she understands the report, and that she can tell you exactly what the report means. Just being told that your Pap smear is "precancerous" or "possibly precancerous" or even just "abnormal" isn't good enough. Don't let ominous-sounding terms stop you from asking questions. In most cases those words *don't* mean cancer, although they may indicate cell changes that could eventually lead to cancer. Keep in mind that many hysterectomies are performed for "suspected cancer"; yet the removed uterus shows no signs of cancer. Don't be frightened into an operation you don't need.

All cytopathologists (experts in the study of diseased cells) use a classification system that provides a continuum from normal to cancerous. To describe cell changes, they use the terms *dysplasia* (which means "abnormal development of cells" that may or may not be cancerous) or *cervical intraepithelial neoplasia* (CIN) which means, simply, "new and abnormal tissue growth" that may or may not be cancerous

How You Can Make Your Pap Smear More Accurate

Lubricants, contraceptive foams and jellies, even semen and blood can mingle with the cells taken during a Pap smear, making it difficult for the lab technician to examine the slide properly.

For best results, avoid using these products for 3 days before your Pap smear. (And use a condom.) Schedule your appointment well after your period has ended.

Don't douche for at least 3 days before your appointment. It can wash away the cells your doctor needs to sample.

A Pap smear can identify bacterial and fungal infections like *Candida* and *Trichomonas*. An infection can make it harder to examine the slide, though, because it can obscure precancerous cell abnormalities or cause cell abnormalities that resemble precancerous conditions. Because of that, you may want to have a second Pap smear after your infection has been treated, but no sooner than 1 month after your first Pap smear.

"among the cells lining the cervix." They may also use a newer term, *squamous* (a flat surface cell) *intraepithelial lesion* (SIL). Using these terms, they rate a smear as having mild, moderate, or severe dysplasia; CIN I, II, or III; low- or high-grade SIL; or invasive cancer.

Find out exactly how your Pap smear was graded. It will help you decide if the treatment your doctor recommends is appropriate. You may also want to request a copy of the pathologist's report. You can always have a second pathologist read your Pap smear, too, if the report seems ambiguous or incomplete.

WHAT YOU NEED TO KNOW IF YOUR PAP SMEAR IS ABNORMAL

• If your Pap smear falls into the "abnormal but benign" category (the old Class 2 Pap), find out exactly what that means. Do you have a bacterial or fungal infection? Inflammation associated with the use of an IUD or exposure to DES? Cell changes that would indicate a viral infection such as herpes or venereal warts? Your lab report should include this information. If it's an infection, your doctor will "treat and repeat." She'll give you medication for the condition and take another Pap smear in about 3 months. (Wait at least a month to have a second Pap smear, since

it takes time for cervical cells to regrow, and a second smear taken too soon after the first may miss abnormalities.)

If your second Pap smear is abnormal, your doctor may be willing to "treat and repeat" again. Or she may want to do further diagnosis as she would for a suspicious Pap smear, although many doctors would contend that's unnecessary.

• If your Pap smear is "clearly abnormal" again, find out exactly what that means. If you have mild dysplasia (CIN I or a low-grade squamous intraepithelial lesion) keep in mind that this condition is of "indeterminate neoplastic potential." That is, it may or may not go on to become cancerous, and it never leads directly to cancer. Up to 40 percent of cases of mild dysplasia disappear without treatment. (They are more likely to regress after a biopsy, which is *not* considered to be treatment.)

Some doctors do not treat mild dysplasia, at least not immediately. They keep tabs on it with Pap smears every 3 months or so. Others will want to do further diagnosis.

How will your doctor decide if you need treatment? If she is aggressive, she may want to do further diagnosis and treatment immediately. If she is conservative, she may simply watch and wait for a time.

Your risk for cervical cancer and your willingness to return for follow-up Pap smears may influence her recommended course of action.

Some doctors feel it is important to treat even mild dysplasia if a Pap smear indicates exposure to the human papilloma virus (HPV). This virus causes venereal warts, some too tiny to be seen. Some forms of the virus carry an increased risk of cancer. And since the virus is transmitted through sexual intercourse, being treated helps stop the spread. Women do seem to develop immunity to the disease, so that after treatment they are unlikely to be reinfected by their mates. Their mates, though, can spread the virus to other women. (They can be treated with little discomfort with a cream that peels the upper layers of skin off their penis.)

- If your Pap smear is "suspicious" (moderate or severe dysplasia; CIN II or III; high-grade squamous intraepithelial lesions; or carcinoma in situ—cancer that has not yet started to spread), it means you have a condition that most doctors believe has a good chance of progressing to invasive cancer unless it is treated. It's true that a few of these cases regress without treatment. The catch, though, is that there's no way for your doctor to identify those lesions.

- And, of course, if your Pap smear indicates invasive cancer, you'll want to take quick action. But even invasive cancer may not mean you need a hysterectomy (see below).

WHAT'S INVOLVED IN TREATMENT?

These days, most doctors follow a clearly abnormal or suspicious Pap smear with a cervical biopsy. They remove bits of tissue from the cervix, using a magni-

---

How Often Should I Have a Pap Smear?

That's a good question. For years, the American Cancer Society recommended that every woman have an annual Pap smear. Then in 1980 it began recommending Pap smears every three years, after two consecutive negative test results. The recommendation for longer screening periods was based on the concept that cervical cancer usually takes many years to progress from a precancerous dysplasia to carcinoma in situ to invasive cancer.

In 1988, however, the American Cancer Society adopted a policy similar to that endorsed by the American College of Obstetricians and Gynecologists, the National Cancer Institute, and the American Medical Association. That policy states: "All women who are, or have been, sexually active, or have reached age 18 should have an annual Pap test and pelvic examination. After a woman has had three or more consecutive, satisfactory, normal annual examinations, the Pap test may be performed less frequently at the discretion of her physician."

What's a good time interval? A study by researchers at the University of Washington, in Seattle, suggests that going more than two years without a Pap smear increases your risk of developing cervical cancer.

In the study, the risk for squamous cell cervical cancer, the most common type, was almost four times higher for women who had Pap tests every three years compared with women who had the test every year. Women who had the test every two years and women who had the test annually had the same risk. And women who hadn't had a Pap test in ten years or more had over twelve times the risk.

Besides the frequency of Pap smears, two other risk factors stood out. Women who had multiple lifetime sex partners or who were younger than age 18 at first sexual intercourse were more likely than women without these risk factors to develop cervical cancer. Such women would be wise to have annual Pap smears, the researchers say.

fying instrument called a colposcope that allows the doctor to view the lesions that need to be sampled. (Don't agree to a "blind" or random biopsy. Their inaccuracy makes them worthless.)

A biopsy can take from 5 to 20 minutes. Since the cervix has few nerve endings, the procedure causes little pain and is done without anesthesia. During the biopsy, bits of tissue about the size of half a grain of rice are removed, using an instrument that resembles a paper punch.

During the colposcopy, your gynecologist should also scrape cells from the cervical canal, a procedure called endocervical curettage. Both the biopsy and curettage tissue samples are sent to a pathologist for microscopic examination. Both colposcopic-directed biopsy and endocervical curettage are considered to be highly accurate ways of diagnosing cervical cancer.

If your biopsy confirms cell changes that you and your doctor decide require treatment, you may have several choices.

Most forms of dysplasia on the surface of the cervix are removed in a simple, in-office procedure that usually requires no anesthesia. The lesions are destroyed by freezing in a procedure called cryosurgery or vaporized with a carbon dioxide laser. Some doctors burn lesions with a cauterizing probe, but since this older treatment can hurt and is more likely to cause the cervical canal to constrict with scar tissue, it's less frequently used nowadays.

Laser surgery is slightly more likely to destroy all the lesions in one treatment. About 5 percent of women who have cryosurgery and 2 percent who have laser surgery will need a second treatment in order to be cured.

If your abnormal cells extend into the cervical canal, your doctor should suggest a cone biopsy (or conization), a surgical procedure in which a cone-shaped piece of tissue is removed from the center of the cervix. Conization should *not* be done prior to obtaining the pathologist's report on your colposcopic biopsy and endocervical curettage. Since it is surgery and involves general anesthesia and a hospital stay, it is usually reserved for cases in which invasive cancer needs to be ruled out.

If your doctor says you need a conization, make sure you understand exactly why he or she thinks this is the best treatment for your condition. If you aren't satisfied that this treatment is necessary, or that lesser treatment might work just as well, get a second, independent opinion.

Cone biopsies can interfere with a woman's fertility and with her ability to carry a child to term. You can get more than one conization, but most doctors don't like to do more than two. (In these cases they will recommend a hysterectomy.) If you do have a

You're Seldom Too Old for a Pap Smear

The women most likely to develop cervical cancer—those aged 60 or older—are also least likely to have regular Pap smears, according to a survey from the Centers for Disease Control and Prevention. Only 52 percent of women aged 60 or older had had a Pap smear the previous year, compared with 81 percent of women aged 18 to 39 and 67 percent of women aged 40 to 59.

Studies suggest that every woman benefits from having at least one Pap smear, no matter what her age. Cervical cancer is two to three times more likely to be found in previously unscreened women over age 65 compared to women aged 65 or younger. Women who have had regular Pap smears during their younger years should have at least two consecutive negative Pap smears between ages 60 and 70, with the option to stop screening at age 70, says the American Geriatrics Society. They base their recommendation on a study from Sweden that shows that the incidence of cervical cancer is low enough in women aged 70 or older who have had at least one normal Pap smear in the previous ten years to recommend discontinuing screening at age 70.

"cone," you should be followed closely enough in the future so that, if abnormal cells return, they are detected early enough to be removed by cryosurgery or laser.

In select cases, conization can be used instead of hysterectomy as a treatment for very early invasive cancer, called microinvasive cancer. To be eligible for this treatment:

- Your cancer should not have penetrated more than 3 mm into the tissue of the uterus. (Some doctors will do conizations up to 5 mm penetration, but this carries more risk that the cancer has spread.)
- The cone should remove all the cancer, not just part of it.
- The edges of the cone should show that the cancer has not spread into the blood vessels.

Simple hysterectomy is still the "treatment of choice" for microinvasive cancer. That's because, even though a fairly large number of women have been treated by conization for this condition, no large, long-term study has followed them to see if the procedure really does cure their cancers.

Are you better off seeing a gynecological specialist for any of these procedures? The specialists, of course, say "Yes!" The general gynecologists say they can do many different procedures. The truth is that almost every doctor tends to specialize, doing some things well and other things not as well. If your doctor is honest with you, he or she will hand you off if it's in your best interest. But it's up to you, the medical consumer, to choose the doctor who will treat you for a particular condition. There are no national figures showing how many conizations or colposcopies the average gynecologist performs in, say, a week. But these are questions you should ask your doctor.

You should certainly see a gynecological oncologist (specializing in cancer) for conization for invasive cancer. You may also want to see this specialist for any kind of conization; he does more "cones" than a general gynecologist and his skill means he will be able to remove the smallest amount of tissue required, which means less damage to the cervix.

Colposcopy and colposcopy-directed biopsy also take some expertise; a doctor can miss lesions or take much longer to do this procedure if he's not highly skilled. Here, as always, it's a good idea to ask your doctor how many of the procedure he performs each week, how long he's been doing it, how he was

trained. If you're uneasy about your doctor's skill in any particular procedure, find another doctor. You may want to call the head of your local hospital's gynecology department. Ask him what doctor he recommends for your procedure. Then ask him if that's because that doctor is the best or if it's because he's the only doctor in town performing the procedure!

Radiation Therapy

Radiation therapy (also called radiotherapy, cobalt treatment, or irradiation) is the use of radioactive materials or high-energy rays to stop cancer cells from growing and multiplying. Radioactive cobalt and high-energy X-ray machines produce ionizing radiation that is used to destroy the cells of a tumor or interfere with its ability to grow. Radiation therapy is often used in conjunction with the surgical removal of a tumor or it may be used in place of surgery when a tumor cannot be removed. It's used to reduce the size of an inoperable tumor that may be causing pain by pressing on the spinal cord or esophagus, as well as pain from brain and bone tumors. Radiation therapy may also be used in conjunction with chemotherapy, especially in the treatment of breast cancer.

EXTERNAL RADIATION TREATMENT

External radiation treatment is similar to having an X ray taken of a broken bone, but the dose of radiation is larger and usually given daily during a 4-to-6-week period. An apparatus called a linear accelerator (a high-powered X-ray machine) is used to develop an invisible beam of electrons that is directed to the tumor site. Linear accelerators are housed in special rooms that are well shielded to prevent the escape of excess radiation.

The linear accelerator looks like something from a science fiction film; however, upon closer examination, it resembles a soup ladle turned upside down, suspended over a table. The beam-generating portion of the machine can be adjusted to a variety of positions to ensure proper placement before treatment begins. A sophisticated mechanism, using motors and gears, positions the arm with pinpoint accuracy prior to treatment. Once the correct coordinates are entered for the treatment, the patient is placed on a hydraulically operated table that is adjusted for proper height and tilt. The accelerator then fires a high-energy beam of electrons at the treatment site.

Before any treatment is given, however, the therapeutic radiologist must calculate the exact dosage of radiation required to treat the patient. This involves determining the intensity of the beam and the time of exposure—a process somewhat like developing photographs, only a lot more complex. Factors such as the size of the patient (thickness of chest, abdomen, etc.) and the location of the tumor must be taken into account. In addition, the patient is literally marked up like a dartboard to help the technicians aim the machine at the exact tumor site.

INTERNAL RADIATION TREATMENT

Internal radiation treatment places radioactive implants inside the body, usually in a body cavity, such as the vagina, or into a tumor of the breast, pituitary, or prostate. The implant is left inside for a few days and the patient remains hospitalized.

Side effects may occur, since the radiation treatment can affect the normal cells surrounding the cancerous site. Some commonly experienced side effects are nausea, vomiting, fatigue, and reddening and blistering of the skin (much like a severe sunburn). Antiemetics may be used to reduce nausea and vomiting, while skin creams may be used to soothe burned skin.

RISKS FROM RADIATION

Exposure to radiation, whether diagnostic (imaging) or therapeutic (treatment) is not without its risks. In fact, the Food and Drug Administration (FDA), the federal agency responsible for ensuring the safety of radiation devices, has stated that calculating the health risks from radiation is a very inexact science, riddled with uncertainty. The FDA, through its Center for Devices and Radiological Health, attempts to set standards for exposure to radiation equipment.

Radiation exposure is measured in "rem," a unit that describes the biological effects on a person from a dose of radiation. One rem equals 1,000 millirems (mrem). To put this in some type of perspective: For the average person exposure to background (naturally occurring) radiation alone amounts to 300 mrem per year, 200 mrem from environmental radon alone.

The exact amount of radiation a person receives from medical sources is dependent on a number of factors: the type of equipment, strength of radiation field generated, duration of exposure, and amount of shielding used. High-level doses of radiation (generally, doses of more than 100 rem), when received by the whole body or large portions of the body, will cause clinical effects known as acute radiation syndrome. As the dose rises above 100 rem, symptoms such as nausea, vomiting, and malaise begin to appear. Higher doses are followed by more serious problems, such as infections, fever, hemorrhage, loss of hair, diarrhea, and loss of body fluids.

The amount of radiation absorbed is the most important factor in determining biological effects. But the same amount of radiation is generally more harmful to children than to adults. The developing embryo in the mother's womb is thought to be the most vulnerable of all to radiation damage.

Therapeutic Radiologists and Radiologic Technicians

A therapeutic radiologist (sometimes called a roentgenologist) is a specialist trained in the use of X rays and other forms of radiant energy to treat disease. In order to become a radiologist, a physician must complete an approved course of study in radiology. Board-certified radiologists have also taken and passed a rigorous written and oral examination administered by the American Board of Radiology.

Radiologic technicians (also known as X-ray technicians) are responsible for preparing patients for radiation treatments, using radiation equipment, and assisting the radiologist in the proper adjustment of equipment. They must complete an approved course of study and, in many states, have a valid license.

Commonly Affected Sites and Side Effects of Radiation Treatment

Abdomen and Pelvis

Bladder irritation (cystitis)

Bloating

Decreased appetite (anorexia)

Nausea and vomiting

Diarrhea

Sexual dysfunction

> **Impotence**
>
> **Menstrual changes**
>
> **Painful intercourse**
>
> **Sterility**

Skin reactions

Arms and Legs

Lhermitte's sign, decreased function

Skin reactions

Weight increase with fluid retention (edema)

Chest and Breast

Decreased appetite (anorexia)

Difficulty in swallowing (esophagitis)

Radiation pneumonitis, difficulty in breathing

Skin reactions

Head and Neck

Difficulty in swallowing (esophagitis)

Disturbance of chewing muscles (trismus)

Dry mouth

Ear inflammation (otitis media)

Eye inflammation (conjunctivitis)

Hair thinning or loss (alopecia)

Mouth sores (stomatitis)

Mucositis

Skin reactions

Taste and smell changes

Tooth decay

Large Areas of Radiation Treatment and/or High Dosage of Radiation

Bone marrow depression

Bleeding, decreased platelet count (thrombocytopenia)

Infection, fewer white cells (leukopenia)

Radiation syndrome (fatigue, malaise, anorexia, diarrhea, nausea and vomiting)

Skin reactions

Weight increase with fluid retention (edema)

Source: Managing the Side Effects of Chemotherapy and Radiation, by Marilyn J. Dodd, R.N., Ph.D., 1987 by Appleton & Lange. Used by permission of the publisher, Prentice Hall Press/A Division of Simon & Schuster, New York.

Four things happen when radiation strikes a cell:

1. It may pass through the cell without doing any damage.
2. It may damage the cell, but the cell partially repairs the damage. (The ability of a cell to repair some of the damage wrought by radiation explains why a given dose of radiation delivered in small amounts over a long period is less damaging than the same dose given all at once.)
3. It may damage the cell so that the cell not only fails to repair itself but also reproduces in damaged form over a period of years.
4. It may kill the cell. The death of a single cell may not be harmful, but serious problems occur if so many cells are killed in a particular organ that the organ no longer can function properly. Incompletely or incorrectly repaired cells may, over time, produce delayed health effects such as cancer, genetic mutations, and birth defects.

Even though therapeutic exposures are very high in comparison with the small amounts used in diagnostic procedures, the risks must be weighed against the benefits. In all cases, it's best to discuss all of your concerns with your radiologist before deciding upon a course of treatment.

Transplants

It used to be that when the heart failed or the lungs ceased to function, death was imminent. But since the middle of this century, organ transplantation has become a way to prolong life for many.

When attempting organ transplantation, three problems need to be overcome:

1. Surgical technique must be highly refined so that the new organ functions properly when placed in the body.
2. The response of the human body's immune system is to reject foreign substances; methods to counteract this response are necessary for organ transplantation to be successful.
3. Suitable organs from donors must be available.

The Network for Organ Sharing is an independent network of hospitals around the country that helps 15,000 people a year receive the organs and tissues they need. Recipients are selected based upon time on a waiting list; medical urgency and blood type; the proper size match for organs other than the kidneys;

and proper tissue match for kidney transplants. For more information on organ transplant procurement programs, see "Organ Donor Programs" in section 9, "Family Health and Resources."

BONE MARROW TRANSPLANTS

Bone marrow transplantation is the treatment of choice for certain types of leukemia, such as chronic myelogenous leukemia (CML), aplastic anemia (failure of bone marrow), and severe combined childhood immune-deficiency syndrome. Bone marrow transplants may also help in some forms of lymphoma, relapsed acute leukemia, and testicular cancer.

Bone marrow is a liquid, not a solid organ. Marrow produces the red and white blood cells and platelets of the bloodstream. In bone marrow transplantation, genetic matching is important. Often the donor is a sibling. The donation of bone marrow is relatively simple compared with solid organ donations. The donor is given a general or spinal anesthesia and needles are inserted in the pelvis to gently withdraw 1 quart of red bone marrow. The donor is discharged within 24 hours.

Transplantation for the recipient requires two steps. First, all the cells in the recipient's bone marrow must be killed over a 7-day period. This is accomplished by giving high doses of chemotherapy and radiation. The actual transplant is much like receiving a blood donation, with 1 quart of marrow dripped into the recipient's bloodstream through a catheter.

The major concern following bone marrow transplantation is graft-versus-host disease (GVH), the condition where a newly transplanted immune system attacks the organs and tissues of the recipient. This condition usually shows up 3 to 5 weeks after the transplantation. Its symptoms are rash, fever, and sometimes diarrhea. GVH can be treated with immunosuppressive medications.

CORNEA TRANSPLANTS

Cornea transplants are performed to save the sight of people who may become blind due to a cloudy cornea (the transparent area covering the front of the eyeball).

These transplants are usually very successful because there are no blood vessels in the cornea, and therefore the body's immune system cannot attack the new cornea. Matching certain characteristics of the donor and the recipient's immune systems also improves the overall outcome of the transplant.

The two types of corneal transplants are partial-thickness and full-thickness grafts. In partial grafts, only the outer layer of the cornea is used. It takes about a month for the transplanted cornea to knit naturally; until that time, the cornea is held in place by sutures.

HEART TRANSPLANTS

In the United States, the most common indicator for heart transplantation is advanced coronary artery disease combined with a history of heart attacks. Transplants are also considered in cases of advanced heart failure and life-threatening arrhythmia. Eighty percent of heart transplant recipients survive the first year, and 70 percent survive five years or more.

Recipients are often limited to those younger than 60 years of age, since these patients have a potentially longer survival rate, and younger people can better tolerate immunosuppressive medicines, especially the side effects, which include the weakening of the skeleton and diabetes. Side effects of the immunosuppressive cyclosporine include high blood pressure and abnormalities of kidney function.

An acceptable donor is one younger than 50 years of age. It is necessary that the major blood group (A, O, B, or AB) of donor and recipient match.

The heart transplant procedure requires careful co-ordination of two operations—one on the donor and one on the recipient. No more than 4 hours should pass between the time the heart is removed from one patient and transplanted into the other. Because of this time constraint, the two coordinating hospitals should be no more than 1,000 to 1,500 miles from each other.

The risk of rejection is greatest during the first month after surgery. Routine heart biopsies are necessary to check for rejection, because no simple blood tests exist that can do this.

The hospital stay following a heart transplant is about 3 weeks. About 75 percent of recipients can eventually return to their previous occupation.

HEART AND LUNG TRANSPLANTS

In some cases a heart-lung transplant is indicated because the lungs have been damaged due to heart dis-ease. In other cases, severe lung diseases alone can necessitate the operation. These diseases include advanced pulmonary hypertension, advanced emphysema, interstitial fibrosis (a scarring of the lungs), and advanced cystic fibrosis.

Only 10 percent of heart donors can provide lungs as well. The typical recipient is younger than 45 years old.

The follow-up to heart-lung transplantation is similar to that following heart transplant surgery. In addition, the respiratory system is monitored for signs of possible pneumonia or lung rejection. Lung rejection is treated with the steroid medication methylprednisolone.

For unknown reasons, heart-lung recipients suffer fewer and less severe episodes of heart rejections than do heart recipients alone.

KIDNEY TRANSPLANTS

Kidney transplants have become routine at major hospitals worldwide. Most kidney transplant recipients have been on dialysis and are tired of the restrictiveness of this method of waste removal. Moreover, dialysis doesn't enable the kidney to perform other functions, such as the production of red blood cells; therefore, patients on dialysis often are anemic. For these people, kidney donation can be the answer.

Since only one functioning kidney is essential for a healthy life, donors are often living relatives of the recipient. When related donors are unavailable, unrelated and cadaver kidneys may be used. Even though using a related donor has the added benefit of a close genetic match, kidney transplant patients must remain on immunosuppressant drugs to prevent rejection of the donor kidney.

During the actual transplantation, the new kidney is usually planted low in the abdomen rather than at the site of the original kidney. This is because it is difficult to attach a new kidney to existing blood vessels. Often one or even both native kidneys remain in the recipient.

One side effect of kidney transplantation is acute tubular necrosis, or ATN, which is the production of little urine. This side effect usually clears up. The hospital stay for the recipient is usually 10 to 14 days.

LIVER TRANSPLANTS

In the past decade, the five-year survival rate for liver transplant patients has grown from 10 percent to more than 50 percent. The liver is the body's largest solid organ and functions as its chemical factory, regulating the levels of chemicals found in the blood. It also plays an all-important role in the digestion of food and the release of energy when the body requires it.

When it begins to fail, one of the first signs is a yellow discoloration of the skin and whites of the eyes called jaundice. This is caused by the liver's inability to adequately filter bilirubin from the bloodstream and excrete it into the bile ducts. Bilirubin is a by-product of a very important function performed by the liver, the breakdown of old red blood cells. Liver failure can be caused by a variety of diseases, medications, or by excessive alcohol and drug abuse.

In liver transplantation, matching blood groups between the donor and recipient are not necessary but are desired. Matching organ size, however, is important. In this case, the donor can either be a living relative or a cadaver.

Liver transplantation is a demanding operation, taking 6 to 18 hours. And recovery is more complicated than for kidney or pancreas recipients. A month or more may pass before the recipient is released from the hospital. During this time, immunosuppressant drugs are administered to lessen the chance of organ rejection. Symptoms of rejection include fever, back pain, and jaundice.

LUNG TRANSPLANTS

In addition to the heart-lung transplant, it has recently become possible to perform single- and double-lung transplants, also known as isolated lung transplantation.

Eighty-five percent of lung transplant recipients are alive after one year, 75 percent after two to three years. Only a few hundred such operations have been performed worldwide since the first isolated lung transplant operation in 1983.

Lungs must be transplanted within 6 hours of being harvested from the donor. In addition, it's very important to prevent obstruction of the airways, which could lead to other complications such as a buildup of fluids and heart failure. Cyclosporine, an immunosuppressant drug, is administered to reduce the risk of tissue rejection.

Methods of checking for lung rejection include lung scan, biopsy, and a laser test that measures blood flow in the lungs.

PANCREAS TRANSPLANTS

Because diabetics are living longer than ever, they are also suffering from diseases brought on from long-term diabetes—diseases such as kidney failure, blindness, and the lack of sensation in the arms and legs that can lead to amputation.

Either the transplantation of an entire pancreas or merely the insulin-producing islet cells can reverse these effects. If an entire pancreas is transplanted, part of the organ's drainage system is also included. Pancreas transplantation is relatively new, with most advances coming in the past decade.

Following surgery, anticoagulants must be taken for several days as well as aspirin for several months thereafter. Blood sugar levels are monitored to determine how well the new pancreas is producing insulin, and also to determine if any rejection is taking place.

6. Medications

INTRODUCTION

Over 80 percent of all office visits end with at least one prescription being written. Medications are an important part of a person's medical care. In some cases, the benefits are the difference between life and death.

Yet most people know little about the medications they take or even about where to get them at the best price. Studies suggest that almost half of all prescriptions filled are never fully used. Consumers report confusion about side effects, shelf life, and even how to read the instructions given to them by a doctor or pharmacist.

In this section, you will learn most of what you will ever need to know about the prescription and nonprescription medications you use. You will also learn ways to lower your costs of drugs and how to use drugs more safely, and will even find a list of drug companies that provide free medications.

Being knowledgeable about pharmaceuticals can make the medications you take far more effective by helping you avoid, or be prepared for, side effects and other problems often associated with drugs.

The Making of a Pharmacist

To be a pharmacist, a person must train at an accredited school of pharmacy, of which there are seventy-two in the United States and Puerto Rico. Basically, there are two professional degrees awarded in pharmacy: the bachelor of science (B.S. Pharmacy) and the doctor of pharmacy (Pharm.D.). The bachelor's degree—which is as far up the education ladder as most pharmacists go—requires five years of collegiate study in courses covering the fields of physiology, biochemistry, biology, and pharmacology. And as more pharmacists step from behind the counter and offer more health and drug therapy information, pharmacy schools are shifting their emphasis toward patient care. In addition, depending upon the particular school, the degree requirements may demand some practical experience outside the classroom, through internships in hospital and community pharmacies.

A rarer breed is the pharmacist with a doctor of pharmacy degree. Although the academic requirements are more intensive than with the B.S., enrollment is growing, in large part due to the expanded role of the pharmacist in the health care system and the chance that the advanced degree will mean even more clout in the marketplace.

Does it matter what degree your pharmacist has? Should you go to the trouble of finding one with a doctorate? Probably not. What does matter is whether your pharmacist holds a valid license. In order to receive one, a graduate in pharmacy must pass an examination given by the board of pharmacy in the state where he or she plans to practice. In order to retain

What a Good Pharmacist Does: A Checklist

- **Does more than merely read a doctor's prescription, fill it, label it, and charge for it. Instead, a good pharmacist is willing and eager to expand the pharmacist's role, beyond that of a "pill counter," to a recognized member of the health care team and a drug information specialist.**
- **Keeps important family medication records called Patient Medication Profiles (see pg. 352) and uses them to help prevent allergic reactions to drugs, dangerous interactions, duplicate medications, and drug abuse.**
- **Advises how to use prescription and nonprescription medication: how and when to take it; what the possible side effects are; what the shelf life is; how to store the medication; and whether there is potential for dangerous interactions with foods and/or other medications.**
- **Answers your questions about the staggering variety of medicines, remedies, tonics, pills, elixirs, lotions, salves, capsules, and powders on the market.**
- **Advises you, when it seems necessary, to seek a medical practitioner's help.**

Glossary of Pharmaceutical Terms

Inevitably, in your consultations with this important health care provider, the pharmacist, unfamiliar words and terms will crop up. Here are some of the most common.

Adverse reaction. Any reaction to a drug that becomes a serious condition or even a hazard in and of itself, and occurs at normal doses.

Bioequivalence. Since the mid-1970s, the Food and Drug Administration has required that generic drugs have the same therapeutic effects as the brand-name drugs when administered to people under the conditions spelled out in the labeling. When this is the case, the drug products are said to be bioequivalent.

Contraindication. Any condition or disease that renders some particular line of treatment improper or undesirable.

Drug-drug interactions. Drugs can affect the activity of each other when more than one drug is taken at a time. The activity of one may be decreased or increased when a second drug is taken, or the combination of two drugs may cause an entirely different effect than is intended.

FDA. The Food and Drug Administration is the federal agency responsible for approving all prescription and nonprescription medicines on the basis of safety, effectiveness, and proper labeling.

Food-drug interactions. Foods can interact with drugs in a variety of ways: by either slowing down or speeding up the time the medication takes to travel to the part of the body where it's needed or by preventing a drug from being absorbed properly. In addition, the natural and artificial chemicals in foods can render drugs useless or even dangerous.

Generic drugs. Every drug has a generic name, usually a condensed version of the original chemical name, which is suggested and filed for by the pharmaceutical company that invented the drug. The manufacturer also registers the drug under the company's own promotional name, and that name is the brand name. For example, acetaminophen is the generic name for the brand-name pain remedies Tylenol, Anacin-3, and Panadol. A generic drug, which does not have to be the same size, shape, or color of the brand-name product, does duplicate the active ingredients of the brand-name drug.

Nonprescription medicine. Any medicine that can be bought without a doctor's prescription. Distribution of nonprescription medicines is unrestricted, and the medicines may be sold, for example, in grocery stores as well as pharmacies.

Over-the-counter (OTC) medicine. The same as nonprescription medicine.

Prescription drugs. Medicines prescribed by a doctor or dentist and dispensed only by them or by a registered pharmacist.

Side effects. Effects on the body apart from the principal action of the medicine. Side effects are usually undesirable, but some cause only minor inconveniences. For example, drowsiness is a side effect of certain antihistamines.

Pharmacy Settings:
Chain Drugstores vs. Independents

Where will you find the best pharmacist? While the independently owned community pharmacy is still a visible, and certainly a viable, part of the American scene—2 out of every 3 prescription drugs are dispensed at such pharmacies, according to the National Association of Retail Druggists—chain stores owned by large national corporations such as Eckerd's, Thrift, Revco, and Walgreen's are steadily making inroads into the market. Another part of the changing scene is the inclusion of pharmacies in supermarkets and discount stores.

As you shop around for a pharmacist for your and your family's needs, and encounter these different settings, you'll probably be wondering if there are advantages of one over the other. Frankly, that's a question for which there's no pat answer—it depends upon the individual pharmacy and its policies, as well as the pharmacist and his or her knowledge and communications skills.

However, there are questions you can ask concerning how business is run at a particular pharmacy, whatever the setting:

- What personalized services are offered? Free home delivery? Convenient hours, especially during evenings and weekends? Arrangements for you to receive emergency medications when the pharmacy is closed or the pharmacist away? Patient Medication Profiles? Patient counseling on drug interactions, side effects, etc.? Help with orthopedic and prosthetic devices or other medical aids? Compliance with your preferences, such as nonchildproof caps, capsules instead of tablets, etc.?
- Is there an area set aside for you to speak privately, if you wish, with the pharmacist?
- Are consumer health education materials available?
- Does the pharmacy have the refill policies that you want? Phone-in refills? Refills available at other locations? Pharmacist willing to contact your physician for you, if necessary?
- Can a rare drug be easily and quickly obtained should your doctor prescribe such for you? Will the pharmacist compound special prescriptions?
- Are the pharmacy's prices competitive with others in your community?
- Does the pharmacy offer a charge account to its customers?
- Does the pharmacy accept your prescription drug insurance?
- Does the pharmacy provide end-of-the-year prescription cost statements for income tax and insurance purposes?
- Does the pharmacy offer a senior citizen discount?
- Is the physical layout convenient? Accessible to the handicapped?

Patient Medication Profile:
What It Is; Why You Need It

By now, you probably have discovered that many considerations come into play when choosing a pharmacist who meets your family's needs. But one of the most important by far is whether the pharmacy has a system that monitors all the drugs your family is taking. Commonly called Patient Medication Profiles or simply Patient Profiles, these systems can aid the pharmacist in preventing medication errors—and, to judge from a study reported in the *British Medical Journal*, we could use all the help we can get: Many doctors don't know the drugs their patients are taking, even when the doctors themselves are prescribing the medications. And neither do the patients. Most cannot accurately describe their drug treatments without their medications at hand.

If this is the case with you and your physician—and it was true in 70 percent of the cases studied—then who's monitoring whether previous medications worked or didn't work? Or keeping track of what medications caused allergic reactions or serious side effects? Who will alert the physician and patient to possible dangerous drug interactions? These are the primary reasons that an up-to-date Patient Medication Profile can be invaluable. While this is a record you may want to keep for yourself, your pharmacist definitely should keep one.

These profiles range from the simple (a card file) to the highly technological (a computerized system that will store and retrieve new and old information and even type labels). Once you've asked around and found a pharmacist who keeps such a record on every customer, ask what information is on it. The American Pharmaceutical Association recommends that a Patient Medication Profile contain the following:

- Your name, address, and phone number
- Your and your family's birthdays (The pharmacist has to know this to check if the dosage is appropriate to the age of the user.)
- Any allergies, reactions, or adverse effects you've demonstrated
- Any drugs that have proved ineffective for you
- A concise health history, including any conditions or diseases that would preclude the use of certain drugs (for example, diabetes, hypertension, or ulcer)
- The over-the-counter, or nonprescription, medicines you take
- The date and number of each prescription filled for you, the name of the drug, its dosage and strength, quantity, directions for use, and price. Also, the prescriber and dispenser of each medication.

Keep in mind that this service will only be useful if you buy all your medicine from the same pharmacy.

the license, many states require the pharmacist to take continuing-education courses. And in the event of misconduct or incompetence, the pharmacist is subject to disciplinary action by the state board.

If you wish to verify that the pharmacist has complied with state licensing requirements, ask him or her to show you the license. It's usually posted on the wall behind the pharmacy counter.

State Pharmacy Boards

These agencies are responsible for regulating the practice of pharmacy within their state, including the administration of licensing examinations and enforcement of the pharmacy practice act. All complaints about pharmacists should be directed to these offices.

Alabama
Board of Pharmacy
One Perimeter Park S., Suite 425
U.S. 280 I-459
Birmingham, AL 35243
205-967-0130

Alaska
Board of Pharmacy
551 Raven View Court
Fairbanks, AK 99712-2514
907-452-2556

Arizona
Board of Pharmacy
5060 N. 19th Avenue, Suite 101
Phoenix, AZ 85015
602-255-5125

Arkansas
Board of Pharmacy
320 W. Capitol, Suite 802
Little Rock, AR 72201
501-324-9200

California
Board of Pharmacy
1020 N Street, Room 448
Sacramento, CA 95814
916-445-5014

Colorado
Board of Pharmacy
1560 Broadway, Suite 1310
Denver, CO 80202-5146
303-894-7750

Connecticut
Board of Pharmacy
State Office Building, Room G1A
165 Capitol Avenue
Hartford, CT 06106
203-566-3917

Delaware
Board of Pharmacy
Jesse S. Cooper Building, Room 205
Federal and Water Streets
Dover, DE 19901
302-736-4708

District of Columbia
Board of Pharmacy
614 H Street N.W., Room 923
Washington, DC 20001
202-727-7468

Florida
Board of Pharmacy
1940 N. Monroe Street
Tallahassee, FL 32399-0775
904-488-7546

Georgia
Board of Pharmacy
166 Pryor Street S.W.
Atlanta, GA 30303
404-656-3912

Hawaii
Board of Pharmacy
P.O. Box 3469
Honolulu, HI 96801
808-548-8542

Idaho
Board of Pharmacy
280 W. 8th Street, Suite 204
Boise, ID 83720
208-334-2356

Illinois
Board of Pharmacy
320 W. Washington Street
Springfield, IL 62786
217-785-0800

Indiana
Board of Pharmacy
One American Square, Suite 1020
Box 82067
Indianapolis, IN 46282
317-232-2960

Iowa

Board of Pharmacy
1209 East Court
Executive Hills W.
Des Moines, IA 50319
515-281-5944

Kansas

Board of Pharmacy
Landon State Office Building, Room 513
Topeka, KS 66612-1220
913-296-4056

Kentucky

Board of Pharmacy
1228 U.S. 127 S.
Frankfort, KY 40601
502-564-3833

Louisiana

Board of Pharmacy
5615 Corporate Boulevard
Baton Rouge, LA 70808-2537
504-925-6496

Maine

Board of Pharmacy
Board of Commissioners of the Profession of Pharmacy
Statehouse Station 35
Augusta, ME 04333
207-582-8723

Maryland

Board of Pharmacy
4201 Patterson Avenue
Baltimore, MD 21215-2299
410-764-4755

Massachusetts

Board of Pharmacy
Leverett Saltonstall Building, 15th Floor, Room 1514
100 Cambridge Street
Boston, MA 02202
617-727-9954

Michigan

Board of Pharmacy
611 W. Ottawa
P.O. Box 30018
Lansing, MI 48933
517-373-0620

Minnesota

Board of Pharmacy
2700 University Avenue W., Room 107
St. Paul, MN 55114-1079
612-642-0541

Mississippi

Board of Pharmacy
C&F Plaza, Suite 1165
2310 Highway 80 W.
Jackson, MS 39204
601-354-6750

Missouri

Board of Pharmacy
P.O. Box 625
Jefferson City, MO 65102
314-751-0091

Montana

Board of Pharmacy
510 First Avenue N., Suite 100
Great Falls, MT 59401
406-761-5131

Nebraska

Board of Pharmacy
301 Centennial Mall S.
P.O. Box 95007
Lincoln, NE 68509
402-471-2115

Nevada

Board of Pharmacy
1201 Terminal Way, Suite 212
Reno, NV 89502
702-322-0691

New Hampshire

Board of Pharmacy
Health and Human Services Building
6 Hazen Drive
Concord, NH 03301
603-271-2350

New Jersey

Board of Pharmacy
1207 Raymond Boulevard, 6th Floor
Newark, NJ 07102
201-648-2433

New Mexico

Board of Pharmacy
University Tower, Suite 400-B
1650 University Boulevard N.E.
Albuquerque, NM 87102
505-841-9102

New York

Board of Pharmacy
Cultural Education Center, Room 3035
Albany, NY 12230
518-474-3848

North Carolina
Board of Pharmacy
602H Jones Ferry Road
P.O. Box 459
Carrboro, NC 27510
919-942-4454

North Dakota
Board of Pharmacy
P.O. Box 1354
Bismarck, ND 58502-1354
701-258-1535

Ohio
Board of Pharmacy
77 S. High Street, 17th Floor
Columbus, OH 43266-0320
614-466-4143

Oklahoma
Board of Pharmacy
4545 N. Lincoln Boulevard, Suite 112
Oklahoma City, OK 73105
405-521-3815

Oregon
Board of Pharmacy
505 State Office Building
P.O. Box 231
Portland, OR 97207
503-229-5849

Pennsylvania
Board of Pharmacy
P.O. Box 2649
Harrisburg, PA 17105-2649
717-783-7157

Puerto Rico
Board of Pharmacy
800 Roberto H. Todd Avenue
P.O. Box 10200
Santurce, PR 00908
809-725-8161

Rhode Island
Board of Pharmacy
304 Cannon Building
3 Capitol Hill
Providence, RI 02908-5097
401-277-2837

South Carolina
Board of Pharmacy
1026 Sumter Street, Room 209
P.O. Box 11927
Columbia, SC 29211
803-734-1010

South Dakota
Board of Pharmacy
P.O. Box 518
Pierre, SD 57501-0518
605-224-2338

Tennessee
Board of Pharmacy
500 James Robertson Parkway, 2nd Floor
Nashville, TN 37219-1149
615-741-2718

Texas
Board of Pharmacy
8505 Cross Park Drive, Suite 110
Austin, TX 78754-4594
512-832-0661

Utah
Board of Pharmacy
160 East 300 South
P.O. Box 45802
Salt Lake City, UT 84145-0802
801-530-6628

Vermont
Board of Pharmacy
Pavilion Office Building
Montpelier, VT 05602-2710
802-828-2875

Virginia
Board of Pharmacy
1601 Rolling Hills Drive
Richmond, VA 23229
804-662-9911

Washington
Board of Pharmacy
1300 S.E. Quincy, EY-20
Olympia, WA 98504
206-753-6834

West Virginia
Board of Pharmacy
236 Capitol Street
Charleston, WV 25301
304-558-0558

Wisconsin
Board of Pharmacy
P.O. Box 8935
Madison, WI 53708
608-266-2811

Wyoming
Board of Pharmacy
1720 S. Poplar, No. 5
Casper, WY 82601
307-234-0294

Pharmacists and Over-the-Counter Drugs

"Why even worry about OTCs?" you ask. "After all, doesn't the mere fact that they're available without a prescription speak for their safety, and doesn't the Food and Drug Administration oversee the effectiveness of over-the-counter remedies as well as prescription drugs?"

First, no drug is harmless and completely safe. Each and every one is a chemical, designed to alter the body's function in some way—for the better, it is hoped. Compared to prescription drugs, yes, OTCs are relatively safe. Nonetheless, OTCs must be used with caution. Some nonprescription drugs are as strong as the medications your doctor prescribes. And, as for the FDA's "stamp of approval" or the agency's ability to remove a suspect drug from the market, keep in mind that ineffective and marginally effective drugs do exist. And unaware consumers are buying them. F. James Grogan, a leading pharmacist/writer, estimates that more than $1 billion is squandered on what he calls "second-rate OTC drugs."

With more than 300,000 OTC products on the market, the choices can be confusing, and as wary a consumer as you may be, in your confusion you may turn to the most visible source of "information" on OTCs—advertising. Frankly, television and magazine ads do not always point you in the most cost-effective direction, nor do their claims ensure that you find the safest, most effective drug for your problem or condition. But a good pharmacist may.

Another reason for finding a pharmacist who can counsel you wisely is that doctors tend to underplay—if not actually dispute—the therapeutic role OTCs can play in your health care. The health care professional right there on the scene, where the OTCs are being sold, is the pharmacist, not the doctor. Whatever your questions may be—and the following are just samples—about whatever category of OTC you're interested in, ask right on the spot.

- **Colds and coughs:** Do I need a decongestant or antihistamine?
- **Antacids:** Are any of them nonconstipative or good for a low-sodium diet?
- **Laxatives:** Which has the least side effects?
- **Pain:** What's preferable—aspirin or acetaminophen? Are "bargain" aspirin okay?
- **Obesity:** Is any one diet aid safer and better than the others? Are any safe?

Just keep in mind that, out of all the questions asked, advice sought, and answers given, you're shopping for a pharmacist who will:

- Be a source of professionally based, unbiased, factual, and honest information on OTCs.

Pharmacists and Over-the-Counter Drugs *(cont.)*

- Help you sort out the good from the poor or downright useless OTCs.
- Tell you if there's no proof that a particular remedy works.
- Keep you posted on any previous prescription-only medicines that are now available over the counter, such as Benadryl, topical hydrocortisone, Tinactin, and Actifed.
- Warn you of the risks or side effects of potentially hazardous drugs.
- Warn you about potentially dangerous interactions between over-the-counter medications and prescription drugs you may be taking.
- Help you use nonprescription remedies wisely and appropriately, according to the label instructions. (If you are taking drug preparations in forms you do not normally use or fully understand—for instance, suppositories or prolonged-release tablets—look for a pharmacist who will provide detailed, perhaps even written instructions.) A lot of pharmacists assume that people can choose the best OTC remedy merely by reading labels, and that they will comply automatically with the manufacturers' recommendations. This is simply not true.

So your job is to find a pharmacist who will be willing to check your nonprescription drug purchases and point out the OTCs that are appropriate and effective for what's ailing you. The entire process goes something like this:

- First, determine what your symptoms are.
- Ask the pharmacist what ingredients are needed to treat your diagnosed condition.
- Work together to find the products containing the needed ingredient(s). (A good pharmacist can help ensure that you don't pay for ingredients you don't need.)
- Choose a safe, effective, and economical product from that list.

OTC drug sales are big business—really big. In 1993 U.S. manufacturers' sales were around $14.2 billion, which was up from the year before when sales topped $13.3 billion, according to the research firm Kline and Company, who predict sales topping $15.2 billion in 1994. And, if the projections of experts are right, the business will get even better: The prediction is a 7 percent increase per year in sales. All the more reason to choose a pharmacist who knows the business.

A word of warning regarding OTCs: In the interest of health, be sure to consult a pharmacist and possibly a physician before buying any OTC preparation for babies, young children, elderly persons, debilitated patients, and/or pregnant or breast-feeding women.

How to Read a Prescription

A standard prescription, written out by a doctor and subsequently filled by a pharmacist, contains several basic facts: the physician's name and address; the patient's name and address; the name of the drug, its strength, and its dosage; any special instructions that the patient must be aware of (whether drug should be taken with food, at bedtime, etc.); the physician's signature and his or her authorization for (or against, as when he or she checks "brand necessary") any generic substitutions of the drug.

The information on most prescriptions, however, is in coded form. Don't let the Latin directions or esoteric shorthand keep you from figuring out what you're supposed to do with the medicine.

Here's a list of some phrases and terms that turn up frequently on prescription sheets:

a.c. = before meals
ad lib. = freely; as needed
AM = morning
b.i.d. = twice a day
c̄ = with
cap = capsule
cc or cm = cubic centimeter
ext = for external use
gtt = drops
h.s. = before bedtime
mg = milligrams
ml = milliliters
noct = at night
non repetat = no refill
pc = after meals
PM = evening
po = by mouth
prn = as needed
qd = once a day
qh = every hour
q.i.d. = four times a day
rep = refill
s = without
sig = label; directions
sig ut dict = take as directed
stat = at once
tab = tablet
t.i.d. = three times a day
top = apply topically
x = times

Safe Use of Medications

Just as medications bought over the counter and in prescription form are not always foolproof cures or effective treatments for particular medical conditions, neither are they always completely safe to use. Specifically, there are risks involved with taking medications that appear to have been tampered with, stored improperly or not stored in their original containers, or are past their expiration date. However, there are steps that you can take to protect yourself and your family from any accidental poisonings.

PRODUCT TAMPERING

Because of the publicity surrounding product tampering cases in the 1980s, manufacturers have made extensive changes in the way OTC medications are packaged and labeled. Inner and outer safety seals have been added to virtually every product to make it easier—for everyone from the store clerk to the consumer—to detect product tampering. In addition, a written warning advises against purchasing or using the product if the safety seal is broken.

Even though manufacturers have added these safety features, it's still the consumer's responsibility to carefully examine the package, preferably before purchasing the product but definitely before ingesting it. Packaging will vary somewhat, depending on the form of medication you are purchasing. In addition to being placed in sealed containers, pills and capsules may also be individually sealed in what is called a blister pack. Look for seals around the caps on liquid medications as well as seals on any packaging containers. Topical medications such as creams and ointments, which are usually packaged in tubes or jars, should have a safety seal on any outer packaging.

Here are a few things to look for when purchasing packaged medications.

- Check to see if the container has been tampered with in any way. If the seal appears to be disturbed in any fashion, don't purchase the product.
- Outer and inner linings that are open, seals that are disturbed or cracked, or holes could indicate product tampering.
- Products with disturbed caps, cotton plugs, and wrapping should be avoided. The contents of the container should be looked at next.
- Pills, capsules, and tablets should not be discolored, colored differently from one another,

crumbly, in different sizes or shapes, deformed, give off an unusual odor, or have smeared or unclear imprints.
- Liquid medications should likewise be checked for uniformity in color, thickness and texture, any unusual odors, and any foreign particles.
- Creams and ointments should be checked for color and texture. Any sign of discoloration or a sandy feeling could indicate a problem.

If you have any suspicions that something might be wrong, don't purchase the product. If you have already purchased a product, return it to the store where it was purchased or contact the manufacturer. Some manufacturers have a toll-free telephone number where consumers may report problems with product packaging.

PROPER STORAGE

You should always store medications in a cool, dry place, in a locked cabinet, and out of the reach of children. The glove box of your car may be fine for maps and notepads, but it definitely isn't the place for medications. Protect your medications from heat, freezing, and moisture. Exposing your medications to the extremes of temperature and moisture could change the chemical makeup of the drug, thereby defeating its therapeutic purpose. If you ingest the medication in this condition, you may also expose yourself to the potential effects of an accidental poisoning.

Store your medications in their original containers including any outside packaging material, especially if it contains dosage information. The original containers are designed to protect medication from moisture and exposure to air.

Do not store different medications in the same bottle. This is an accident waiting to happen. And don't think that you can tell one pill from the other by color. Some pills and capsules resemble one another, causing you to forget which medications you mixed.

EXPIRATION DATE

Always check the expiration date on the medications in your home medicine cabinet. Manufacturers put those expiration dates on the products so you won't accidentally take something that is no longer safe and effective and could actually harm you.

The expiration date of medications will vary somewhat. For example, cold tablets are usually good for two to three years, while vitamins and minerals may retain their potency for up to six years. Use the expiration date on your medications as sort of a "window," or time frame. It doesn't mean that on the date shown, usually expressed as month and year, the product automatically loses its potency. It does mean that after that date, the product could begin to deteriorate and lose its effectiveness.

If you have any doubts as to the expiration date of a particular medication, you may contact the manufacturer or discard the medication. It's always a good idea to replace any medications that are old, appear strange or discolored, or give off an unusual odor.

OTHER SAFETY PRECAUTIONS

Always read the label before taking or giving any medication. Taking the wrong dosage could result in an unexpected side effect or problem. Use child-resistant containers for all medications. Never leave your medications unattended when children are present; it only takes a matter of seconds for an accident to happen.

When dealing with medications, whether OTC or prescription, it's always best to err on the side of safety and double-check all packaging, safety seals, and dosage instructions. If a problem does arise, call your physician or pharmacist immediately, and if necessary contact your nearest poison control center.

Shelf Life of Medications

Important to the safe and effective use of prescription and nonprescription drugs is knowing when a drug has gone beyond its expiration date. The shelf life of medications varies, and often it is hard to tell from the look, smell, or flavor of a drug that it is past its prime. While aspirin smells like vinegar when it is no longer fresh and some liquids take on a different color, become cloudy, or separate and form solid "gunk" at the bottom of the container, other medications give no visible or olfactory clues.

The good news is that many prescription drugs now show their expiration dates on their labels—and, of course, the containers show the dates that the drugs were originally filled. Generally, too, the expiration dates for nonprescription remedies can be found on the box, bottle, or tube—although, unfortunately, these can be hard to read.

A good rule of thumb to remember is the adage "When in doubt, throw it out." Don't forget, too, that

(1) medications whose labels are lost or unreadable should be discarded; (2) a savvy consumer will record the date that all over-the-counter medications are purchased and first opened; and (3) the pharmacist can be a big help in determining how long to keep medications.

Here is the shelf life for some popular drugs.

Cold tablets	1–2 years
Laxatives	2–3 years
Minerals	6 years or more
Nonprescription painkiller tablets	1–4 years
Prescription antibiotics	2–3 years
Prescription antihypertension tablets	2–4 years
Travel sickness tablets	2 years
Vitamins	6 years or more

Mail-Order Drugs

In light of the high cost of prescription drugs, consumers can save time and money by ordering them through mail-order companies and discount pharmacies. A mail-order pharmacy can offer substantial savings on prescription and nonprescription, or over-the-counter, drugs, and it's easy to see why:

- First, the drugs usually cost less through the distribution houses because the drugs are bought in bulk (at about 10 percent less than the average wholesale price), so drug prices to the consumer usually exclude the retail markup.
- And since the drugs are sold to consumers in volume (that is, quantities that last several months) there are fewer dispensing and administration fees.
- Plus, whenever possible the distribution houses substitute generic drugs, which are traditionally less costly than brand-name drugs.

No one mail-order pharmacy has the lowest prices across the board, but usually a consumer can expect to pay less for some drugs through a mail-order pharmacy than through a local pharmacy or drugstore. When deciding where to purchase any prescription drugs, the consumer should shop around at local pharmacies as well as mail-order pharmacies, because the prices may vary. The consumer should keep in mind, too, that the specific dosage and type of drug and the frequency with which the consumer must take it indicate whether a mail-order service is the best way to obtain drugs.

If a consumer takes a wide range of drugs whose dosages change, requires a small quantity of drugs, or needs the drugs right away, mail-order pharmacies may not be a viable option. Mail-order pharmacies deliver the drugs with a delay of sometimes up to 3 weeks, and do not offer the same amount of personal attention and service a consumer would find at a local pharmacy. Consumers who benefit economically from these companies are usually those who order large quantities of a specific drug—that is, drugs taken regularly for a chronic health condition such as arthritis.

On the whole, mail-order pharmacies do offer safe and effective delivery of drugs: They have a long-standing safety record and most double- and triple-check their orders. There are no more incidences of mistakes made in filling orders at mail-order pharmacies than there are at local pharmacies. However, consumers should always investigate the practices of the mail-order pharmacy they choose: Check its reputation with the Better Business Bureau and find out what other services the mail-order pharmacy has to offer. Some mail-order pharmacies offer customers information concerning drug interactions and side effects with their order, toll-free telephone access to a pharmacist and to a prescription refill service, a catalog service for OTC drugs, and special services for the blind and hearing-impaired.

Although the services of some mail-order companies are only available to members of certain organizations, there are also mail-order pharmacies that are open to anyone. Before deciding on a mail-order pharmacy, consumers should also check their health insurance or with their employer to see if mail-order drugs are covered.

Mail-Order Pharmacies
Action-Mail Order: 800-452-1976
AARP: 202-872-4700 (available to members only)
Family Pharmaceuticals: 800-922-3444
Medi-Mail: 800-331-1458
National Pharmacies: 202-347-8800 (available to members only)
Pharmail: 800-237-8927

Generic Drugs

A generic drug (the name of which is usually a condensed version of the drug's original chemical name) is one whose active ingredients duplicate those of the brand-name product. The name of the generic drug is designated by drug experts and approved by governmental agencies.

Typically, the process from brand-name drug to generic version goes like this: Brand-name, or pioneer, drugs are made by pharmaceutical companies (innovator companies) who spend much time and money developing, researching, and clinically testing the new drug. After Food and Drug Administration (FDA) approval of the new drug, the innovator company has a patent for the drug for seventeen years, which gives the company the right to name the drug and ensures it a monopoly on the sale, marketing, and advertisement of the drug itself. The seventeen years also allow the innovator company to recoup the exorbitant costs incurred while researching and developing the new drug.

When the drug comes off patent, generic drug companies may manufacture generic versions of the pioneer drug. About fifteen drugs a year come off patent. Drugs that have recently come off patent include Lopressor, Tenormin, Corgard, Xanax, and Dobutrex (in 1993) and Tagamet, Mezlin, and Bricanyl (in 1994). Drugs that will come off patent in 1995 include Minipress, Pipracil, Talwin, Capoten, and Oraflex. It is calculated that 94 percent of brand-name drugs will be available in generic form in 1995.

Why this explosion of generics onto the market? The movement can be traced, in part, to 1984, before which time generic drug manufacturers' efforts to make generic drugs were somewhat thwarted by the FDA's regulations requiring that the generic version of the drug undergo the same rigid testing and approval procedures as the pioneer drug went through. However, a law passed in Congress (the Drug Price Competition and Patent Term Restoration Act) stipulated that generic drugs need not go through all the orginal testing, done initially by the innovator company, to see if the active ingredient of the drug is safe and has therapeutic value for the general populace.

Instead, what the generic drug manufacturer must prove is that the generic version is bioequivalent to the brand-name drug. A generic drug is termed bioequivalent if the active ingredient of the drug is absorbed into the bloodstream at the same rate and at the same extent as the brand-name drug's absorption rate. After showing bioequivalency, the generic drug manufacturer includes in the drug various excipients, such as inert fillers, preservatives, coloring agents, and binders, in order to further distinguish their generic version. Because generic drug manufacturers are at liberty to choose the fillers they ultimately use in their drug, it is not always known what kind of side effects or allergic reactions are possible for the recipi-

What About Safety?

The subject of generic drug efficacy and safety has been questioned ever since a 1989 scandal afflicted the generic drug industry. In August of that year the Food and Drug Administration was roundly chastised by the federal Department of Health and Human Services' Office of the Inspector General for failing to keep close rein on its generic review process. Three former employees of the FDA's generic drug division pleaded guilty to accepting illegal payments from drug manufacturers in exchange for handling drug applications more quickly, three generic drug company officers were indicted on bribery charges, and the FDA began investigating eleven generic drug firms implicated in faulty or fraudulent practices. By September 1989, 26 drugs had been recalled and suspensions issued for 141 others.

After the discovery of the scandal, the FDA undertook extensive measures to investigate the practices of generic drug manufacturers and to ensure the overall safety of generic drugs for the consumer. The FDA rigorously tested existing generic drugs and promptly removed the questionable generic drug manufacturers and their drugs from the market. Now generic drugs are not only under the careful eye of the FDA but are also scrutinized by the innovator drug companies. The innovator drug companies, whose brand-name products are continually competing with the generic versions, hold independent drug tests or "defensive biostudies" on generics to prove that their pioneer drugs are superior.

A Matter of Substitution or Safety?

The battle over generic drugs may have as much to do with substitution as with safety, and the fact that doctors aren't happy with what they see as a loss of autonomy and control when pharmacists substitute generics for brand-name drugs.

Most states have repealed their antisubstitution laws, under which if a doctor prescribed a certain brand of a drug, the pharmacist could not substitute the generic version, even if it cost less and was the chemical twin of the prescribed brand. Now pharmacists nearly everywhere can fill a prescription with a generic, but the process varies depending on whether the state's substitution law is permissive or mandatory. Half require the doctor to write "dispense as written," "brand necessary," or words to that effect, and in most of the other states the doctor must sign on either one of two signature lines—one line allows the pharmacist to substitute, the other to dispense only as written.

Several state legislatures are considering bills that would change prescription forms and procedures to actually encourage substitution. Doctors would have to write out the words "brand medically necessary" or some such phrase. In the handful of states that currently require the handwritten phrase, surveys have found that doctors just do not bother to do that.

Find out what your state's law is concerning the substitution of a generic drug. These laws strengthen the role (and responsibility) of the consumer *and* the pharmacist in decision-making.

10 Commonly Prescribed Drugs and Their Generic Versions

Brand Name/Generic Name	Prescribed For
Premarin/conjugated estrogens	estrogen
Amoxil/amoxicillin	antibiotic
Zantac/ranitidine hydrochloride*	ulcer
Lanoxin/digoxin	heart
Synthroid/levothyroxine sodium	thyroid hormone
Procardia/nifedipine	heart
Xanax/alprazolam	anxiety
Vasotec/enalapril maleate	hypertension
Cardizem/diltiazem hydrochloride	heart
Ceclor/cefaclor	antibiotic

*Generic to be available in 1995.

ent due to the inclusion of these fillers. And because the FDA allows a certain small variance rate in bioequivalency testing, the potency of various generic drugs may differ among themselves, which in turn could lead to problems if a person switches between different brands of the generic drug.

Generic drugs are usually less expensive than their brand-name equivalents—on the average, 30 percent cheaper, even 50 to 70 percent cheaper than the more expensive medicines—because their manufacturers do not go to the expense of advertising them, nor do they sink money into inventing new products.

With the ever-climbing costs of health care and of prescription drugs, more and more consumers are

Therapeutic Substitution

Depending on who you are and how you look at the issue, therapeutic substitution is either a way that pharmacists, with their superior knowledge of medicines, can fine-tune your doctor's orders to ensure that you get the best drug for your problem at the best price—or a dangerous encroachment on physicians' prescribing privileges and a threat to your health.

A big step beyond generic substitution, therapeutic substitution (pharmacists prefer to call it therapeutic *interchange*) allows a pharmacist to switch an entirely different drug believed by the pharmacist to be therapeutically similar to the drug prescribed by the physician. This practice differs from generic substitution in that the drug dispensed is not a generic version of the prescribed drug, but is one with an entirely different chemical composition.

As you can imagine, organized medicine is on the warpath against therapeutic substitution. True, it is standard practice in many hospitals, but doctors fear its spread to the corner drugstore and health care settings beyond the hospital, specifically health maintenance organizations (HMOs) and nursing homes. The worst-case scenario here, say the doctors, is that cost-slashing budgeteers will try to save money without regard for patient well-being and substitute cheaper drugs in the pharmacy without telling the doctors who care for HMO patients.

The director of the American Medical Association's division of drugs and toxicology, interviewed in the April 10, 1989, *Medical World News,* summed up organized medicine's position on extending therapeutic substitution to large HMOs: an "acceptable and sensible" arrangement only if practiced with physicians' knowledge and consent.

Some 40 percent of HMOs have substitution practices and prescribe from an approved formulary, according to the trade group for HMOs, Group Health Association of America. The country's largest HMO, Kaiser Permanente, has used therapeutic substitution from an approved formulary for more than fifteen years.

Does therapeutic substitution threaten the health of consumers? Does it undermine the system of checks and balances that conscribe the traditional roles of physician and pharmacist? Or does therapeutic substitution benefit consumers by involving pharmacists in determining the most effective drug with the least possible side effects at the most economical cost? No doubt the debate will rage on as more and more HMOs adopt the practice of therapeutic substitution to help contain ever-rising pharmaceutical costs. But the question really comes down to how much of a factor cost should be in drug selection. That's a question you should take up with your physician and your pharmacist anytime a drug is prescribed for you.

The medical profession, staunchly opposed to therapeutic substitution, maintains that therapeutic decisions reached by physicians are based on a complex body of medical information relevant to a specific patient—make sure this is indeed the case with you.

choosing to purchase generic drugs. In 1991 consumers spent $5.5 billion on generic drugs, and by 1995 the annual figure is expected to have risen to $15 billion. Generic drug manufacturing is quite a profitable business; once thought of as inferior to brand-name drugs, generic drugs challenge their brand-name counterparts in price. In fact, because the generic drug industry is so profitable, 80 percent of generic drug manufacturers are actually innovator drug companies.

37 MOST COMMON NONPRESCRIPTION (OTC) DRUGS AND THEIR POSSIBLE SIDE EFFECTS

Category/Type of Drug (recommended by % of pharmacists) (Top Brand Name) Possible side effects of the top brand (caused by overdosage, extended or improper use, allergic reactions, a chronic or special health condition)

1. Adult Cough Medications (100%) (Robitussin) Dizziness, headache, nausea, rash, vomiting
2. Adult Cold Preparations (99.7%) (Drixoral) Drowsiness, excitability in children; higher dosages: dizziness, nervousness, sleeplessness
3. Antidiarrheals (99%) (Imodium A-D) Allergic reaction; overdosage: CNS (central nervous system) depression, constipation, nausea
4. Children's Cold Preparations (99%) (Dimetapp) Drowsiness, excitability in children; higher dosages: dizziness, nervousness, sleeplessness
5. Children's Cough Medications (99%) (Robitussin) See no. 1, Adult Cough Medications
6. Athlete's Foot/Jock Itch Remedies (98%) (Tinactin) Irritation
7. Ibuprofens (98%) (Advil) Allergic reaction, heartburn, stomach pain, upset stomach
8. Throat Lozenges (98%) (Chloraseptic) Allergic reaction
9. Acetaminophens (97%) (Tylenol) Allergic reaction; overdosage: hepatic toxicity leading to diaphoresis, nausea, vomiting
10. Antacids (97%) (Mylanta) people with kidney insufficiency: CNS depression, other symptoms of hypermagnesemia; prolonged use for normophosphatemic patients: anorexia, hypophosphatemia, malaise, muscle weakness, osteomalacia
11. Stool Softeners/Other Products (97%) (Colace) Bitter taste, nausea, throat irritation, rash
12. Bulk Laxatives (94%) (Metamucil) Allergic reaction, minor bloating and gas
13. Hemorrhoidal Preparations (94%) (Anusol) Allergic reaction, burning; symptoms to discontinue use: irritation, pain, swelling, redness
14. Canker Sore/Cold Sore Remedies (93%) (Zilactin) Mild stinging
15. Vaginal Antifungals (92%) (Monistat 7) symptoms to discontinue use: fever, pain, vaginal discharge
16. Aspirins (91%) (Bayer) Allergic reaction, heartburn, nausea, stomach pain, vomiting
17. Flu Remedies (91%) (Thera-Flu) overdosage: dizziness, drowsiness, excitability in children, nervousness, sleeplessness
18. Pediculicides (90%) (Nix) Asthmatic episodes/breathing difficulty in susceptible persons, itching, redness, swelling
19. Toothache/Teething Remedies (88%) (Orajel)*
20. Topical Anesthetics (88%) (Americaine) Allergic reaction
21. Allergy Relief Products (84%) (Chlor-Trimeton) Drowsiness, excitability in children; higher dosages: dizziness, nervousness, sleeplessness
22. Eardrops (84%) (Debrox)*
23. Suntan/Sunscreen Products (82%) (Presun) Allergic reaction; symptoms to discontinue use: irritation, rash
24. Pregnancy Test Kits (81%) (EPT)*
25. Asthma Relief Products (78%) (Primatene) Loss of appetite, nausea, nervousness, sleeplessness, tremor
26. Irritant or Stimulant Laxatives (75%) (Dulcolax) Abdominal cramps, discomfort
27. Acne Preparations/Treatments (74%) (Oxy-5 or -10) Allergic reaction, burning, drying, or peeling of skin, irritation, itching, redness, swelling
28. Thermometers (73%) (B-D)*
29. Diet Aids/Programs (61%) (Slim-Fast)*
30. Contact Lens Solutions (55%) (Bausch & Lomb) Allergic reaction
31. Saline Laxatives (52%) (Fleet) Abdominal pain, burning sensation, cramping, rectal discomfort; symptoms to discontinue use: nausea, vomiting
32. Ovulation Test Kits (51%) (First Response)*
33. Antiplaque/Gingivitis Rinses (44%) (Plax)*
34. Fluoride Rinses (39%) (ACT)*
35. Denture Cleansers (36%) (Efferdent)*
36. Toothpaste (35%) (Crest)*
37. Occlusives (33%) (Johnson & Johnson)*

* No harmful side effects listed. Read label and use as directed.

50 MOST COMMONLY PRESCRIBED DRUGS, THEIR GENERIC EQUIVALENTS AND SIDE EFFECTS

Name of Drug (generic equivalent) (Other Brand Names when available) Common side effects

1. Premarin (conjugated estrogens) Abdominal cramps, abnormal vaginal bleeding, bloating, breast swelling and tenderness, depression, dizziness, enlargement of benign tumors in the uterus, fluid retention, gallbladder disease, hair loss from the scalp, increased body hair, migraine headaches, nausea, vomiting, sex-drive changes, skin darkening, skin rash or redness, swelling of wrists and ankles, vaginal yeast infection, weight gain or loss, yellow eyes and skin
2. Amoxil (amoxicillin) (Larotid, Polymox, Trimox, Wymox) Agitation, anemia, anxiety, changes in behavior, confusion, diarrhea, dizziness, hives, hyperactivity, insomnia, nausea, rash, vomiting, weight gain or loss, yellow eyes and skin
3. Zantac (metolazone) (Diulo) Anemia, abdominal bloating, blood clots, blurred vision, chest pain, chills, constipation, depression, diarrhea, dizziness, fainting, fatigue, gout, headache, hepatitis, high blood sugar, hives, impotence, inflammation of the skin, joint pain, loss of appetite, low potassium levels, sodium levels, muscle spasms, nausea, rapid heartbeat, rash, sensitivity to light, upset stomach, vertigo, vomiting, yellow eyes and skin
4. Lanoxin (digoxin) Apathy, blurred vision, change in heartbeat, diarrhea, dizziness, headache, loss of appetite, lower-stomach pain, nausea, psychosis, weakness, yellow vision
5. Synthroid (levothyroxine) (Levothroid, Levoxine) Side effects are rare—however, if excessive dosage, symptoms are: changes in appetite, diarrhea, fever, headache, increased heart rate, irritability, nausea, sleeplessness, sweating, weight loss
6. Procardia (nifedipine) (Adalat) Cough, dizziness, headache, heartburn, light-headedness, low blood pressure, mood changes, muscle cramps, nasal congestion, nausea, nervousness, shortness of breath, sore throat, swelling of arms, legs, hands, and feet, tremors, weakness, wheezing
7. Xanax (alprazolam) Abdominal discomfort, abnormal muscle tone, cramps and spasticity, agitation, allergies, anxiety, blurred vision, chest pain, confusion, constipation, decreased/increased sex drive, depression, diarrhea, dizziness, dry mouth, fainting, fatigue, headache, hyperventilation, increased/decreased appetite, increased/decreased salivation, infection, lack of coordination, low blood pressure, menstrual problems, nausea, rapid heartbeat, rash, ringing in the ears, skin inflammation, speech difficulties, stiffness, sweating, tiredness or sleepinesss, tremors, upper respiratory infections, weight gain or loss
8. Vasotec (enalapril) Abdominal pain, allergic reactions, angina pectoris, angioedema, asthma, blood clots, blurred vision, bronchitis, confusion, constipation, cough, decreased urination, depression, diarrhea, difficulty in breathing, sleeping, and digestion, dizziness, dry eyes and mouth, excessive perspiration, fainting, fatigue, fluid in lungs, hair loss, headache, heart palpitations, hepatitis, herpes zoster, hives, impotence, inflammation of the mouth and tongue, itching, lack of muscle coordination, loss of appetite and smell, low blood pressure, muscle cramps, nausea, nervousness, pinkeye, pneumonia, rash, red skin, ringing in the ears, runny nose, sleepiness, sore throat and hoarseness, stroke, taste alteration, tearing, tingling (pins and needles), upper respiratory infection, upset stomach, vertigo, vomiting, weakness, wheezing
9. Cardizem (diltiazem hydrochloride) Abnormally slow heartbeat, dizziness, fluid retention, flushing, headache, nausea, rash, weakness
10. Ceclor (cefaclor) Diarrhea, hives, itching
11. Seldane (terfenadine) Change in bowel habits, cough, dizziness, dry mouth, nose, or throat, headache, hives, itching, nausea, nervousness, rash, sore throat, stomach and intestinal problems, vomiting
12. Naprosyn (naproxen) Abdominal pain, bruising, constipation, diarrhea, difficult breathing,

50 Most Commonly Prescribed Drugs, Their
Generic Equivalents and Side Effects (CONT.)

Name of Drug (generic equivalent) (Other Brand Names when available) Common side effects

dizziness, drowsiness, headache, hearing changes, heartburn, indigestion, inflammation of the mouth, itching, light-headedness, nausea, rapid heartbeat, red or purple spots on the skin, ringing in the ears, skin eruptions, sweating, swelling due to fluid retention, thirst, vertigo, visual changes

13. Calan (verapamil hydrochloride) (Calan SR, Isoptin, Isoptin SR, Verelan) Congestive heart failure, constipation, dizziness, fatigue, fluid retention, headache, low blood pressure, nausea, rash, shortness of breath, slow heartbeat

14. Mevacor (lovastatin) Abdominal cramps/pain, altered sense of taste, blurred vision, constipation, diarrhea, dizziness, gas, headache, heartburn, indigestion, itching, muscle cramps/pain, nausea, rash, weakness

15. Ortho-Novum 7/7/7 See no. 40, Ortho-Novum

16. Augmentin (generic ingredients: amoxicillin, clavulanate potassium) Diarrhea, itching or burning of the vagina, nausea or vomiting, skin rashes or hives

17. Prozac (fluoxetine hydrochloride) Abnormal dreams, agitation, anxiety, bronchitis, chills, diarrhea, dizziness, drowsiness and fatigue, hay fever, inability to fall asleep, increased/decreased appetite, light-headedness, nausea, nervousness, sweating, tremors, weakness, weight loss, yawning

18. Capoten (captopril) Abdominal pain, constipation, cough, diarrhea, dizziness, dry mouth, fatigue, hair loss, headache, inability to sleep, labored breathing, loss of appetite and taste, nausea, peptic ulcer, rash, stomach irritation, tingling (pins and needles), vomiting

19. Proventil (INHL/RFL) (albuterol sulfate) (Ventolin) Aggression, agitation, cough, diarrhea, dizziness, excitement, general body discomfort, headache, heartburn, increased appetite and blood pressure, indigestion, irritability, labored breathing, light-headedness, muscle cramps, nausea, nervousness, nightmares, nosebleed, overactivity, palpitations, rash, ringing in the ears, shakiness, sleepless-

ness, stomachache, stuffy nose, throat irritation, tooth discoloration, tremors, vomiting, wheezing, worsening bronchospasm

20. Trimox See no. 2, Amoxil

21. Tagamet (cimetidine) Agitation, anxiety, breast development in males, depression, diarrhea, disorientation, dizziness, hallucinations, headache, impotence, mental confusion, psychosis, sexual dysfunction, sleepiness

22. Provera (medroxyprogesterone acetate) Acne, anaphylaxis, blood clots, bleeding between menstrual periods, breast tenderness or sudden flow of milk, cervical erosion or secretion changes, depression, drowsiness, fever, fluid retention, headache, hives, insomnia, itching, jaundice, menstrual flow changes, nausea, rash, skin discoloration, weight gain/loss

23. Tenormin (atenolol) Diarrhea, dizziness, fatigue, headache, light-headedness, low blood pressure, nausea, slow heartbeat, vertigo

24. Dyazide (generic ingredients: hydrochlorothiazide, triamterene) Abdominal pain, anemia, blurred vision, breathing difficulty, change in potassium level, constipation, diabetes, diarrhea, dizziness, dry mouth, fatigue, fluid in lungs, headache, hives, impotence, irregular heartbeat, kidney failure, kidney stones, muscle cramps, nausea, rash, sensitivity to light, strong allergic reaction, tingling (pins and needles), vertigo, vision changes, vomiting, weakness, worsening of lupus, yellow eyes and skin

25. Amoxicillin (Manufacturer: Biocraft) See no. 2, Amoxil

26. Lopressor (metoprolol tartrate) Depression, diarrhea, dizziness, itching, rash, shortness of breath, slow heartbeat, tiredness

27. Cipro (ciprofloxacin hydrochloride) Abdominal pain/discomfort, diarrhea, headache, nausea, rash, restlessness, vomiting

28. Ventolin (INHL/RFL) See no. 19, Proventil

29. Micronase (glyburide) (Diabeta) Bloating, heartburn, nausea

30. Dilantin (phenytoin sodium) Decreased coordination, involuntary eyeball movement,

50 Most Commonly Prescribed Drugs, Their Generic Equivalents and Side Effects (*cont.*)

Name of Drug (generic equivalent) (Other Brand Names when available) Common side effects

mental confusion, slurred speech, unsteady movement

31. Vicodin (generic ingredients: hydrocodone bitartrate, acetaminophen) (Anexsia, Lortab, Norcet, Zydone) Dizziness, light-headedness, nausea, sedation, vomiting

32. Coumadin (warfarin sodium) Hemorrhage

33. Lasix (furosemide) Anemia, constipation, cramping, diarrhea, dizziness, fever, headache, high blood sugar, inflammation of the lymph or blood vessels and the pancreas, itching, loss of appetite, low potassium, muscle spasms and cramps/pain, nausea, rash, reddish or purplish spots on the skin, restlessness, ringing in the ears or hearing loss, sensitivity to light, skin inflammation, stomach or mouth irritation, vertigo, vision changes, vomiting, weakness, yellow eyes and skin

34. Triphasil See no. 40, Ortho-Novum

35. IBU (ibuprofen) (Advil, Rufen) Abdominal cramps, abdominal discomfort, bloating and gas, constipation, diarrhea, dizziness, fluid retention and swelling, headache, heartburn, indigestion, itching, loss of appetite, nausea, nervousness, rash, ringing in ears, stomach pain, vomiting

36. Lopid (gemfibrozil) Abdominal pain, acute appendicitis, constipation, diarrhea, eczema, fatigue, headache, indigestion, nausea, rash, vertigo, vomiting

37. Voltaren (diclofenac sodium) Abdominal bleeding, pain/cramps, swelling, constipation, diarrhea, dizziness, fluid retention, gas, headache, indigestion, itching, nausea, peptic ulcer, rash, ringing in the ears

38. Darvocet-N (generic ingredients: propoxyphene napsylate, acetaminophen) (Darvon-N: contains propoxyphene napsylate only) Drowsiness, dizziness, nausea, sedation, vomiting

39. Amoxicillin (Manufacturer: Warner-Chilcott) See no. 2, Amoxil

40. Ortho-Novum (Other oral contraceptives brand names include Demulen, Levlen, Loestrin, Lo/Ovral, Modicon, Nordette, Norethin, Norinyl, Ovcon, Ovral, Triphasil) Abdominal cramps, acne, appetite changes, bleeding in spots during a menstrual period, bloating, blood clots, breast tenderness or enlargement, cataracts, chest pain, depression, difficulty in breathing, dizziness, fluid retention, gallbladder disease, growth of face, back, chest, or stomach hair, hair loss, headache, heart attack, high blood pressure, inflammation of the large intestine, kidney trouble, liver tumors, lumps in the breast, menstrual pattern changes, migraine, muscle, joint, or leg pain, nausea, nervousness, premenstrual syndrome, secretion of milk, sex-drive changes, skin rash or discoloration, stomach cramps, stroke, unexplained bleeding in the vagina, vaginal discharges and infections, visual disturbances, vomiting, weight gain or loss, yellow skin or whites of eyes

41. Tylenol w/Codeine (generic ingredients: acetaminophen, codeine phosphate) (Phenaphen w/Codeine) Dizziness, light-headedness, nausea, sedation, shortness of breath, vomiting

42. Propoxyphene NAP w/APAP See no. 38, Darvocet-N

43. Glucotrol (glipizide) Constipation, diarrhea, dizziness, drowsiness, headache, hives, itching, low blood sugar, nausea, sensitivity to light, skin rash and eruptions, stomach pain

44. Diabeta See no. 29, Micronase

45. Zestril (lisinopril) (Prinivil) Chest pain, cough, diarrhea, difficulty in breathing, dizziness, fatigue, headache, low blood pressure, nausea, rash, vomiting, weakness

46. Pepcid (famotidine) Constipation, diarrhea, dizziness, headache

47. Theo-Dur (theophylline) Convulsions, diarrhea, disturbances of heart rhythm, fluid retention, flushing, frequent urination, hair loss, headache, heart pounding, irritability, low blood pressure, muscle twitching, nausea, nosebleed, rapid breathing, rash, restlessness, sleeplessness, stomach pain, vomiting

48. Hismanal (astemizole) Diarrhea, dizziness, drowsiness, dry mouth, fatigue, headache,

50 Most Commonly Prescribed Drugs, Their
Generic Equivalents and Side Effects (CONT.)

Name of Drug (generic equivalent) (Other Brand Names when available) Common side effects

increase in appetite, inflammation of the eyelids, joint pain, nausea, nervousness, sore throat, stomach and intestinal pain, weight gain

49. Triamterene w/HCTZ See no. 24, Dyazide
50. Inderal (generic ingredient: propranolol hydrochloride) Abdominal cramps, constipation, decreased sexual ability, depression, diarrhea, difficulty in breathing, disorientation, dry

eyes, fever with sore throat, hair loss, hallucinations, headache, light-headedness, low blood pressure, lupus erythematosus, nausea, rash, reddish or purplish spots on the skin, short-term memory loss, slow heartbeat, tingling, tiredness, trouble sleeping, upset stomach, visual changes, vivid dreams, vomiting, weakness

Drug Companies That Provide Free Medication

A poor person who suffers from chronic illnesses necessitating lifesaving drugs—anything from cancer to severe anemia—may be eligible to receive free medications from the drug manufacturers.

The drug companies do not generally advertise such programs, so it is up to consumers to contact the manufacturers of the drugs they need and ask if such programs for indigent people are offered. Usually the drug manufacturer requires a doctor's consent and proof of the patient's financial hardship.

The following companies provide medicine for the poor through patient assistance programs. Most require that patients meet certain income requirements. A few allow annual family incomes as high as $35,000 to $40,000.

Abbott Laboratories/Ross Laboratories
202-637-6889; 800-922-3255

Adria Laboratories Inc.
614-764-8100

Allergan Prescription Pharmaceuticals
800-347-4500, extension 6219

Amgen Inc.
800-272-9376

Boehringer Ingelheim
203-798-4131

Bristol-Myers Squibb
800-736-0003

Burroughs-Wellcome
919-248-4418

Ciba-Geigy
908-277-5849

Genentech Inc.
800-879-4747

Glaxco Inc.
800-452-9677

Hoechst-Roussel
800-776-4563

Hoffman–La Roche Inc.
800-526-6367

ICI/Stuart
302-886-2231

Immunex Corp.
206-587-0430

Johnson & Johnson (Ortho Biotechnology)
908-704-5232

Johnson & Johnson (Janssen Pharmaceuticals)
908-524-9409

Eli Lily and Co.
317-276-2950

Marion Merrell Dow
816-966-4250

Merck Sharp Dohme
215-540-8600

Norwich-Eaton
607-335-2079

Parke-Davis
201-540-2000

Pfizer Pharmaceuticals
800-869-9979

Sandoz Pharmaceuticals
800-937-6673

7. Medical Equipment

INTRODUCTION

For people with disabilities and other handicapping conditions, adaptive and durable medical equipment can be the difference between dependency and independence. Over the last few decades, with the great advancements that have been made in medical technology, equipment and devices have been manufactured that have opened up the world for people who might otherwise have been confined to their homes by physical barriers.

In this section, the major equipment available for individuals with physical disabilities is reviewed. Also discussed is durable medical equipment, such as walkers and canes. You will also learn about the available prostheses that have revolutionized the way people with disabilities can function and maneuver.

Being disabled used to mean a life of confinement. But today, with the available equipment and technology, most people with handicapping conditions have a better opportunity for a productive and fulfilling life.

Adaptive Equipment for the Disabled

Today disabled persons have a wide range of helpful machines, building structures, and gadgets to aid them in gaining access to buildings, in communicating, and in leading an unhampered lifestyle, thanks in large part to the enactment of the Americans with Disabilities Act in 1990.

HOME COMPUTERS, ROBOTIC DEVICES, AND LOCOMOTIVE EQUIPMENT

At home, the disabled person can be greatly aided by the use of a computer or robotic devices. A computer can help the disabled person to communicate, operate household functions (such as turning on lights), and allow the person to work and shop at home. Computers come in a variety of styles and work capacities but can be set up to be voice-activated or controlled by one hand, a foot, or a head nod. Other devices, such as a mouse, mouth stick, or a light pen, can facilitate the operation of a computer by a disabled person who cannot use a keyboard.

Other electronic machines, such as a voice synthesizer, will translate the printed word to the spoken word, and machines that can transcribe standard written characters into braille enable visually impaired individuals to communicate. Telecommunications devices for the deaf (TDDs) allow deaf persons to see the spoken conversation on a display screen and to type back responses on a keyboard. Some TDDs have printers as well as external signalers to alert deaf persons to incoming calls. Various models of listening devices, amplifiers, and artificial larynxes help hearing or vocally impaired individuals.

Robotic devices can make performing such tasks as lifting and moving items or eating and drinking easier to accomplish for the disabled person. Other locomotive equipment and aids for people with disabilities include wheelchairs (available in many styles and sizes and motorized or operated manually), canes, crutches, and walkers (for partially ambulatory individuals), and Seeing Eye dogs (for visually impaired individuals).

MODIFICATIONS IN THE HOME

Modifications in the home that aid in accommodating a disabled person include lowering the counters and cabinets, making appliances easily accessible for a wheelchair-bound person to use, designing wider doorways, and installing toilet and shower grab bars. Beds and toilets can be lowered or heightened to the disabled person's specifications. Kitchen utensils and crockery can be specially equipped with handles, barriers, and grips to facilitate hand manipulation, drinking, and eating. Lifts can be installed for the purpose of traveling up stairs, getting into a tub, and sitting in and operating a car.

MODIFICATIONS IN THE WORKPLACE

In the workplace, certain modifications can be made so that people who have a variety of limitations and disabilities can be allowed to work. Structural changes such as desk heights, doorway widths, and the installation of ramps can give disabled persons the freedom to move about the workplace. Specialized equipment, such as a TDD or a machine to transcribe braille characters, can be installed to give hearing- and visually impaired workers an opportunity to work. Disabled persons may choose to work for a company from their own home, through the use of computers and modems linked to the company's computer system.

The Americans with Disabilities Act

With the passage of the Americans with Disabilities Act (ADA) on July 26, 1990, disabled persons are entitled to have access to public buildings (use of ramps and other access areas specifically designated for those with disabilities) to use telecommunications devices (for hearing- and speech-impaired individuals), and to have the same number and quality of public services that a nondisabled person receives (transportation, state and governmental services). Additionally, employers cannot discriminate against a qualified person with a disability.

The Americans with Disabilities Act stipulates that public accommodations (restaurants, hotels, theaters, doctors' offices, pharmacies, stores, museums, parks, libraries, and so on) must be made accessible to persons with disabilities. If physical barriers exist in these public places, the barriers must be taken down, altered, or replaced with physical structures that provide the disabled with easy access. Elevators are required in buildings that have three or more stories or have more than 3,000 square feet of floor, and hotels that offer public transportation must provide this service to disabled persons as well.

Concerning employment, the ADA states that employers cannot discriminate against a qualified disabled person (in hiring or in promotion) and cannot screen out disabled applicants solely on the basis of their disabilities. Effective in July of 1994, employers who have as few as fifteen employees must also provide "reasonable accommodation" to disabled workers in the way of modifying equipment or job restructuring.

Further, public transportation, including bus and rail cars and bus and train stations, must be made accessible to disabled persons (Amtrak stations must be made accessible by July 26, 2010). Transit authorities must provide special transportation services to disabled persons who cannot use fixed-route bus services. Governments, both state and local, cannot discriminate against qualified disabled persons, and their facilities, services, and communications must also be made accessible. Telephone companies must provide telecommunications devices and service for the hearing-impaired.

In legal matters, although individuals can bring private lawsuits to obtain court orders to stop discrimination, money damages cannot be awarded. Individuals can file complaints with the Attorney General, who in turn can file discrimination lawsuits and obtain money.

RESOURCES FOR SERVICES FOR THE DISABLED

Regional Disability and Business Technical Assistance Centers (DBTACs)
800-949-4232 V/TDD

Region 1 (CT, ME, MA, NH, RI, VT)
New England DBTAC
145 Newbury Street
Portland, ME 04101
207-874-6535 V/TDD

Region 2 (NJ, NY, PR, VI)
Northeast DBTAC
United Cerebral Palsy Association of New Jersey
354 S. Broad Street
Trenton, NJ 08608
609-392-4004 V
609-392-7044 TDD

Region 3 (DE, DC, MD, PA, VA, WV)
Mid Atlantic DBTAC
Independence Center of Northern Virginia
2111 Wilson Boulevard, Suite 400
Arlington, VA 22201
703-525-3268 V/TDD

Region 4 (AL, FL, GA, KY, MS, NC, SC, TN)
Southeast DBTAC
**United Cerebral Palsy Association, Inc./
National Alliance of Business**
1776 Peachtree Street, Suite 310 North
Atlanta, GA 30309
404-888-0022 V
404-888-9098 TDD

Region 5 (IL, IN, MI, MN, OH, WI)
Great Lakes DBTAC
University of Illinois at Chicago/UAP
1640 W. Roosevelt Road M/C627
Chicago, IL 60608
312-413-7756 V/TDD

Region 6 (AR, LA, NM, OK, TX)
Southwest DBTAC
Independent Living Research Utilization/The Institute for Rehabilitation and Research
2323 S. Shepherd Street, Suite 1000
Houston, TX 77019
713-520-0232 V
713-520-5136 TDD

Region 7 (IA, KS, MO, NE)
Great Plains DBTAC
University of Missouri at Columbia
4816 Santana Drive
Columbia, MO 65203
314-882-3600 V/TDD

Region 8 (CO, MT, ND, SD, UT, WY)
Rocky Mountain DBTAC
Meeting the Challenge, Inc.
3630 Sinton Road, Suite 500
Colorado Springs, CO 80907-5072
719-444-0252 V/TDD

Region 9 (AZ, CA, HI, NV, Pacific Basin)
Pacific DBTAC
Berkeley Planning Associates
440 Grand Avenue, Suite 500
Oakland, CA 94610
510-465-7884 V
510-465-3172 TDD

Region 10 (AK, ID, OR, WA)
Northwest DBTAC
Washington State Governor's Committee
P.O. Box 9046
Olympia, WA 98507-9046
206-438-3168
206-438-3167 TDD

Materials Development Projects

Employment

Cornell University
School of Industrial and Labor Relations
106 Extension
Ithaca, NY 14853-3901

International Association of Machinists Center for Administration, Rehabilitation, and Employment Services
1300 Connecticut Avenue N.W., Suite 912
Washington, DC 20036

Public Accommodation/Accessibility

Barrier Free Environments, Inc.
Water Garden
Highway 70 W.
P.O. Box 30634
Raleigh, NC 27622

Federal Contacts for ADA Information

Equal Employment Opportunity Commission
1801 L Street N.W.
Washington, DC 20507
800-USA-EEOC V
202-663-4494 TDD

U.S. Department of Justice
Civil Rights Division
Coordination and Review Section
P.O. Box 66118
Washington, DC 20035-6118
202-514-0301 V
202-514-0381 TDD
202-514-0383 TDD

U.S. Architectural and Transportation Barriers
Compliance Board
1331 F Street N.W., Suite 1000
Washington, DC 20004-1111
800-USA-ABLE V
202-272-5449 TDD

The President's Commission on Employment of People
with Disabilities
1331 F Street N.W., 3rd Floor
Washington, DC 20004-1107
202-376-6200 V
202-376-6205 TDD

Other Organizations and Services for the Disabled

American Coalition of Citizens with Disabilities
1200 15th Street N.W., Suite 201
Washington, DC 20005
202-785-4265

Disabled American Veterans
P.O. Box 14301
Cincinnati, OH 45250
606-441-7300
Disabled hotline 800-332-2399

Job Accommodation Network
West Virginia University
P.O. Box 6123
Morgantown, WV 26506
800-526-7234

National Home Business Network for the Disabled
P.O. Box 368
Weatherford, TX 76086

National Organization on Disability
910 16th Street N.W.
Washington, DC 20037
202-293-5960
202-293-5968 TDD

Special Needs Catalogs

AT&T Special Needs Center
2001 Route 46, Suite 310
Parsippany, NJ 07054
800-233-1222

Accent Buyer's Guide
Accent Special Publications
P.O. Box 700
Bloomington, IL 61702

Access to Recreation
2509 Thousand Oaks Boulevard, Suite 430
Thousand Oaks, CA 91360
800-634-4351
805-498-7535

Adaptive Communication Systems
P.O. Box 12440
Pittsburgh, PA 15231
412-264-2288

Bristol-Myers Co.
Guide to Consumer Product Information
P.O. Box 14177
Baltimore, MD 21268

Consumer Care Products, Inc.
Sheboygan Falls, WI 53085

Dorothy O'Callaghan
P.O. Box 19083
Washington, DC 20036

Hydra-Fitness
P.O. Box 599
Belton, TX 76513-0599
800-433-3111

IBM National Support Center for Persons
with Disabilities
2500 Windy Ridge Parkway
Marietta, GA 30067
800-426-2133

Kemp & George
2515 E. 43rd Street
Chattanooga, TN 37422
800-343-4012

Radio Shack Catalog for People with Special Needs
At local Radio Shack stores or from:
300 One Tandy Center
Fort Worth, TX 76102

Special Toys 4 Special Kids
11834 Wyandot Circle
Westminster, CO 80234

Swedish Rehab
100 Spence Street
Bay Shore, NY 11706
800-645-5272

Durable Medical Equipment

Durable medical equipment is equipment that can stand repeated use, is primarily and customarily used to serve a medical purpose, generally is not useful to a person in the absence of illness or injury, and is appropriate for use at home.

Durable medical equipment that consumers use at home, for their own personal use or for certain disabilities or health conditions, is varied and diverse. Consumers may use home health equipment, such as breathing aids and other respiratory equipment and monitors, treatment-oriented equipment (dialysis, pain control), functional aids (ostomy products, feeding mechanisms), and daily living and ambulatory aids (beds, lifts, wheelchairs, walkers).

These home care products are designed to aid, assist, and help the individual at home. Insurance may cover the cost of these products if a doctor orders them and provided they are a medical necessity. Medicare covers 80 percent of the cost of durable medical equipment, with the beneficiary responsible for 20 percent copayment. Depending upon your needs, you may either rent or purchase medical equipment. The decision to rent or purchase should be made after consulting with your physician and reviewing your insurance coverage. The cost of the equipment and length of time it will be needed are factors affecting the decision to rent or purchase.

ACTIVITIES OF DAILY LIVING

Equipment to aid and facilitate daily living activities include specialized beds and bedroom equipment, lifts, wheelchairs, crutches, walkers, canes, and various gadgets. Beds can be specially equipped with bed rails and can be electrically or manually adjusted in position and in height. Special bed pillows (designed to give support to the head, neck, and shoulders), trays, tables, body pillows (for bedsores), and mattresses can also be used to increase the comfort of the bedridden individual.

Lifts, used for the bath or elsewhere around the house, can be helpful in moving an individual from a wheelchair or bed to another location. Stair glides or lifts allow a disabled individual to have access to upper and lower levels.

Wheelchairs come in many different styles, widths, and heights and can be manually controlled or can be motorized and controlled by a hand or chin joystick or by a breath-activated control. Other types of scooters, wheelchair/recliners, wheelchair cushions and commode attachments, and portable wheelchair ramps and carriers can increase the mobility and/or comfort of the individual. Crutches, walkers, and canes, which are available in different styles, improve the mobility of partially ambulatory individuals.

Such varying styles of equipment include walkers that can be equipped with wheels, canes that can have a four-pronged base, and crutches that can be placed under the arm or attached to the forearm. Other personal aids to assist the individual in and around the house include reaching and gripping devices, specially adapted grips for utensils, and specially designed plates and cups.

Functional aids—those aids designed to assist the individual perform bodily functions as well as other activities—include ostomy products, enteral pumps, and various types of commodes, waste management devices, and other bath aids. Individuals who have had an ostomy—surgery to make an artificial opening in the body to allow the release of feces from the bowel or urine from the bladder (e.g., ileostomy, colostomy, uterostomy)—have surgically created stomas (artificial openings). These people must use ostomy products, such as collection pouches and drainage bags, ostomy adhesives, cleansers, ointments, and deodorants, and peristomal coverings.

Enteral nutrition pumps deliver nutritional liquids to the individual by way of the small intestine. Enteral pumps can be portable, have safety mechanisms and alarms in them, and use IV (intravenous) stands, enteral feeding tubes, and enteral feeding bags.

There are various styles, shapes, and kinds of commodes that an individual can use at home. Commodes can be backless, be set up like a chair, or have armrests and adjustable seat heights. Disposable waste systems, such as a collection bag used in conjunction with a commode, are also available.

Bathing can be made much safer with the use of sturdy bath and shower seats, grab bars and guardrails, and bathtub transfer benches, which help people move in and out of the bathtub. Handheld shower heads are convenient for patients to use in conjunction with bath seats or bathtub transfer benches.

DIALYSIS EQUIPMENT

Dialysis machines filter wastes and other toxic substances from an individual's blood when the person's kidneys are no longer able to function. Dialysis, in the form of hemodialysis and peritoneal dialysis, can be done at home, offering the patient a less expensive treatment method and a more independent lifestyle. Equipment supply houses can provide complete information on the exact specifications for modifications in household plumbing needed to accommodate home dialysis machines.

Hemodialysis uses a kidney machine, which removes impurities from the blood. The blood is diffused across a semipermeable membrane, separated in large and small particles, and filtered with a dialysate (a solution of nutrients). Blood is pumped from and delivered back to the patient through access devices (fistulas or shunts) located on either the lower leg or the forearm.

Peritoneal dialysis utilizes the patient's own peritoneum (the membrane that covers the wall of the abdomen) as the dialyzing semipermeable membrane needed to clean and filter the blood. A type of peritoneal dialysis that can be done at home is continuous ambulatory peritoneal dialysis (CAPD).

PAIN EQUIPMENT

The transcutaneous electrical nerve stimulation (TENS) unit delivers electrical impulses, through electrodes placed on the skin, to the individual in order to control pain. The electrical impulses act as an alternative stimulus for the brain and, in effect, block the pain messages of the brain. These small, portable units easily attach to a belt and can be activated as necessary.

RESPIRATORY EQUIPMENT

Respiratory equipment used for oxygen therapy in the home can take the form of oxygen concentrators, liquid oxygen with oxygen cylinders, and mechanical ventilators. Other breathing aids, such as nebulizers/compressors, air purifiers, and portable aspirators (suction machines), can also help an individual in a home environment.

Oxygen concentrators isolate regular oxygen from the air and deliver it in prescribed amounts to the individual. Oxygen concentrators are available in stationary and portable models. Liquid oxygen, available in immobile as well as portable units, can deliver a continuous flow of oxygen to the individual or can release it periodically. Cannulas, masks, and other regulators administer and control desired amounts of oxygen to the individual.

There are two types of ventilators: negative and positive. Negative ventilators, or "iron lungs," create a negative external pressure around the chest which forces air into the lungs and expands the chest. Popular in the 1950s for treating polio patients, negative pressure ventilator use has been largely replaced by positive pressure ventilators. Positive pressure ventilators create a high-pressure gradient by introducing a high-pressure gas in the individual's lungs. The individual, breathing through a tracheal tube, can be totally supported by the machine or can initiate each breath and then have the machine assist (called intermittent positive pressure breathing, or IPPB).

Other breathing aids such as CPAP—continuous positive airway pressure—provide individuals afflicted with sleep apnea with constant airflow pressure through a facial mask. Nebulizers (with compressors), devices used to disseminate a mixture of liquid (in the form of a spray) and gas to an individual for aerosol therapy, are machines that are effective in treating a variety of respiratory disorders (allergies and asthma, for example). Air purifiers and portable aspirators (suction devices that remove mucus and other fluids) can aid the respiratory function of an individual at home.

For more information on the types of durable medical equipment available, look no further than ordinary community resources. With the growth in home care and the need for medical equipment, many community pharmacies have added a complete line of medical equipment. In addition, they may also have specialists who can advise you on the types of equipment you need and arrange for special fittings for personal care products.

Also contact medical and surgical supply houses in your area and request their catalog of home care equipment. You may find listings for these companies in the business pages of your telephone directory under the listing "Hospital Equipment and Supplies."

Prostheses

Prostheses are artificial substitutes for missing body parts, such as limbs, joints, organs, and nerves. Biomedical engineering—sometimes known as bionics—is the application of engineering principles, combined with the knowledge of physiology, to help design and manufacture these devices.

Three types of materials are commonly used by bioengineers in the design of prostheses: metals, ceramics, and polymers.

Metals, because of their strength, make good temporary or long-term implants, such as bone plates, nails, and screws. They are also used to make electrodes and to seal implantable energy packs.

Ceramics are often powders that, when mixed with a liquid, can be shaped and fired at high temperatures. They are known for their ability to resist heat. One example is Bioglass, a glasslike material so close to bone that the body does not reject it as a foreign object.

Polymers are long chains of repeating molecular structures. They can be classified as either elastomers (stretchable rubbers) or rigid plastics. Polymers can be custom-made to exhibit a variety of properties, more than any other bioengineering material. Polymers can include acrylics, which are used to make artificial eyeballs, or polyurethanes, which are suitable for various joints or artificial-heart components.

In addition to the most common prostheses listed below, various researchers have developed artificial, high-tech devices to help restore failed vision and hearing as well as to stimulate damaged nerves.

ARTIFICIAL HEARTS AND HEART COMPONENTS

Artificial hearts. Artificial hearts (or more precisely, mechanical pumping devices) have been developed through several programs within the United States, including the University of Utah, Pennsylvania State University–Hershey, and the Cleveland Clinic Foundation.

The now banned Jarvik-7 artificial heart was developed through the Utah program, and was implanted in a few patients who were in the final stages of heart failure. It used a stainless-steel mold and was made of a polyurethane called Biomer. The heart's interior was reinforced with Dacron mesh, with each ventricle having a polyurethane base and a Velcro patch to hold it inside the chest.

To date, none of the artificial hearts developed is truly a self-contained device. Most must be powered from outside sources, which means the patient must be tethered to the power pack.

The National Heart, Lung and Blood Institute estimates that a totally implantable artificial heart will not be ready until early in the twenty-first century. Until then, development is going forward on what is called a left ventricular assist device. This device is designed to assist the natural heart with pumping action until a heart transplant can be performed.

Heart valves. The heart contains four valves. Any artificial valves implanted must not cause clots and must allow blood to flow freely while also closing tightly and quickly. The two categories of artificial valves are biological valves and mechanical valves. Biological, or natural valves are often taken from pigs; they cause less clotting than mechanical valves but do not last as long. Mechanical valves use suture rings composed of metal or plastic coated with Dacron, Teflon, or Biolite carbon.

Pacemakers. Heart function depends on electrochemical impulses that regulate heartbeat. When this function is impaired, an artificial pacemaker may be implanted. These systems include a pulse generator consisting of circuitry and a power source attached to a wire that has a tiny electrode at its tip.

ARTIFICIAL JOINTS

Finger joints. Finger joints damaged by disease, usually rheumatoid arthritis or osteoarthritis, can be replaced surgically by artificial joints made of metal, plastic, or silicone rubber. The operation can relieve pain and restore some movement to hands whose cartilage, bone, and joint lining have been destroyed. In the procedure, an incision exposes the joint, and the ends of the diseased bone and the diseased cartilage are cut away. The artificial joint is inserted into the bone ends. The skin and tissue are sewn up and the finger is immobilized in a splint until the wound has healed in about 10 days, at which time physical therapy can begin.

Hip joints. Replacement of a diseased or damaged hip joint is the oldest and most frequently performed type of joint replacement surgery. The new ball-and-socket joint approximates normal motion and range of movement. The ball-and-shaft portion fits into the femur and the socket fits into the pelvis. In this procedure, the diseased tissues of the joint socket and the hollow center of the thighbone are removed and the cavities cleaned.

An acrylic cement made of powder and liquid is squirted into the pelvic bone and pressed into the porous tissue until it hardens. More cement is poured into the thighbone after its ball joint has been removed. The artificial stem is placed into the bone until it adheres.

Knee joints. The knees are both the largest and most often injured joints of the human body. Artificial knee joints try to approximate the vast movements of this joint: its movements from side to side and its ability to circle around a moving axis. These prostheses are divided into two types: those that include artificial ligaments and those that rely on the remaining natural ligaments. An example of the latter is the total condylar knee. Two examples of knee joints are the hinge joint, which rotates on a hinge, and the less radical resurfacing of the joint using a peg or similar device to replace the ligaments.

Artificial joints have been developed for the wrist, hand, elbow, shoulder, ankle, and toe, but are not yet as successful or as extensively used as knee, hip, and finger replacements.

ARTIFICIAL LIMBS

Artificial limbs must provide a controllable imitation of human movement. Since the natural human arm and leg can perform a variety of movements, often simultaneously, these are particularly difficult prostheses to design. The following are popular types of artificial arms and legs.

Conventional *mechanical arms* rely on a system of cables and pulleys that require much concentration. Ten to 15 percent of amputees use mechanical arms, but only about 1 percent do so successfully.

The *Utah Arm* is the only prosthetic elbow and hand that relies only on electricity. It is made of a flexible plastic of glass-reinforced nylon and carbon fibers. Electrodes on the arm's socket have circuits that can be individualized. The electrodes can "read" the biceps and triceps or the shoulder's deltoid muscles. A microcomputer in the elbow tells a battery when to power a particular movement.

The *Otto Bock Hand* is the oldest and most reliable powered hand. It uses batteries that are inside the forearms with on/off switches inside the palms. The hand can open and close at various speeds and can be fine-tuned. The Otto Bock Greifer is a type of claw attachment that can replace the hand for heavy-duty work.

MIT Knees is the term given to a variety of passive and passive/powered artificial legs. Passive legs can only absorb energy; powered/passive legs can produce mechanical power. New, computer-controlled legs allow amputees to walk upstairs foot over foot by transferring information from a natural leg to a prosthetic leg.

The *Seattle Foot* has a leaf spring inside to give the wearer a more natural, diving-board effect when he walks. This foot is designed for active amputees who play sports, and the foot can be added to most artificial legs.

ARTIFICIAL TEETH

Dentures, appliances that replace missing teeth, consist of an acrylic (tough plastic) or metal base with mounted teeth made of acrylic or porcelain. Impressions are made of the upper and lower gums and filled with plaster of Paris when they harden, forming a model from which accurately shaped denture baseplates can be created.

The patient must bite onto wax-rimmed plates to enable the dentist to measure the relationship between upper and lower jaw. A temporary wax denture is fitted into the patient's mouth to allow the dentist to make adjustments to the position of the teeth. When the bite and appearance of the wax model are satisfactory, the wax is replaced with metal and finished polished dentures are fitted.

Dentures in the lower jaw stay in place by resting on gum ridges. Suction holds dentures to the upper jaw. Fitting usually occurs several months after extraction to enable the gums to heal and shrink. Full dentures replace all the teeth. Partial dentures replace only the teeth that are missing.

Tooth implants are a method of attaching false teeth to the bone instead of relying on partial dentures or bridgework. A hole is drilled into the upper or lower jaw and an implant, or stem, made of titanium alloy is inserted into the hole.

A few months later, the bone grows back to fasten the stem securely to the bone. The false tooth is usually screwed into the stem 3 to 4 months after the stem is implanted. Metal frames anchored to the bone in back and at the front of the mouth can also be used as implants, especially in patients who are missing all their lower teeth.

8. Insurance

INTRODUCTION

Nothing in health care is more confusing than health insurance. Today more than ever before, insurance is a profusion of terms and options, some of which were never heard of a decade ago. Managed care, health maintenance organizations, Medicare, and Medicaid are just four types of insurance products that create havoc in the average consumer's mind.

In this section, almost everything you need to know about health insurance is covered. If you are a Medicare beneficiary, you can review what is and is not covered. You can learn about diagnosis-related groups (DRGs), which explains how hospitals are paid for your care. If you work for a large corporation, find out how your employer is exempt from most state insurance laws and what that means to your rights. If you are considering joining an HMO, you will learn about the fifty largest ones and how to contact them.

Health insurance need not be as complicated as most of us think it is. With the information found in this section, you will better understand your current insurance program and your health insurance options.

Health Insurance

TYPES OF POLICIES

Before you attempt to purchase any insurance policy, you should be familiar with the myriad and often mysterious terms associated with the business (covered later in this section) *and* you should know the difference between the different types of insurance. Here's a rundown on each type:

Hospital insurance provides coverage for inpatient and outpatient hospital services. For inpatient services this insurance usually specifies the number of days of hospitalization the policy covers and specifies dollar limits on total benefits payable.

Medical/surgical insurance is divided into two portions: The medical portion pays for doctor visits to the hospital and may pay for office visits. Other medical services covered include drugs, X rays, anesthesia, and laboratory tests performed outside the hospital. The surgical portion covers the surgeon's fees, whether the surgery was performed in the hospital, the doctor's office, or an ambulatory

surgical center. (An ambulatory surgical center is a medical facility where surgical procedures are performed on an outpatient basis. It may be a freestanding center or a facility associated with a hospital but is separate from it.)

Major medical insurance is often referred to as catastrophic insurance because it protects against the high cost of medical care associated with a serious illness or accident. Before benefits are paid, this type of insurance usually requires you to pay a yearly deductible, typically ranging from $100 to $500, although deductibles vary from one policy to another. After the deductible is met, major medical insurance pays up to a certain percentage of covered expenses while you pay the remaining percentage. A typical coinsurance arrangement is 80 percent paid by your insurance company and 20 percent by you.

Once your out-of-pocket expenses reach a certain amount, many major medical policies protect you from further outlays of cash. This is known as a stop-loss provision. Your insurance company pays the remaining covered expenses up to the maximum limit. Because of such a provision, and the protection major medical insurance offers, if you can afford *only* one type of health insurance, you should consider purchasing a major medical policy.

It is important to remember that major medical insurance is usually cheaper than hospital or medical/surgical insurance because of the sometimes large deductibles these policies carry.

Comprehensive insurance is a term applied to an insurance plan that combines hospital, medical/surgical, and major medical coverage in one policy. It usually requires a deductible and copayment up to a stop-loss limit just like major medical insurance. A comprehensive policy may have lifetime benefits of $1 million to $5 million.

OTHER TYPES OF INSURANCE

The confusion surrounding the purchase of health insurance too often results in the inefficient outlay of health dollars. And the best way to avoid that is to buy only what you need. The following types of insurance provide coverage for very limited services or conditions; therefore, we do not recommend them as substitutes for what you really need: basic hospital, medical/surgical, or major medical insurance.

Questions to Ask Before You Select Any Policy

These questions should help you evaluate the coverage provided by the policies you are comparing.

Hospital Insurance

- Does the policy pay indemnity benefits or service benefits? (Service benefits tend to be more complete and are preferable.)
- Does the policy cover the daily room and board rate of the hospitals in your area? (To get those rates call your community hospitals or your state's hospital association.)
- How many days of hospitalization does the policy cover? (If less than 30 days, this may not be the best policy you can buy.)
- Does the policy have a waiting period before hospital benefits are provided? (We do not recommend hospital policies with waiting periods of 7 days or longer.)
- Does the policy cover preexisting conditions? (Some conditions may be excluded for a period of time, then covered later.)
- Does the policy pay for prescription medicines and other services such as X rays and laboratory tests?
- Does the policy cover the costs associated with surgery, such as charges for the operating, recovery, and other specialty rooms?
- Does the policy cover specialty care, such as intensive care, coronary care, and burn care? (Specialty care can cost as much as thousands of dollars a day. Avoid any policy that doesn't pay at least a portion of this cost.)
- Does the policy cover inpatient and outpatient psychiatric care?
- Does the policy cover outpatient services, either at a hospital or at a freestanding ambulatory care center? (Coverage of such services is definitely a plus.)
- Does the policy cover the expenses associated with an emergency department or urgicare center visit?
- Does the policy require you to use one particular hospital, or do you have a choice?
- Does the policy pay anything toward the services you receive in a hospital that does not have an agreement with your insurance company? (Sometimes an insurance company will pay a portion of expenses arising out of treatment in what are called noncontracting facilities.)
- Does the policy require a deductible and copayments? (The less you pay out of pocket, the better.)
- Can the policy be renewed? (We recommend a guaranteed-renewable policy and one that also guarantees that the premium will not change during the life of the contract.)
- Can the benefits be changed at the discretion of the company? (If so, such a policy should be avoided.)

Medical/Surgical Insurance

- Does the policy require a deductible and copayments? (We recommend policies for which you do not have to pay out of your own pocket for such basic services.)

- How much does the policy pay toward doctor visits when you are in the hospital? (Check with your doctor to find out if this amount covers his or her usual fee.)
- How many visits does the policy cover when you are in the hospital? (If you have an extended illness, your benefits could be used up quickly.)
- Does the policy cover home visits by your doctor or office visits? If so, how many of each type?
- Does the policy cover diagnostic tests performed in a doctor's office?
- Does the policy cover outside laboratory services for the tests ordered by your doctor?
- Does the policy cover second opinions?
- Does the policy have a surgical schedule that pays one lump sum regardless of the surgeon's fee, or does it pay the "usual, customary, and reasonable" fee of the surgeons in your area? (Policies that pay benefits in line with surgeons' fees in your area are preferable.)
- Does the policy pay for your surgeon to bring in a consultant on your case?
- Does the policy cover the cost of an assistant surgeon? (Pay close attention to this because some policies pay only for the primary surgeon.)
- Does the policy cover surgical procedures performed in the ambulatory care unit of a hospital or a freestanding ambulatory care center? (Increasing numbers of insurance companies are recognizing the potential for cost containment in same-day, or outpatient, surgery. Look for a policy that has this benefit.)
- Can you pay the premium on an annual basis?
- Can the policy be renewed? (Once again, a guaranteed-renewable policy is best.)

Major Medical Insurance

- What is the maximum dollar amount of coverage provided by the policy? (Ideally, you are trying to find a policy with unlimited benefits, but maximum benefits in the range of $1 million to $2 million are good.)
- Does the policy have a deductible that you can afford? (Major medical policies usually have much higher deductibles than basic hospital and medical/surgical insurance.)
- Does the deductible apply to a benefit period—for example, one year—or does it apply each time you file a claim? (To avoid excessive out-of-pocket expenses, choose a policy with a yearly deductible rather than a per-incident deductible.)
- Are the coinsurance/copayment provisions of the policy at least 80 percent/20 percent? (This arrangement is a common one among major medical policies.)
- Does the policy restore any portion of the maximum benefits once you are well and can submit medical evidence to establish your improved health? (Some policies do this provided you have not made claims for a certain period of time.)
- What is the stop-loss amount at which point you stop paying anything toward your medical expenses? (This amount is very important to know, since it determines your maximum out-of-pocket expense. This may be as low as $1,000 or as high as $5,000.)
- Does the policy cover all hospital and doctor expenses associated with your care, or are there services excluded?
- Can the policy be renewed? (Find one that is guaranteed-renewable.)

Accident. Very limited in coverage—and for this reason not the best insurance for your money—accident insurance excludes illness but does cover medical expenses resulting from an accident.

Dental. Dental insurance usually covers routine dental care as well as crowns, bridges, and root canals. Some policies do cover orthodontic work, but not if it is for cosmetic purposes. Because the premium for dental insurance is very high, your best opportunity to acquire dental insurance is probably through an employer-provided group plan. We have more to say about this type of insurance later.

Disability income insurance. While technically not health insurance, but nevertheless often included in health insurance benefits packages, this insurance provides you with income when you are unable to work because of illness or accident. (If your disability was the result of a job-related accident, you are probably covered by your state's workers' compensation insurance.)

You may purchase disability income insurance policies on a long- or short-term basis, but you should know that these policies usually have a waiting period, anywhere from 7 to 14 days or longer, before any benefits are paid. The longer the waiting period, the lower the premium.

Depending upon the provisions of the policy, the degree of your disability could have a significant impact on whether you receive benefits. The more common types of disability are:

- Occupational disability: defined as a person's inability to perform the duties of his or her occupation.
- General disability: defined as a person's inability to perform the duties of any occupation for which he or she may be suited as a result of education, training, or experience.
- Combination disability: defined in terms of a specified time during which a person is unable to perform the duties of his or her occupation.

Disease-specific. This insurance usually covers one disease—for example, cancer or heart disease. Not only does disease-specific insurance pay limited benefits, but it also may duplicate what you already have or are about to purchase. For these reasons your money is better spent on more comprehensive types of insurance.

Long-term care. This insurance is also known as nursing home insurance, since it generally covers the services provided in skilled, intermediate, and custodial care nursing homes. Today there are more than 1.5 million policies in force. However, some policies cover services provided only by a skilled nursing facility—an institution that offers nursing services similar to those provided in a hospital. The most important point to remember is that benefits will be paid only if you receive skilled nursing care, the need for which must be certified by a physician as being medically necessary. If you should no longer require care at the skilled level, your benefits may cease. Some of the newer policies provide coverage for intermediate or custodial care facilities; however, you must carefully examine the benefits to determine when the policy will cover these services.

Travel. Usually sold at airports or through automobile clubs and some credit card companies, this insurance offers to pay a certain amount of money if you are injured or killed as a result of an accident while traveling. The benefits are for a limited time only and probably duplicate coverage that you already have or are about to purchase. Not really health insurance, travel insurance is more a form of life insurance, with the money paid out not necessarily intended to pay for the cost of medical services.

Employee Retirement Income Security Act (ERISA)

WHAT IS ERISA?

ERISA, or Employee Retirement Income Security Act of 1974, is a set of laws governing how employers are to administer health insurance benefits, particularly hospital and physicians' services benefits, for exempt salaried employees under a company's health and welfare benefits plan. This legislation requires an employer to provide its employees with a written report on the financial status of any health and welfare benefits it offers.

The annual report must include the names of the plan's trustees, and the business address and telephone number of the plan administrator. It must also clearly explain the duties and responsibilities of those charged with operating the plan.

Trustees of the plan have what is called a fiduciary responsibility to act prudently and in the interests of the plan participants and beneficiaries. This means that the trustees ensure that the plan is properly funded and that its financial resources are not used in a wasteful manner.

Shopping Tips

1. Do not buy more insurance than you need for yourself and your family. Duplicate policies only mean duplicate premium expenses. And if you make a claim against both insurance companies, don't expect to collect twice. The companies will invoke the coordination of benefits clause in your plan and only pay up to their contractual obligations.

2. Check the rating of the insurance company to determine its financial condition. Companies such as A. M. Best, Duff & Phelps, Moody's, and Standard & Poor rate insurance companies according to their financial stability and ability to pay claims. (Check your library for publications by these companies.)

3. Check with your state's insurance department to determine if a particular company is authorized to sell its policies in your state. Also check on the particular plan to determine if it has been approved for sale by the insurance commissioner.

4. Make sure the salesperson clearly explains the policy's schedule of benefits, and you fully understand the contract. This includes waiting periods, exclusions, periods of noncoverage, and preexisting conditions. (The time to discover that a service isn't covered is *before* you sign the contract, not *after*.)

5. Don't purchase a policy with excessively high deductibles and stop-loss limit. Individual deductibles of $2,500 to $3,000 and family deductibles of up to $5,000 may cost you more in out-of-pocket expenses than they return in benefits. Shop for a stop-loss limit under $5,000.

6. Purchase group insurance if at all possible. Group plans are generally less expensive and in some cases may offer more complete coverage than individual plans. (Join a social, fraternal, or alumni group if it will help you purchase insurance at lower rates.)

7. Consider joining a health maintenance organization (HMO) if one in your area has an open enrollment period. You may discover that you get twice the coverage for the same amount of premium and lower deductibles and copayments. (In some cases you may not have any deductible or copayment with an HMO.)

8. Always answer the insurance application as honestly as you can. Incomplete answers could leave you open to having your insurance policy canceled, thereby making it more difficult for you to purchase subsequent insurance.

9. Always pay your premium by a check made out to the company, not the salesperson. Also inquire about any discount for paying your premiums on an annual basis. (The next best thing is to pay quarterly.)

10. Always take advantage of the 30-day "free look" period offered by your insurance company. If, before the 30 days have expired, you discover that the policy is not right for you or your family, you may return it and receive a full refund of your premium.

Key Insurance Terms

As we all know, the medical profession has its specialized language. But beyond that, long after you've left the doctor's office or passed through a hospital's doors, you must be conversant in another kind of lingo—health-insurance-speak. Too often, instead of saying things the simple, comprehensive way, insurance companies fall back on a system of cumbersome codes that often only insiders understand.

Here, in straightforward language, are the meanings of common health insurance terms.

Accumulation period—the number of days during which the insured person must incur eligible medical expenses at least equal to the deductible in order to receive a benefit.

Allocated benefits—benefits for which the maximum amount payable for specific services is itemized in the insurance contract.

Ambulatory benefits—benefits available to you for health care services received while not confined to a hospital bed as an inpatient; for example, outpatient care, emergency room care, home health care, preadmission testing.

Ambulatory surgical center—a medical facility that performs outpatient surgical procedures.

Application—a signed statement of facts that an insurance company uses to decide whether to sell you a policy.

Assignment—an agreement in which you instruct your insurance company to pay the hospital, doctor, or medical supplier directly for services you receive and at the payment rate established by the insurer.

Benefits—the amount of money or services an insurance company will pay or provide under the provisions of the policy.

Cancellation—the termination of a policy before it would normally expire.

Claim—a notification by you, your doctor, or your hospital to your insurance company stating that you have received a medical service and are requesting payment in accordance with the policy.

COBRA—the Consolidated Omnibus Reconciliation Act of 1985 which requires employers to offer continuation of group-health insurance coverage to certain employees and dependents for 18 to 36 months after they leave their companies' employ.

Coinsurance/copayment—a cost-sharing requirement in many health insurance policies in which you, the insured, assume a portion or percentage of the costs of covered services. The most common cost-sharing provision has you responsible for 20 percent of covered expenses while the insurer pays the remaining 80 percent.

Conditionally renewable clause—a provision that permits a policyholder to renew a policy up to a certain age limit, such as 65, provided all conditions of the insurance contract have been met.

Conversion clause—a provision in a group policy that provides the insured person with the opportunity to purchase individual coverage in the event the group policy is terminated.

Coordination of benefits—a practice insurance companies use to avoid duplication of payment when a person is covered by more than one policy.

Covered expense—a medical expense that you incur and the insurance company agrees to pay.

Custodial care facility—a facility that provides

Key Insurance Terms *(cont.)*

round-the-clock room and board to aged or handicapped persons who require personal care, supervision, or assistance in daily activity.

Deductible—the amount you, the policyholder, must pay before an insurance plan pays for any portion of the cost.

Disability insurance—insurance that pays you a portion of your salary when you are sick or injured and unable to work.

Disease-specific insurance—insurance that provides benefits should you develop a specific illness such as cancer, heart disease, poliomyelitis, encephalitis, or spinal meningitis.

Effective date—the date insurance begins; the first day you can file a claim and have benefits paid.

Eligibility—determination of whether an applicant qualifies for coverage for health care rendered.

Employer mandate—a requirement that employers provide or arrange health insurance coverage for employees. Typically, such proposals require coverage of workers' families, too.

Exclusions—specific conditions or circumstances under which a policy will not provide benefits. The specific services excluded from a policy may be found in the policy's schedule of benefits.

Explanation of benefits—a statement from an insurance company itemizing the medical services you received and the amount of insurance coverage provided for each service.

Fee for service—an arrangement under which doctors or other health care providers are paid separately for each service they perform. Some economists say this method of payment may give doctors an incentive to provide more services than they need.

First-dollar coverage—a policy with no deductible that covers the first dollar of your expenses.

Free look—a period of time—usually 10 to 30 days—during which you may return the policy and receive a full refund of any premium paid.

Grace period—a period of time—usually 30 or 31 days—after the date a premium is due during which the policy remains in force and the premium may still be paid without penalty.

Group insurance—insurance, usually issued through employers and unions, that covers a group of persons.

Guaranteed-renewable clause—a provision that guarantees the policyholder the right to renew as long as premiums are paid on time. While the insurance is in force, the company cannot raise the premium unless all policyholders have their premiums raised at the same time.

Health insurance purchasing cooperative (HIPC)—an entity that buys insurance coverage and medical care for a large number of people, including employees of small businesses.

Health maintenance organization (HMO)—an prepaid group health plan, which provides a range of services in return for fixed monthly premiums.

Home health care—care rendered in a patient's home, such as nursing services, therapy, or medications.

Hospital insurance—insurance that covers costs of hospital care resulting from injury or illness.

Key Insurance Terms *(cont.)*

Indemnity benefits—a fixed dollar payment for a specific health care service, such as $100 a day for hospitalization. Should the cost of care be more than your policy pays, you are responsible for the difference.

Indemnity policy—insurance that pays a specified amount of money each day or week that you are in the hospital and that pays a set amount for medical and surgical procedures.

Individual insurance—a policy that you purchase yourself and that is not part of a group plan. The policy covers you and, usually, your dependents.

Individual practice association (IPA)—a prepaid health care plan that is offered to groups of people by physicians in private practice.

Inpatient—someone who is officially admitted and occupies a hospital room while receiving hospital care, including room, board, and general nursing care.

Inside limit—a provision that limits insurance payment for any type of service, regardless of the actual cost of the service.

Intermediate care facility—a facility that provides health care and services to persons who do not require the care and services of a hospital or a skilled nursing facility.

Lapsed policy—an insurance policy that has been canceled for nonpayment of premiums.

Level of care—the type and intensity of treatment necessary to adequately and efficiently treat your illness or condition.

Major medical insurance—insurance that offsets the large expenses of a severe and prolonged illness or injury.

Managed care—a method of delivering, supervising, and coordinating health care, often through HMOs and other networks of doctors and hospitals. The purpose is to eliminate inappropriate services, control costs, and assure access to effective treatments.

Managed competition—a health policy that combines free-market forces with government regulation. Large groups of consumers and businesses buy health care from organized networks of doctors and hospitals, which are supposed to compete by offering low prices and high quality.

Medicaid—a government program that provides assistance to the poor.

Medical/surgical insurance—insurance that covers some of the fees of physicians and surgeons for care provided in the hospital, office, or home and covers part of the cost of laboratory tests performed outside the hospital.

Medicare—the government's medical insurance program for people aged 65 and older and for the disabled.

Medicare-approved amount—a dollar figure approved by Medicare that will be either the usual and customary charge, the prevailing charge, or the actual charge (whichever is lowest) and is the amount Medicare pays the doctor.

Medicare assignment—an agreement by a physician or medical provider to accept the Medicare-approved amount as payment in full for services rendered to a Medicare beneficiary.

Optionally renewable clause—a provision that gives an insurance company the right to cancel the coverage at any anniversary or, in some cases, at any premium due date. The company may not cancel the coverage between such dates.

Key Insurance Terms *(cont.)*

Outpatient—someone who is not officially admitted as an inpatient to a hospital, who receives hospital care (for example, laboratory work and X rays) without occupying a hospital bed or receiving room, board, or general nursing care.

Period of noncoverage—provisions that specify periods when the insurance contract is not in force.

Policy—the legal document issued by the insurance company to you, the policyholder, that outlines the conditions and terms of the insurance. Also called the contract.

Policy limit—the maximum benefits an insurance company will pay under a particular policy.

Preexisting condition—an injury occurring, disease contracted, or physical/mental condition that existed prior to issuance of a health insurance policy. Usually, benefits will not be paid for services related to preexisting conditions, although many insurance companies cover these conditions after a certain waiting period.

Preferred provider organization (PPO)—an organization of doctors and hospitals that provides medical services to groups of people at discounted rates. Members of the groups agree to use only the "preferred" providers.

Premium—the amount you pay—monthly, quarterly, semiannually, or annually—to purchase the insurance and keep it in force.

Prepaid plan—a plan that provides medical services to a group of persons who pay for the services in advance in the form of a monthly fee. Health maintenance organizations and individual practice associations are prepaid plans.

Provider—a new term used to describe doctors, nurses, hospitals, pharmacists, and anyone else who provides health care.

Renewal Clause—a clause that indicates the provisions under which the policy may or may not be renewed. Since many individual health insurance policies are written for a limited time, usually one year, they must be renewed at the end of each term. The provisions you are most likely to encounter are:

Guaranteed-renewable: The company guarantees your right to renew your policy to a specific age, commonly 65. (Medicare supplemental insurance is usually not purchased until age 65, with some policies renewable for life.) A guaranteed-renewable policy may also have a guaranteed premium which will not be raised during the term of the policy.

Conditionally renewable: You may renew your policy until you reach a certain age, usually 65, provided you have complied with the other conditions of your policy.

Optionally renewable: The company may decline to renew your policy on the anniversary date.

Rider—a document that amends the policy. It may increase or decrease benefits, waive the condition of coverage, or in any other way amend the original contract.

Schedule of benefits—the list of medical services that a particular insurance policy will cover or the maximum amounts payable for certain conditions.

Key Insurance Terms *(cont.)*

Skilled nursing facility (SNF)—a facility that provides skilled nursing care and related services for patients who require inpatient medical or nursing care.

Stop-loss provision—a provision that limits your out-of-pocket expenses to a set amount, after which the insurance policy pays all expenses up to the plan's maximum benefits.

Surgical schedule—a list of cash allowances that are payable for various types of surgery, with maximum allowances based upon the severity of the operation.

Tax cap—a limit on federal tax breaks for health insurance. The term can apply to employers or employees or both.

Third-party payer—an organization (such as an insurance company) that reimburses medical care providers (such as hospitals and medical practitioners) for services provided to policyholders.

Usual, customary, and reasonable—a charge for medical care that is consistent with the going rate for identical or similar services in the same geographic area.

Waiting period—the length of time an employee must wait from his or her date of employment or application for insurance coverage to the date his or her insurance goes into effect.

Workers' compensation insurance—an insurance program, usually established by the state, that provides benefits to employees who are injured in the course of their employment.

WHAT IS THE RESPONSIBILITY OF THE EMPLOYER?

Under ERISA, the employer is responsible for providing participants of the company's plan with all documents pertaining to the plan, and also agrees to pay all claims made by beneficiaries. If the employee's right to a benefit is denied, he or she is entitled to a written explanation of the reason for the denial, which may then be appealed. In addition, the employer agrees not to discriminate against any employee who files an appeal when a claim is rejected or ignored.

WHAT IS THE EMPLOYEE ENTITLED TO?

All participants in the plan are entitled to examine, free of charge, all documents pertaining to the plan under ERISA regulations; to obtain copies of all of these documents upon written request to the plan administrator (a small fee for the copies may be charged); and to receive a summary of the plan's annual financial report, free of charge. If these rights are not provided, the employee has the option of filing suit in a federal court.

According to the provisions found in ERISA, all requests for financial materials from the plan must be fulfilled within 30 days. If the plan fails to provide the materials requested, the employee or beneficiary may file suit in federal court.

Under ERISA, the employee or his or her dependents shall receive hospital and physicians' benefits upon the presentation of his or her medical benefits identification card to the hospital or physician. The hospital or physician will submit a claim for covered services directly to the insurance company for direct payment. If the hospital or physician refuses to submit the claim to the insurance company, the employee should obtain an itemized bill or receipt from the provider. The employee writes the group and agreement numbers, appearing on the insurance identification card, directly on the bill or receipt and submits it to the insurance company for payment.

Employees can obtain more information on their ERISA rights from their employer's human resources department or benefits department. If you have specific questions pertaining to your rights under ERISA that have not been answered by your employer, contact the nearest office of the United States Labor-Management Services Administration,

Department of Labor (consult the blue pages of your telephone directory under U.S. Government Offices).

Consolidated Omnibus Reconciliation Act (COBRA)

WHAT IS COBRA?

The Consolidated Omnibus Budget Reconciliation Act (COBRA) of 1986 is designed to provide laid-off or terminated employees, as well as other qualified employees, an opportunity to maintain their medical coverage in the event that it otherwise might be lost.

Specifically, employers must offer to employees who are about to lose their jobs and to dependents who are about to lose their coverage the same health care benefits offered to "similarly situated" active employees.

The law applies to all employers except churches, the federal government, the District of Columbia, and employers with fewer than twenty employees.

WHO IS ELIGIBLE?

Situations (also known as qualifying events) that provide continued coverage for employees, their spouses and dependents under COBRA include termination of employment or reduction of hours, death, divorce or legal separation, eligibility for Medicare, and loss of dependent status by a child. Those who would have previously been uninsured due to these situations now have time to seek insurance while retaining their previous coverage.

Current employees, former employees, and retirees are all covered employees. Partners, directors, agents, and independent contractors who are covered by a plan will be covered employees if the employer maintains a plan that covers any common law employees.

To be eligible for COBRA coverage, the employee must not previously have been eligible for Medicare and must be a resident of the United States.

WHAT IS THE RESPONSIBILITY OF THE *EMPLOYER?*

Any type of group health plan maintained by the employer that provides medical care to employees (even if the involvement in that plan is minimal) must comply with COBRA. "Medical care" is defined under COBRA as the diagnosis, cure, and treatment or prevention of disease, or transportation primarily for and essential to medical care.

Included are drug and alcohol treatment programs, health clinics, and any other facilities or programs intended to alleviate a health problem. Excluded are programs available to all employees regardless of their condition, and first-aid care.

The plan administrator must give notice of COBRA rights to all qualified employees and their spouses. The plan administrator must also distribute notice to new employees when they are eligible.

In general, the continuation coverage offered to a qualified beneficiary must be identical to the coverage provided to active employees, their dependents, and their spouses. Therefore, the employer cannot calculate the premium for continuation coverage separately from the premium for active employee coverage.

An employer who does not provide the choice of continued coverage for its employees will not be permitted to take the tax deduction for its contributions to the plan.

WHAT IS THE RESPONSIBILITY OF THE *EMPLOYEE?*

Once an employee has been notified of his COBRA continuation rights, he has 60 days to decide whether he wants to continue his coverage. If he elects to include his family members who qualify as beneficiaries under COBRA, they are bound by that decision. However, each family member who is a qualified beneficiary must be offered the chance to make an independent choice among the following options: receiving COBRA coverage, receiving core coverage, or switching coverage during an open enrollment period.

The employee is responsible for making premium payments under the COBRA plan. If these payments are not made, coverage can be terminated before its full term. Coverage will also be terminated if the employee becomes covered by another group health plan; however, Congress is now considering legislation—titled the Technical Corrections Bill—that would eliminate this reason for ending COBRA coverage. Finally, COBRA coverage will end if the beneficiary becomes eligible for Medicare.

The 10 Largest Blue Cross and Blue Shield Plans

The following Blue Cross and Blue Shield plans from a Blue Cross Blue Shield Association Survey in 1992 are ranked, in descending order, according to their total enrollment.

1. Empire Blue Cross and Blue Shield
   622 3rd Avenue
   New York, NY 10017
2. Pennsylvania Blue Shield
   1800 Center Street
   P.O. Box 890089
   Camp Hill, PA 17089-0089
3. Blue Cross and Blue Shield of Michigan
   600 Lafayette Street E.
   Detroit, MI 48226-2998
4. Blue Cross of Western Pennsylvania
   5th Avenue Place
   Pittsburgh, PA 15222
5. Blue Cross of California
   21555 Oxnard Street
   Woodland Hills, CA 91367
6. Blue Cross and Blue Shield of Illinois
   233 N. Michigan Avenue
   P.O. Box 1364
   Chicago, IL 60690
7. Blue Cross and Blue Shield
   of New Jersey
   33 Washington Street
   P.O. Box 420
   Newark, NJ 07102
8. Blue Cross and Blue Shield
   of Massachusetts
   100 Summer Street
   Boston, MA 02110
9. Independence Blue Cross
   1901 Market Street
   Philadelphia, PA 19103
10. Blue Cross and Blue Shield of Virginia
    2015 Staples Mill Road
    P.O. Box 27401
    Richmond, VA 23279

Source: Blue Cross/Blue Shield Association, Chicago.

WHAT IS THE PERIOD OF COVERAGE?

The coverage period begins with the date of the qualifying event, and the period of continuation coverage may vary according to the nature of the qualifying event. The period is 36 months for widows, divorced spouses, spouses of Medicare-eligible employees, and dependent children no longer dependent under the plan. The period is 18 months for employees who have reduced hours or whose employment has been terminated. (Allowances are made if more than one qualifying event occurs during the first continuation period, but the period is never longer than 36 months from the date of the first qualifying event.)

The structure of the plan year depends on the employee's labor contract; for nonunion employees, the plan year would typically begin the first of the new year. For union members, the plan typically begins the first of the year following the expiration of the previous agreement.

WHAT IS THE COST TO BENEFICIARIES?

Employees are responsible for making monthly payments for their COBRA coverage, which includes the base cost of the plan plus administrative fees. This currently amounts to approximately 107 percent of the basic premium cost. For example, if the basic premium for family coverage is $300 per month, under COBRA the employer may charge up to $321 per month ($300 × 1.07).

For more information on COBRA, contact your employer, human resources department, or your benefits department.

State Insurance Departments

The state insurance department is responsible for regulating all aspects of the insurance industry. This includes approving policies, licensing agents, and investigating fraudulent claims. All complaints involving insurance companies or agents should be made to this office.

Alabama
Alabama Insurance Department
Retirement Systems Building
135 S. Union Street
Montgomery, AL 36130-3401
205-269-3550

Alaska
Alaska Division of Insurance
Department of Commerce and Economic Development
State Office Building
333 Willoughby Avenue
Mail to: P.O. Box D
Juneau, AK 99811
907-465-2515

Arizona
Arizona Insurance Department
3030 N. 3rd Street
Phoenix, AZ 85012
602-255-5400

Arkansas
Arkansas Insurance Department
University Tower Building, Room 400
12th Street and University Avenue
Little Rock, AR 72204
501-371-1325

California
California Department of Insurance
3450 Wilshire Boulevard, Suite 201
Los Angeles, CA 90010
213-736-2572

Colorado
Colorado Division of Insurance
Department of Regulatory Agencies
First Western Plaza Building, Room 500
303 W. Colfax Avenue
Denver, CO 80204
303-866-6274

Connecticut
Connecticut Insurance Department
State Office Building, Room 425
153 Market Street
Hartford, CT 06106
203-297-3800

Delaware
Delaware Insurance Department
Rodney Building, Suite 100
841 Silver Lake Boulevard
Dover, DE 19903
302-736-4251
800-282-8611

District of Columbia
District of Columbia Insurance Administration
Department of Consumer and Regulatory Affairs
613 G Street N.W., 6th Floor
Washington, DC 20001
202-727-7424

Florida
Florida Department of Insurance
The Capitol, Plaza Level II
Tallahassee, FL 32399-0300
904-488-3440

Georgia
Georgia Office of Commissioner of Insurance
Floyd Memorial Building, West Tower
2 Martin Luther King Jr. Drive
Atlanta, GA 30334
404-656-2056

Hawaii
Hawaii Insurance Division
Department of Commerce and Consumer Affairs
110 Richards Street
Honolulu, HI 96813
808-586-2790

Idaho
Idaho Department of Insurance
State Capitol Building
500 S. 10th Street
Boise, ID 83720
208-334-2250

Illinois
Illinois Department of Insurance
Bicentennial Building
320 W. Washington Street
Springfield, IL 62767
217-782-4515

Indiana
Indiana Department of Insurance
311 W. Washington Street
Indianapolis, IN 46204-2787
317-232-2385

Iowa
Iowa Division of Insurance
Department of Commerce
Lucas State Office Building
East 12th and Grand Avenue
Des Moines, IA 50319
515-281-5705

Kansas
Kansas Insurance Department
420 W. 9th Street
Topeka, KS 66612
913-296-7081

Kentucky
Kentucky Department of Insurance
Public Protection and Regulation Cabinet
Fitzgerald Building
229 W. Main Street
Mail to: P.O. Box 517
Frankfort, KY 40602
502-564-3630

Louisiana
Louisiana Department of Insurance
Insurance Building
950 N. 5th Street
Mail to: P.O. Box 94214
Baton Rouge, LA 70804-9214
504-342-5900

Maine
Maine Bureau of Insurance
Department of Professional and Financial Regulation
Statehouse Station 34
Augusta, ME 04333
207-582-8707

Maryland
Maryland Insurance Division
Department of Licensing And Regulation
Stanbalt Building
501 St. Paul Place
Baltimore, MD 21202
410-333-2520

Massachusetts
Massachusetts Division of Insurance
240 Friend Street
Boston, MA 02114
617-727-7189

Michigan
Michigan Insurance Bureau
Department of Licensing and Regulation
Ottawa Building North
611 W. Ottawa Street
Mail to: P.O. Box 30220
Lansing, MI 48909
517-373-9273

Minnesota
Minnesota Department of Commerce
Metro Square Building, Room 500
7th and Robert Streets
St. Paul, MN 55101
612-296-6848

Mississippi
Mississippi Insurance Department
Walter Sillers State Office Building
550 High Street, Room 1804
Mail to: P.O. Box 79
Jackson, MS 39205
601-359-3569

Missouri
Missouri Company Regulations
Division of Insurance
Department of Economic Development
Harry S. Truman State Office Building, Room 630
301 W. High Street
Mail to: P.O. Box 690
Jefferson City, MO 65102
314-751-4126

Montana
Montana State Auditor Office
P.O. Box 4009
Helena, MT 59604
404-444-2040

Nebraska
Nebraska Department of Insurance
State Office Building
301 Centennial Mall S.
Mail to: P.O. Box 94699
Lincoln, NE 68509
402-471-2201

Nevada
Nevada Insurance Division
Department of Commerce
1665 Hot Springs Road
Mail to: Capitol Complex
Carson City, NV 89710
702-687-4270

New Hampshire
New Hampshire Insurance Department
169 Manchester Street
Concord, NH 03301
603-271-2261

New Jersey
New Jersey Division of Administration
Department of Insurance
20 W. State Street, CN-325
Trenton, NJ 08625
609-292-5363

New Mexico
New Mexico Department of Insurance
495 Old Santa Fe Trail
Pasco de Peralta
Mail to: P.O. Drawer 1269
Santa Fe, NM 87504-1269
505-827-4500

New York
New York Insurance Department
160 West Broadway
New York, NY 10013
212-602-0429

North Carolina
North Carolina Agent Services and Consumer Division
Department of Insurance
Dobbs Building
430 N. Salisbury Street
Mail to: P.O. Box 26387
Raleigh, NC 27611
919-733-7349

North Dakota
North Dakota Insurance Department
State Capitol, 5th Floor
Bismarck, ND 58505-0320
701-224-2440

Ohio
Ohio Department of Insurance
2100 Stella Court
Columbus, OH 43215-0566
614-644-2658

Oklahoma
Oklahoma Insurance Department
State Insurance Building
1901 N. Walnut Boulevard
Mail to: P.O. Box 53408
Oklahoma City, OK 73152-3408
405-521-2828

Oregon
Oregon Insurance Division
Department of Commerce
21 Labor and Industry Building
Salem, OR 97310
503-378-4271

Pennsylvania
Pennsylvania Division of Consumer Affairs
and Enforcement
Department of Insurance
1321 Strawberry Square
Harrisburg, PA 17120
717-787-5173

Puerto Rico
Puerto Rico Office of the Insurance Commissioner
Cobian's Plaza
1607 Ponce de León Avenue, Stop 23
Mail to: P.O. Box 8330
Fernández Juncos Station
Santurce, PR 00910
809-722-8686

Rhode Island
Rhode Island Department of Business Regulation
Director and Insurance Commissioner
233 Richmond Street, Suite 237
Providence, RI 02903-4237
401-277-2223

South Carolina
South Carolina Department of Insurance
1612 Marion Street
Mail to: P.O. Box 100105
Columbia, SC 29202-3105
803-737-6117

South Dakota
South Dakota Division of Insurance
Department of Commerce and Regulation
Insurance Building
910 E. Sioux Avenue
Pierre, SD 57501
605-773-3563

Tennessee
Tennessee Department of Commerce and Insurance
Volunteer Plaza
500 James Robertson Parkway
Nashville, TN 37243-0565
615-741-2241

Texas

Texas State Board of Insurance
State Insurance Building
333 Guadalupe Street
P.O. Box 149104
Austin, TX 78714-9104
512-463-6468

Utah

Utah Insurance Department
3110 State Office Building
Salt Lake City, UT 84114-1201
801-530-3800

Vermont

Vermont Department of Banking and Insurance
State Office Building
120 State Street
Montpelier, VT 05602
802-828-3301

Virgin Islands

Virgin Islands Office of the Lieutenant Governor
Lieutenant Governor's Office Building
18 Kongen Gade
Charlotte Amalie
St. Thomas, VI 00802
809-774-2991

Virginia

Virginia Bureau of Insurance
State Corporation Commission
Jefferson Building
1220 Bank Street
Mail to: P.O. Box 1157
Richmond, VA 23209
804-786-7694

Dental Insurance

Although not yet as prevalent as medical insurance, dental insurance is becoming more popular, with at least 1 person out of 4 now covered under some sort of plan. Virtually all dental insurance plans are group policies, not individual ones, and as such may cover a substantial part of your dental bill. Just remember that dental insurance does not cover everything. In fact, it sometimes covers the least expensive treatment, and for this reason and others it's important that you find a good "match" between your particular insurance plan, if you have one, and your dentist. Don't go through the entire process of selecting a dentist before you find out if he or she will cooperate with the restrictions imposed by your insurance plan. Here are a few tips.

• The first thing to do is get a copy of the brochure that details your plan and go over it so you know what your benefits are, what the deductible is, and if there are any exclusions and limitations.

• Then, in your shopping around and interviewing, ask a few questions: Will the dentist file your claim for you? Will the dentist agree to accept as 100 percent payment the amount that your insurance company "allows" for specific procedures? You will probably find that many of the dentists you talk to will accept whatever your insurance company pays for "the basics"—such as cleaning and polishing, X rays, and simple extractions.

• Crowns, bridges, dentures, orthodontic and periodontic work, and oral surgery are another matter, however. It's not easy to find a dentist who accepts as 100 percent payment what the insurance company "allows" for these more complicated dental services. Generally, dental insurance plans—unless they're particularly good and top-of-the-line policies—tend to limit their coverage for these procedures, or even exclude them entirely.

• The difference between what the dentist charges and what your plan pays will be your out-of-pocket expenses. If keeping these to a minimum is a priority with you, then select the dentist who agrees to accept your plan's payments for the majority of procedures.

Washington
Washington Office of the Insurance Commissioner
Insurance Building, Room 200
Mail to: Mail Stop AQ-21
Olympia, WA 98504
206-753-7301

West Virginia
West Virginia Department of Insurance
2100 Washington Street E.
Charleston, WV 25305
304-558-3394

Wisconsin
Wisconsin Office of the Commissioner of Insurance
Loraine Building
121 E. Wilson
Madison, WI 53702
608-266-0102

Wyoming
Wyoming Insurance Department
Herschler Building, 3rd Floor
122 W. 25th Street
Cheyenne, WY 82002
307-777-7401

Health Maintenance Organizations (HMOs)

Health maintenance organizations (HMOs), no longer the obscure alternative to conventional group medical insurance plans they once were, now boast 39 million subscribers nationwide. Likely to be multistate operations owned by large businesses, HMOs come in a variety of forms, but with some elements in common:

- HMO members (usually called subscribers) receive comprehensive medical care for a fixed (or prepaid, meaning paid before you receive the services) monthly premium. The plan generally covers physician fees and services, hospitalization and surgery, home health care, outpatient surgery, some nursing home services, and preventive care such as routine checkups and immunizations.
- The services are provided by an organized group of medical professionals who receive a fixed monthly payment per subscriber, regardless of the services rendered (or not rendered, whatever the case may be). In essence, the HMO requires that physicians live within a budget because the HMO receives the same payment per subscriber per month regardless of the medical and hospital services used. If the services provided to the subscriber group exceed the monthly budget, then the HMO loses money. As you can see, this runs counter to the traditional fee-for-service system, which in effect encourages overutilization: The more services a physician provides or orders, the bigger the payment.
- Subscribers, for the most part, are limited to those physicians, hospitals, and other medical providers approved by the HMO. In the classic HMO plan, you agree to give up an unlimited choice of doctors in exchange for economical health care. The first thing you do is choose a primary care physician (either a family practitioner, general practitioner, pediatrician, internist, or obstetrician-gynecologist) from the HMO's selected list. You receive all medical care from that doctor, who also decides whether you get a test or procedure, see a specialist, or go into the hospital. In HMO jargon this physician is your "gatekeeper" to the rest of the medical system.

This idea of being locked into the approved list of providers has discouraged many people from joining HMOs, but, according to a report from a Minnesota-based research firm, InterStudy, as many as a quarter of the nation's 556 HMOs offer subscribers the opportunity to go to non-HMO doctors under certain circumstances.

Be aware, however, that freedom may carry a price tag. It is quite possible that when you use doctors outside the HMO network you will be required to pay a part of your medical bill (similar to a copayment in a traditional plan) and perhaps even meet a set dollar amount (in other words, a deductible) before the HMO will begin cost sharing.

On the other hand, if you find this lock-in provision daunting and downright discouraging, bear in mind one important fact: Classic free choice plans—you choose whom to go to and your company pays—are vanishing. In 1992 the Health Insurance Association of America reported that only 8 percent of all conventional insurance plans fit this description. So any squeamishness about joining an HMO solely because of a "lock-in" restriction may be unnecessary as fewer and fewer plans of any kind—traditional or managed care—offer free choice.

Managed Care

At one time managed care meant a health maintenance organization (HMO); today it can mean any type of medical coverage that limits your ability to pick and choose doctors and hospitals. This is in sharp contrast to the fee-for-service system in which you pick your personal or family doctor and also have some say in the selection of specialists and hospitals. Over the years critics have charged that the fee-for-service system is nothing more than a blank check for doctors and hospitals, with no allowance for control over utilization or cost. Things are changing, however, as consumers, business executives, and politicians search for ways to reduce health care expenditures. What appears to be emerging is a system designed to not only reduce spending for medical care but also manage the level and extent of care you receive.

Managed care means that you will use only those doctors, including specialists, and hospitals who belong to the managed care network. Your right to self-referral will be severely curtailed and you will need to obtain approval for many specialized diagnostic and treatment procedures. Should you receive medical care (other than emergency) from a provider not in the network, you will be subject to higher out-of-pocket expenditures, in the form of deductibles and copayments.

You may already be in a form of managed care plan and not realize it. Insurance companies who once sold straight indemnity plans, those with the most freedom of choice, have now added a utilization component that requires prior approval for certain services. Another aspect of these plans is a more thorough review to determine if the care you received was appropriate. If, in the opinion of your insurance company, the care you received was not appropriate, your doctor or the hospital could receive a reduced reimbursement.

Other forms of managed care plans are preferred provider organizations (your choice is limited to a list of providers), exclusive provider organizations (your choice is limited to one organization of providers), and managed indemnity plans (a traditional health insurance plan that requires prior approval for some services). Given the rapid changes occurring in the field of managed care, you are likely to see any number of variations on these basic systems.

Managed care is also being touted as a major component of the national health care reform package. According to the proposed plan, each state would have one or more so-called health alliances that would make arrangements with providers to deliver services. In order to be ready for this new system, physicians and hospitals are busy forming what are called physician hospital organizations, or PHOs. If you obtain your medical coverage from one of these alliances, your choice of providers will be limited to those in the PHO. These organizations will be expected to deliver quality care while reducing unnecessary utilization.

A Few Cautions Concerning Medicare HMOs

• **Carefully consider the benefits that will be provided by the HMO. Do they equal or exceed what you presently receive through Medicare Parts A and B and your Medicare supplemental insurance?**

• **Do you have a choice in the selection of your primary care physician? Are you required to give up your present physician if you join the HMO?**

• **Does the monthly fee or premium you would pay to the HMO equal or exceed the cost of your Medicare supplemental insurance?**

• **Do you fully understand the procedures for enrolling in and withdrawing from the HMO?**

HMOs are organized in several ways:

Staff model. The HMO hires physicians to work on a salary-plus-bonus basis at the HMO's own multi-specialty clinic or hospital. They see only HMO subscribers. The classic organizational model for an HMO, the staff model is the progenitor of all other plans.

Group model. The HMO contracts with separately incorporated physician groups whose practitioners see only HMO subscribers but who continue to practice in their own offices or clinics.

Individual practice association (IPA). The HMO contracts with private practice physicians who agree to see some HMO subscribers along with their regular fee-paying patients in their own offices or clinics. Now the most popular HMO model, the IPA has grown more rapidly than any other type in recent years. One explanation proffered for this unprecedented rise is the heated competition between private practitioners and HMOs, resulting in physicians forming their own HMOs or joining existing ones.

Network model. The HMO contracts with two or more independent group practices, generally unrelated and located in different geographical locations. Along with the HMO subscribers, the physicians continue to see their regular fee-paying patients.

MEDICARE HMOS

Only since 1985 have HMOs been interested in enrolling significant numbers of older Americans. That year the Health Care Financing Administration (HCFA) opened the door for Medicare beneficiaries to enroll in HMOs. It also became possible for retiring employees who already belong to HMOs through their employers to retire into Medicare HMO programs. If you are nearing or already at Medicare age, you need to know some facts unique to Medicare HMO programs:

• HMO Medicare coverage is a supplement to, not a substitute for, your Medicare coverage. When you join the HMO, you do not give up your Medicare Part A hospital insurance or Part B medical insurance coverage. You continue to pay your Part B premium as you always did and continue to be covered. The HMO program is supplemental, or "wraparound," insurance, which covers the costs of hospital and/or medical services not covered by Medicare. Think of an HMO plan as competing with other Medicare supplemental insurance plans for your business. You do not have to give up Medicare to join an HMO, nor do you give up any part of your monthly Social Security check to an HMO.

• You may be required to pay the HMO a monthly premium for coverage of hospital and medical expenses over and above basic Medicare coverage. Depending on the costs of medical care in your area and the particular HMO and options you pick, the individual HMO premium may range from nothing to around $100 a month. Some company retirement plans contribute to the HMO monthly payments. An HMO premium may seem high, but you should remember that you are likely to spend 15 percent or more of your annual income on medical care. The premium, in contrast to traditional Medicare supplemental insurance, picks up many out-of-pocket expenses that you would otherwise have to pay.

The proper comparison of two insurance plans is always this: *Compare premiums plus out-of-pocket costs for one plan to premiums plus out-of-pocket costs for the other.*

The Medicare HMO plan will cover all basic Medicare services and some additional services, usually including: deductible for hospital and skilled nursing services; deductible and copayment for physician services in hospital and office settings; diagnostic and rehabilitation services and prescription drugs (sometimes an extra fee).

- You will receive all your medical and hospital care from the HMO delivery system. So be sure you understand the HMO and are comfortable with its benefits and limitations.
- An HMO cannot deny you membership because of any medical condition unless you have end stage renal disease (chronic kidney failure) or are receiving hospice benefits.

Furthermore, HMOs cannot require you to have a medical examination as a condition of enrollment.

- If you join the HMO and don't like it, you may withdraw at any time for any reason and return to your previous Medicare benefits. To withdraw you simply fill out a withdrawal form, which can take up to 30 days to process. Until you receive a letter clearly indicating reinstatement in Medicare, you are still covered by the HMO for all medical care needs. An HMO can drop you only if you move out of its service area or if it documents that you are completely uncooperative with its administrative rules—you don't pay your monthly premium, you permit misuse of your membership card, and so on.
- All your medical and hospital claims will be sent to the HMO to process and pay on your behalf. Although you will have to pay for a few services as specified in your HMO contract, most will be handled on your behalf. You periodically will receive a printout from the HMO of all claims paid during the period.

IS AN HMO THE BEST SETTING FOR YOU?

The array of insurance plans available to the average American, employed or not, may be bewildering at times. Do you go HMO? PPO? Or IPA? Maybe traditional health insurance is for you. Fee-for-service versus prepaid? Rather than land mines with the potential to blow your budget to smithereens, think of the myriad of options as opportunities to get the most for your medical dollar. The good news here is that doctors, hospitals, and insurance companies are fiercely competing for your business. They need you. And you need to find the highest-quality medical care at the most reasonable cost.

It is possible to make an informed choice—simply follow the steps outlined here to consider *eligibility, coverage,* and *costs.* But first keep in mind these guidelines:

- The only purpose of health insurance is to protect you and your family against large out-of-pocket medical expenses.
- HMOs usually offer more comprehensive hospital and medical benefits than traditional health insurance, without the costly deductibles and copayments. HMOs can save you money—up to 28 percent—compared with conventional health insurance. Your premiums may be a little less or about the same. And HMO subscribers do not submit claims, so there is little or no paperwork to complete.
- The biggest drawbacks we have touched on already: the lock-in restriction whereby subscribers can use only designated providers, and the fact that a physician's authorization (the "gatekeeper" philosophy again) is needed before nonemergency services in order to have the HMO cover the cost of such services. As to problems with convenience and care, anecdotes abound: There's been talk of out-of-the-way, inconveniently located offices and clinics, long waits for appointments, superficial, even perfunctory examinations, and the tendency to undertreat problems by limiting access to expensive diagnostic tests.

Now to what you need to consider before you make an informed choice.

Eligibility
Nearly everyone joins an HMO through an employer, and HMOs market primarily to companies with at least ten employees. Check with your personnel office or supervisor if you're not sure whether an HMO is offered. While you probably have no control over

which HMO your employer asks you to join, you usually do get to say yes or no. During the annual "open enrollment" period, you can choose whether to stay enrolled in your current health insurance plan or sign up with an HMO or PPO. If you become dissatisfied with your choice, you probably will not be able to change until the next year's enrollment period.

Coverage

The government requires federally qualified HMOs to cover a comprehensive range of benefits; HMOs that are not federally qualified have no such requirement. So, first check to see if the HMO you are considering is federally qualified, and if it is, these benefits will be covered:

- All hospital inpatient services with no limits on costs or days
- Hospital outpatient diagnostic and treatment services, including rehabilitation services with some limitations
- Skilled nursing home and home health services
- Short-term detoxification for substance abuse
- Medical treatment and referral for alcohol and drugs
- Preventive care

To get a list of federally qualified HMOs throughout the country, write: Department of Health and Human Services Office of Prepaid Health Care, HCFA Office of Compliance, Security Boulevard, Baltimore, MD 21207; or call 410-966-7626.

Other services are not required but may be covered, if the HMO so chooses: prescription drugs; vision care; dental care; long-term rehabilitation; intermediate nursing care; durable medical equipment; prosthetics; and chiropractic care. HMOs often offer a prescription drug or vision care "rider" separate from the main policy and at additional cost. Only a few HMOs cover dental care.

If the plan is a PPO or nonqualified HMO, and therefore without benefit requirements, check the benefit package. Be aware that some HMOs are beginning to offer "low-option plans," with deductibles, copayments, and fewer benefits—in short, return to concepts similar to those in traditional health insurance.

Costs

You must consider two types of expenses when estimating the total cost of your health insurance: the monthly premium contribution you pay regardless of the amount of services you use and the out-of-pocket costs you pay based on services you use.

First, determine what your annual premium contribution will be if you join an HMO versus a traditional plan. It may be zero if your employer chooses to pay the full premium. According to a KPMG Peat Marwick survey, the average monthly premiums in 1992 for the various types of plans stacked up as follows:

Single (or individual) coverage

Traditional plan	$154
HMO plans	$148
PPO	$157

Family coverage

Traditional plan	$384
HMO plans	$377
PPO	$412

Ask about other out-of-pocket expenses you will be required to pay. It is not uncommon, for instance, to have copayments on office visits, prescription drugs, emergency room services, urgent care services, and mental health benefits.

Next, examine all the important medical and hospital services not covered or only partially covered by the HMO and traditional plans, and liberally estimate what your annual out-of-pocket costs will be. Your annual expense under each plan will be a combination of your premium contribution and your estimated out-of-pocket expenses.

You may find that the HMO is a good buy, and the PPO only slightly better than traditional health insurance. Important to note is the fact that the amount an HMO saves you increases as you use more medical services. In other words, the cost advantage of HMOs becomes evident when you most need to depend on your medical insurance—when you or someone in your family suffers a serious accident or illness.

HMO Medical Care and the Question of Quality

After all the scribbling and calculating we have had you do regarding matters of eligibility and cost, now sharpen your pencil and get ready to tackle the question of quality. At this point you may have concluded that an HMO provides excellent benefits at an economical cost, but that you will join the HMO only if it

More Questions You Should Ask

Believe it or not, you're not yet ready to decide whether an HMO is the best setting for your money until you have more information in hand:

Is the HMO the multispecialty clinic type or office-based? You may want the convenience of a large facility where you can visit your primary physician, consult a specialist, have your laboratory or radiology tests done, and go to the pharmacy—all under one roof. Or you may want the quieter, more personal confines of a physician's private office, especially if you have an established rapport with this physician.

How long has the HMO been in business? A number of HMOs, particularly in oversupplied cities, are in failing financial health, so an HMO's experience is a critical point. Two or three years may be adequate, but less than that probably not.

Is the HMO the entity you will want to treat you when you are sick? Whether it's a clinic or private office, visit the facility and observe closely. Do the physical environment and medical equipment look clean, modern, and cared for? Does the staff treat patients and visitors courteously and professionally? Does the HMO adhere to its appointment schedule or are a lot of appointments backed up? Patient confidentiality prevents HMOs from releasing subscribers' names, but ask your friends if they belong to the HMOs in your area. Are they satisfied with the performance?

What is the travel time to the primary care facility and/or hospital? Consider this for when you or a family member is very sick and others are having to make repeated trips to visit.

How are appointments for both routine and urgent care made? How long will it take to be seen? If you are sick, you should not have to wait more than a day or two to see your physician, although some HMOs ask people to wait up to a week or two if the medical problem does not require immediate attention.

What do you do when you need emergency care? Ideally, an HMO will want you to use its emergency center or an affiliated hospital's emergency room for immediate treatment. However, as you know (and you hope the HMO realizes), not every emergency situation is so strategically and conveniently orchestrated. Some HMOs (and even some traditional insurance plans) establish complicated rules for their subscribers who seek emergency care during night and weekend hours or away from home (in HMO jargon, "outside the service area"). While it is reasonable and proper to have you call your primary physician first, if that doctor or his/her backups do not respond quickly, you should be able to use the closest available emergency service with full confidence that the HMO will pay the bill. Routine or nonemergency care outside the HMO service area may not be covered.

Voluntary Accrediting Organizations

The following organizations set standards for HMOs, make periodic on-site visits to determine if standards are being met, and issue certificates of accreditation (usually good for three years). Any one of these groups should be able to tell you the accreditation status of a particular HMO. But a few words of caution: HMOs pay for the privilege of the on-site inspection in the hope, of course, that they will be granted accreditation, so one might argue a potential conflict of interest here, not to mention self-promotion. Then there's the matter of an absence of consumer participation in the setting of standards as well as in the accrediting process itself—accrediting teams are comprised of health professionals, and not consumers.

While the accreditation status of an HMO is not 100 percent indicative of the quality of care it delivers, it is a good starting point.

Accreditation Association for Ambulatory Healthcare
9933 Lawler, Suite 512
Skokie, IL 60077-3702
708-676-9610

Joint Commission on the Accreditation of Healthcare Organizations
One Renaissance Boulevard
Oakbrook Terrace, IL 60181
708-916-5600

National Committee for Quality Assurance
1350 New York Avenue N.W., Suite 700
Washington, DC 20005
202-628-5788

provides medical care that is as good as or better than what you now receive.

Regarding the obvious question—HMO quality versus fee-for-service plan quality—let us say this. The results of various studies over the last twenty-five years can be summed up in one sentence: There is no evidence that you will end up healthier or sicker by being treated in an HMO system as opposed to the traditional system. Just as there are good *and* bad fee-for-service providers, the same holds true for HMO providers.

What is quality medical care? In our opinion it includes these elements:

- Technically competent medical treatment provided by properly trained and credentialed professionals in clean, modern, well-equipped facilities
- Accessible and convenient services provided without bureaucratic hassles or unreasonable delays

- Personal care respectful of the dignity and intelligence of you and your family
- Coordinated care in which your primary care physician links all specialty or hospital services you need into one sensible treatment plan
- Measurement of the results of treatment to evaluate whether the medical system achieves its goal of curing your illness, relieving your pain, or assisting in your rehabilitation

CHOOSING AN HMO PLAN: SOME FINAL CONSIDERATIONS

- Consider your primary care physician.

A good relationship with your primary care physician is imperative in an HMO setting, since he/she is the person responsible for all your medical services and the gatekeeper to specialty and hospital care. Ask to interview prospective physicians before joining the HMO. (Most HMOs and PPOs will not allow this until after you have enrolled, but insist upon it.)

What formal qualifications should you look for in selecting the doctor? Even though no amount of analysis is foolproof, a good place to start is the doctor's education and credentials. We also recommend you interview the potential candidate(s) and, at the least, talk about such matters as type of practice, his/her telephone accessibility, his/her commitment to prevention and health promotion, how the HMO monitors and controls quality of care, among other things. Fortunately, if you are not satisfied with your final choice, it does not have to be final. Any good HMO will allow you to select a different doctor, although some require a month's notice to process the switch.

• Consider the backup system of hospital and specialty care.

Which hospital(s) will your primary care physician use? Is the hospital a community hospital or major medical center? What is its reputation for quality and service? Find out if your primary care physician will remain fully involved in your care throughout a hospital stay.

What about specialized hospital or rehabilitation programs? If you need a specialized service (for example, physical rehabilitation or mental health counseling), find out how and with whom the HMO contracts for such services.

What are the HMO's rules about specialty referrals? Look at the HMO physician list and see if all major specialties are represented. Make sure it is the physician's responsibility, not yours, to ensure that the paperwork on referrals from your primary care doctor to specialists is completed.

What formal programs does the HMO have to help assure high-quality care? A good HMO will cover the costs of a second opinion on elective surgery, monitor the necessity of every hospital admission, and track infection, complication, and mortality rates. The HMO will periodically audit their physicians' medical charts and have a rigorous protocol for the investigation of subscriber complaints.

THE MERITS OF HEALTH MAINTENANCE ORGANIZATIONS

Now to recap: The big advantage of an HMO, given our assumptions about what a consumer typically wants, is that all but a trivial portion of care is prepaid. There are no worries about having cash to go to the hospital. There are no service-specific charges, so there is no need to negotiate with the doctor about accepting assignment. There are far fewer, or no, forms to fill out. One payment covers everything.

Depending on the costs of medical care in your area and the particular HMO and options you pick, the individual HMO premium may range from nothing to around $100 a month. An HMO premium may seem high, but remember that you are likely to spend 15 percent or more of your income on medical care. In contrast to traditional so-called Medigap coverage, the HMO premium picks up many out-of-pocket expenses that you would otherwise have to pay. More important is the peace of mind knowing that this is the *only* cost, except for nominal copayments. As we've said before, the proper comparison of two insurance plans is always this: *Compare premiums plus out-of-pocket costs for one plan to premiums plus out-of-pocket costs for the other*.

Get exact figures from the HMOs that you are considering—including the average out-of-pocket costs for their Medicare members—but bear in mind that HMO benefit packages differ to some degree. Medicare requires the low-option plan in Medicare-approved HMOs to be at least equal to Medicare benefits, *without* the Medicare copayments and deductibles. Compare these to 15 percent of your annual income. Depending on your income, the HMO may save you anywhere from nothing (a break-even situation, but with added peace of mind) to a lot.

A big issue with HMOs is freedom of choice of doctors and hospitals. A number of alternatives that look like HMOs in some respects have emerged in recent years. *Preferred provider organizations* (PPOs) have closed panels of doctors like HMOs, but not quite: For an extra fee you can go to the doctor or hospital of your choice; the PPO just covers less of the cost to you if you stray from the preferred providers. Generally, a PPO's benefits are not as generous as those of an HMO but a little better than a traditional fee-for-service plan—Blue Cross and Blue Shield, for example.

PPOs are just one variety of *competitive medical plans* (CMPs) with which the Health Care Financing Administration has been experimenting. Basically, CMPs are prepaid plans that do not have to meet the very stringent (and costly) federal requirements for Medicare HMOs. They receive a set amount, based on the average cost of treating a Medicare beneficiary in the counties they serve, adjusted for local wage and

The 50 Largest HMOs (1991)

The following HMOs are ranked, in descending order, according to their enrollment.

1. **Kaiser Foundation Health Plan, Inc.**
Northern California Region
1950 Franklin Street
Oakland, CA 94612
415-987-1000

2. **Kaiser Foundation Health Plan, Inc.**
Southern California Region
393 E. Walnut
Pasadena, CA 91101
818-405-5000

3. **Health Insurance Plan of Greater New York**
220 W. 58th Street
New York, NY 10019
212-373-5100

4. **Health Net**
21600 Oxnard Street
Woodland Hills, CA 91367
818-719-6732

5. **HMO PA—U.S. Healthcare**
980 Jolly Road
P.O. Box 1109
Blue Bell, PA 19422
215-628-4800

6. **Pacificare, Inc.**
5995 Plaza Drive
Cypress, CA 90630
714-952-1121

7. **Medica**
5601 Smetana Drive
P.O. Box 1587
Minneapolis, MN 55440
612-936-1200

8. **Harvard Community Health Plan**
75 Mt. Auburn Street
Cambridge, MA 02138
617-495-2010

9. **Group Health Cooperative of Puget Sound**
521 Wall Street
Seattle, WA 98121
206-448-5600

10. **U.S. Healthcare, Inc.**
S. 61 Paramus Road
Paramus, NJ 07652
201-843-6200

11. **Health Alliance Plan of Michigan**
2850 W. Grand Boulevard
Detroit, MI 48202
313-872-8100

12. **Bay State Health Care**
101 Main Street
Cambridge, MA 02142
617-868-7000

13. **Kaiser Foundation Health Plan of the Northwest**
3600 N. Interstate Avenue
Portland, OR 97227
503-280-2050

14. **Californiacare**
21555 Oxnard Street, 9th Floor
Woodland Hills, CA 91367
818-703-2602

15. **Blue Choice**
150 E. Main Street
Rochester, NY 14647
716-454-1700

16. **FHP, Inc.**
9900 Talbert Avenue
Fountain Valley, CA 92708
714-963-7233

17. **HMO Illinois**
2001 Midwest Road, Suite 300
Oak Brook, IL 60521
708-620-3000

18. **Group Health, Inc.**
2829 University Avenue S.E.
Minneapolis, MN 55414
612-623-8400

19. **CIGNA Medical Group Healthplan**
9808 Scranton Road, Suite 400
San Diego, CA 92121
619-457-5361

20. **Keystone Health Plan East, Inc.**
251 St. Asaph Road
Bala Cynwyd, PA 19004
215-668-1230

21. **M.D. Individual Practice Association, Inc.**
4 Taft Court
Rockville, MD 20737
301-762-8205

22. **Foundation Health, A California Health Plan**
3400 Data Drive
Rancho Cordova, CA 95670
916-631-5000

23. **Kaiser Foundation Health Plan of Mid-Atlantic States, Inc.**
4200 Wisconsin Avenue N.W.
Washington, DC 20016
202-364-3300

24. **Kaiser Foundation Health Plan of Colorado**
10350 E. Dakota Avenue
Aurora, CO 80012
303-344-7500

25. **Medcenters Health Plan, Inc.**
5050 Excelsior Boulevard,
Suite 401
Minneapolis, MN 55416
612-927-2050

26. **Humana Medical Plan, Inc. (South Florida)**
1505 N.W. 167th Street
Miami, FL 33169
305-623-2100

27. **HMO Blue**
492 Old Connecticut Path
Framingham, MA 01701
508-935-2900

28. **Humana-Michael Reese HMO**
2545 S. King Drive
Chicago, IL 60616
312-808-3810

29. **TakeCare Corporation**
2300 Clayton Road, Suite 1000
Concord, CA 94520
415-246-1300

30. **Sanus/New York Life Health Plan**
271 Madison Avenue
New York, NY 10016
212-683-7799

31. **Kaiser Foundation Health Plan of Ohio**
1300 E. 9th Street, Suite 1100
Cleveland, OH 44114
216-621-5600

The 50 Largest HMOs (1991) *(cont.)*

The following HMOs are ranked, in descending order, according to their enrollment.

32. **Chicago HMO Ltd.**
540 N. Lasalle Street
Chicago, IL 60610
312-751-4460

33. **Heritage National Healthplan**
1910 E. Kimberly Road
Davenport, IA 52807
319-344-4400

34. **Pilgrim Health Care, Inc.**
10 Accord Executive Drive
P.O. Box 200
Norwell, MA 02061
617-871-3950

35. **Kaiser Foundation Health Plan, Inc.**
Hawaii Region
711 Kapliolani Boulevard
Honolulu, HI 96813
808-834-5333

36. **U.S. Healthcare**
1981 Marcus Avenue, Suite E-111
Lake Success, NY 11042
516-326-9320

37. **Health Options, Inc.**
8665 Baypine Road, Suite 300
Jacksonville, FL 32256
904-731-7967

38. **AV-MED Health Plan**
8930 N.W. 39th Avenue
Gainesville, FL 32606
904-372-8400

39. **HealthPlus, Inc.**
6611 Kenilworth Avenue
Riverdale, MD 20737
301-277-6520

40. **ChoiceCare**
655 Eden Park Drive, Suite 400
Cincinnati, OH 45202
513-784-5200

41. **Western Ohio Health Care Plan**
6601 Centerville Business Parkway
P.O. Box 591208
Miamisburg, OH 45459
513-439-9355

42. **Independent Health**
220 White Plains Road
Tarrytown, NY 10591
914-631-0939

43. **Kaiser Foundation Health Plan of Georgia, Inc.**
3355 Lenox Road N.E.,
Suite 1000
Atlanta, GA 30326
404-233-0555

44. **Physicians Health Plan of Ohio, Inc.**
3650 Olentangy River Road
Columbus, OH 43214
614-442-7140

45. **Compcare Health Services Insurance Corporation**
501 W. Michigan Street
Milwaukee, WI 53201
414-226-6744

46. **Comprecare Healthcare Services, Inc.**
12100 E. Iliff Avenue
P.O. Box 441170
Aurora, CO 80044
303-695-6685

47. **HIP/Rutgers Health Plan**
1 World's Fair Drive
Somerset, NJ 08873
908-560-9898

48. **Rush Health Plans**
33 E. Congress Parkway, Suite 600
Chicago, IL 60605
312-922-9338

49. **CareAmerica Health Plans, Inc.**
20520 Nordhoff Street
Chatsworth, CA 91311
818-407-2206

50. **Group Health Association, Inc.**
4301 Connecticut Avenue N.W.
Washington, DC 20008
202-364-2003

---

price differences. For this they are supposed to offer medical care. Depending on the cost of the care in the area and the options available within an individual CMP, they can be as generous as an HMO but should not offer less than the standard Medicare benefits.

For people who travel a good deal, a major disadvantage of HMOs is their reluctance to cover health care outside of their service area for other than severe emergencies. If your HMO is in North Dakota and you are vacationing in Florida, you can expect that an emergency room visit for something serious will be covered but not a visit to a local doctor for a cold. On the other hand, many HMOs offer a toll-free number to call for preapproval of treatment. And because of consumer demand, many HMOs have loosened their requirements.

Joining an HMO is not forever. You may decide that, no matter how great the savings and peace-of-mind factor, HMOs are just not for you. Don't worry. You have the right to drop out, and you will be covered by Medicare just as before. You can give one a try without any fear—assuming, of course, that your area has an HMO that accepts Medicare patients.

Medicare

Medicare is the federal insurance plan for persons aged 65 and over (and some disabled people under 65) who are eligible for Social Security or Railroad Retirement benefits. It is run by the Health Care Financing Administration of the U.S. Department of Health and Human Services. Social Security Administration (SSA) offices across the country take applications for

Medicare and provide information about the program. Review the general eligibility requirements presented here to determine if you qualify for the program. All specific questions regarding your eligibility should be directed to the SSA office in your area.

WHO MAY APPLY FOR MEDICARE, AND WHO'S ELIGIBLE

Anyone who thinks they are in one of the groups that Medicare covers can apply for inclusion in the program. In fact, if there is any doubt at all in your mind as to whether you are eligible, or in the mind of the representative of Social Security at the Social Security Administration office where you apply for Medicare, you should apply. It is better to apply and get a decision than to be turned down when you really are eligible.

THE BASIC COVERAGE GROUPS

Medicare was originally intended for "the elderly"— those aged 65 or older. It now covers:

- The elderly—those who are aged 65 or older
- Those who are permanently and totally disabled
- Those who have end stage renal disease, the medical term for kidney disease that is severe enough to require dialysis or a transplant

Of course, things are not really this simple. Most, but not all, of the nation's elderly are covered. The permanently and totally disabled are covered, but only if they meet the Social Security Administration's current definition of "permanently and totally disabled" and have received Social Security disability payments for at least two years. Those with end stage renal disease are covered, but only if they meet the current definition of the disease. For most people, becoming eligible is just a matter of turning 65 and applying. For a few, it can be a frustrating process involving lawyers, appeals, and a lot of expense and anguish. The following information applies to the general eligibility requirements. All questions regarding your specific eligibility for Medicare should be directed to your local Social Security Administration office.

ELIGIBILITY REQUIREMENTS FOR MEDICARE COVERAGE

Everyone who is eligible for Medicare, in any of the coverage groups, has to be a citizen of the United States, either by birth or naturalization, or an alien admitted for permanent residence who has resided in the United States for at least five years.

They must also have attained age 65. If they are not yet 65, they must be disabled, or be suffering from end stage renal disease. A common misconception is that you will be covered if you are receiving Social Security payments. *This is not true unless you meet the requirements above.* The requirements for Social Security and Medicare are different. For example, it is possible to start receiving Social Security payments at 62, but you will not be covered by Medicare until you reach age 65.

In addition, to be eligible for Medicare, you must be entitled to payments under the Social Security Act or the Railroad Retirement Act. This means, in general, that you must have worked for at least ten years (or, alternatively, 6 quarters out of the last 13 quarters) in a job that was covered under the Social Security Act, or be covered based on the earnings record of someone who is covered.

The language we use daily makes almost no distinction between "eligible" (for something) and "entitled" (to something.) The Social Security and Medicare laws use the words differently. You are "eligible" for Medicare as soon as, and whenever, you meet the eligibility requirements that apply to you. You are "entitled" to Medicare only after you have applied and are officially determined (sometimes after a session in court, pitting you against the federal government) to be eligible.

If this sounds somewhat confusing, it is; however, we've done our best to keep the language simple. We tried substituting "receiving Social Security payments" for "entitled," but that doesn't work because you can be entitled and not be receiving payments (for example, if you continue working after age 62 and make enough to reduce your Social Security payments to zero).

The following translation of the legalese is the best we can do; the important thing to keep in mind is that in order to receive Medicare, *you must apply*. There's only one exception to this: If you are already entitled to Social Security payments and turn age 65, you are enrolled in (and entitled to) both parts of Medicare, unless you advise the Social Security Administration that you do not want Part B. There are two exceptions to the exception. You're not automatically enrolled, even if you're receiving checks, if (1) you are entitled to Medicare on the basis of government employment or (2) you are residing outside the United States. Otherwise, you *must apply*. The upshot is: *If you want it, apply for it.*

THE WORK REQUIREMENT

A quarter is one-fourth of a year, or 3 months. While you can be covered with as few as 6 quarters worked, the majority of Social Security recipients have worked for the ten-year (40-quarter) period the Social Security Act specifies. There is an alternative requirement for persons who have died or attained age 62 without having 40 quarters. (Death prior to age 62 is relevant because it is possible to be entitled to Medicare on the earnings record of someone who has died.) Finally, it is also possible to be covered if you have worked for 6 out of the last 13 quarters, ending with the one in which one becomes entitled to Social Security benefits. The eligibility conferred under the last option, however, can be lost. Eligibility under the first two is permanent.

The alternative requirement is this: The person must have one quarter of coverage for each year elapsing after 1950 or the year they reached age 21, whichever is later, and the year before the year in which they attained age 62 or died, whichever is earlier. Alternatively, they can have 6 quarters in the 13-quarter period (three years and 3 months) in which they become entitled to Social Security payments. A minimum of 6 quarters is always required.

This last option can be thought of as a "window" of eligibility that is linked to the month you apply for, and are found eligible for, Social Security. Obviously, if you wait to apply until you have no longer worked for 6 out of the last 13 quarters, counting backward from the quarter in which the application occurs, you can lose your eligibility under this option. The following tables may help make this a bit clearer.

Social Security (and Medicare) Eligibility Alternatives: Quarters of Coverage Required

Option 1	*Option 2*	*Option 3*
40 quarters, regardless of when earned	One quarter for each calendar year after age 21 or 1950, until age 62, whichever results in lower requirement	Six out of last 13 quarters

For a quarter in which you worked to count for Medicare (and Social Security) purposes, you must have earned a certain amount during the quarter. You must also have earned it from an employer covered under Social Security. Prior to 1979, you had to earn at least $250 each quarter; beginning in 1979 that amount increased to $260 and has increased every year since. Here are the earnings per quarter required since 1979:

$290 in 1980	$470 in 1988
$310 in 1981	$500 in 1989
$340 in 1982	$520 in 1990
$370 in 1983	$540 in 1991
$390 in 1984	$570 in 1992
$410 in 1985	$590 in 1993
$440 in 1986	$620 in 1994
$460 in 1987	

The exception that allows fewer than 40 quarters of coverage applies primarily to individuals who returned to, or entered, the work force late in life and became disabled or died before age 62, and aliens who have entered the United States and have resided here for at least five years. (Aliens must be *legal residents* for five years to receive Medicare, but their work counts toward coverage as soon as they start working.) Let's look at some examples:

Marge Smith, who has never worked before, starts working in the first quarter of 1985, because her husband is disabled, and she works continuously. She was born in 1926, became 21 in 1947, and will become age 62 in 1988. She needs 37 quarters of coverage (because the number of years after 1950 and before 1988 is 37), or 6 out of the 13-quarter period before her entitlement to Social Security payments. Although she is 62 in 1988, she does not yet have 13 quarters. She first becomes eligible for Social Security payments after the first quarter of 1989 (in April). She is covered at this point, and will be eligible for Medicare when she becomes 65, *but she should apply for Social Security now to be entitled to Medicare.* (If her husband is covered, she can be entitled based on his earnings record.)

Why should Marge apply now? Because if she stops work and more than 7 quarters go by before she applies, *she will no longer meet the alternative 6-out-of-the-last-13-quarters requirement* for getting Medicare. The connection with entitlement to Social Security is what makes the magic work, because it sets the point from which one starts counting backward.

> John Smith, their son, attained age 21 in 1983. He becomes disabled in 1988. He started working in 1984, right after he graduated from college, and worked continuously until 1988. He needs 6 quarters. (He has, of course, 4 for each of the years 1984, 1985, 1986, and 1987, a total of 16; he needs 4 to be covered by the formula above (one each for 1984–87), but the minimum is 6. He is covered, because he has at least 6 quarters. He will be eligible for Medicare when he has been entitled to Social Security disability payments for two years.

John meets the minimum-of-6-quarters requirement *and* the 6-out-of-the-last-13 requirement. He has to meet *both* to be entitled to Social Security. He is *not* eligible for Medicare until he has been entitled to Social Security for two years.

> Victoria Smith-Jones, Marge Smith's English cousin, enters the country as a lawfully admitted alien in the first quarter of 1988, because her cousin Marge's situation is difficult, and the two want to be together. She was born in 1926 and will become age 62 in 1988. She has a job waiting for her and works continuously. She needs 37 quarters of coverage (because the number of years after 1950 and before 1988 is 37), or 6 out of the 13-quarter period before her entitlement to Social Security payments. She becomes eligible for Social Security pay-

> ments at age 62, as does Marge, and is wise enough to apply to protect her eligibility for Medicare, but she is not actually eligible for Medicare until she has resided in the U.S. for five years. She meets this requirement in the first quarter of 1993. She is *eligible* for Social Security (and *entitled* to it) in the second quarter of 1992, but is not eligible for Medicare until the first quarter of 1993, after she has lived in the U.S. for five years. The fact that she became 65 in 1991 is not relevant here, because Victoria is an alien.

For reasons known only to Congress, the five-year residency requirement applies to Part B of Medicare, not Part A. An alien can qualify for Part A as soon as he or she is entitled to Social Security, but must wait five years for Part B, regardless of entitlement.

The requirement of 40 quarters of covered work has been scaled back, as we've shown in the examples above, for people whom Congress knew could not have worked so long. These include most of the disabled, and most of those with end stage renal disease. (From now on, we'll use the word "disabled" to mean those who meet the current legal definition of "permanently and totally disabled." We understand that this definition excludes many people who cannot, in fact, obtain work.)

Do not assume that you do not meet this requirement. Many people do not know about the alternative ways of becoming eligible, and erroneously think that they must have worked for 40 continuous quarters. This is not always true, as we've seen.

Another reason not to assume that you are not eligible is that you may be eligible based on the earnings record of someone who is covered. For example, widows and widowers are covered if they were married to their spouses at least one year before the death of the spouse. Divorced persons are eligible if they were married to the covered person for at least ten years. Also:

- *Wives* are eligible if their husband is covered and they have attained age 65.
- *Divorced wives* are eligible if they were married to the person on whose earnings record they are

covered, have attained age 65, and have not re-married.

- *Husbands* are eligible under the same conditions as wives.
- *Divorced husbands* are eligible under the same conditions as divorced wives.
- *Widows and widowers* are eligible if they are over 65.
- *Mothers and fathers* of covered children are eligible if they have attained the age of 65.
- *Surviving parents* of children eligible for Social Security who were receiving at least one-half of their support from their child at the time of the child's death or disability are eligible when they reach age 65.

You now have to deal with a division of labor in the federal government. Until you have been determined to be eligible for Medicare, you are the responsibility of the Social Security Administration, which makes eligibility determinations for both Medicare and Social Security benefits. Once you are eligible for Medicare, you will deal with the Health Care Financing Administration (HCFA), which runs Medicare and Medicaid. (For the sake of brevity and avoidance of alphabet soup, we'll use "Medicare" to refer to HCFA from now on, unless there's a clear need to distinguish the program from those who run it.) For the moment, please believe us when we say that we are not trying to confuse Social Security issues with Medicare issues. Until you are found eligible for Medicare, the two are tied together in a Gordian knot. Most of the advice we give on Medicare will also help you preserve or increase your benefits under Social Security. Right now, we want to give you some information (and encouragement) about:

What to Do If You Are Not Eligible Now

Remember: You cannot get Medicare unless you are eligible for Social Security. (There is an option to purchase Medicare as insurance if you're not eligible. We discuss that later.) In order to make sure you are eligible for Medicare, qualify for Social Security. (And if you're a resident alien, make sure you meet the five-year requirement.)

You are likely to be found ineligible only if you don't meet the age, alien residency, or work requirement. Only time will cure the first two.

If the reason that you are found not to be eligible is that you do not have enough covered work, there's only one answer: more work, earning at least $590 (for 1993) in each quarter, until you meet either the standard test or the alternative. The standard test, as we discussed above, is 1 quarter of work for each of the years after the year you turned 21 and before the year you turned 62 or became disabled (in the eyes of Social Security). The standard is 40 for most of us. The alternative is 6 out of the last 13 quarters before you apply for Social Security. But you should eliminate the possibility that you've been found ineligible due to an error.

Make Sure Your Earnings Record Is Right

You can obtain your Personal Earnings and Benefit Estimate Statement every three years by requesting Form 7004-PC from your local Social Security office, or calling 800-234-5772. It's important that your earnings are properly credited to your account, and not to another person's account. If you discover a mistake, act quickly, because you have only a limited amount of time to make corrections.

If your earnings record does not show that you have enough covered quarters to be covered now, the first thing to do is make sure that the record is accurate. It can be in error regarding *whether or not* there were any earnings in a quarter. This can affect your eligibility for Social Security and Medicare. It can also be in error about the *amount* you earned. This can affect your eligibility for both programs *and* the amount of your Social Security benefits.

To straighten out an earnings record that has errors in it, Social Security has to check it against other records that are correct. This is where the hard part begins. Ideally, you will have all the paycheck stubs or pay envelopes that were ever issued to you, and you will have all of your federal, state, and local tax returns for your entire working life. You will have the name and address of all of your former employers. None of them will have shut down, moved, or changed their names. If all of this is true, straightening out your earnings record will be a snap.

The foregoing is almost never true, of course. Fortunately, all you usually have to provide is information on the last five years of earnings, which are typically the highest-earning years (your SSA payment is based on the "high five"). Those five years contain 20 of the 40 quarters you need to show that you worked, so all that is necessary is proving that you worked some in 20 other quarters.

Personnel at your local SSA district office can help you straighten out your earnings record. SSA has specialists in this at regional offices if the local office can't help you, and your case can be sent to them as a last resort. The problem is that all of this will take *time*. For this reason, it is important to start early before you need Medicare.

If you are unable to qualify for Medicare by virtue of working under the Social Security system, you still have the option of purchasing Medicare. Persons who are age 65 and who do not otherwise qualify for Medicare can purchase Medicare coverage just like private insurance. The 1994 premium for the combined Part A (hospital insurance) and Part B (doctor insurance) is $286.10 per month.

If you purchase Medicare, you will still have to purchase supplemental insurance to have a package that really protects you against the financial effects of illness.

You are permitted to purchase Part B of Medicare (doctor insurance) if you are a resident of the United States, are 65 or over, and either a citizen or an alien lawfully admitted for permanent residence who has resided in the U.S. for the last five years. (It is under this rule that *everyone* enrolls in Part B.) If you are not eligible for Part A of Medicare, enrolling for Part B entitles you to purchase it. So you have to buy Part B to get Part A. Examples:

> Victoria Smith-Jones's brother Cedric is entranced by Victoria's letters about life in the U.S., and decides to move here in late 1988. He is lawfully admitted for permanent residence. Being independently wealthy, he decides not to work. He loses most of his fortune in the 1992 stock market crash and can no longer afford his extremely expensive medical insurance. He is 65 in early 1993, and discovers that he is not eligible for Medicare because he has never worked. (Anywhere. Anytime.) He decides to purchase Medicare. He calls his local Social Security office, establishes that he is not eligible but does meet the re-

quirements for purchase, and requests that an application to purchase Part B and Part A be sent to him, and signs up.

> Amber Smith Citron, aged 66, Marge's sister, was married to her former husband, Harold Citron, for nine years and 361 days. She would be eligible for Medicare on his earnings record had she been married to him for ten years. She has been working, and will have worked for 6 out of the last 13 quarters, counting from the first quarter of 1989. But she is worried about medical expenses now. She meets the requirements of age (65 or older), citizenship, and current U.S. residence, and, like Cedric, signs up to purchase Medicare. Unlike Cedric, she will be eligible in early 1989. When she is eligible, she will no longer pay the Part A premium and will pay a reduced Part B premium.

HOW AND WHEN TO APPLY

Once more: Being between ages 62 and 65 does not *entitle* you to Medicare. Being 65 or older does not *enroll* you for Medicare. It may take action on your part when you turn 65. Some people are automatically enrolled, others are given notices that they need to enroll. Automatic enrollment and notification are administrative actions of the Social Security Administration, *not* requirements of the law. The categories of those who are enrolled automatically have changed, and could change again. *If you want Medicare, apply for it.* The worst that can happen is that you'll find out your enrollment is already taken care of. The present situation is as follows:

• If you are 65 or older and have been receiving Social Security or Railroad Retirement benefits, you will automatically be enrolled for participation in Parts A and B (the hospital and doctor insurance portions of Medicare). You will receive a notice and your card about 3 to 4 months before your sixty-fifth birthday. Your card will *not* be valid until you turn 65. You are covered for Medicare even if you do not have your card; the hospital can bill under your Social Security number even if you do not have the card. You can obtain a Temporary Notice of Medicare Eligibility from your Social Security office.

- If you are 65 or older when you apply for Social Security benefits, you will automatically be enrolled as part of the application process for Social Security. Your card will be sent to you in the mail automatically. You are covered for Medicare even if you do not have your card if you are over 65 and have been found eligible for Social Security.
- End stage renal disease patients are automatically enrolled if they are receiving Social Security disability benefits; otherwise, they must apply.

If you enrolled for Social Security and began receiving benefits before you were 65, *you must take action to enroll in Medicare*. Formerly, persons were notified by mail when they were eligible to enroll. This service has been dropped as a cost-cutting measure. You will have to keep track of the time yourself. You can apply for Part B Medicare coverage *to begin on your sixty-fifth birthday* anytime between 3 months before your sixty-fifth birthday and 3 months after. If you apply later than this, your Part A (hospital insurance) coverage will begin on the date you apply, not on your birthday. Your "personal enrollment period," as SSA calls it, is these 7 months. The following table may help.

Month in Which 65th Birthday Occurs:	Earliest Month to Apply:	Latest Month to Apply:
January 1995	October 1994	April 1995
February 1995	November 1994	May 1995
March 1995	December 1994	June 1995
April 1995	January 1995	July 1995
May 1995	February 1995	August 1995
June 1995	March 1995	September 1995
July 1995	April 1995	October 1995
August 1995	May 1995	November 1995
September 1995	June 1995	December 1995
October 1995	July 1995	January 1996
November 1995	August 1995	February 1996
December 1995	September 1995	March 1996
January 1996	October 1995	April 1996
February 1996	November 1995	May 1996
March 1996	December 1995	June 1996

Enrolling in Medicare Part B

If you do not apply for Part B (doctor insurance) when you apply for Part A, you will not be eligible to apply until the next general enrollment period, which runs from January 1 to March 31 of each year. Your premium will be raised 10 percent for each year you wait to apply. In addition, you will not have coverage begin until July 1 of the year you enroll.

We recommend that you apply for Part B coverage at the time you apply for Part A, if you can afford it. Failure to take Part B will make any supplemental insurance you buy harder to obtain, will make your premium higher, and may make supplemental insurance harder to get. The Part B premium is tax-deductible just like any other medical insurance premium.

Glossary of Medicare Terms

Medicare, a federal medical benefits program for people aged 65 and older and for certain permanently disabled younger people, is probably the largest and the most expensive single program that the federal government runs. It is also one of the most complex. And because it is so big and confusing, the more the Medicare beneficiary knows, the better he can determine the kind of experience he'll encounter with the program and whether he gets the maximum benefit from it.

As with most government programs, Medicare has a lingo all its own. Familiarize yourself with these common terms and you'll make a giant step toward cutting through the bureaucratic red tape that envelops Medicare.

Administrative law judge (ALJ)—an official charged with making decisions in administrative matters, as opposed to civil or criminal law.

Ambulatory surgery—a large, though limited, range of procedures using operative and anesthesia techniques that allow the patient to recuperate at home, rather than in the hospital, immediately following the operation.

Approved charge—the amount that Medicare has determined is appropriate for payment to a physician for a service, based on his and his colleagues' histories of charge.

Assignment—a process in which a Medicare beneficiary agrees to have Medicare's share of the cost of a service paid directly to a doctor or other provider, and the provider agrees to accept the Medicare-approved charge as payment in full.

Medicare pays 80 percent of the cost, the beneficiary 20 percent.

Balance billing limit—the maximum fee a nonparticipating physician may charge a Medicare beneficiary for any medical service provided. In 1995 this amount is limited to 115 percent of the Medicare-approved amount.

Carriers—private organizations, usually insurance companies, that have contracts with the Health Care Financing Administration to process claims under Part B (doctor insurance) of Medicare.

Case law—the body of court decisions that establishes binding interpretations of the law passed by legislative bodies.

Competitive medical plan—an arrangement for prepaid care that is not as restricted as a health maintenance organization (HMO) in benefits offered, premium calculation, and the like.

Conversion clause—a provision found in group health insurance plans that gives individuals the right to convert their coverage to individual coverage with the same insurance company.

Coordination of benefits—a process in which insurers cooperate to make sure that they do not, together, pay more than 100 percent of the amount billed for any medical service. It also prevents a person from collecting twice for the same service.

Copayment—portion of the cost of care an insured person is required to pay, while the insurance usually, but not always, pays for the major part of the cost.

Deductible—amount that must be paid by an insured person before an insurance plan pays for any portion of the cost.

Department of Health and Human Services—the federal department charged generally with the administration of national "welfare" programs. Formed from the old Department of Health, Education, and Welfare when the Department of Education was split off.

Diagnosis-related groups (DRG) system—a method of paying hospitals based on the average cost of treating patients with statistically similar conditions.

Doctor of Chiropractic—a holder of the degree of doctor of chiropractic (D.C.), a school of medicine that places almost exclusive reliance on manipulation for alignment of the skeleton, plus exercise and nutrition. Chiropractors are eligible to participate in the Medicare program.

Doctor of medicine—a holder of the degree of medical doctor (M.D.), the dominant school of medicine in the United States. Medical doctors are eligible to participate in the Medicare program.

Doctor of osteopathy—a holder of the degree of doctor of osteopathy (D.O.), a school of medicine that emphasizes, but not exclusively, proper alignment of the skeleton. Osteopathic doctors are eligible to participate in the Medicare program.

Durable medical equipment—medical equipment that is intended to be used over and over again, usually by the patient or a caregiver, rather than being used once or a few times and discarded. Examples are wheelchairs, hospital beds, and oxygen tanks.

Earnings record—the record of amounts earned by each individual for whom Social Security taxes were paid; maintained by the Social Security Administration.

End stage renal disease—kidney disease that is severe enough to require lifetime dialysis or a kidney transplant. End stage renal disease patients are eligible for Medicare and may be eligible for Social Security payments if found to be disabled.

Explanation of Benefits (EOB)—a summary of how an insurance company paid a claim to a provider or the insured person. The EOB shows how much the provider billed, how much the provider was reimbursed, and what portion of the claim is the responsibility of the insured. The EOB also tells the insured how to file an appeal in the event payment for a service is disallowed.

Explanation of Medicare Benefits (EOMB)—a form sent to a Medicare beneficiary after a claim is paid, indicating the date and type of service received, name of the provider, Medicare-approved amount, payment to the provider, and the amount owed by the Medicare beneficiary. The EOMB also tells the Medicare beneficiary how to file an appeal in the event payment for a service is disallowed.

Federal judicial districts—major divisions of the United States that are under the jurisdiction of a single federal appeals court. The federal district courts make laws that establish precedents that the Social Security Administration and Medicare must follow, but these precedents have binding force only within the judicial district, unless Congress aligns laws with them or the Supreme Court makes them the law of the land by upholding them when an appeal from the federal district court decision is filed.

Freedom of choice options—arrangements under which members of a health maintenance organization or other prepaid plan can use physicians who are outside the panel of participating doctors, if they wish to do so. Additional payment is usually involved. This applies to Medicare beneficiaries enrolled in health maintenance organizations or competitive medical plans.

General enrollment period—the time from January 1 to March 31 of each year when anyone eligible for Part B of Medicare can enroll in it.

General medical/surgical floors—the areas of a hospital in which patients who do not require special treatment are cared for.

Health Care Financing Administration (HCFA)—the part of the U.S. Department of Health and Human Services that operates Medicare and, together with the states, Medicaid.

Health maintenance organization (HMO)—an entity that combines the functions of insurer and provider of care, giving most necessary care for a prepaid fee and placing an emphasis on prevention and careful assessment of medical necessity. When an HMO has a contract with the Health Care Financing Administration, it is permitted to offer its services to Medicare beneficiaries and collect a monthly fee from Medicare.

Home health agency—an agency approved by Medicare for the delivery of home health services to Medicare beneficiaries.

Home health care—care rendered in a patient's residence by employees of a home health agency or other approved provider of such care.

Hospice—a facility that provides medical care in a homelike setting for the terminally ill.

Immigration and naturalization records—records maintained by, or issued by, the U.S. Departments of State and Interior which show that an alien has legally entered the United States or become a citizen. These records may be used to determine eligibility for both Social Security and Medicare.

Individual enrollment period—the time, running from 3 months before one's sixty-fifth birthday to 3 months after, during which one can enroll in Part B of Medicare without a premium increase for delayed enrollment.

Individual practice association (IPA) health maintenance organization—a health maintenance organization that is staffed by physicians in private practice who continue to maintain their own offices and see both HMO and non-HMO patients.

Inpatient—(n.) someone admitted to the hospital for care; (adj.) pertaining to care given in a hospital.

Intensive care unit—the unit in a hospital in which people whose life support requires constant monitoring, or who require close and constant observation, are cared for.

Intermediaries—private organizations, usually insurance companies, that have contracts with the Health Care Financing Administration to process claims under Part A (hospital insurance) of Medicare.

Intermediate care facility—an institution that provides less intensive care than a skilled nursing facility. Patients are generally more mobile, and rehabilitation therapies are stressed.

Medicaid—a federal/state program, established by Title XIX of the Social Security Act, that provides medical care to the poor. Each state maintains eligibility requirements, which are available from the state department of welfare.

Medically needy—eligible for Medicaid, not because of absolute lack of income, but because income, less accumulated medical bills, is below state income limits for the Medicaid program.

Medical necessity—the state of being thought to be required by the prevailing medical consensus, or a determination made by a doctor that a Medicare beneficiary needs a particular service.

Medical necessity determination—a formal judgment, usually made for purposes of insurance payment, that a treatment was or was not medically necessary. Medicare will pay only for services that are deemed to be medically necessary.

Medicare discharge rights—also called "An Important Message from Medicare." This notice advises Medicare beneficiaries what to do in the event they are given a notice of noncoverage by a provider. It spells out the appeals process available to a Medicare beneficiary when he/she does not agree with the determination made by the provider.

Medicare insured group—an experimental approach to providing care to Medicare beneficiaries in which a traditional provider of retiree benefits, such as a corporation or union welfare plan, takes over responsibility for all care to those 65 or over in return for a set payment from Medicare.

Medicare-participating physician—a doctor who has agreed to accept assignment on all claims from all Medicare beneficiaries in return for certain incentives.

Medicare supplemental insurance—also called Medigap insurance because it covers the gaps in the Medicare system such as the Part A and B deductibles and copayments. Only policies meeting the standards developed by the National Association of Insurance Commissioners may be advertised and sold as Medigap policies.

Notice of noncoverage—an official notice to a Medicare beneficiary that the provider has reason to believe that Medicare will no longer pay for the services provided. This is not an official determination by Medicare, but permits the beneficiary to request an official determination by the peer review organization. The provider is responsible for filing the request for review with the peer review organization.

Notice of utilization—the official determination made by a peer review organization when a Medicare beneficiary requests a review to determine if the provider was correct in issuing a notice of noncoverage for services. If a beneficiary receives a negative response, he/she may then file an appeal with the peer review organization.

Outliers—cases that fall outside the statistical norms of the DRG system, either in total cost or in days of hospitalization required. Medicare makes additional payments for outliers if the peer review organization approves.

Out-of-area care—care that is given to a member of a health maintenance organization when the member is outside the service area of the HMO. This is an issue largely because federal laws for HMO certification require the definition of a service area. Depending on the HMO, arranging for out-of-area care can be a problem.

Out-of-pocket limit—an amount no more than which an insured individual is required to pay, after which his insurance policy pays all costs for the services it covers, regardless of other provisions. Also called a stop-loss limit.

Outpatient surgery—surgery performed without admission to a hospital, even though the surgery may be performed in the hospital.

Outpatient treatment—treatment at a hospital, or in a setting outside a hospital, that does not require admission or temporary residence in the hospital.

Packed red cells—blood cells that have been separated from the plasma, and are transfused separately. Medicare Parts A and B cover this service.

Patient Self-Determination Act—a provision of the Medicare law that requires hospitals to advise all Medicare patients of their right to make patient care decisions. In order to make health care decisions—including the right to accept or refuse treatment and the right to execute advance directives—all adult individuals must be provided with written information about their rights under state law.

Peer review organization (PRO)—any one of a group of doctors that has a contract with the Health Care Financing Administration to evaluate the medical necessity of care rendered to Medicare beneficiaries under the Medicare program, and to investigate the quality of care in providers serving Medicare beneficiaries. The peer review organization is responsible for issuing the notice of utilization when a Medicare beneficiary appeals a notice of noncoverage.

Permanently and totally disabled—a term of art under the Social Security Act, applying to those persons who meet the definition of disability in the act, and qualify for Social Security payments and Medicare on that basis.

Power of attorney—a legal document giving one person the power to act as the representative of another in certain situations, which can be defined in the power of attorney document.

Preferred provider organization (PPO)—an arrangement in which patients are "locked in" to a group of providers, usually by restrictions on payment for services provided by those not in the group of providers, in return for discounts or expanded services. A wide variety exists: Some resemble traditional insurance plans; some resemble health maintenance organizations.

Primary diagnosis—the chief medical reason for an encounter with a health care provider or admission to a hospital; used by Medicare to determine payment for the services received.

Prospective payment—payment made before a service is rendered, and accepted as payment in full by the provider; the opposite of fee-for-service payment. Medicare DRGs are an example of a prospective payment system.

Protocol—a written plan for caring for a particular condition, intended as a guideline to physicians, and usually adopted by a medical institution such as a clinic, hospital, or health maintenance organization. May be used to help determine medical necessity of services provided to Medicare beneficiaries.

Provider—a generic term for any person (for example, a doctor) or entity (for example, a home health agency or a hospital) approved to give care to Medicare beneficiaries and to receive payment from Medicare.

Qualified Medicare beneficiary (QMB)—a low-income Medicare beneficiary who is eligible to have his/her Medicare Part B premium paid for by Medicaid. The beneficiary must have income at or below the national poverty level ($7,608 for an individual, $10,092 for a family of two), and resources worth less than $5,000 (individual) or $6,000 (family of two).

Quarter of coverage—one-fourth of a calendar year during which a person earns enough, in employment covered by Social Security, to have the quarter counted toward the number needed (usually 40) to ensure entitlement to Social Security and Medicare.

Recovery room—the place in a hospital where patients are brought after surgery for close observation until they are ready to be taken to their floors or special care units.

Registered nurse (RN)—generally, the highest trained of nurses, one licensed by a state to provide general nursing services after passing a qualifying examination; may or may not hold collegiate degree.

Respirator—a medical device that takes over breathing functions for patients who are permanently or temporarily unable to breathe on their own.

Secondary diagnosis—a condition that exists in addition to the one that is the chief reason for an encounter with a health care provider or admission to a hospital; plays an important role in helping to determine the payment under Medicare Parts A and B.

Service area—the geographical region in which a health maintenance organization or other prepaid health care plan has agreed to provide services.

Sheltered, or custodial, care—care that is primarily nonmedical. Residents of sheltered or custodial care facilities do not require constant attention from nurses and aides but do need assistance with one or more daily activities, or no longer want to be bothered with keeping up a house. The social needs of residents are met in a safe, secure environment free of as many anxieties as possible.

Skilled nursing facility—an institution that offers nursing services similar to those given in a hospi-
tal, to aid recuperation of those who are seriously ill. Distinguished from intermediate care and custodial care, which may meet some minor medical needs but are intended primarily to support elderly and disabled individuals in the tasks of daily living.

Social health maintenance organizations—experimental programs that try to provide for the medical and social needs of the elderly and disabled in one prepaid package. So far these have not been too successful because they were more expensive than was hoped.

Social Security Administration (SSA)—the part of the U.S. Department of Health and Human Services that operates the various programs funded under the Social Security Act and determines eligibility for Medicare.

Social Security number—a unique number assigned to each individual by the Social Security Administration for tax and benefits purposes. Also used as a unique personal identifier by many other government programs and private enterprises.

Social Security office—local offices of the Social Security Administration, found throughout the country, which take applications for Social Security and Medicare and handle processing of Medicare requests for reconsideration and appeals.

Special care units—portions of a hospital organized and staffed to take care of one kind of (usually serious) problem, such as a cardiac care unit, intensive care unit, burn unit, and so on.

Specialist—a physician who has elected to practice, and usually has special training in, some branch of medicine other than primary care, such as surgery, or who has an exclusive focus in one area of primary care, such as allergy, gastroenterology, or ear, nose, and throat care. Especially in urban areas, specialists are expected to have certification from specialty societies or boards that they have had adequate training in the specialty.

Staff model health maintenance organization—a health maintenance organization staffed by doctors who are its employees and are not in individual or group practice.

Supplemental security income (SSI)—a program that provides small stipends to the elderly, blind, and disabled who for one reason or another are not eligible for other, more generous welfare programs.

Swing beds—hospital beds approved by Medicare for use as hospital or skilled nursing facility beds, depending on demand.

Usual, customary, and reasonable reimbursement system—a means of determining payments to doctors based on statistical profiles of their and their colleagues' history of charges.

Utilization review committee (URC)—a group of doctors in a hospital who review lengths of hospital stays and treatments to make sure that they are medically necessary.

Waiver of liability—a legal removal of an individual's responsibility to pay for a treatment in an instance where Medicare or Medicaid does not pay for it.

State Medicare Part B Carriers

These are the insurance companies that process Medicare Part B (doctor and outpatient services) for the federal agency that administers the Medicare program. You would contact the carrier in your state with questions concerning claims submitted or claims paid.

Alabama
Medicare/Blue Cross–Blue Shield of Alabama
P.O. Box 830-140
Birmingham, AL 35283-0140
205-988-2244
800-292-8855

Alaska
Medicare/Aetna Life and Casualty
200 S.W. Market Street
P.O. Box 1998
Portland, OR 97207-1998
503-222-6831
800-547-6333
Customer service site in Oregon.

Arizona
Medicare/Aetna Life and Casualty
P.O. Box 37200
Phoenix, AZ 85069
602-861-1968
800-352-0411

Arkansas
Medicare/Arkansas Blue Cross and Blue Shield
P.O. Box 1418
Little Rock, AR 72203-1418
501-378-2320
800-482-5525

California
For counties of Imperial, Los Angeles, Orange, San Diego, San Luis Obispo, Santa Barbara, Ventura:
Medicare/Transamerica Occidental Life Insurance Co.
Box 50061
Upland, CA 91785-0061
213-748-2311
800-675-2266

For rest of state:
Medicare Claims Department
Blue Shield of California
Chico, CA 95976
In area codes 209, 408, 415, 707, 916
916-743-1583
800-952-8627
In area codes 213, 619, 714, 805, 818
714-824-0900
800-848-7713

Colorado
Medicare/Blue Cross and Blue Shield of Colorado
Claims: P.O. Box 173560
Correspondence/Appeals: P.O. Box 173500
Denver, CO 80217
800-332-6681 in Colorado outside of metro area
303-831-2661 in metro Denver

Connecticut
Medicare/The Travelers Insurance Co.
538 Preston Avenue
P.O. Box 9000
Meriden, CT 06454-9000
800-982-6819
203-728-6783 in Hartford
203-237-8592 in the Meriden area

Delaware
Medicare/Pennsylvania Blue Shield
P.O. Box 890200
Camp Hill, PA 17089-0200
800-851-3535

District of Columbia
Medicare/Pennsylvania Blue Shield
P.O. Box 890100
Camp Hill, PA 17089-0100
800-233-1124

Florida
Medicare/Blue Shield of Florida, Inc.
P.O. Box 2525
Jacksonville, FL 32231
904-355-3680
800-333-7586
For fast service on simple inquiries including requests for copies of explanation of Medicare benefits notices, requests for Medpard directories, brief claims inquiries (status or verification on receipt), and address changes: 800-666-7586

Georgia

Medicare/Aetna Life and Casualty
P.O. Box 3018
Savannah, GA 31402-3018
912-920-2412
800-727-0827

Hawaii

Hawaii Medicare/Aetna Life and Casualty
P.O. Box 3947
Honolulu, HI 96812
808-524-1240
800-272-5242

Idaho

Equicor, Inc.
3150 N. Lakeharbor Lane, Suite 254
P.O. Box 8048
Boise, ID 83703-6219
208-342-7763
800-627-2782

Illinois

Medicare/Blue Cross and Blue Shield of Illinois
P.O. Box 4422
Marion, IL 62959
312-938-8000
800-642-6930

Indiana

Medicare Part B/Associated Insurance Companies, Inc.
P.O. Box 7073
Indianapolis, IN 46207
317-842-4151
800-622-4792

Iowa

Medicare/IASD Health Services Inc.
(D/B/A Blue Cross and Blue Shield of Iowa)
636 Grand
Des Moines, IA 50309
515-245-4785
800-532-1285

Kansas

For counties of Johnson, Wyandotte:

Medicare/Blue Cross and Blue Shield of Kansas City
P.O. Box 419840
Kansas City, MO 64141-6840
816-561-0900
800-892-5900

For rest of state:

Medicare/Blue Cross and Blue Shield of Kansas
P.O. Box 239
Topeka, KS 66601
913-232-3773
800-432-3531

Kentucky

**Medicare-Part B/Blue Cross and Blue Shield
of Kentucky**
100 E. Vine Street
Lexington, KY 40507
606-233-1441
800-999-7608

Louisiana

Arkansas Blue Cross and Blue Shield
Medicare Administration
P.O. Box 95024
Baton Rouge, LA 70895-9024
800-462-9666
504-529-1494 in New Orleans
504-272-1242 in Baton Rouge

Maine

Medicare/Blue Shield of Massachusetts/Tri-State
P.O. Box 1010
Biddeford, ME 04005
207-282-5689
800-492-0919

Maryland

For counties of Montgomery, Prince Georges:

Medicare/Pennsylvania Blue Shield
P.O. Box 890100
Camp Hill, PA 17089-0100
800-233-1124

For rest of state:

Maryland Blue Shield, Inc.
1946 Greenspring Drive
Timonium, MD 21093
410-561-4160
800-492-4795

Massachusetts

Medicare/Blue Shield of Massachusetts, Inc.
1022 Hingham Street
Rockland, MA 02371
617-956-3994
800-882-1228

Michigan

Michigan Medicare Part B/Blue Cross and Blue Shield
P.O. Box 2201
Detroit, MI 48231-2201
800-482-4045 in area code 313
800-322-0607 in area code 517
800-442-8020 in area code 616
800-562-7802 in area code 906
313-225-8200 in Detroit

Minnesota

For counties of Anoka, Dakota, Fillmore, Goodhue, Hennepin, Houston, Olmsted, Ramsey, Wabasha, Washington, Winona:

Minnesota Medicare/The Travelers Insurance Co.
8120 Penn Avenue S.
Bloomington, MN 55431
612-884-7171
800-352-2762

For rest of state:

Medicare/Blue Shield of Minnesota
P.O. Box 64357
St. Paul, MN 55164
612-456-5070
800-392-0343

Mississippi

Medicare/The Travelers Insurance Co.
P.O. Box 22545
Jackson, MS 39225-2545
601-956-0372
800-682-5417 in Mississippi
800-227-2349 outside Mississippi

Missouri

For counties of Andrew, Atchison, Bates, Benton, Buchanan, Caldwell, Carroll, Cass, Clay, Clinton, Daviess, DeKalb, Gentry, Grundy, Harrison, Henry, Holt, Jackson, Johnson, Lafayette, Livingston, Mercer, Nodaway, Pettis, Platte, Ray, St. Clair, Saline, Vernon, Worth:

Missouri Medicare/Blue Shield of Kansas City
P.O. Box 419840
Kansas City, MO 64141-6840
816-561-0900
800-892-5900

For rest of state:

Medicare/General American Life Insurance Company
P.O. Box 505
St. Louis, MO 63166
314-843-8880
800-392-3070

Montana

Medicare/Blue Cross and Blue Shield of Montana
2501 Beltview
P.O. Box 4310
Helena, MT 59604
406-444-8350
800-332-6146

Nebraska

Medicare Part B/Blue Cross and Blue Shield of Nebraska
P.O. Box 3106
Omaha, NE 68103-0106
913-232-3773
800-633-1113
Customer service site in Kansas.

Nevada

Medicare/Aetna Life and Casualty
P.O. Box 37230
Phoenix, AZ 85069
602-861-1968
800-528-0311

New Hampshire

Medicare/Blue Shield of Massachusetts/Tri-State
P.O. Box 1010
Biddeford, ME 04005
207-282-5689
800-447-1142

New Jersey

Medicare/Pennsylvania Blue Shield
Box 400010
Camp Hill, PA 17140-0010
800-462-9306

New Mexico

New Mexico Medicare/Aetna Life and Casualty
P.O. Box 25500
Oklahoma City, OK 73125-0500
800-423-2925
505-843-7771 in Albuquerque

New York

For counties of Bronx, Kings, New York, Richmond:

Medicare B/Empire Blue Cross and Blue Shield
P.O. Box 2280
Peekskill, NY 10566
212-490-4444

For counties of Columbia, Delaware, Dutchess. Greene, Nassau, Orange, Putnam, Rockland, Suffolk, Sullivan, Ulster, Westchester:

Medicare B/Empire Blue Cross and Blue Shield
P.O. Box 2280
Peekskill, NY 10566
800-442-8430

For county of Queens:

Medicare/Group Health, Inc.
P.O. Box 1608, Ansonia Station
New York, NY 10023
212-721-1770

For rest of state:

Medicare Blue Shield of Western New York
7-9 Court Street
Binghamton, NY 13901-3197
607-772-6906
800-252-6550

North Carolina

Equicor Inc.
P.O. Box 671
Nashville, TN 37202
919-665-0348
800-672-3071

North Dakota

Medicare/Blue Shield of North Dakota
4510 13th Avenue S.W.
Fargo, ND 58121-0001
701-282-0691
800-247-2267

Ohio

Medicare/Nationwide Mutual Insurance Co.
P.O. Box 57
Columbus, OH 43216
614-249-7157
800-282-0530

Oklahoma

Medicare/Aetna Life and Casualty
701 N.W. 63rd Street
Oklahoma City, OK 73116-7693
405-848-7711
800-522-9079

Oregon

Oregon Medicare/Aetna Life and Casualty
200 S.W. Market Street
P.O. Box 1997
Portland, OR 97207-1997
503-222-6831
800-452-0125

Pennsylvania

Medicare/Pennsylvania Blue Shield
Box 890065
Camp Hill, PA 17089-0065
800-382-1274

Puerto Rico

**Puerto Rico Medicare/Seguros de
Servicio de Salud de Puerto Rico**
Call Box 71391
San Juan, PR 00936
800-462-7015 in Puerto Rico
800-474-7448 in U.S. Virgin Islands
809-749-4900 in San Juan metro area

Rhode Island

Medicare/Blue Shield of Rhode Island
444 Westminster Mall
Providence, RI 02901
401-861-2273
800-662-5170

South Carolina

**Medicare Part B/Blue Cross and Blue Shield
of South Carolina**
Fontaine Road Business Center
300 Arbor Lake Drive, Suite 1300
Columbia, SC 29223
803-754-0639
800-868-2522

South Dakota

Medicare Part B/Blue Shield of North Dakota
4510 13th Avenue S.W.
Fargo, ND 58121-0001
701-282-0691
800-437-4762

Tennessee

Equicor, Inc.
P.O. Box 1465
Nashville, TN 37202
615-244-5650
800-342-8900

Texas

Medicare/Blue Cross and Blue Shield of Texas, Inc.
P.O. Box 660031
Dallas, TX 75266-0031
214-235-3433
800-442-2620

Utah

Medicare/Blue Shield of Utah
P.O. Box 30269
Salt Lake City, UT 84130-0269
801-481-6196
800-426-3477

Vermont

Medicare/Blue Shield of Massachusetts/Tri-State
P.O. Box 1010
Biddeford, ME 04005
207-282-5689
800-447-1142

Virgin Islands

**Virgin Islands Medicare/Seguros de Servicio de Salud
de Puerto Rico**
Call Box 71391
San Juan, PR 00936
800-474-7448 in U.S. Virgin Islands
809-778-2665 in St. Croix
809-774-3898 in St. Thomas

THE 25 MOST COMMON DIAGNOSIS-RELATED GROUPS (DRGS)

Diagnosis-related groups, or DRGs, are used to classify the services delivered in hospitals. Developed for Medicare, they are now being used by other insurance companies to determine the payment a hospital should receive for a particular service. There are 477 individual DRGs. The 25 most common and the average payment for each are listed below.

DRG number	DRG name	Total number of discharges	Average length of stay (days)	Average total charge per discharge
127	Heart failure and shock	604,169	7.76	$7,721
89	Simple pneumonia and pleurisy with complications (age greater than 17)	376,640	8.79	8,451
14	Specific cerebrovascular disorders	349,539	10.63	9,727
140	Angina pectoris	341,499	4.48	4,615
430	Psychoses	278,687	22.02	11,344
209	Major joint and limb reattachment procedures	274,354	10.47	17,545
182	Esophagitis, gastroenteritis, and misc. digestive disorders with complications (age greater than 17)	257,898	6.25	5,790
296	Nutritional and misc. metabolic disorders with complications (age greater than 17)	212,583	8.38	7,262
138	Cardiac arrhythmia and conduction disorders with complications	186,314	5.88	6,235
96	Bronchitis and asthma with complications (age greater than 17)	179,211	7.13	6,711
174	Gastrointestinal hemorrhage with complications	166,448	6.95	7,500
88	Chronic obstructive pulmonary disease	165,344	7.62	7,652
320	Kidney and urinary tract infections with complications (age greater than 17)	163,391	8.46	7,539
121	Circulatory disorders with acute myocardial infarction and cardiovascular complications, patient discharged alive	143,524	9.64	12,065
148	Major small and large bowel procedures with complications	141,394	15.88	24,238
79	Respiratory infections and inflammations with complications (age greater than 17)	138,653	11.94	12,999
416	Septicemia	136,583	10.43	11,544
15	Transient ischemic attack	134,266	5.48	5,039
462	Rehabilitation	130,073	20.76	16,667
112	Vascular procedures except major reconstruction without pump	129,173	6.09	15,778
410	Chemotherapy	126,275	3.72	5,026
124	Circulatory disorders except acute myocardial infarction with cardiac catheterization and complex diagnoses	123,924	5.77	9,364
210	Hip and femur procedures except major joint with complications (age greater than 17)	117,757	13.07	14,718
143	Chest pain	115,777	3.38	3,882
243	Medical back problems	106,916	7.18	5,356

Source: "The 15 Most Common Diagnosis-Related Groups," *Managed Healthcare News,* Feb. 1993. Health Care Investment Analysts, Baltimore, Maryland. Used with permission.

Virginia

For counties of Arlington, Fairfax; cities of Alexandria, Falls Church, Fairfax:

Medicare/Pennsylvania Blue Shield
P.O. Box 890100
Camp Hill, PA 17089-0100
800-233-1124

For rest of states:

Medicare/The Travelers Insurance Co.
P.O. Box 26463
Richmond, VA 23261
804-254-4130
800-552-3423

Washington

Mail to your medical service bureau. If you do not know which bureau handles your claim, mail to:

King County Medical Blue Shield
P.O. Box 21248
Seattle, WA 98111-3248
800-422-4087 in King County
206-464-3711
800-572-5256 in Spokane
509-536-4550
800-552-7114 in Kitsap
206-377-5576
206-597-6530 in Pierce
206-352-2269 in Thurston
Others: Call collect if out of calling area.

West Virginia

Medicare/Nationwide Mutual Insurance Co.
P.O. Box 57
Columbus, OH 43216
614-249-7157
800-848-0106

Wisconsin

Medicare/WPS
Box 1787
Madison, WI 53701
800-362-7221
608-221-3330 in Madison
414-931-1071 in Milwaukee

Wyoming

Blue Cross and Blue Shield of Wyoming
P.O. Box 628
Cheyenne, WY 82003
307-632-9381
800-442-2371

Medicaid

WHAT IS IT?

Medicaid, the joint federal and state health insurance plan for low-income individuals, was created by an act of Congress with the passage of Public Law 89-97, the Social Security Amendments of 1965. This legislation was initially intended to create the Medicare program, a health insurance plan for those Americans 65 years of age or older. However, some last minute wrangling between the House and Senate led to the inclusion of financial grants to states for the medical assistance program, and what became known as Medicaid.

The states have considerable flexibility in structuring their programs, which vary substantially from state to state. In addition to medical coverage for low-income individuals, the Medicaid program also covers children, the elderly poor, and the blind and disabled. Aside from California, which calls its program MediCal, the program is known in most states as Medicaid or medical assistance.

The Health Care Financing Administration (HCFA), the federal agency that administers the Medicaid program, estimated that some 33 million people would receive benefits in 1994, with expenditures in excess of $160 billion. In addition, a recent HCFA study projects that Medicaid's portion of national health expenditures, currently around 11.3 percent, could increase to nearly 21 percent by the year 2000. The program's national expenditures on health care in the year 2000 is expected to exceed $1.5 trillion.

Under Medicaid, states receive matching payments from the federal government ranging from 50 to 83 percent, depending upon state per-capita income. This means that the federal government pays a greater share of a poorer state's Medicaid budget than does the state itself.

WHO IS COVERED?

As noted earlier, Medicaid is intended for certain groups within the general population. The major groups within the state—termed the "categorically needy," in Medicaid jargon—that must be covered under Medicaid are:

• Recipients of Aid to Families with Dependent Children (AFDC), a federal/state cash assistance program for which the states set eligibility standards

- The aged, blind, and disabled receiving cash assistance from the federal supplemental security income (SSI) program or eligible for Medicaid under more restrictive state criteria. (The consumer must check the specific eligibility requirements of his or her state.)
- Pregnant women and children under age 6 whose family income does not exceed 133 percent of the federal poverty line. For example, if the federal poverty line is $10,000, a family could earn $13,300 and still be eligible for coverage under the Medicaid program.

In addition, states have the option to cover numerous other groups of medically needy people (termed "medically needy," in Medicaid jargon), of which the largest numbers are residents of long-term care facilities (also called nursing homes). States are also given the option of extending coverage to pregnant women and infants whose family income does not exceed 185 percent of the poverty line. Using the previous example, this figure would be an income up to $18,500 per year. Those eligible for this coverage most likely have an infant with serious medical problems, the cost of which exceeds the family's ability to pay.

WHAT IS COVERED?

The Medicaid law, and subsequent federal regulations, mandate a basic list of services that must be included in any state Medicaid program. These services are:

Inpatient hospital services

Outpatient hospital services

Physician services

Medical and surgical services of dentists

Laboratory and X-ray services

Nursing facility services for individuals 21 and over

Home health care for persons eligible for nursing facility services

Family planning services and supplies

Rural health clinic services

Federally qualified health center services

Nurse-midwife services

Services of certified pediatric or family nurse practitioners

Early and periodic screening, diagnostic, and treatment services for children under 21 and treatment for conditions identified in screening

Assurance of the availability of necessary transportation

In addition to these mandated services, states have the option of offering up to thirty-two more categories of care, such as podiatric and chiropractic services, private duty nursing, and physical therapy. Definitions and limitations on eligibility for services are available from local welfare offices.

In some cases, a low-income Medicare beneficiary may be eligible to have the state Medicaid program pay for his or her Part B premium, and in most cases the Part B deductibles and copayments. This person is deemed a qualified Medicare beneficiary, or QMB. The exact extent of coverage is determined by that individual's income in relation to the federal poverty line.

WHO IS ELIGIBLE?

How do you find out if you are eligible for one of the Medicaid programs? By visiting the local office of your state's welfare department and submitting an application for the program. Some people may feel embarrassed at the thought of having to visit a welfare office; however, it is the official state agency for accepting and processing Medicaid applications. Only the state can determine if a person meets the criteria for any of the specific Medicaid programs.

Just because you submit an application does not mean that you will automatically be eligible for both the categorically needy and medically needy programs. The medically needy program is designed for people with limited income and assets who incur unusually large medical expenses, whereas the categorically needy program provides income assistance, in addition to medical assistance.

As we go to press, the Clinton Administration is proposing the first major change to the Medicaid program in a quarter century. Under health care reform currently proposed, Medicaid would only cover welfare and supplemental security income (SSI) recipients. These are the categorically needy as distinguished from the medically needy. All other recipients, the so-called medically needy, will receive their medical care from the plans offered by the health alliances.

Glossary of Medicaid Terms

Medicaid is a health care program—officially known as Title XIX of the Social Security Act—for low-income individuals and families. Medicaid was established at the same time as Medicare and is administered by the states, who establish eligibility requirements based upon federal guidelines. Medicaid is available to specific classes of low-income individuals, as well as the aged, blind, and permanently disabled. The following terms are used by those who administer Medicaid eligibility or payment or who provide medical services.

AABD (Aid to Aged, Blind, and Disabled)—a program designed for the aged, blind, and disabled who are eligible for financial assistance under Medicaid.

AB (Aid to the Blind)—a program designed for the blind who are eligible for financial assistance under Medicaid.

AFDC (Aid to Families with Dependent Children)—a program of financial assistance designed for low-income families who meet Medicaid eligibility guidelines.

APTD (Aid to the Permanently and Totally Disabled)—a program of financial assistance and social services designed for the permanently and totally disabled who meet Medicaid eligibility guidelines.

Capitation payment—a monthly payment made by the state Medicaid agency to physicians, hospitals, laboratories, and other health care providers to cover the cost of medical services provided to Medicaid recipients. The capitation payment is made whether or not the Medicaid recipient receives any medical services.

Categorically needy—those individuals or families who are eligible for Medicaid and who meet financial eligibility requirements for Aid to Families with Dependent Children (AFDC), Supplemental Security Income (SSI), or an optional state supplement.

Coinsurance—a cost-sharing requirement under a health insurance policy which provides that the insured will assume a portion or percentage of the costs of covered services. For example, the insurance company pays 80 percent of the cost of a service and the insured pays 20 percent.

Copayment—a type of cost-sharing under Medicaid that requires the recipient to pay a specified flat amount per unit of service or unit of time, with Medicaid paying the remainder of the cost. Medicaid recipients pay the first $5 toward the cost of office visits, laboratory tests, or prescription medications. For example, if a typical office visit to a physician costs $25, the Medicaid recipient pays $5 and Medicaid pays the remaining $20.

Covered services—the specific services and supplies for which Medicaid will provide reimbursement. Covered services under the Medicaid program consist of a combination of mandatory and optional services within each state.

Customary, prevailing, and reasonable charges—method of reimbursement used which limits payment to the lowest of the following: the physician's actual charge, the physician's median charge in a recent two-year period (customary), or an amount large enough to cover 75 percent of all charges submitted in that same time period (prevailing).

Customary charge—the charge a physician or supplier usually bills his or her patients for furnishing a particular service or supply.

Deductible—an amount of money that must be paid by an insured person before an insurance company will pay claims filed against it. For example, a deductible may be $250 for an individual and $500 for a family, after which the insurance company begins to pay benefits.

Department of Health and Human Services—the federal agency that establishes the guidelines and provides the funding to the states for the administration of the Medicaid program.

Diagnosis related groups (DRGs)—a method of paying hospitals based on the average cost of treating patients with similar conditions.

Early and periodic screening, diagnosis, and treatment (EPSDT)—a program specifically targeted at pediatric and adolescent age groups. It is designed to bring about early screening, detection, and treatment of acute and chronic conditions.

Essential spouse—a spouse who is living with an aged, blind, or disabled individual receiving cash assistance and whose needs were included in determining the amount of cash payment to the aged, blind, or disabled individual under Old Age Assistance (OAA), Aid to the Blind (AB), Aid to the Permanently and Totally Disabled (APTD), or Aid to Aged, Blind, and Disabled (AABD); and who is determined essential to the individual's well-being.

Expenditure—an amount of money paid by a state agency for the covered medical expenses of eligible Medicaid recipients.

Family planning services—medical and related counseling services provided to individuals for the purpose of enabling such individuals to determine freely the number or spacing of their children. Such services must be furnished or prescribed under the supervision of a physician and may include diagnosis, treatment, drugs, supplies, or devices.

Federal financial participation—federal matching funds received by the states to assist in the funding of the Medicaid program. Each state receives an amount of matching funds equal to the federal government's share of the state Medicaid budget.

Fiscal agent—a contractor that processes or pays vendor claims on behalf of the Medicaid agency.

Fiscal year—any twelve-month period for which annual accounts are kept. The federal government's fiscal year extends from October 1 to the following September 30.

Health Care Financing Administration (HCFA)—the federal agency that administers the Medicaid/Medicaid program.

Health insuring organization—an organization that (1) pays for medical services provided to recipients in exchange for a premium or subscription charge paid by the state Medicaid agency; and (2) assumes an underwriting risk.

Health maintenance organization (HMO)—a health care organization that is both an insurer and provider of medical care, delivering comprehensive health care to members for a fixed monthly fee. HMOs may be sponsored by hospitals, physicians, insurance companies or unions.

Home health agency—a public agency or private organization that is primarily engaged in providing skilled nursing services and other therapeutic services in the patient's home, and that meets certain conditions designed to ensure the health and safety of the individuals who are furnished these services.

Home health services—services provided in a patient's residence by employees of a home health agency or other approved provider of home health care. All services must be ordered by a physician and delivered under a plan established and periodically reviewed by a physician. The services are provided on a visiting basis and include: part-time or intermittent skilled nursing care; physical, occupational, or speech therapy; medical social services, medical supplies and appliances (other than drugs and biologicals); home health aide services, and services of interns and residents.

Inpatient hospital services—items and services such as bed and board, nursing and related services, diagnostic and therapeutic services, and medical or surgical services furnished to a patient who has been admitted to a hospital and who occupies a bed.

Intermediate care facility—an institution furnishing health-related care and services to individuals who do not require the degree of care provided by hospitals or skilled nursing facilities as defined under Title XIX (Medicaid) of the Social Security Act.

Laboratory and radiological services—professional and technical laboratory and radiological services ordered by a licensed practitioner and provided in an office or similar facility (other than a hospital outpatient department or clinic) or by a qualified laboratory.

Medically needy—individuals or families who need financial assistance with medical expenses even though their incomes exceed current poverty guidelines. These individuals and families are eligible for coverage up to the limits set in the state's Medicaid plan.

Medicare principles—rules of reasonable cost-based reimbursement used by Medicare.

OAA (Old Age Assistance)—a program designed for the financial assistance of the needy aged who meet income and resources eligibility.

Other practitioners' services—health care services of licensed practitioners other than physicians and dentists such as chiropractors, podiatrists, nurse-practitioners, nurse-midwives, and licensed therapists.

Outpatient hospital services—services furnished to outpatients by a participating hospital for diagnosis or treatment of an illness or injury.

Portable X ray—a radiograph taken with portable equipment, usually in the patient's place of residence, under the general supervision of a physician.

Prescribed drugs—drugs dispensed by a licensed pharmacist on the prescription of a practitioner licensed by law to administer such drugs, and drugs dispensed by a licensed practitioner to his own patients. This does not include medications that are covered by the practitioner's bill, or drugs covered by a hospital's bill.

Prevailing charge—the charge that would cover 75 percent of the customary charges made for similar services in the same locality.

Psychiatric hospital—an institution primarily engaged in providing, under the supervision of a physician, psychiatric services for the diagnosis and treatment of mental illnesses.

Qualified HMO—an HMO that has been determined by the Public Health Service to be a qualified HMO under Section 1310(d) of the Public Health Service Act.

Reasonable charge—the reasonable charge is the lowest of: the actual charge billed by the physician or supplier; the charge the physician or supplier customarily bills his or her patients for the same service; and the prevailing charge which most physicians or suppliers in that locality bill for the same service. Increases in the physicians' prevailing charge levels are recognized only to the extent justified by an index reflecting changes in the costs of practice and in general earnings.

Reasonable cost—the reasonable cost is based on the actual cost of providing such services, including direct and indirect costs of providers, and excluding any costs which are unnecessary in the efficient delivery of services covered by the insurance program.

Recipient—an individual who has been determined to be eligible for Medicaid and who has used medical services covered under Medicaid.

Rural health clinic—an outpatient facility that is primarily engaged in furnishing physicians' and other medical and health services and that meets certain other requirements designed to ensure the health and safety of the individuals served by the clinic. The clinic must be located in an area with a shortage of personal health services, or as a health personnel shortage area, and has filed an agreement with the Secretary of the Department of Health and Human Services not to charge any individual or other person for items or services for which such individual is entitled to have payment made by Medicaid/Medicare, except for the amount of any deductible or coinsurance amount applicable.

Skilled nursing facility (SNF)—a facility that is specially staffed and equipped to provide intensive nursing and rehabilitative care to patients. Care is provided by licensed nurses or licensed therapists under the supervision of doctors. Distinguished from intermediate care and custodial care facilities which are intended primarily to support elderly and disabled individuals in the tasks of daily living.

Skilled nursing facility services—all services furnished to inpatients of a formally certified skilled nursing facility that meets standards required by the Secretary of Health and Human Services. For example, injections of medications, catheterizations, physical therapy, and other forms of rehabilitation.

Spend-down—refers to a method by which an individual establishes Medicaid eligibility by reducing gross income and resources through incurring medical expenses until net income (after medical expenses) meets Medicaid financial requirements.

State buy-in—a program made available to state Medicaid agencies, by the federal government, whereby the state purchases Supplementary Medical Insurance (Medicare Part B) for needy eligible individuals. The state pays the monthly Part B premium and also picks up the cost of deductibles and copayments for eligible recipients.

State plan—a comprehensive, written commitment by a Medicaid agency to administer or supervise the administration of a Medicaid program in accordance with federal requirements.

Supplemental Security Income (SSI)—a program of income support for low-income aged, blind, and disabled persons established by Title XVI of the Social Security Act.

State supplemental payment (SSP)—an additional payment made by the states to recipients of Supplemental Security Income (SSI). States that had been making higher payments to individuals under their previous programs of cash assistance were required to pay the difference between the SSI benefit and the previous payment. This difference is known as SSP.

Third-party liability—under Medicaid, third-party liability exists if there is any entity (including other government programs or insurance) which is or may be liable to pay all or part of the medical cost of injury, disease, or disability of an applicant or recipient of Medicaid.

Usual, customary and reasonable charges—method of reimbursement used under Medicaid which is consistent with the going rate or charge in certain geographical areas for identical or similar services.

Vendor—an institution, agency, organization, or individual practitioner which provides health or medical services.

Source: U.S. Department of Health and Human Services, Health Care Financing Administration, Intergovernmental Affairs Office, Medicaid Bureau.

State Medicaid Offices

These offices are responsible for administering the Medicaid program. They provide information on eligibility requirements and extent of program coverage in the individual state.

Alabama
Alabama Medicaid Director
Alabama Medicaid Agency
2500 Fairlane Drive
Montgomery, AL 36130
205-277-2710

Alaska
Alaska Medicaid Director
Alaska Department of Health and Social Services
Division of Medical Assistance
P.O. Box H-07
Juneau, AK 99811
907-465-3355

Arizona
Arizona Medicaid Director
Arizona Health Care Cost Containment System
801 E. Jefferson Street
Phoenix, AZ 85034
602-234-3655

Arkansas
Arkansas Medicaid Director
Department of Human Services
Information and Referral
P.O. Box 1437, Slot 1100
Little Rock, AR 72203-1437
501-682-8292

California
California Medicaid Director
Department of Health Services
Referral Office For Medi-Cal
714-744 P Street
Sacramento, CA 95814
916-322-5824

Colorado
Colorado Medicaid Director
Department of Social Services
Division of Medical Services
1575 Sherman, 10th Floor
Denver, CO 80203-1714
303-866-5901

Connecticut
Connecticut Medicaid Director
Department of Human Resources
Medical Care Administration
110 Bartholomew Avenue
Hartford, CT 06106
203-566-2934

Delaware
Delaware Medicaid Director
Department of Health and Social Services
Division of Economic Services
Biggs Building
Delaware State Hospital
P.O. Box 906
New Castle, DE 19720
302-421-6139

District of Columbia
Washington D.C. Medicaid Director
Office of Health Care Financing
D.C. Department of Human Services
1331 H Street N.W., Suite 500
Washington, DC 20005
202-727-0735

Florida
Florida Medicaid Director
Department of Health and Rehabilitative Services
Medicaid Program Office
Provider and Consumer Relations Office
Building 6, Room 260
1317 Winewood Boulevard
Tallahassee, FL 32399
904-488-8291

Georgia
Georgia Medicaid Director
Georgia Department of Medical Assistance
2 Martin Luther King Jr. Drive S.E.
Atlanta, GA 30334
404-656-4479

Hawaii
Hawaii Medicaid Director
Department of Human Services
Health Care Administration Division
820 Mililani Street, Room 817
Honolulu, HI 96813
808-548-3855

Idaho
Idaho Medicaid Director
Department of Health and Welfare
Bureau of Medical Assistance
450 W. State Street, 6th Floor
Boise, ID 83720
208-334-5794

Illinois
Illinois Medicaid Director
Illinois Department of Public Aid
Division of Medical Programs
201 S. Grand Avenue E.
Springfield, IL 62743-0001
217-782-2570

Indiana
Indiana Medicaid Director
Indiana Department of Public Welfare
Medical Assistance Unit
100 N. Senate Avenue, Room 701
Indianapolis, IN 46204
317-232-6865

Iowa
Iowa Medicaid Director
Bureau of Medical Services
Department of Human Services
Hoover State Office Building
Des Moines, IA 50319-0114
515-281-8794

Kansas
Kansas Medicaid Director
Department of Social and Rehabilitative Services
Division of Income Maintenance
Docking State Office Building, Room 624-South
Topeka, KS 66612
913-296-3981

Kentucky
Kentucky Medicaid Director
Cabinet For Human Resources
Department of Medicaid Services
275 E. Main Street
Frankfort, KY 40621
502-564-4321

Louisiana
Louisiana Medicaid Director
Department of Health and Human Resources
Office of Family Security
P.O. Box 91030
Baton Rouge, LA 70804-9030
504-342-3891

Maine
Maine Medicaid Director
Department of Human Services
Statehouse Station 11
Augusta, ME 04333
207-289-2674

Maryland
Maryland Medicaid Director
Medical Assistance Division
Office of Income Maintenance
Department of Human Resources
201 W. Preston Street
Baltimore, MD 21201
410-225-6535

Massachusetts
Massachusetts Medicaid Director
Department of Public Welfare
180 Tremont Street
Boston, MA 02111
617-574-0205

Michigan
Michigan Department of Social Services
Citizen's and Legislative Inquiry
For referral to local agency:
517-373-0707
800-638-6414

Minnesota
Minnesota Department of Human Services
Health Care and Residential Programs
Metro Square Building
444 Lafayette Road
St. Paul, MN 55155
612-296-2766

Mississippi
Mississippi Medicaid Director
Department of Public Welfare
Division of Medicaid
239 N. Lamar Street, Suite 801
Jackson, MS 39201-1311
601-359-6050

Missouri
Missouri Medicaid Director
Department of Social Services
Division of Medical Services
P.O. Box 6500
Jefferson City, MO 65102
314-751-6922
800-392-1261

Montana
Montana Medicaid Director
Department of Social and Rehabilitation Services
Economic Assistance Division
111 Sanders Street
P.O. Box 4210
Helena, MT 59604
406-444-4540

Nebraska
Nebraska Medicaid Director
Department of Social Services
301 Centennial Mall S., 5th Floor
Lincoln, NE 68509
402-471-9330

Nevada
Nevada Medicaid Director
Department of Human Resources
Nevada Welfare Division
Medicaid Section
2527 N. Carson Street
Carson City, NV 89710
702-687-4378

New Hampshire
New Hampshire Medicaid Director
New Hampshire Division of Health and Human Services
Department of Human Services—Office of Economic Services
6 Hazen Drive
Concord, NH 03301
603-271-4353
800-852 3345

New Jersey
New Jersey Medicaid Director
Department of Human Services
Division of Medical Assistance and Health Services
7 Quakerbridge Plaza, CN-712
Trenton, NJ 08625
609-588-2600
609-588-2602

New Mexico
New Mexico Medicaid Director
Department of Human Services
Medical Assistance Division
P.O. Box 2348
Santa Fe, NM 87504-2348
505-827-4315

New York
New York Medicaid Director
State Department of Social Services
Division of Medical Assistance
10 Eyck Office Building
40 N. Pearl Street
Albany, NY 12243
518-474-9132
800-342-3715

North Carolina
North Carolina Medicaid Director
Department of Human Resources
Division of Medical Assistance
1985 Umstead Drive
Raleigh, NC 27603
919-733-2060

North Dakota
North Dakota Medicaid Director
North Dakota Department of Human Services
Medical Services
State Capitol
Bismarck, ND 58505
701-224-2321

Ohio
Ohio Medicaid Director
Department of Human Services
Benefits Administration
30 E. Broad Street, 31st Floor
Columbus, OH 43266-0423
614-466-3196

Oklahoma
Oklahoma Medicaid Director
Department of Human Services
Medical Services Division
P.O. Box 25352
Oklahoma City, OK 73125
405-557-2539

Oregon
Oregon Medicaid Director
Department of Human Resources
Senior Services Division
203 Public Service Building
Salem, OR 97310
503-378-2263

Pennsylvania

Pennsylvania Medicaid Director
Department of Public Welfare
Health and Welfare Building, Room 515
Harrisburg, PA 17105-2675
717-787-1870

Puerto Rico

Puerto Rico Medicaid Director
Office of Economic Assistance to the Medically Indigent
Building A, Call Box 70184
San Juan, PR 00936
809-765-9941

Rhode Island

Rhode Island Medicaid Director
Department of Human Services
Division of Medical Services
600 New London Avenue
Cranston, RI 02902
401-464-3575

South Carolina

South Carolina Medicaid Director
Department of Social Services
Division of Medicaid Eligibility
P.O. Box 8206
Columbia, SC 29202-8206
803-253-6100

South Dakota

South Dakota Medicaid Director
Department of Social Services
Office of Medical Services
700 Governor's Drive
Pierre, SD 57501
605-773-3495

Tennessee

Tennessee Medicaid Director
Department of Health and Environment
Bureau of Medicaid
729 Church Street
Nashville, TN 37219
615-741-0213

Texas

Texas Medicaid Director
Department of Human Services
Office of Services to the Aged and Disabled
P.O. Box 149030
Austin, TX 78714-9030
512-450-3050

Utah

Utah Medicaid Director
Utah Department of Health
Bureau of Medical Payments
Medicaid Information Unit
288 North 1460 West
Salt Lake City, UT 84116
801-538-6155

Vermont

Vermont Medicaid Director
Vermont Agency of Human Services
103 S. Main Street
Waterbury, VT 05676
802-241-2880
802-241-2220

Virgin Islands

Virgin Islands Medicaid Director
Bureau of Health Insurance and Medical Assistance
Knud Hansen Complex
Charlotte Amalie
St. Thomas, VI 00802
809-774-4624

Virginia

Virginia Medicaid Director
Virginia Department of Medical Services
Division of Medical Social Services
Eligibility and Appeals Section
600 E. Broad Street, Room 1300
Richmond, VA 23219
804-786-7933

Washington

Washington Medicaid Director
Department of Social and Health Services
Community Services Offices
See blue pages of local telephone directory for listing of local office.

West Virginia

West Virginia Medicaid Director
West Virginia Department of Human Services
Client Services
1900 Washington Street E.
Charleston, WV 25305
304-558-7867

Wisconsin

Wisconsin Medicaid Director
County Department of Social Services
See blue pages of local telephone directory for listing of local office.
800-362-3002 Recipient hotline
608-266-4279 in Madison area

Wyoming

Wyoming Medicaid Director
Department of Health and Social Services
Division of Public Assistance and Social Services
Hathaway Building, 3rd Floor
Cheyenne, WY 82002
307-777-7531

State Welfare Offices

These agencies are responsible for administering public assistance programs, including direct financial payments and Medicaid. All inquiries concerning eligibility should be directed to local offices of the welfare department.

Alabama

Department of Welfare
Department of Human Resources
James East Folsom Administrative Building
64 N. Union Street
Montgomery, AL 36130-1801
205-261-3190

Alaska

Department of Welfare
Division of Public Assistance
Department of Health and Social Services
Alaska Office Building, Room 309
P.O. Box H-07
Juneau, AK 99811-0640
907-465-3347

Arizona

Department of Welfare
Division of Family Support
Department of Economic Security
1400 W. Washington Street
P.O. Box 6123
Phoenix, AZ 85005
602-255-3596

Arkansas

Department of Welfare
Division of Economic and Medical Services
Department of Human Services
Donaghey Building, Room 316
7th and Main Streets
P.O. Box 1437
Little Rock, AR 72201
501-682-8375

California

Department of Welfare
Department of Social Services
State Office Building 9
744 P Street
Mail Station 17-11
Sacramento, CA 95814
916-445-2077

Colorado

Department of Welfare
Services to Families and Children
Department of Social Services
State Social Services Building, 3rd Floor
1575 Sherman Street
Denver, CO 80203-1714
303-866-5981

Connecticut

Department of Welfare
Department of Income Maintenance
110 Bartholomew Avenue
Hartford, CT 06106
203-566-2008

Delaware

Department of Welfare
Division of Economic Services
Department of Health and Social Services
CT Building
Delaware State Hospital
1901 N. DuPont Highway
P.O. Box 906
New Castle, DE 19720
302-421-6734

District of Columbia

Department of Welfare
Commission On Social Services
Department of Human Services
609 H Street N.E., 5th Floor
Washington, DC 20002
202-727-5930

Florida

Department of Welfare
Bureau of Quality Assurance
Division of Economic Services
Department of Health and Rehabilitation Services
Building 6, Room 432
1317 Winewood Boulevard
Tallahassee, FL 32399
904-487-1597

Georgia
Department of Welfare
Division of Family and Children Services
Department of Human Resources
878 Peachtree Street N.E., Room 421
Atlanta, GA 30309
404-894-6386

Hawaii
Department of Welfare
Family and Adult Services Division
Department of Human Services
Queen Liliuokalani Building
1390 Miller Street
P.O. Box 339
Honolulu, HI 96809
808-548-5908

Idaho
Department of Welfare
Bureau of Medical Assistance
Division of Welfare
Department of Health and Welfare
Towers Building
450 W. State Street
Boise, ID 83720
208-334-6630

Illinois
Department of Welfare
Department of Public Aid
Harris II Building
100 S. Grand Avenue E.
Springfield, IL 62704
217-782-6716

Indiana
Department of Welfare
State Office Building, Room 701
100 N. Senate Avenue
Indianapolis, IN 46204
317-232-4705

Iowa
Department of Welfare
Bureau of Economic Assistance
Department of Human Services
Hoover State Office Building, 5th Floor
1300 E. Walnut Street
Des Moines, IA 50319-0114
515-281-8629

Kansas
Department of Welfare
Income Maintenance and Medical Services
Department of Social and Rehabilitation Services
Docking State Office Building, Room 624-S
915 Harrison Street
Topeka, KS 66612
913-296-6750

Kentucky
Department of Welfare
Department of Social Insurance
Human Resources Cabinet
Human Resources Building
275 E. Main Street
Frankfort, KY 40621
502-564-3703

Louisiana
Department of Welfare
Office of Eligibility Determinations
Department of Social Services
755 Riverside N.
P.O. Box 94065
Baton Rouge, LA 70804-4065
504-342-3947

Maine
Department of Welfare
Bureau of Income Maintenance
Department of Human Services
Human Services Building
Whitten Road
Statehouse Station 11
Augusta, ME 04333
207-289-2415

Maryland
Department of Welfare
Social Services Administration
Department of Human Resources
Saratoga State Center, Room 578
311 W. Saratoga Street
Baltimore, MD 21201
410-333-0103

Massachusetts
Department of Welfare
Deputy Commission, Support Services
180 Tremont Street, 13th Floor
Boston, MA 02111
617-574-0213

Michigan
Department of Welfare
Department of Social Services
Commerce Center
300 S. Capitol Avenue
P.O. Box 30037
Lansing, MI 48909
517-373-2000

Minnesota
Department of Welfare
Department of Human Services
444 Lafayette Road
St. Paul, MN 55155-3818
612-296-2701
612-296-2702

Mississippi
Department of Welfare
515 E. Amite Street
P.O. Box 352
Jackson, MS 39205
601-354-0341

Missouri
Department of Welfare
Division of Family Services
Department of Social Services
Broadway State Office Building
221 W. High Street
P.O. Box 88
Jefferson City, MO 65103
314-751-4247

Montana
Department of Welfare
Economic Assistance Division
Department of Social and Rehabilitation Services
SRS Building, Room 205
111 Sanders Street
P.O. Box 4210
Helena, MT 59604
406-444-4540

Nebraska
Department of Welfare
Department of Social Services
State Office Building
301 Centennial Mall S.
P.O. Box 95026
Lincoln, NE 68509-5026
402-471-3121

Nevada
Department of Welfare
Department of Human Resources
2527 N. Carson Street
Carson City, NV 89710
702-885-4128

New Hampshire
Department of Welfare
Division of Human Services
Department of Health and Human Services
Health and Welfare Building
6 Hazen Drive
Concord, NH 03301-6521
603-271-4321
800-852-3345 in New Hampshire

New Jersey
Department of Welfare
Department of Human Services
6 Quakerbridge Plaza, CN-716
Trenton, NJ 08625
609-588-2401

New Mexico
Department of Welfare
Human Services Department
1105 St. Francis Drive
Santa Fe, NM 87502
505-827-8720

New York
Department of Welfare
Department of Social Services
10 Eyck Building, 16th Floor
40 N. Pearl Street
Albany, NY 12243
518-474-9475

North Carolina
Department of Welfare
Division of Social Services
Department of Human Resources
Albemarle Building, Room 813
325 N. Salisbury Street
Raleigh, NC 27611
919-733-3055

North Dakota
Department of Welfare
Public Assistance
Department of Human Services
State Capitol
Bismarck, ND 58505
701-224-2332

Ohio
Department of Public Assistance
Division of Public Assistance
Department of Human Services
State Office Tower, 27th Floor
30 E. Broad Street
Columbus, OH 43266-0423
614-466-4815

Oklahoma
Department of Welfare
Family Support Division
Department of Human Services
Sequoyah Memorial Office Building
2400 N. Lincoln Boulevard
P.O. Box 25352
Oklahoma City, OK 73125
405-521-3076

Oregon
Department of Welfare
Adult and Family Services Division
Department of Human Resources
Public Service Building, Room 417
Capitol Mall
Salem, OR 97310
503-378-6142

Pennsylvania
Department of Welfare
Health and Welfare Building, Room 333
Forster Street and Commonwealth Avenue
P.O. Box 2675
Harrisburg, PA 17105
717-787-2600

Puerto Rico
Department of Welfare
Department of Social Services
Old Naval Base, Isla Grande
Building 10, 2nd Floor
P.O. Box 11398
Santurce, PR 00910
809-721-4624
800-722-7400

Rhode Island
Department of Welfare
Department of Human Services
Aime J. Forand Building
600 New London Avenue
Cranston, RI 02920
401-464-2121

South Carolina
Department of Welfare
Office of Audits, Investigations and Support Services
Department of Social Services
North Tower Complex
1535 Confederate Avenue
P.O. Box 1520
Columbia, SC 29202-1520
803-734-6188

South Dakota
Department of Welfare
Department of Social Services
Richard F. Kneip Building
700 Governor's Drive
Pierre, SD 57501
605-773-3165

Tennessee
Department of Welfare
Office of Family Assistance
Department of Human Services
Citizens Plaza Building
400 Deaderick Street, 15th Floor
Nashville, TN 37219
615-741-5463

Texas
Department of Welfare
Department of Human Services
John H. Winters Human Services Building
701 W. 51st Street
P.O. Box 2960
Austin, TX 78769
512-450-3040

Utah
Department of Welfare
Office of Assistance Payments Administration
Department of Social Services
Social Services Building
120 North 200 West
P.O. Box 45500
Salt Lake City, UT 84145-0500
801-538-3970

Vermont
Department of Welfare
Department of Social Welfare
Human Services Agency
Waterbury Office Complex, Building A
103 S. Main Street
Waterbury, VT 05676
802-241-2852

Virgin Islands
Department of Welfare
Income Maintenance Program
Department of Human Services
Barbel Plaza S.
St. Thomas, VI 00802
809-774-2299 ext. 220

Virginia
Department of Welfare
Department of Social Services
Blair Building, Suite G
8007 Discovery Drive
Richmond, VA 23229-8699
804-662-9236

Washington
Department of Welfare
Division of Income Maintenance
Department of Social and Health Services
Office Building 2, 3rd Floor
12th Avenue and Franklin Street
Mail Stop OB-31C
Olympia, WA 98504
206-753-3080

West Virginia
Department of Welfare
Department of Human Services
State Office Building 6, Room B-617
1900 Washington Street E.
Charleston, WV 25305
304-558-8290

Wisconsin
Department of Welfare
Bureau of Economic Assistance
Division of Community Services
Department of Health and Social Services
Wilson Street State Office Building
One W. Wilson Street, Room 358
P.O. Box 7851
Madison, WI 53707
608-266-3035

Wyoming
Department of Welfare
Division of Public Assistance and Social Services
Department of Health and Social Services
Hathaway Building, 3rd Floor
2300 Capitol Avenue
Cheyenne, WY 82002-0710
307-777-6068

Department of Veterans Affairs

The Department of Veterans Affairs (VA) is the successor to the independent agency the Veterans Administration and was made the fourteenth cabinet department in 1989. The Department of Veterans Affairs, whose central office is in Washington, D.C., is headed by the Secretary of Veterans Affairs and is made up of several suborganizations, which include the National Cemetery System, the Veterans Benefits Administration, and the Veterans Health Administration. Higher officials of the VA are appointed by the President of the United States and are subject to Senate approval.

The VA ensures medical and hospital services as well as various types of benefits for veterans and their families. Benefits include health care (medical centers, nursing home care units, outpatient clinics), life insurance plans and centers, education assistance, rehabilitation concerning vocations, compensation for military service (for disabilities and in cases of death), and pension payments.

WHO IS ELIGIBLE?

Veterans of all military, naval, and air service are eligible for benefits from the Department of Veterans Affairs. To be eligible for medical services from the Veterans Health Administration, however, certain service-connected criteria must be met. Veterans can write, call, or visit any regional VA office for information concerning their eligibility for benefits. Or veterans may obtain information and application forms from local veterans organizations and from the American Red Cross. A complete list of offices and representatives follows this discussion.

VETERANS HEALTH ADMINISTRATION

The Veterans Health Administration, the largest health care system in the United States, operates 171 medical centers with 64,763 beds, 191 outpatient centers, 128 nursing homes, 36 residential living centers, and numerous community and outreach clinics. It's staffed by more than 200,000 employees and has recorded more than 900,000 hospital admissions and more than 20 million outpatient visits. Total spending for medical care in the Veterans Health Administration is expected to exceed $15 billion in 1994.

HOSPITAL AND OUTPATIENT CARE

Hospital care and some outpatient care can be obtained by any veteran who has sustained a service-connected disability and whose condition originated or was aggravated during active service. Restrictions and exact conditions of eligibility apply:

- Veterans who were discharged dishonorably cannot receive care.

- Veterans can be treated in VA medical centers only for those medical conditions incurred while in active service.
- Veterans with service-connected disabilities can receive different benefits according to their disability ratings (a medical determination as to the extent of disability and expressed as a percentage such as 100 percent, 70 percent, 50 percent, etc., disabled).

Hospital care is also available to category A veterans: veterans who receive a pension; veterans who are eligible for Medicaid; veterans exposed to ionizing radiation (atom bomb tests) and Agent Orange; former prisoners of war; veterans of World War I or earlier conflicts; and other low-income veterans.

Hospital care, outpatient services, prescription drugs, and medicines are all available for: any medical disability of veterans of World War I; veterans who receive regular allowances for aid and attendance or who are housebound; veterans who have service-connected disabilities rated at 50 percent or more; and veterans who were prisoners of war. These veterans are also entitled to receive ambulatory care, outpatient treatment and home health services, special adaptive equipment, prosthetic appliances (for loss of limbs, hands, feet, etc.), or special aids for sight impairment (a guide dog, for example).

Dental Services

Complete dental care is provided for veterans with service-connected dental disabilities, prisoners of war (for 6 months or more), or veterans who have service-connected disabilities rated at 100 percent. Dental care (dental examination and onetime dental treatment) is available to a veteran who has had at least 180 days of service and who has a dental condition that developed or was aggravated during active service and existed at the time of discharge.

Pharmacy Services

Prescription medications are available to veterans in a VA treatment program and who have a VA-doctor-written prescription filled at a VA pharmacy. Veterans receiving aid and attendance or household benefits and veterans on the fee-basis program may have non-VA physicians write prescriptions to be filled at a VA pharmacy.

Other Benefits and Allowances

Other medical benefits include travel allowances to VA medical centers and eyeglasses (for those veterans with category A entitlement). Compensation for disability for veterans and their dependents, special monthly compensation for certain veterans, medical care for the spouse and children of certain disabled veterans, and alcohol and drug treatment for veterans are also provided by the VA health system.

Other health-related benefits for veterans include health insurance programs, burial benefits, and death benefits. The VA offers several insurance plans—plans specifically tailored to World War I veterans, World War II veterans, Korean conflict veterans, service-disabled veterans, and World War II/Korean conflict veterans with service-connected or non-service connected disabilities.

Also available, among various other group insurance programs, is a group life insurance that covers reservists, National Guard members, and ROTC members. The VA also provides burial benefits, such as reimbursement for burial expenses, a burial allowance, a burial flag, optional interment in a national cemetery, and a headstone or marker. These benefits are provided for the surviving spouse and children of war veterans or veterans who died in a VA medical facility or who were entitled to VA compensation or pension. Death benefits of certain veterans also extend to the surviving spouse and children: Educational assistance and compensation is available to family members.

Resources for Veterans' Services

Listed below are some useful addresses and phone numbers of national VA offices and other organizations that provide assistance to veterans. An asterisk (*) denotes private veterans services organizations that assist the veteran with claims for benefits.

General Information

Veterans Affairs Department
810 Vermont Avenue N.W.
Washington, DC 20420
202-535-8165

Benefits, Compensation, Insurance, and Pensions

Veterans Benefits Administration
810 Vermont Avenue N.W.
Washington, DC 20420
202-535-8026
Insurance hotline 800-669-8477

*American Legion National Organization
1608 K Street N.W.
Washington, DC 20006
202-861-2711

*American Red Cross
Military/Social Services
18th and D Streets N.W.
Washington, DC 20006
202-639-3586

*Army and Air Force Mutual Aid Association
Fort Meyer
Arlington, VA 22211
703-522-3060
800-336-4538

*Disabled American Veterans
807 Maine Avenue S.W.
Washington, DC 20024
202-554-3501

Burial Benefits

Veterans Affairs Department
Compensation and Pension Service
810 Vermont Avenue N.W.
Washington, DC 20420
202-233-2264

State Workers' Compensation Offices

These agencies are responsible for providing financial support to workers who are injured on the job. All inquiries concerning industries covered by workers' compensation should be directed to these offices.

Alabama
Workers' Compensation
Department of Industrial Relations
602 Madison Avenue
Montgomery, AL 36130
205-242-2868

Alaska
Workers' Compensation
Department of Labor
P.O. Box 25512
Juneau, AK 99802
907-465-2790

Arizona
Workers' Compensation
State Compensation Fund
3031 N. 2nd Street
Phoenix, AZ 85012
602-631-2000

Arkansas
Workers' Compensation
Justice Building, 2nd Floor
Little Rock, AR 72201
501-682-3930

California
Workers' Compensation
Department of Industrial Relations
Wing A, 5th Floor
395 Oyster Point Boulevard
South San Francisco, CA 94080
415-737-2600

Colorado
Workers' Compensation
Division of Labor
Department of Labor and Employment
1120 Lincoln Street, 13th Floor
Denver, CO 80203
303-894-7530

Connecticut
Workers' Compensation
1890 Dixwell Avenue
Hamden, CT 06514
203-789-7783

Delaware
Workers' Compensation
Division of Industrial Affairs
Department of Labor
820 N. French Street
Wilmington, DE 19801
302-571-2877

District of Columbia
Workers' Compensation
Office of Workers' Compensation
Department of Employment Services
1200 Upshur Street N.W., 3rd Floor
Washington, DC 20011
202-576-6265

Florida
Workers' Compensation
Labor and Employment Security Department
301 Forest Building
Tallahassee, FL 32399
904-488-2514

Georgia
Workers' Compensation
State Board of Workers' Compensation
1 CNN Center, Suite 1000
Atlanta, GA 30303
404-656-2034

Hawaii
Workers' Compensation
Disability Compensation Division
Labor and Industrial Relations Department
830 Punchbowl Street
Honolulu, HI 96813
808-548-5414

Idaho
Workers' Compensation
State Insurance Fund
1215 W. State Street
Boise, ID 83720
208-334-2370

Illinois
Workers' Compensation
Illinois Industrial Commission
100 W. Randolph Street, Suite 8-272
Chicago, IL 60601
312-814-6555

Indiana
Workers' Compensation
402 W. Washington Street, W196
Indianapolis, IN 46204
317-232-7103

Iowa
Workers' Compensation
Division of Industrial Services
Department of Employment Services
1000 E. Grand
Des Moines, IA 50319
515-281-5934

Kansas
Workers' Compensation
Department of Human Resources
600 Merchants Bank Tower
Topeka, KS 66612
913-296-3441

Kentucky
Workers' Compensation
Workers' Claims
The 127 Building
U.S. 127 S.
Frankfort, KY 40601
502-564-3070

Louisiana
Workers' Compensation
Office of Labor
P.O. Box 94094
Baton Rouge, LA 70804
504-925-4221

Maine
Workers' Compensation
Statehouse Station 27
Augusta, ME 04333
207-289-3751

Maryland
Workers' Compensation
6 N. Liberty Street, Room 940
Baltimore, MD 21201
410-333-4775

Massachusetts
Workers' Compensation
Industrial Accident Board
600 Washington Street, 7th Floor
Boston, MA 02111
617-727-4300

Michigan
Workers' Compensation
Bureau of Workers' Compensation
Department of Labor
P.O. Box 30016
Lansing, MI 48909
517-373-3480

Minnesota
Workers' Compensation
Department of Labor and Industry
444 Lafayette Road
St. Paul, MN 55101
612-296-6490

Mississippi
Workers' Compensation
1428 Lakeland Drive
Jackson, MS 39216
601-987-4200

Missouri
Workers' Compensation
Labor and Industrial Relations Department
722 Jefferson Street
P.O. Box 58
Jefferson City, MO 65102
314-751-4231

Montana
Workers' Compensation
State Compensation and Mutual Fund Insurance
Department of Administration
5 S. Last Chance Gulch
Helena, MT 59601
406-444-6518

Nebraska
Workers' Compensation
State Capitol, 13th Floor
P.O. Box 94967
Lincoln, NE 68509
402-471-2568

Nevada
Workers' Compensation
State Industrial Insurance System
515 E. Musser Street
Carson City, NV 89714
702-687-5220

New Hampshire
Workers' Compensation
Department of Labor
19 Pillsbury Street
Concord, NH 03301
603-271-3174

New Jersey
Workers' Compensation
Department of Labor
John Fitch Plaza, CN-381
Trenton, NJ 08625
609-292-2414

New Mexico
Workers' Compensation
Labor and Industrial Commission
180 Randolph S.E.
Albuquerque, NM 87106
505-841-6000

New York
Workers' Compensation
Executive Office
Workers' Compensation Board
180 Livingston Street
Brooklyn, NY 11248
718-802-6666

North Carolina
Workers' Compensation
Industrial Commission
Department of Economic and Community Development
430 N. Salisbury Street
Raleigh, NC 27603
919-733-4820

North Dakota
Workers' Compensation
Workers' Compensation Bureau
4007 N. State Street
Bismarck, ND 58501
701-224-3800

Ohio
Workers' Compensation
246 N. High Street
Columbus, OH 43266
614-466-1935

Oklahoma
Workers' Compensation
1915 N. Stiles
Oklahoma City, OK 73105
405-557-7600

Oregon
Workers' Compensation
Department of Insurance and Finance
Labor and Industries Building
Salem, OR 97310
503-378-3304

Pennsylvania
Workers' Compensation
Department of Labor and Industry
3607 Derry Street, 4th Floor
Harrisburg, PA 17120
717-783-5421

Puerto Rico
Workers' Compensation
State Insurance Fund
P.O. Box 365028
San Juan, PR 00936
809-781-0122

Rhode Island
Workers' Compensation
610 Manton Avenue
Providence, RI 02909
401-272-0700

South Carolina
Workers' Compensation
P.O. Box 1715
Columbia, SC 29202
803-734-5744

South Dakota
Workers' Compensation
Division of Labor and Management
Department of Labor
Kneip Building
Pierre, SD 57501
605-773-3681

Tennessee
Workers' Compensation
Department of Labor
501 Union Building
Nashville, TN 37243
615-741-2395

Texas
Workers' Compensation
Texas Compensation Commission
200 E. Riverside Drive
Austin, TX 78704
512-448-7900

Utah
Workers' Compensation
Industrial Commission
160 East 300 South
Salt Lake City, UT 84111
801-530-6800

Vermont
Workers' Compensation
Department of Labor and Industry
7 Court Street
Montpelier, VT 05602
802-828-2286

Virgin Islands
Workers' Compensation
Department of Labor
P.O. Box 890
Christiansted
St. Croix, VI 00820
809-773-1994

Virginia
Workers' Compensation
Workers' Compensation Commission
P.O. Box 1794
Richmond, VA 23214
804-367-8666

Washington
Workers' Compensation
Department of Labor and Industries
234 General Administration Building
Mail Stop HC-901
Olympia, WA 98504
206-753-6307

West Virginia
Workers' Compensation
Division of Workers' Compensation
P.O. Box 3051
Charleston, WV 25332
304-344-2580

Wisconsin
Workers' Compensation
Division of Workers' Compensation
Industrial and Labor Human Relations
P.O. Box 7901
Madison, WI 53707
608-266-6841

Wyoming
Workers' Compensation
Department of Employment
122 W. 25th Street
Cheyenne, WY 82002
307-777-7441

9. Family Health and Resources

INTRODUCTION

Health care is too important to leave completely in the hands of others. Regardless of how well trained or competent your health care professional may be, most responsibility falls on your shoulders. And most of us are quite competent in handling much of our own health care needs.

It has been estimated that up to 80 percent of all health care is self-care. That means most of the time we take care of our own minor medical problems, regulate our own nutrition, and protect ourselves from accidents and injuries. Yet, while we may not have a health care professional in our home to supervise our activities, we generally act out of information we have learned from a wide range of sources.

In this section, you will find facts, figures, information, and resources to help you and your family take charge of your health. From recommended daily dietary allowances to home remedies, in this section you have a complete family guide to maintaining health.

Basic Medical Supplies for the Home

Self-care activities run the gamut from home treatment of a twisted ankle with ice and rest to preparing for major surgery or managing a terminal illness. And the program can start with something as simple as a well-stocked medicine cabinet and the knowledge to monitor signs and symptoms and treat injuries and illnesses. The medicine cabinet should not be easily accessible to small children or placed in areas of the house where temperatures fluctuate. While one cannot store every medication for every illness, there are ten basic elements that one should include in a home medicine cabinet:

1. Any prescription medications one may take
2. Pain relievers such as aspirin or aspirin substitutes. (Unless directed by your doctor, children should never be given aspirin because of its association with Reye's syndrome.)
3. Ipecac to induce vomiting. (Never administer without your doctor's advice.)
4. Antacid for gastrointestinal distress
5. Antidiarrheal medication
6. Petroleum jelly for dry skin and skin irritations
7. Laxative
8. Salt (a natural antiseptic)
9. Thermometer (rectal thermometer recommended for children under age 3)
10. First-aid kit: antibiotic ointment; antiseptic solution (hydrogen peroxide); ice pack; gauze; adhesive and gauze pads; bandages; cotton and cotton-tipped swabs; hydrocortisone cream; scissors; soap; tissues; tweezers; first-aid manual.

Every first-aid area should also have a list of essential phone numbers in case of an emergency: local police, fire, and ambulance, Poison Control Center, and family physician.

The 22 Most Important Home Medical Tests

Home medical testing has made it possible for people to take better care of themselves and thus remain healthier. The availability of sophisticated and reliable equipment has added a whole new emphasis on home medical tests. It's easy to forget that just a few short years ago, home testing was limited to taking body temperature.

Nowadays, computer-controlled devices are used to monitor heart rate and respiration, blood pressure, and blood sugar. Mechanical equipment can be used to measure the percentage of body fat, examine an eardrum for an infection, or illuminate a sinus cavity. Other chemical-based tests use specially treated paper, in the form of dipsticks, to test blood and urine.

Home medical testing is not designed to replace professional medical care; however, it can help you determine when you need professional care.

Not only are there more home testing products on the market, but they are also more widely available. You'll find home tests at pharmacies, where they may be displayed in special sections, in health and beauty stores, in supermarkets, and through mail-order companies. Home medical tests can give you the information you need to make informed decisions about your medical care and your overall health.

When used properly, home medical tests enable you to determine, monitor, and screen for various illnesses and conditions. Certain precautions, however, are worth noting. Here are some consumer tips issued by the U.S. Food and Drug Administration. Keep these suggestions in mind when using all self-care test products.

1. Before you buy, note the expiration date for kits that contain chemicals. Don't buy a test if the expiration date is past.
2. Follow storage instructions. Keep containers tightly capped. Avoid moisture, light, and extremes of heat and cold. Keep out of reach of children.
3. Read and study the package insert. Make sure you understand the test and how to use it. Follow instructions exactly. Do not skip steps. If the test is timed, use a clock or a watch to be precise.
4. Note special precautions such as avoiding certain food, drugs, or vitamins before testing. Take the test at the recommended time, if any is specified.
5. Some tests use colors to indicate results. If you are color-blind, have someone who can discern color help you interpret test results.
6. Some tests require collecting urine. Always collect urine in a clean, dry container. Soap or other residue can cause faulty test results.
7. Know what to do if test results are positive, negative, or unclear.
8. If you have questions about a test, consult a pharmacist or other health care professional. Also check the package insert for a telephone number you can call.

The following section describes what we consider to be the twenty-two most important home medical tests. Some of these tests require special equipment, while others do not. We'll describe the test, tell you how it's conducted, and suggest where it might be available.

BODY TEMPERATURE

Monitoring the body's temperature is probably the easiest home test there is, and one you've most likely done hundreds of times. Before we detail the various thermometers available for home testing, we should say this about so-called normal body temperature: 98.6°F (37°C) is a standard that was based on a German study of more than 1 million people in 1868. According to a study published in the *Journal of the*

American Medical Association in 1992, today's thermometers are quicker and more accurate. Doctors in the U.S. measured oral temperatures up to four times a day over a 3-day period in healthy men and women, and the average was 98.2°. The authors concluded that 98.9° overall should now be regarded as the upper limit of the normal oral range in healthy adults aged 40 and younger.

The most common types of thermometers are:

Oral glass bulb. The most popular type of thermometer and probably found in every home. Usually filled with mercury or some other heat-sensitive chemical. The mercury-filled thermometer appears to have a silver streak in the center, while the other chemical appears red.

Electronic thermometer. A heat-sensitive metal tip is placed in the mouth and a computer chip electronically reads and displays the temperature in digital form. This is probably the most expensive type of thermometer.

Disposable thermometer. This thermometer is used once and discarded. It uses specially treated, heat-sensitive paper that either displays the actual temperature or changes color to indicate a fever is present.

Plastic strip thermometer. A plastic strip is placed against the forehead to take a temperature reading. Some of these temperature strips may be left on the forehead to continually monitor the presence of a fever. These strips may display the temperature or change color to indicate a fever.

You can find a special infant pacifier thermometer that even changes color when the baby's temperature rises. Pharmacies, health and beauty stores, and supermarkets carry thermometers.

PULSE MEASUREMENT AND FITNESS TESTING

Electronics has made it possible to monitor several body functions at the same time with a unit that is no larger than a personal stereo. It measures heart rate in average beats, oxygen uptake, calories expended, and elapsed time. It is used to calculate target heart rates and can also calculate a fitness index based on age, sex, weight, and oxygen use.

This is one self-monitoring device that has more than one use, and may be especially important to someone with a cardiac condition. Ask your doctor or pharmacist about the availability of the newest entry in the pulse-monitoring field.

VISION TESTING

Most forms of vision testing can be performed in the home using eye charts akin to what you find in the doctor's office. You can screen yourself for visual acuity, astigmatism, color blindness, and macular degeneration. Many of the charts used for home vision testing are available at pharmacies, health and beauty stores, and through mail-order companies.

Visual acuity. The Snellen chart is what you see in doctors' offices. It has the large letters at the top and the smaller letters at the bottom. If you can read the ⅜-inch letters at 20 feet, your visual acuity is said to be 20/20.

Astigmatism. This chart is somewhat like the face of a clock with all the numbers connected by parallel lines (12 to 6, 9 to 3, and so forth). The effect is a star burst with all lines crossing in the center. When looking at the chart, all the lines should appear uniformly dark.

Color blindness. Home testing for color blindness is done using a multicolored chart in which a number has been hidden among the many colors. It is most often keyed to red and green or blue and yellow. A color-blind person would not be able to distinguish the number.

Macular degeneration. The Amsler Grid Test is used to detect macular degeneration. The test consists of a grid with tiny squares and a dot at the center of the chart. Your ability to stare at the dot and see the smaller squares is very important. If any of the lines appear wavy or disappear, you should consult your eye care professional.

EAR EXAMINATION

Young children often have more than their share of earaches and other ear problems. That's why parents can benefit from learning how to use the otoscope, a handheld lighted instrument with a magnifying lens and a viewing cone, to monitor the health of the ear canal and the eardrum. The otoscope is a rather simple piece of equipment as medical equipment goes. Using it is not that difficult and with a little effort you can become skilled at it. You'll need some time and a willing patient.

You'll need to learn to identify the basic structure of the ear and eardrum, as well as the symptoms of ear infections. This includes identifying the normal color and shape of the eardrum, the location of the bones of the middle ear, and the signs of pressure behind the eardrum.

Otoscopes can be purchased at most pharmacies and through mail-order companies.

SELF-EXAM FOR DENTAL PLAQUE

Dental plaque is the unseen enemy of teeth and a major cause of tooth decay and gum disease. The best way to get rid of plaque is through proper daily brushing and flossing of the teeth. However, since plaque is virtually invisible, you need help in finding it: special plaque-disclosing tablets, such as Red-Kote or X-pose. After your regular brushing and flossing, chew one of the tablets and make sure you thoroughly mix it with your saliva. As the tablet dissolves, it leaves behind a red stain that adheres to the plaque. You may need a small light and dental mirror to complete your examination. The darkest areas are those with the most plaque and other debris. Regular use of the plaque-disclosing tablets will help you in your battle against tooth decay and gum disease. Dental disclosing tablets and other dental self-care tools are available from dentists and pharmacies.

HOME BLOOD PRESSURE MONITORING

High blood pressure is often called a silent killer, because unlike other diseases it often remains hidden. You don't get a rash or sore spot, so you may have it but not know it. However, you can learn to monitor your own blood pressure.

You'll need a blood pressure cuff, or sphygmomanometer (*sfig-mo-muh-NOM-itur*) as it is called, and a little practice. Blood pressure cuffs generally come in two varieties, manually operated cuffs and computerized cuffs. They both work the same way. It's just that the manual cuff requires a bit more work because you need to learn how to inflate the cuff, listen for the heartbeat, and read the blood pressure gauge. The computerized model does all the work for you.

Blood pressure home monitoring kits are available at most pharmacies, health and beauty stores, and through mail-order companies.

HOME CHOLESTEROL TEST

Health-conscious consumers now have the option of testing their cholesterol level at home, thus bypassing a trip to the doctor and laboratory. The Food and Drug Administration has approved an at-home cholesterol test that provides your total cholesterol reading in as few as 15 minutes.

Developed and manufactured by ChemTrak, Inc., of Sunnyvale, California, the cholesterol self-test device—the AccuMeter—is marketed by American Home Products and is available in pharmacies. The test kit comes complete with instructions and illustrations, showing you how to obtain your blood sample and use the AccuMeter.

For best results, it's recommended that you obtain the blood sample from your finger using the lance supplied with the kit. According to the manufacturer, this procedure is relatively painless. After you've pricked your finger, gently apply pressure to help form the drop of blood. Now place the blood sample on the test strip located on the AccuMeter. After a minute or two the blood separates into its components and is then ready to be read by the AccuMeter. The test is complete in about 15 minutes when the total cholesterol level is displayed. This particular test is not capable of determining your HDL and LDL cholesterol levels. (High-density lipoprotein, or HDL, is the carrier of cholesterol believed to transport cholesterol away from the tissues and to the liver, where it can be excreted. Low-density lipoprotein, or LDL, is the main carrier of harmful cholesterol in the body. Your total cholesterol level is the sum of HDL and LDL.)

The instructions cite the National Cholesterol Education Program's recommendations that a total cholesterol reading of 200 or less is desirable, 200 to 239 is borderline high, and 240 and above is high. You are cautioned, however, against jumping to any conclusions based upon a single test. For best results, it is recommended that you establish a baseline cholesterol reading by repeating the test several times. Consumers with questions about the home cholesterol test kit may call the manufacturer toll-free at 800-927-7776.

SELF-TESTING FOR LUNG FUNCTION

Self-tests for lung functions can be performed with or without special equipment. There are six generally recognized self-tests that you can perform at home, the first two of which do not require special equipment.

Match test. Hold a lighted match about 6 inches from your mouth, take a deep breath, and then exhale as forcefully as you can. If you can blow the match out without any problems, chances are you don't have any serious lung problems.

Forced Expiratory Test. You'll need a stopwatch to count the seconds it takes to exhale all of your breath. Take a deep breath and, with your mouth open, exhale as fast as you can. The normal time is between 2 and 6 seconds. If it takes you longer than that, you may need additional testing.

For the following tests, you will need a peak flow meter (a device that measures the amount of air you exhale) and a spirometer (an instrument that measures the amount of air entering and leaving the lungs).

Peak Expiratory Flow Rate. Take a deep breath and blow into the mouthpiece of the peak flow meter, which registers in liters the volume of air leaving your lungs. Repeat this test three times to establish a baseline. Any decrease in the amount of air exhaled could indicate a potential problem and should be closely monitored.

Forced Vital Capacity (FVC) and *Forced Expiratory Volume in 1 Second.* Use the spirometer for these tests. Take a deep breath and then blow into the mouthpiece of the spirometer for as long and hard and fast as you can. This measures how much air you can expel from your lungs after a deep breath. Some spirometers will also calculate your forced expiratory volume in 1 second. This is a measure of how long it takes to expel at least 75 percent of your normal lung capacity in 1 second. If your measurement is less than 75 percent, it could indicate the need for further testing.

Maximum Voluntary Ventilation (MVV). The purpose of this test is to measure the maximum volume of air that you can inhale and exhale in 1 minute. You'll need two things for this test: a spirometer and the forced vital capacity reading from your earlier test. Hold the spirometer in your hand, and inhale and exhale as fast as you can for 15 seconds. Note the reading on the spirometer and multiply it by 4. This gives you your MVV for 1 minute. You should repeat this process at least three times in order to determine your average MVV. The exact amount of air you are able to inhale and exhale is dependent on your age, body size, lung capacity, and general state of health. Your MVV should be about fifteen to twenty times greater than your FVC reading. If your MVV falls short of this range, then it could indicate that you need to seek professional assistance for a complete pulmonary workup.

Peak flow monitors and spirometers may be purchased at pharmacies and through mail-order companies.

URINALYSIS

Simple-to-use home urinalysis products make it easy to monitor the workings of many body systems: the endocrine system, kidneys, liver, gallbladder, blood, spleen, bone marrow, and pancreas.

You'll need what are called dipsticks to perform the urinalysis. Dipsticks are specially treated papers that contain chemicals that react to the various components of urine. You can monitor the acidity (pH) and density (specific gravity) of urine, or you can check for blood, ketones (an indication of possible diabetes), and glucose.

Multiple-purpose dipsticks make it possible to perform a series of tests with one urine sample. There are also single-purpose dipsticks that monitor such things as glucose, vitamin C, and protein. Urine dipstick tests are available from pharmacies and through mail-order companies.

SELF-TESTING FOR URINARY TRACT INFECTIONS

Urinary tract infections (UTIs) are diseases that affect the kidneys, ureters, bladder, and urethra. When the urinary system has an infection, it can be downright painful and uncomfortable and, if left untreated, can lead to serious kidney disease. Self-tests for urinary tract infections can help identify the culprits causing the problem.

Three types of tests determine the presence of a urinary tract infection: cultures, leukocyte dipsticks, and nitrite dipsticks.

Cultures. You place a sample of the urine on a specially prepared slide or tube. If a bacterium is present, it should grow in the medium.

Leukocyte dipstick. This test checks the urine for the presence of white blood cells, which may indicate that an infection is present, since an increase in white blood cells indicates that the body is fighting an infection.

Nitrite dipstick. This test looks for nitrites that are not normally present in the urine. A certain type of bacteria converts the nitrates in our diet to nitrites, and if nitrites are in the urine, then an infection may also be present.

Dipstick tests are available from pharmacies and through mail-order companies.

OVULATION AND PREGNANCY SELF-TEST

These two self-tests are listed together (but sold separately) because in a sense you can't have one without the other. Ovulation testing enables women to track their periods of maximum fertility and use that information to control their reproductive activities. Pregnancy testing enables women to confirm whether or are not they are pregnant.

Ovulation testing is accomplished with a urine sample and a specially treated dipstick that detects the presence of a luteinizing hormone excreted during ovulation. The dipstick is placed in the urine and observed for any color change. Comparing the color to the guide supplied with the test kit will indicate whether or not the hormone is present.

Pregnancy testing is similar in that it also looks for a hormone that is produced only when a woman is pregnant. A urine sample is collected and mixed with a special reagent solution (a chemical that helps to identify the hormone). After it has been mixed, a special dipstick is used to test the solution. Changes in color indicate whether or not the woman is pregnant. Because there is always the chance of a mistake, it is advisable to repeat any pregnancy test.

Home tests for ovulation and pregnancy are available in most pharmacies, health and beauty stores, and even some supermarkets.

HOME BLOOD GLUCOSE MONITORING

People with diabetes naturally have the most pressing need for blood glucose monitoring; however, even if you aren't diabetic, you may want to consider home blood glucose monitoring. This is especially true if there's any evidence of diabetes in your family. Home glucose monitoring enables diabetics to take control of their lives and take precautions against secondary illnesses, such as kidney disease, blindness, nerve damage, and heart disease.

The glucose monitors of today are very sophisticated and quite accurate, a far cry from the early chemical dipsticks that many diabetic people used. Two popular methods for monitoring glucose are reagent pads and glucose meters. The reagent pad changes color depending on the amount of glucose in the blood, while the meter reads a strip of specially treated paper and produces a digital display.

A variety of equipment is available, from finger stick devices to glucose meters, and most of it can be found in the self-care section of pharmacies.

HOME THROAT CULTURES

Sore throats are generally associated with the cold and flu season and are caused by viruses. Another type of sore throat, however, is caused by a bacteria known as streptococcus, or "strep" for short. This type of sore throat, if not properly diagnosed and treated, can lead to other illnesses.

The only way to determine if a sore throat is caused by this bacteria is to take a throat specimen and culture it. If strep is present, it will grow in the culture.

Performing a throat culture test is a two-step process. Your physician can supply you with the specimen collection kit and show you how to collect the specimen. The collection kit is basically a large cotton swab that is swept through the throat from side to side. Once you've collected the specimen, you then return it to the physician or a laboratory.

The laboratory will grow the culture in a special oven and report the results to your physician. Because of the special equipment involved, you can't do the full test at home. By taking the specimen yourself, however, you save the cost of an additional visit to the doctor.

SELF-TEST FOR BREATH ALCOHOL

This type of test is very important if you're planning a night on the town and don't want to end up with a driving while intoxicated (DWI) citation on your driving record. Research has shown that alcohol enters the bloodstream very quickly and, before you know it, your blood alcohol level is over the legal limit.

There are two basic types of monitors with which to check your blood alcohol level.

Balloon test. The balloon test is probably the best known of the breath alcohol monitors. It consists of a balloon mouthpiece and a glass tube filled with specially treated crystals. As you blow into the balloon, your breath flows over the crystals, which change color according to the level of alcohol present.

Electronic breath meter. This type of monitor works on the same principle as the balloon test. As you blow through the mouthpiece of the meter, it automatically measures the amount of alcohol that is present. The display will signal whether or not your blood alcohol level is at or near the legal limit.

Breath alcohol monitors are available from pharmacies and through mail-order companies.

HOME SCREENING FOR BOWEL CANCER

Colorectal cancer is called the silent cancer because people are reluctant to discuss it publicly. Yet it is responsible for some 60,000 cancer deaths each year. The home screening test for colorectal cancer is designed to detect the presence of hidden (occult) blood in the stool.

The advantage of using the home screening kit for colorectal cancer is that you can do it in the privacy of your home. In addition, when colorectal cancer is detected early, the chance of recovery is much better. There are three basic types of home screening kits.

Stain method. A small stool specimen is collected and placed on a specially treated piece of paper. The presence of occult blood is determined after a staining solution is applied to the specimen. The stain will adhere to the occult blood.

Toilet paper test. Special toilet paper is used and then sprayed with a chemical disclosing agent. If occult blood is present, the paper will turn blue.

Pad test. This is probably the easiest test to use, since it only requires dropping a test pad in the toilet after a bowel movement. If occult blood is present, the pad will change color.

Home screening tests for colorectal cancer are available from pharmacies, health and beauty stores, and through mail-order companies.

HOME TEST FOR PINWORMS

Pinworms usually infect children; however, no one is immune from these intestinal parasites. The most commonly observed symptom is itching in the anal area, especially at night.

You don't need much more than a flashlight to conduct this test, since it's primarily one of observation. If you don't observe the worms, you may want to check for worm eggs, and for that you'll need a tape test.

It's best to check for pinworms at night when they are most active and the threadlike adult worm can be observed. You simply shine the light over the anal area and note the presence or absence of worms. If there are no worms present, you may also want to check for worm eggs.

The pinworm egg test is done using a sticky tape that is pressed over the anal area and collects the eggs. Because they are microscopic in size, you can't observe them with the naked eye, so in most cases you will have to take the tape to your doctor or a laboratory.

Medication to combat pinworms is available from pharmacies or your doctor.

VAGINAL SELF-EXAM

The vaginal self-exam is intended to enable women to learn more about their bodies and become better informed on the subject of gynecological health. Through routine examination and monitoring they can learn how to spot indications of infections, irritations, or discharges. This information can then be used in conjunction with the professional care they are receiving.

You'll need the following equipment to perform a vaginal self-exam: flashlight or other suitable light, a handheld mirror, and a vaginal speculum (an instrument with two duck-billed blades that open to allow the viewing of the vaginal walls and cervix).

The examination is best done with your knees bent and the feet spread apart. The mirror should be placed in front of the vagina and should have a long handle so it's easy to reach. The speculum is then inserted into the vagina with the blades closed. After insertion, carefully turn the handle and open the blades. With the mirror positioned in front of the vagina, shine the light into the mirror and reflect the light into the vagina.

It's a good idea to use the self-exam information that's included with the speculum kit, since this describes the normal appearance of the vagina and cervix. Any irregularities should be noted and mentioned to your health care professional.

Vaginal self-exam kits are available from pharmacies, women's health centers, and through mail-order companies.

BREAST SELF-EXAM

The breast self-exam is one of the best ways to protect yourself from breast cancer and put your mind at ease. The other two ways are a breast exam by a doctor or someone trained to do it and a breast X ray (mammogram).

Why do the breast self-exam? According to the American Cancer Society, there are many good reasons for doing the breast self-exam (BSE) each month. One reason is that breast cancer is most easily treated and cured when it is found early. Another is that if you do BSE every month, it will increase your skill and confidence when doing the exam. When you get to know how your breasts normally feel, you will quickly be able to feel any change. Another reason—it's easy to do. Remember: BSE could save your breast—and save your life. Most breast lumps are found by women themselves, but, in fact, most lumps in the breast are not cancer. Be safe, be sure.

When to do BSE? The best time to do BSE is about a week after your period, when breasts are not tender or swollen. If you do not have regular periods or sometimes skip a month, do BSE on the same day every month.

How to do BSE. Here is the protocol as recommended by the American Cancer Society.

1. Lie down and put a pillow under your right shoulder. Place your right arm behind your head.
2. Use the finger pads of your three middle fingers on your left hand to feel for lumps. Your finger pads are the top third of each finger.
3. Press firmly enough to know how your breast feels. If you're not sure how hard to press, ask your doctor or nurse. Or try to copy the way your doctor uses the finger pads during a breast exam. Learn what your breast feels like most of the time. A firm ridge in the lower curve of each breast is normal.
4. Move around the breast in a set way. You can choose either a circle, an up and down line, or a wedge. Do it the same way every time. It will help you to make sure that you've gone over the entire breast area, and to remember how your breast feels each month.
5. Now examine your left breast using right-hand finger pads.
6. If you find any changes, see your doctor right away.

For added safety, you might want to check your breasts while standing in front of a mirror, right after you do your BSE each month. See if there are any changes in the way your breasts look, dimpling of the skin, or changes in the nipple, redness or swelling. You might also want to do an extra BSE while you're in the shower. Your soapy hands will glide over the wet skin, making it easy to check how your breasts feel.

TESTICULAR SELF-EXAM

Men have finally discovered something women have known for quite some time—the value of self-examination for cancer. Women have learned to do self-examination for breast cancer, and it has paid off in the number of cancers that have been detected early. Cancer experts tell us that early detection of cancer leads to early treatment and increased chances of survival.

This is especially true when dealing with testicular cancer, a form of male cancer that can be detected through self-examination. At one time a confirmed diagnosis meant almost certain death, but today—with early detection—the recovery rate is roughly 90 percent.

Most tumors found in the testicles are malignant and spread rapidly; in half of all cases, the cancer invades other parts of the body, usually the lungs or abdominal lymph tissue. Because doctors are concerned with the spread of cancer cells throughout the body, they aggressively pursue the cancer with surgery, radiation, and chemotherapy. You may avoid subjecting yourself to such an ordeal by learning a simple self-exam technique.

Examining yourself for testicular cancer is relatively easy and doesn't require more than 3 minutes of your time once a month. Every man should be able to spare at least 3 minutes a month for this important health check. Here's how to get started:

1. It's best to do the exam following a warm bath or shower.
2. Make sure the scrotal skin is relaxed.
3. Examine one testicle at a time.
4. Roll each testicle between the thumb and fingers of both hands.
5. Massage the surface lightly and check for any irregularities or anything that seems strange (you may feel the epididymis, which runs up the back of the testicle, but that's normal).
6. If you find any bumps or hard lumps, contact your doctor.

SELF-TEST FOR ERECTION PROBLEMS

The test most often used to detect erection problems is the Nocturnal Penile Tumescence Stamp Test, or NPT. Impotence, the inability to achieve an erection, may be caused by physical or psychological factors, or a combination of both.

The NPT test can help determine whether or not a man's ability to achieve an erection is physical or psychological. It is considered normal for a man to have one to four erections during periods of deep sleep known as rapid eye movement sleep. This information led to the development of the stamp test.

This test is relatively easy to perform, and the only thing you need is a roll of stamps. You may use postage stamps or you can order a roll of specially designed stamps for this purpose. You will need a strip of four to six stamps and a total of twelve to eighteen stamps for the 3-night test.

You select the first strip of stamps and place them around the penis before going to bed. Upon awakening, examine the stamps to determine if they are broken or if there are any perforations between stamps. If the stamps are broken or perforated in any way, it probably means that you had an erection sometime during your sleep. In any event, it's recommended that you repeat the test for 3 consecutive nights.

Additional information on the stamp test and tests for impotence can be obtained from any trained sex counselor. Ask your pharmacist for information on the availability of stamps for the NPT test.

SINUS TRANSILLUMINATION

At one time or another, nearly everyone has experienced some sort of sinus problem. The all-too-familiar pain around the eyes, the stuffy nose, and the ever-present headache are all reminders of the discomfort brought on by sinus problems.

You can save yourself some time and money if you learn how to conduct an examination of your own sinuses using a flashlight. Both the maxillary (the sinuses below your eyes and either side of your face) and frontal (those above your eyes) can be examined. This type of examination is known as transillumination, a fancy way of saying that you're going to shine a light through your sinuses.

In addition to the flashlight, you'll need a darkened room and a mirror. Once in the room, stand in front of the mirror, open your mouth, and carefully insert the flashlight. Then close your mouth around the flashlight so that no light escapes. With all that light in your mouth it should be easy to see your maxillary sinuses. Clear sinuses will appear bright, while congested sinuses will be cloudy.

Examine your frontal sinuses by placing the light just under the bony ridge above your eyes. You may find a penlight is better suited for examining the frontal sinuses. Once again, compare the amount of light that is visible from each sinus to determine whether it is clear or congested.

SELF-TEST FOR BODY FAT COMPOSITION

You don't need to be an Olympic athlete to be interested in your body fat composition. Researchers who study fitness have developed some general guidelines on the subject of fat to body weight percentages.

Using the standard of 19 percent body fat for men and 22 percent for women, you can test yourself to determine how well you measure up to these standards. The researchers also note that the percentage of body fat for athletically inclined men and women should be 15 and 18 percent respectively.

The easiest form of body fat testing you can do is the skinfold thickness test. You'll need a special caliper to measure the thickness of the skinfolds taken on various parts of the body. The best location to do a skinfold test is the forearm or the area below the shoulder blade. You pinch the skin and pull it away from the body until you have a fold of skin that can be measured with the caliper. Place the caliper over the fold and slowly close it. When you can't close it any further, take the reading from the scale on the caliper. Record this reading on the chart supplied with the caliper kit. Use the body fat tables that come with the calipers to make a determination of your percentage of body fat.

Body fat composition kits are available from pharmacies and through mail-order companies. You might even check with fitness clubs in your area.

Home Remedies

Home remedies, using products that are easily obtained and found in many households, are the cornerstone of medical self-care. Whether termed folk medicines or self-care, home remedies were the main way of treating illnesses until the advent of modern medicine. Proponents assert that even today, however, home remedies can offer relief when expensive doctor visits and prescriptions don't. And many of them do not have the unpleasant side effects and adverse reactions of today's prescription medications.

Here are some home remedies that can be very soothing for some of the bumps, bruises, headaches, and stomachaches of life.

HOME REMEDIES FOR 25 COMMON ILLS

Bruises. To help avoid a nasty bruise when you've been bumped hard, immediately apply an ice pack to constrict the blood vessels and reduce swelling. If no ice is available, a pack of frozen vegetables will do. Use the ice pack as long as it is comfortable. After the first day, you can switch to heat treatments to bring blood back into the area and promote healing. Persistent, severe pain may indicate a bone fracture.

Hives. Take an over-the-counter antihistamine, but be sure to read the label first. Some antihistamines cause drowsiness, making it inadvisable to drive or operate other large machinery. If shortness of breath occurs, get to the nearest emergency room.

Cooling your mouth after eating hot peppers. Drink a glass of milk. Casein, a protein in milk, binds to the mouth's temperature receptors, edging out the spicy oil in hot peppers.

Bee stings. Quickly apply meat tenderizer; it contains papain, which helps to break down the proteins present in insect venom. Remove the stinger by scraping across the sting with a knife or other firm object. Do not use your fingers to remove the stinger, since you could accidentally squeeze the venom sack, releasing more venom into the wound. Take an antihistamine to reduce pain and swelling; apply an ice pack to further reduce swelling.

Mosquito bites. Apply ice to the bite; it may help reduce inflammation and swelling. Dissolve 1 tablespoon of Epsom salts in a quart of water, chill, and then place on the bite, using a cloth.

Poison ivy. Immediately rinse the affected area with rubbing alcohol followed by water. Wash your clothing to deactivate poison ivy's itch-causing urushiol oil. If you break out in a rash, try any of the following: calamine lotion, zinc oxide, witch hazel, baking soda, or Burow's solution (aluminum acetate).

Athlete's foot. Daub the infected area with vinegar morning and night, and during the day if your sched-

Home Remedies at Your Fingertips

Found in probably every household, the following products are also useful as home remedies. Some of these products are commercial nonprescription medications, while others are common household products. When using household products for medicinal purposes, be sure to read the label for proper dosing and usage. If there's any doubt as to the proper mixture or application, *do not use the product.* Consult a self-care or first-aid guide for additional information.

Acetaminophen—a painkiller and fever reducer for persons allergic to aspirin.

Alcohol—a mild antiseptic or germ killer used topically.

Ammonia—for fainting, used as "smelling salts" by holding an open container under the victim's nose so vapor can be inhaled. Ammonia can also be used as a counterirritant and to neutralize insect bites.

Baking soda—used to neutralize acid burns.

Benzalkonium chloride—a detergent-type cleanser and disinfectant for treating wounds.

Boric acid—a weak germ and fungus killer, used as dusting powder.

Burned toast—used as a substitute for activated charcoal (see *Universal antidote*) to absorb poisons.

Calamine lotion—used for sunburn and minor thermal (heat) burns that do not result in blisters.

Chloride of lime (bleaching powder)—a disinfectant. Avoid direct contact with the wound.

Coffee—used as a stimulant in shock cases if the victim is conscious and bleeding internally.

Egg white—used as a demulcent to soothe the stomach and retard absorption of a poison.

Epsom salts—dissolved in warm water, can be used in treating wounds and to make wet dressings for them.

Flour—made into a thin paste, can be used as a demulcent to soothe the stomach and retard absorption of a poison.

Hydrogen peroxide—a germ killer when in direct contact with bacteria.

Milk—used as a demulcent to soothe the stomach and retard absorption of a poison.

Milk of magnesia—used as a substitute for magnesium oxide (see *Universal antidote*). Milk of magnesia is also used in small doses as an antacid for stomach upset.

Mineral oil—used as drops to treat thermal (heat) burns of the eye. May also be taken internally as a stool softener to promote easier passage.

Oil of cloves—used for temporary relief of a toothache.

Olive oil—used as drops to treat thermal (heat) burns of the eye. Olive oil is also used as an emollient to soften skin.

Petrolatum (Vaseline)—a skin softener and protective ointment used on wound dressings.

Powdered mustard (dry mustard)—used as an emetic (to induce vomiting). Dissolve 1 to 3 teaspoonfuls in a glass of warm water.

Salt (table salt)—used as an emetic. Dissolve 2 teaspoonfuls in a glass of warm water. (Clean seawater can be used if an emetic or a wound cleanser is needed for an accident near an ocean beach.)

Soapsuds (not detergents)—used as an emetic and as an antidote for poisoning by certain metal compounds, such as mercuric chloride. **Soap and clean water can also be used to cleanse wounds.**

Starch, cooked—made into a thin paste as a demulcent to soothe the stomach and retard absorption of a poison.

Tea—made strong, used as a substitute for tannic acid. Tea is also used as a stimulant in shock cases when appropriate.

Universal antidote—recommended as an antidote for poisoning when the poison cannot be identified. The universal antidote is made by mixing ½ ounce activated charcoal, ¼ ounce magnesium oxide, and ¼ ounce tannic acid in a glass of water.

Vinegar (acetic acid)—used to neutralize alkali burns.

---

ule permits. Vitamin E oil applied to the infected area is an additional remedy many find helpful. There are over-the-counter preparations specially formulated for athlete's foot as well.

Bad breath. A simple remedy is brushing your teeth, gums, and surface of the tongue with a thin paste of baking soda and water.

Bear in mind that many times bad breath results from sinus conditions or serious dental conditions, for which you should seek professional care.

Common cold. Vitamin C is helpful in preventing a cold, but once a cold is established, garlic tea is a good remedy. Boil 4 cups of water and remove from heat. Add freshly crushed garlic cloves to the water and let steep. Drink while quite hot. Adding crushed garlic to a vaporizer may also relieve the nasal congestion often associated with a head cold.

Dandruff. More than one home remedy exists for dandruff. You might try applying one or two capfuls of apple cider vinegar to your scalp after a shower. Next, take a small portion of castor oil and rub it vigorously into your scalp and comb your hair. A second remedy involves the vitamin PABA (para-aminobenzoic acid), a member of the B-complex vitamins. A suggested dosage is 100 mg of PABA per day. Supplement this with a natural shampoo and a vinegar rinse.

Cracked skin. Cracked skin often responds to zinc supplements. Experts suggest that a person take 10 mg three times a day; it may take a month or more until results are seen. Another remedy is vitamin E oil. A few drops rubbed into cracked skin each day often brings results within a week.

Headaches. Vitamin B_6 (pyridoxine), at a recommended dosage of 100 mg a day, has been reported to help relieve migraine headaches. For sinus headaches, you might try taking niacin three times a day for a total of 100 mg.

Indigestion. One simple cause of indigestion is eating too much. Smoking can also add to the problem. But if neither overeating nor smoking is the culprit, simple remedies are available. Try drinking mint tea to aid in digestion. Papaya enzymes, available in health food stores, can also help.

Leg cramps. If you suffer from chronic, nighttime leg cramps, orally taking dolomite and bonemeal before retiring has been known to help. Sometimes bonemeal alone can bring relief. If you have recurring leg cramps, it may be a sign that you are deficient in potassium. Adding foods such as bananas, oranges, potatoes, and tomatoes to your diet may provide the potassium you require.

Shingles. Increase your intake of vitamins C and E. Liberally apply vitamin E oil to the sores.

Acne. Fifty milligrams of zinc three times a day has been helpful in some cases. For others, acidophilus, a beneficial bacterium, can clear up severe acne cases. Acidophilus is available in tablets, capsules, and liquid form.

Sore throat. Severe sore throats should be seen by a doctor to rule out strep infection. For common sore throats, however, several types of hot teas and gargles are recommended. One tea recipe calls for hot water, honey, lemon, and a dash of red pepper. One gargle cure calls for ¼ cup of vinegar in 1 cup of water, with a dash each of black pepper and salt. Heat the mixture before gargling.

Constipation. A high-fiber diet is known to be of vital importance to this condition. Make sure your daily intake includes foods like beans and peas, potatoes and carrots, whole-wheat bread, other whole-grain products, dried and fresh fruits, nuts, berries, seeds, and vegetables. Bran is a concentrated form of fiber; make sure your diet includes it.

Swimmer's ear. A few drops of warm vinegar in the ear canal can restore its proper pH balance (a measure of acidity or alkalinity) and prevent the growth of the bacteria responsible for the infection.

Warts. Try rubbing liberal amounts of vitamin E oil on the affected area. You might also want to take garlic-parsley tablets.

Yeast infections. Lactobacillus acidophilus, which is found in yogurts that contain living "viable" cultures, can help eliminate yeast infections. A similar recommendation is to eat plain yogurt, combined with doses of acidophilus pills, available at health food stores. For particularly troublesome cases, another suggested remedy is the application of plain acidophilus yogurt directly into the vagina.

Diaper rash. Liquid lecithin and vitamin E oil are both reportedly effective when commercial ointments and cornstarch fail to work.

Hemorrhoids. In severe cases see your doctor; sometimes surgery is necessary. For lesser cases, rutin tablets, a bioflavonoid found in health food stores, may help ease the pain and swelling. Rutin is found naturally in buckwheat, oranges, and lemons, but not in sufficient amounts to provide rapid relief. Sitz baths may also be used to relieve the discomfort and pain of hemorrhoids as well as speed healing.

Boils. Hot compresses can help bring the boil to a natural head, allowing it to rupture and drain. Poultices, a favorite Pennsylvania Dutch folk remedy, are made from either warm milk and flour or bread crumbs and honey. The warm mixture is spread between layers of soft fabric and placed over the boil. Vitamin E applied directly to the boil is also recommended.

Chicken pox. An oatmeal bath may often relieve the itching that accompanies chicken pox. First, cook 1 to 2 cups of oatmeal and put it into a cloth bag made from two thicknesses of an old sheet. Float this in a tub of warm water, swishing it around until the water becomes silky. Let your child play in the water, making sure the water covers all the sores.

Measurements and Equivalents

If your doctor told you that you had a cyst 2 centimeters long, would you know precisely how large that cyst is? If your prescription said to take 5 milliliters of liquid medicine before each meal, would you know how much to pour? The medical system doesn't always function with the consumer's convenience in mind. Some of us are conversant in the metric system, while others prefer to have explanations given in the plain old American system of measurements. The list below highlights metric measurements and gives you useful household equivalents.

Weights—Metric System

1 kilogram (kg)	= 1,000 grams
1 gram (g, gm)	= 1,000 milligrams
1 milligram (mg)	= 1,000 micrograms

Weight Equivalents (approximate)

65 milligrams	= 1 grain (gr.)
28.35 grams	= 1 ounce (oz.)
0.454 kilograms	= 16 ounces;
(454 grams)	1 pound (lb.)
1 kilogram	= 2.2 pounds

Linear Measurement Equivalents (approximate)

1 millimeter (mm)	= 0.04 inch (in.)
1 centimeter (cm)	= 0.4 inch
2.5 centimeters	= 1 inch
30.5 centimeters	= 1 foot (ft.)
1 meter	= 39.37 inches

Liquid Measurements—Metric System

1 liter (l)	= 1,000 milliliters (ml) or 100 centiliters or 10 deciliters
1 deciliter (dl)	= 100 milliliters or = 10 centiliters
1 centiliter (cl)	= 10 milliliters

Liquid Measurement Equivalents (approximate)

4.7 milliliters	= 1 household teaspoon (tsp.)
5 milliliters	= 1 medical teaspoon
8 milliliters	= 1 dessert spoon
15 milliliters	= 1 tablespoon (tbsp.); ½ fluid ounce
30 milliliters	= 1 fluid ounce
60 milliliters	= 1 wineglass
120 milliliters	= 1 teacup
240 milliliters	= 8 fluid ounces; 1 cup
500 milliliters	= 1+ pint
1,000 milliliters	= 1+ quart

Temperature Equivalents

Centigrade Degrees		Fahrenheit Degrees
0	Freezing	32.0
36.0		96.8
36.5		97.9
37.0		98.6
37.5		99.5
38.0		100.4
38.5		101.3
39.0		102.2
39.5		103.1
40.0		104.0
40.5		104.9
41.0		105.8
100.0	Boiling	212.0

Temperature Conversion Formulas

To convert degrees Fahrenheit to degrees Centigrade, subtract 32, then multiply by 0.555.

To convert degrees Centigrade to degrees Fahrenheit, multiply by 1.8, then add 32.

Home Injuries

Each year millions of people are injured in their homes while they are using the stairs, bathing, or operating electrical appliances, power tools, or housewares. The following tables display the approximate number of injuries reported while using certain appliances and furnishings found in most homes.

Number of Injuries Caused by Appliances

Item	Number of Injuries
Televisions	31,479
Ranges	29,273
Refrigerators	26,680
Fans	21,126
Irons	17,326
Telephones/accessories	16,004
Vacuum cleaners	14,633
Stereo/hi-fi equipment	12,770
Air conditioners	11,611
Washing machines	11,038
Heaters	10,005
Ovens (conventional)	9,860
Food slicers/choppers	9,803
Microwave ovens	7,546
Dishwashers	7,251

Number of Injuries Caused by Utensils/Housewares

Item	Number of Injuries
Knives	416,580
Drinking glasses	132,656
Tableware/accessories	116,796
Cookware	33,030
Pens/pencils	31,330
Scissors	30,787
Waste containers	25,993
Pins/needles	25,345
Manual cleaning equipment	21,890
Lightbulbs	12,163
Toothpicks/hors d'oeuvres picks	7,560
Candles, candleholders	5,254
Laundry baskets	5,173
Kitchen gadgets	4,613
Kitchen mixing bowls	4,541

Number of Injuries Caused by Tools and Hardware

Item	Number of Injuries
Nails, screws, tacks	241,859
Ladders	116,810
Hammers	50,036
Lawn mowers	47,149
Chain saws	44,619
Knives (utility)	31,944
Bench/table saws	30,091
Unpowered garden tools	27,755
Hatchets/axes	18,270
Pliers, wirecutters, wrenches	17,292
Welding equipment	15,374
Hoists, lifts, trucks	15,052
Power mowers	27,755
Portable circular saws	11,732
Handsaws	8,409

Leading Causes of Accidental Deaths

Each year more than 80,000 Americans lose their lives in various types of accidents, ranging from motor vehicle collisions to accidental poisonings. And accidents inflict another 9.1 million disabling injuries. The sad truth is that many of these deaths and injuries could be avoided if people would be more safety-conscious and take a few precautions.

On average, eliminating all accidents would add only about a year to the hypothetical U.S. life expectancy, according to the National Center for Health Statistics. But if the people who were killed in accidents had somehow been able to avoid their fatal encounters, they would have added an average twenty-three to thirty-eight years to their lives.

According to figures compiled by the National Safety Council, motor vehicle accidents account for half of all accidental deaths reported. While traffic accidents kill upwards of 40,000 people annually, the good news is that the number of traffic deaths has decreased 20 percent over the past two decades.

Accidental falls, especially by the elderly, are responsible for the next highest number of accidental deaths. As we age, bones become brittle and lose their strength, making them more susceptible to fractures. A fall that would only cause scrapes and bruises in a young person can be deadly for the elderly. Most deaths are attributed to complications associated with the fractures, such as blood clots.

The National Safety Council compiled the following list of the leading causes of accidental deaths in 1991 (the most recent year available).

1. Motor vehicle accidents (43,500 deaths)
2. Falls (anywhere) (12,200)
3. Poisoning from solids or liquids (5,600)
4. Drowning while swimming, boating, etc. (4,600)
5. Fires, burns (4,200)
6. Suffocation by an ingested object (2,900)
7. Accidents with firearms (1,400)
8. Poisoning by gases (such as carbon monoxide) (800)
9. Miscellaneous (air transport, hypothermia, accidental strangulation, etc.) (12,800)

Number of Injuries Caused by Furniture and Furnishings

Item	Number of Injuries
Tables	332,775
Beds	263,323
Chairs	234,613
Tableware and accessories	116,796
Cabinets, shelves, racks	110,099
Sofas, couches, davenports	101,004
Desks, chests, bureaus	98,084
Rugs and carpets	76,086
Furniture	48,246
Bunk beds	42,969
Bedsprings and bed frames	40,249
Benches	26,131
Waste containers	25,993
Cabinet or door hardware	22,946
Screen doors	14,358
Runners, throw rugs	11,893
Step stools	7,903

Number of Injuries Caused by Structures or Fixtures

Item	Number of Injuries
Stairs, steps	1,004,427
Floors and flooring materials	682,355
Doors	277,555
Ceilings and walls	227,618
Windows and window glass	146,114
Bathtubs and showers	139,434
Fences and fence posts	122,111
Handrails, railings, banisters	40,765
Toilets	34,593
Sinks	20,879
Fireplaces	19,651
Screen doors	14,358
Faucets and spigots	6,227

Source: 1991 National Electronic Injury Surveillance System (NEISS). National Injury Information Clearinghouse, Room 625, 5401 Westbard Avenue, Washington, DC 20207.

Accidental Poisonings and How to Prevent Them

Accidental poisonings are medical emergencies that require immediate attention and first aid. In accidental poisonings a harmful agent is swallowed, inhaled, or consumed. A poison, virtually any substance that disrupts the normal functions of the body, can also be injected or absorbed into the body's system. Even though poisonings occur frequently in the home, poisons are not restricted to household cleaners and the like. Poisons can be medications, gases and fumes, petroleum products, ingested plants, snake venom, insect stings, and food that has spoiled or been improperly prepared. Types of food poisoning include botulism (ingestion of spore-produced toxins usually found in canned foods), and salmonella and staphylococcus poisonings (ingestion of bacteria in old, spoiled, improperly prepared or handled food).

In order to effectively help a victim of an accidental poisoning, it is important to recognize the signs and symptoms of a poisoning. The victim may be unconscious, become suddenly ill, exhibit unusual behavior, or be found near a harmful chemical or poison. Other signs and symptoms include burns or stains on the victim's mouth, breath that smells like chemicals, or burns or stains around or near the victim (clothes, furniture). The victim may be vomiting or having difficulty in breathing. The victim may experience headaches, fever, chills, stomach pain, dizziness, nausea, drowsiness, loss of appetite, and pain and swelling in the throat.

Once an accidental poisoning has been recognized, the local or regional Poison Control Center (PCC) should be contacted. If the PCC number is not known, a local hospital emergency room, paramedics, or a physician can be consulted. The PCC or other contact will instruct how to handle the poisoning emergency. Be prepared to give the victim's age, the type and quantity of poison that has been taken (if known), how much time has elapsed since the ingestion of the poison, and whether or not the victim is unconscious or has vomited. When medical assistance arrives, have the poison on hand, its label or original container, and a sample of the victim's vomit for the medical personnel to examine.

The emergency procedures you can take on your own vary according to the victim's state (whether conscious or unconscious) and the type of suspected poison. For example:

- The poison can be diluted by giving the victim a glass of water or milk (only if he or she is conscious). However, if a petroleum product (kerosene, gasoline) has been ingested, the victim should be given a glass of water, not milk.
- Vomiting should be induced (but, again, only if the victim is conscious). To induce vomiting, give the victim syrup of ipecac or tickle the back of the victim's throat. In the event that the victim is unconscious or is having convulsions, the victim should not be given liquids nor be made to vomit. If the poison's identity is not known, is a strong alkali or acid (detergent, cleaner), or is a petroleum product, vomiting should not be induced. Further damage to the esophagus and throat or inhalation of harmful fumes can result if the victim is made to vomit substances with corrosive materials or strong alkalis and acids.
- The victim's breathing and heartbeat should be monitored. Keep the victim's airway open and loosen any tight or restrictive clothing. The victim can be placed on his or her side or facedown on his or her stomach, keeping the head lower in relation to the rest of the body, in order to prevent the victim from reingesting or breathing in the harmful substance.

In all cases of suspected poisonings, proper medical assistance should be sought.

The best way to prevent accidental poisonings is to make sure that harmful substances are clearly labeled as poisons and are stored and kept in a secure, locked cabinet or on a high shelf. Drugs, medicines, and harmful chemicals should be stored in child-resistant containers and kept out of the reach of children. It is also important to properly store and take careful inventory of all household products (cleaners, detergents, aerosol products, cosmetics, medications, etc.) and of outdoor/garage materials (weed and insect killers, paints, gasoline, motor oils, etc.) so that the home will be safeguarded against accidents involving poisons.

According to the American Association of Poison Control Centers (AAPCC), 92 percent of accidental poisonings occur in the home. The remaining 7 percent of poisonings occur in the workplace, health care facilities, schools, or other settings. Children younger than 13 account for 64.3 percent of all accidental poisonings, with boys having a slightly higher rate of poisoning than girls. However, after the age of 13, female teenagers and adult women have a higher incidence of accidental poisoning than their male counterparts.

The AAPCC also provided the following information on the types of substances involved in accidental poisonings as well as those substances responsible for the largest number of accidental deaths.

Substances Involved in Accidental Poisonings

Cleaning substances
Analgesics (pain relievers)
Cough and cold preparations
Plants
Venom of poisonous insects/snakes
Pesticides (including rodenticides)
Topicals (medications applied to the skin)
Hydrocarbons
Foreign bodies
Antimicrobials (antibiotics)
Sedatives/hypnotics/antipsychotics
Chemicals
Food poisoning
Alcohols
Vitamins

Substances Responsible for Accidental Deaths

Antidepressants
Analgesics
Stimulants and "street" drugs
Cardiovascular drugs
Alcohols
Gases and fumes
Asthma therapies
Chemicals
Pesticides (including rodenticides)
Cleaning substances

Source: 1992 Annual Report of the American Association of Poison Control Centers Toxic Exposure Surveillance System. AAPCC, 3800 Reservoir Road N.W., Washington, DC 20007.

Poison Control Centers Operating Toll-Free Numbers

Staffed by people who are familiar with poisons and poisonings, a poison control center functions more like a library than a hospital or treatment center. Use it as a resource for general information as well as information on prompt and proper information in an emergency.

If a number is not listed for your state, contact the hospitals serving your area.

Alabama

Alabama Poison Center
809 University Boulevard E.
Tuscaloosa, AL 35401
800-462-0800

Regional Poison Center
Children's Hospital of Alabama
1600 7th Avenue S.
Birmingham, AL 35233
800-292-6678

Alaska

Anchorage Poison Center
Providence Hospital
3200 Providence Drive
P.O. Box 196604
Anchorage, AK 99519-6604
800-478-3193

Arizona

Arizona Poison and Drug Information Center
University of Arizona
Arizona Health Science Center, Room 320-K
1501 N. Campbell Avenue
Tucson, AZ 85724
800-362-0101
602-626-6016 in Tucson

Arkansas

Arkansas Poison and Drug Information Center
University of Arkansas for Medical Sciences
College of Pharmacy, Slot 522
4301 W. Markham Street
Little Rock, AR 72205
800-482-8948

California

For counties of Fresno, Kern, Kings, Madera, Mariposa, Merced, Tulare:
Fresno Regional Poison Control Center
Fresno Community Hospital and Medical Center
Fresno and R Streets
P.O. Box 1232
Fresno, CA 93715
800-346-5922

For counties of Los Angeles, Ventura, Santa Barbara:
Los Angeles County Regional Poison Control Center
1925 Wilshire Boulevard
Los Angeles, CA 90057
800-777-6476

For counties of Imperiale, San Diego:
San Diego Regional Poison Center
University of California
San Diego Medical Center
225 Dickinson Street, MC 8925
San Diego, CA 92103-8925
800-876-4766

For San Francisco area:
San Francisco Bay Area Regional Poison Control Center
San Francisco General Hospital
1001 Potrero Avenue, Room 1E86
San Francisco, CA 94110
800-523-2222 in area codes 415, 510, and 707

For counties of Monterey, San Benito, San Luis Obispo, Santa Clara, Santa Cruz:
Santa Clara Valley Medical Center
Regional Poison Center
751 S. Bascom Avenue
San Jose, CA 95128
800-662-9886

University of California at Davis Medical Center
Regional Poison Control Center
2315 Stockton Boulevard, Room 1511
Sacramento, CA 95817
800-342-9293

For counties of Inyo, Mono, Orange, Riverside, San Bernardino:
University of California at Irvine
Regional Poison Center
101 The City Drive, Route 78
Orange, CA 92668
800-544-4404

Colorado

Rocky Mountain Poison and Drug Center
645 Bannock Street
Denver, CO 80204-4507
800-332-3070 in Colorado
303-629-1123 in Denver
800-525-5042 in Montana
800-446-6179 in Las Vegas

Connecticut

Connecticut Poison Control Center
University of Connecticut
Health Center
Farmington, CT 06030
800-343-2722

Florida

Florida Poison Information Center at Tampa General Hospital
Davis Island
P.O. Box 1289
Tampa, FL 33601
800-282-3171

Georgia
Georgia Regional Poison Control Center
Grady Memorial Hospital
80 Butler Street S.E.
Box 26066
Atlanta, GA 30335-3801
800-282-5846

Hawaii
Hawaii Poison Center
Kapiolani Memorial Center for Women and Children
1319 Punahou Street
Honolulu, HI 96826
800-362-3585

Idaho
Idaho Emergency Medical and Poison Control Center
St. Alphonsus Regional Medical Center
1055 N. Curtis Road
Boise, ID 83706
800-632-8000

Illinois
For central and southern Illinois:
Central and Southern Illinois Regional Poison Resource Center
St. John's Hospital
800 E. Carpenter Street
Springfield, IL 62769
800-252-2022

For Chicago and northeastern Illinois:
Chicago and Northeastern Illinois Regional Poison Control Center
Rush-Presbyterian-St. Luke's Medical Center
1753 W. Congress Parkway
Chicago, IL 60612
800-942-5969 in area codes 312, 708, 815, and 309

Indiana
For northern Indiana, northern Ohio, central and southern Michigan:
Indiana Poison Control Center
Methodist Hospital of Indiana
1701 N. Senate Boulevard
P.O. Box 1367
Indianapolis, IN 46206
800-382-9097

Iowa
For Iowa, Minnesota, Nebraska:
Poison Control Center
University of Iowa Hospitals and Clinics
200 Hawkins Drive
Iowa City, IA 52242
800-272-6477

Variety Club Poison and Drug Information Center
Iowa Methodist Medical Center
1200 Pleasant Street
Des Moines, IA 50309
800-362-2327

Kansas
Mid-America Poison Center
University of Kansas Medical Center
3900 Rainbow, Room B-400
Kansas City, KS 66160
800-332-6633

Kentucky
Kentucky Regional Poison Center
Kosair Children's Hospital
P.O. Box 35970
Louisville, KY 40232-5070
800-722-5725
502-589-8222 in metropolitan Louisville and southern Indiana

Maine
Maine Poison Control Center
Maine Medical Center
22 Bramhall Street
Portland, ME 04102
800-442-6305

Maryland
Maryland Poison Center
University of Maryland School of Pharmacy
20 N. Pine Street
Baltimore, MD 21201
800-492-2414

Massachusetts
Massachusetts Poison Control System
300 Longwood Avenue
Boston, MA 02115
800-682-9211

Michigan
Blodgett Regional Poison Center
Blodgett Memorial Medical Center
1840 Wealthy Street S.E.
Grand Rapids, MI 49506
800-632-2727
800-356-3232 Hearing-impaired

For Michigan, northern Ohio, northern Indiana:
Bronson Poison Center
Bronson Methodist Hospital
252 E. Lowell Street
Kalamazoo, MI 49007
800-442-4112

Minnesota

Excluding counties of Anoka, Carver, Hennepin, Scott:
Minnesota Regional Poison Center
St. Paul–Ramsey Medical Center
640 Jackson Street
St. Paul, MN 55101
800-222-1222

Missouri

For Missouri, western Illinois, and Topeka, KS:
Cardinal Glennon Children's Hospital
Regional Poison Center
1465 S. Grand Boulevard
St. Louis, MO 63104
800-366-8888

Montana
Rocky Mountain Poison and Drug Center
645 Bannock Street
Denver, CO 80204-4507
800-525-5042

Nebraska
For Nebraska and Wyoming:
The Poison Center
Children's Memorial Hospital
8301 Dodge Street
Omaha, NE 68114
800-955-9119

New Hampshire
New Hampshire Poison Information Center
Dartmouth/Hitchcock Medical Center
One Medical Center Drive
Lebanon, NH 03756
800-562-8236

New Jersey
New Jersey Poison Information and Education System
Newark Beth Israel Medical Center
201 Lyons Avenue
Newark, NJ 07112
800-962-1253

New Mexico
New Mexico Poison and Drug Information Center
University of New Mexico, North Campus
Albuquerque, NM 87131
800-432-6866
505-843-2551 in Albuquerque

New York
For all counties except Onondaga:
Central New York Poison Control Center
University Hospital at Syracuse
750 E. Adams Street
Syracuse, NY 13210
800-252-5655

Hudson Valley Regional Poison Center
Nyack Hospital
North Midland Avenue
Nyack, NY 10960
800-336-6997

For counties of Chemung, Livingston, Monroe, Ontario, Schuyler, Seneca, Steuben, Wayne, Yates:
Life Line/Finger Lakes
Regional Poison Control Center
University of Rochester Medical Center
601 Elmwood Avenue, Box 321
Rochester, NY 14642
800-333-0542

Western New York Regional Poison Control Center
Children's Hospital of Buffalo
219 Byrant Street
Buffalo, NY 14222
800-888-7655

North Carolina
Duke University Poison Control Center
P.O. Box 3007 DUMC
Durham, NC 27710
800-672-1697

For counties of Alamance, Forsyth, Guilford, Randolph, Rockingham:
Triad Poison Center
Moses H. Cone Memorial Hospital
1200 N. Elm Street
Greensboro, NC 27401-1020
800-722-2222

Western North Carolina Poison Center
Memorial Mission Hospital
509 Biltmore Avenue
Asheville, NC 28801
800-542-4225

North Dakota
North Dakota Poison Information Center
St. Luke's Hospital
720 4th Street N.
Fargo, ND 58122
800-732-2200

Ohio
Akron Regional Poison Control Center
Children's Hospital Medical Center of Akron
281 Locust Street
Akron, OH 44308
800-362-9922

Central Ohio Poison Control Center
Children's Hospital
700 Children's Drive
Columbus, OH 43205
800-682-7625

For counties of Ashtabula, Columbiana, Mahoning, Trumbull; and Lawrence and Mercer counties in Pennsylvania:
Mahoning Valley Poison Center
St. Elizabeth Hospital Medical Center
1044 Belmont Avenue
Youngstown, OH 44501
800-426-2348

Regional Poison Control System and Drug and Poison Information Center
University of Cincinnati Medical Center
231 Bethesda Avenue, M.L. 144
Cincinnati, OH 45267-0144
800-872-5111

Western Ohio Poison and Drug Information Center
Children's Medical Center
One Children's Plaza
Dayton, OH 45404
800-762-0727

Oklahoma
Oklahoma Poison Control Center
Children's Hospital of Oklahoma
940 N.E. 13th Street
Oklahoma City, OK 73104
800-522-4611
405-271-5454 in Oklahoma City

Oregon
Oregon Poison Center
Oregon Health Services University
3181 S.W. Sam Jackson Park Road
Portland, OR 97201
800-452-7165

Pennsylvania
Central Pennsylvania Poison Center
University Hospital
Milton S. Hershey Medical Center
University Drive
Hershey, PA 17033
800-521-6110

In Pennsylvania area codes 814 and 412; also for southwestern New York and northwestern Ohio:
Northwest Regional Poison Center
St. Vincent's Hospital
232 W. 25th Street
Erie, PA 16544
800-822-3232

Susquehanna Poison Center
Geisinger Medical Center
N. Academy Road
Danville, PA 17822-2005
800-352-7001

South Carolina
Palmetto Poison Center
University of South Carolina
College of Pharmacy
Columbia, SC 29208
800-922-1116

South Dakota
For South Dakota, Iowa, Minnesota, Nebraska:
McKennen Poison Control Center
800 E. 21st Street
P.O. Box 5045
Sioux Falls, SD 57117-5045
800-952-0123
800-843-0505

For South Dakota, Minnesota, North Dakota, Wyoming:
St. Luke's Midland Poison Control Center
305 S. State Street
Aberdeen, SD 57401
800-592-1889

Tennessee
Middle Tennessee Regional Poison/Clinical Toxicology Center
501 Oxford House
1161 21st Avenue S.
Nashville, TN 37232
800-288-9999 in area code 615 only

Texas
North Texas Poison Center
Parkland Hospital
5201 Harry Hines Boulevard
P.O. Box 35926
Dallas, TX 75235
800-441-0040

Utah
Intermountain Regional Poison Control Center
50 N. Medical Drive
Salt Lake City, UT 84132
800-456-7707

Virginia
For central, northern, and western Virginia:
University of Virginia Blue Ridge Poison Center
Blue Ridge Hospital, Box 67
Charlottesville, VA 22901
800-451-1428

Virginia Poison Center
Virginia Commonwealth University
Box 522, MCV Station
Richmond, VA 23298
800-552-6337

Washington
Central Washington Poison Center
Yakima Valley Memorial Hospital
2811 Tieton Drive
Yakima, WA 98902
800-572-9176

Mary Bridge Poison Center
Mary Bridge Children's Hospital
317 S. K Street
Tacoma, WA 98405-0987
800-542-6319

Seattle Poison Center
Children's Hospital and Medical Center
4800 Sand Point Way N.E.
P.O. Box C-5371
Seattle, WA 98105-0371
800-732-6985

Spokane Poison Center
St. Luke's Hospital
S. 711 Cowley
Spokane, WA 99202
800-572-5842

West Virginia
West Virginia Poison Center
West Virginia University
School of Pharmacy
3110 MacCorkle Avenue S.E.
Charleston, WV 25304
800-642-3625

Wyoming
See Nebraska; South Dakota.

Diet and Nutrition

Diet refers to the types of foods we eat, the various combinations we use for our meals or snacks. Nutrition, on the other hand, is the science and study of the food we eat and the role it plays in maintaining good health and well-being.

WHAT IS GOOD NUTRITION?

Good nutrition is eating the right types of food to adequately fuel the body for the activities of daily living. Without proper nutrition, we would not be able to work, learn, or play.

Food is the fuel that keeps the body healthy and enables all of the body's systems to function properly. That fuel is furnished by calories, the energy contained in the food we eat. Each cell must be nourished in order to perform the job for which it was designed. Without the proper nutrients, our muscles would have no strength, and we would not be able to walk, let alone run and lift heavy objects.

When we eat foods with the proper nutrients, we feel better, look better, and generally enjoy better health.

WHAT ARE NUTRIENTS?

Nutrients are substances that provide nourishment and are essential for body functions. These include carbohydrates, fats, minerals, proteins, and vitamins. Two other necessary elements, although not nutrients, are fiber and water.

Carbohydrates are a food group that includes starches and sugars, the main sources of fuel for the body. Whole grains, potatoes, cereals, pasta, dried peas and beans, vegetables, and fruits are sources of carbohydrates.

Fats provide energy for metabolism and are the building blocks of cells. There are three types of fats: saturated (found in meat and dairy products), mono-saturated (found in olive oil and avocados), and polyunsaturated (found in fish and vegetables).

Minerals are used by the body to build bones, teeth, blood, and tissue. Dairy products, dried fruits, green vegetables, lean meats, and poultry are some sources of minerals.

Proteins contain substances called amino acids that are vital to the growth and repair of all body tissue. Dairy products, dried fruits, dried peas and beans, eggs, fish, lean meats, and poultry are excellent sources of proteins.

Vitamins are nutrients that are essential for the proper functioning of the body and its components, brain, bones, muscles, nerves, and skin. Dairy products, fruits, vegetables, and whole grains are good sources of vitamins.

Fiber is undigested vegetable matter that passes through the digestive tract, and is an essential part of a healthful diet. Without a sufficient amount of fiber, the intestinal tract may not perform properly, leading to constipation, diverticular disease (inflammation of the bowel), and other disorders.

Water is essential for life, since the body is composed of about 60 percent water. Water is essential to the maintenance of the correct chemical balance of the body and contributes to blood volume.

WHAT IS A HEALTHFUL DIET?

Quite simply, a healthful diet is one that provides you with all the nutrients your body needs to maintain good health and enable you to lead an active lifestyle. However, maintaining such a diet is sometimes easier said than done.

The U.S. Department of Agriculture (USDA) recommends the following considerations when choosing a healthful and enjoyable diet: eat a variety of foods; maintain the proper weight; choose a diet low in fat, saturated fat, and cholesterol; choose a diet with plenty of vegetables, fruits, and grain products; use sugars in moderation; use salt and sodium in moderation; and if you drink alcoholic beverages, do so in moderation.

New USDA dietary guidelines divide foods into six groups and recommend that you eat a certain number of servings each day—except for the fats, oils, and sweets groups, which they suggest you use sparingly. The new food groups are (1) fats, oils, and sweets, (2) milk, yogurt, and cheese, (3) meat, poultry, fish, dry beans, eggs, and nuts, (4) vegetables, (5) fruits, and (6) bread, cereal, rice, and pasta.

These new groups are arranged in the form of a pyramid (see illustration), with the most healthful and nutritious foods serving as the base. You should care-fully eat your way up the pyramid by closely following the recommended servings.

DO YOU NEED TO LOSE WEIGHT?

At any given time, 50 million Americans are on a diet. Of these, the majority gain back the weight they've lost within two years. Being overweight is a health hazard—an especially significant factor in heart disease—yet recent studies suggest that the yo-yo effect of dieting, the losing and gaining of weight, may be as bad as weighing too much in the first place.

The Body Mass Index (BMI) combined with your waist-to-hip ratio is a good way to determine if what you weigh is bad for your health. To find your Body Mass Index, multiply your weight in pounds by 700. Divide that figure by your height in inches. Take that figure and divide by your height in inches again. This final figure is your BMI.

Now determine your waist-to-hip ratio. To do this, take a tape measure and measure the circumference of your waist at its narrowest point and with your stomach relaxed. Next, measure the circumference of your hips at their widest part, where the buttocks protrudes the most. Divide the waist measurement by the hip measurement.

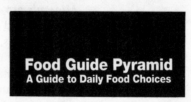

Food Guide Pyramid
A Guide to Daily Food Choices

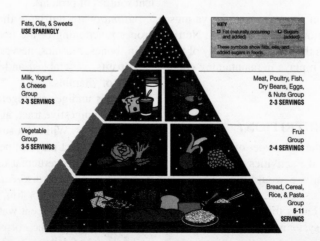

Fats, Oils, & Sweets
USE SPARINGLY

KEY
▢ Fat (naturally occurring and added)   ▢ Sugars (added)
These symbols show fats, oils, and added sugars in foods.

Milk, Yogurt, & Cheese Group
2-3 SERVINGS

Meat, Poultry, Fish, Dry Beans, Eggs, & Nuts Group
2-3 SERVINGS

Vegetable Group
3-5 SERVINGS

Fruit Group
2-4 SERVINGS

Bread, Cereal, Rice, & Pasta Group
6-11 SERVINGS

If your BMI is 25 or less, your risk for heart disease is very low to low; if your BMI is between 25 and 30, your risk is low to moderate; if your BMI is 30 or above, your risk is moderate to very high.

To get a more accurate idea of what your personal BMI means, certain risk factors must be taken into account.

High-risk factors include: being male; being under 40 with a BMI above 25; a waist-to-hip ratio greater than .80 for women or .95 for men; a sedentary lifestyle; smoking; high blood pressure; total blood cholesterol more than 200 mg/dl; HDL ("good" cholesterol) less than 35; type II (adult-onset) diabetes; personal or family history of heart disease.

Low-risk factors include: being female; waist-to-hip ratio less than .80 for women or .95 for men; regular exercise; normal blood pressure; total blood cholesterol less than 200 mg/dl; HDL more than 45; no personal or family history of heart disease.

DIET AND NUTRITION RESOURCES

American Dietetic Association
Consumer Nutrition Hotline
216 W. Jackson Boulevard, Suite 800
Chicago, IL 60606
800-366-1655

Beech-Nut Nutrition, Inc.
Checkerboard Square
Consumer Affairs, 1-B
St. Louis, MO 63164
800-523-6633

HCF Foundation
High Carbohydrate Fiber
University of Kentucky
800 Rose Street
Lexington, KY 40536
800-727-4423

Meat and Poultry Hotline
U.S. Department of Agriculture
Room 1165 S, FSIS
Washington, DC 20250
800-535-4555

Seafood Hotline
U.S. Department of Health and Human Services
Food and Drug Administration
Rockville, MD
800-FDA-4010

Exercise

Research shows the value of exercise in preventing, slowing down, or modifying various diseases and disorders. The variety of disorders linked to inactivity is both broad and startling. Here is a list of how exercise can benefit those suffering from certain ailments.

Coronary heart disease. Lack of exercise is one of eleven factors listed by the American Heart Association that predisposes a person to heart disease. Endurance (aerobic) exercises help reduce other risk factors, such as stress, high blood pressure, and elevated blood fats (high cholesterol).

Overweightness and obesity. The link between inactivity and excess fat is widely recognized. Overweightness is a factor in heart disease, diabetes, and cancer and a suspected factor in other disorders.

Low-back pain. Eighty percent of those suffering from low-back pain can find relief from their discomfort through exercises that improve the elasticity and strength of tense, weakened muscles.

Reducing emotional tension. Exercise is effective in combating tension. One research study discovered that a 15-minute walk reduced neuromuscular tension in a group of men over age 50 more effectively than a dosage of tranquilizers.

Greater productivity and job performance. Aerobic exercise improves endurance and stamina, important factors in any endeavor.

Other benefits. Research supports theories that regular exercise promotes greater self-sufficiency. Other benefits include extended youthfulness, sounder sleep, and less sexual tension.

Activities and the Calories They Consume
(for a person weighing approximately 150 pounds)

Activity	Calories Expended per Hour
Rest and light activity:	**50–200**
Lying down or sleeping	80
Sitting	100
Typing	110
Driving	120
Standing	140
Housework	180
Shining shoes	185

Fit Tips

1. **Be a discriminating exerciser. Choose exercises that are right for your body and meet your own unique exercise goals.**
2. **Know what you are doing and why you are doing it. Stretch or strengthen for a purpose and choose aerobic activities that are right for you.**
3. **Avoid unsafe exercise positions.**
4. **Make discriminate choices about exercise clothes, shoes, and equipment you select.**
5. **Make sure exercise clothes allow you freedom of movement and help keep your body at the right temperature.**
6. **Choose comfortable shoes that meet the needs of your unique feet and the activity you will be performing. If you have flat feet, you will probably need a broader-fitting shoe that will also control side-to-side movements of your feet. If you have high-arched feet, you will probably need a shoe that provides extra cushioning.**

Source: "Fit Tips," in If It Hurts, Don't Do It, by Peter Francis, Ph.D., and Lorna Francis, Ph.D. Rocklin, Calif.: Prima Publishing and Communications, 1988. 916-786-0426. $10.95.

Moderate activity:	200–350	Vigorous activity:	over 350
Bicycling (5 ½ mph)	210	Baseball pitching	360
Walking (2 ½ mph)	210	Ditch-digging (hand shovel)	400
Cleaning car	220	Ice-skating (10 mph)	400
Gardening	220	Chopping or sawing wood	400
Laundry (outside drying)	220	Bowling (continuous)	400
Canoeing (2 ½ mph)	230	Walking (4 mph)	400
Shopping	230	Tennis	420
Washing floors	230	Dancing (square or folkdancing)	430
Golf (foursome)	250	Lawn-mowing (hand mower)	430
Lawn-mowing (power mower)	250	Shoveling snow	450
Painting (house)	290	Hiking	460
Fencing	300	Waterskiing	480
Rowing a boat (2 ½ mph)	300	Hill-climbing (100 feet per hour)	490
Swimming (¼ mph)	300	Aerobics (high-impact)	500
Calisthenics	300	Basketball	500
Walking (3 ¼ mph)	300	Football	500
Badminton	350	Skiing (10 mph)	600
Horseback riding (trotting)	350	Squash and handball	600
Square-dancing	350	Dancing (rock and roll)	630
Volleyball	350	Bicycling (13 mph)	660
Roller-skating	350	Walking (6 mph)	675
Stacking heavy objects (boxes, logs)	350	Rowing (machine)	720
		Scull-rowing (race)	840
		Running (10 mph)	900

DANGERS AND RISK FACTORS IN EXERCISE

Exercise is certainly beneficial, but risk factors and possible dangers must be taken into account. It is important to make aerobic conditioning a priority before attempting anaerobic activities. Aerobic exercises are low-intensity activities such as swimming, biking, and walking that are sustained for 15 to 30 minutes. These activities help build heart and lung capacity, while anaerobic (without oxygen) activities do not. Anaerobic exercises include weight training and sprinting and unplanned activities such as shoveling snow or running to catch a bus.

It is dangerous to participate in anaerobic activities if the heart is not conditioned or if high blood pressure is a factor.

Exercise precautions should be practiced for those suffering from asthma and other allergies. Asthmatics need to monitor their exercise program, especially in cold weather. Exercise-induced anaphylaxis is a condition brought on by exercising in hot or cold weather. It begins with an all-over itch and can progress to hives, choking, fainting, and gastrointestinal problems. One-half of those who get this condition have asthma, hay fever, or eczema, and two-thirds have a family history of allergy. Food allergy plays a role. Often the anaphylaxis manifests itself only after the afflicted person exercises after having eaten a food he or she is sensitive to, such as shellfish.

Even without a predisposition toward allergies, special care should be taken when exercising in hot or cold weather. In the summer months, avoid exercising during the heat of the day. Wearing white, loose-fitting clothing helps to deflect sunlight, and clothing made of 100 percent cotton absorbs perspiration and keeps you cool. Drink fluids, but not ice-cold ones. Drinks such as Gatorade are formulated to replenish the salts your body loses during physical activity.

If proper precautions are taken, you can avoid heatstroke and heat exhaustion. Heatstroke is a medical emergency requiring immediate treatment by a doctor. Its symptoms include faintness, dizziness, headache, nausea, and a feeling of giddiness. The body temperature is usually 104 degrees or higher, the pulse is rapid and the skin flushed.

Heat exhaustion takes longer to develop than heatstroke. Its symptoms include weakness, heavy perspiration, nausea, and a feeling of giddiness. Treatment is resting in a cool place and drinking cool liquids.

In winter, dress warmly and dryly, wearing multiple layers to help trap warm air. And layering helps you to add or take off clothing as conditions change; the layering of hands and feet is a protection against frostbite, too. Drink fluids, but avoid alcohol. If hypothermia (body temperature of 95 degrees or below) develops, get to a warm shelter and drink warm liquids. Early symptoms of hypothermia include shivering and a sense of euphoria.

Note: Those with cardiopulmonary problems may develop angina (chest pains) more quickly in the cold.

EXERCISE AND INJURIES

The RICE program is recommended for those times a muscle is pulled or a bruise occurs. RICE is an acronym for rest, ice, compression, and elevation.

1. Rest: Stop exercising. Continued motion forces more blood into damaged tissue.
2. Ice: Apply ice to the injury to minimize swelling. Use ice continuously for the first 15 minutes, then apply it 10 minutes on and 10 minutes off during the first hour. Don't apply the ice directly to your skin. Put a towel between your skin and the ice.
3. Compression: Wrap an elastic bandage over the injury to help prevent local fluid accumulation. The wrap should be snug but not so tight as to cut off circulation.
4. Elevation: If the injury is to one of the extremities, raise the injured area above chest level. This helps to facilitate blood flow back into the heart and prevents accumulation of fluid due to gravity.

Consult a doctor after beginning RICE if you suffer traumatic injury to a joint, severe pain, pain in a joint or bone persisting more than 2 weeks, or infection.

EXERCISE INSTRUCTORS

When choosing an exercise program, it is important the instructor is qualified. In recent years aerobic exercises done to music have risen in popularity. Several organizations offer highly respected instructor-certification programs. These include IDEA Foundation, Aerobics and Fitness Association of America (AFAA), and American College of Sports Medicine (ACSM). All these programs require certification in CPR. Some require a written exam in physiology and anatomy in addition to the ability to put together a sound exercise routine. The American College of Sports Medicine requires a bachelor's degree or equivalent in an allied health field as well.

Current research suggests that middle-impact aerobics and step aerobics eliminate the stress of low- and high-impact aerobic programs. Step aerobics emphasize a series of up/down patterns on steps ranging from 4 to 12 inches in height. For people who like to jump, high-impact programs can be practiced if care is taken to land with a minimum of stress, bending knees slightly and coming down on the ball of the foot and then rolling onto the heel.

A number of celebrities and exercise gurus have produced exercise videos that can be bought or rented for home use. It is best to check with your doctor before beginning a home exercise program.

Immunizations

Preventing serious illnesses and diseases is better than having to fight them once they strike. We know from historical accounts that smallpox was a scourge until the latter part of the twentieth century. Thankfully, the first steps toward defeating this dreaded disease began with early experimentation with immunization, the use of vaccines to prevent disease.

Vaccines have now been developed that prevent such childhood diseases as influenza, mumps, measles, polio, and whooping cough. Prior to vaccinations, most of these diseases were like rites of passage for every child—a part of growing up.

Vaccinations, however, are not unique to children. Some are intended for adolescents, young adults, and senior citizens. (See the accompanying immunization chart.)

Vaccines help the body build immunity to the viruses that cause many diseases. Once a sufficient number of antibodies have built up, the body, in a manner of speaking, "remembers" the invader and, if it should reenter the body, the antibodies are there to meet it and destroy it. Such is the role of immunizations.

For information on immunizations, contact your local or county health department.

WHAT IS IMMUNIZATION?

Immunization is the injection or implantation of a vaccine, microorganism, antibody, or antigen into the body in order to protect against, treat, or study a disease. A vaccine is a preparation introduced into the body to prevent a disease by stimulating the body's own natural antibodies against it and building the body's immunity to, or inability to contract, that disease.

HOW IS IT ACCOMPLISHED?

Vaccines are generally administered via injection, either intramuscularly (IM) or subcutaneously (under the skin—SC). Some, such as the polio vaccine, can be received orally. Vaccines contain a very small amount of the disease—just enough for the body to recognize it and produce antibodies to defend against it. Once the antibodies are produced, the body is protected from the disease, even when exposed to it. Some vaccinations, such as that for tetanus and diphtheria (Td), require repeated doses, or "boosters," at scheduled intervals (for example, the Td booster is recommended every ten years) to ensure the body's defense against it.

WHY IS IMMUNIZATION IMPORTANT AT DIFFERENT AGES?

According to the U.S. Department of Health and Human Services, successful childhood immunization alone will not necessarily eliminate specific disease problems. Many of the remaining outbreaks of specific diseases now occur in older adolescents and adults. Persons who escaped natural infection or were not immunized with vaccines and toxoids against diphtheria, tetanus, measles, mumps, rubella, and poliomyelitis may be at risk of these diseases and their complications. (See the reference chart on the next page for more immunization information).

Immunizations for Infants, Children, Adolescents, and Adults

Vaccine	Schedule and Dosage	Age Groups	Precautions/Contraindications	Special Considerations
Tetanus-diphtheria toxoid (Td)	2 doses IM 4 weeks apart; 3rd dose 6–12 months after 2nd dose; booster every 10 years	Adolescents beginning at 14–16 years and all adults	Except in the 1st trimester, pregnancy is not a contraindication. History of a neurologic reaction or immediate hypersensitivity reaction following a previous dose. Such individuals should not be given further routine or emergency doses of Td for 10 years.	Tetanus prophylaxis in wound management
Diphtheria, pertussis, tetanus (DPT)	The Centers for Disease Control and Prevention recommends infant DPT immunization be given on the following schedule: 6 weeks of age; 10–14 weeks; 14–22 weeks; 9–17 months; and again between 4 and 6 years of age.	Infants from 2 months to 6 years of age	Encephalopathy within 7 days of administration of previous dose of DPT. Fever of 105° or greater within 48 hours following first vaccination. Collapse or shocklike state within 48 hours of receiving prior dose of DPT. Seizures within 3 days of receiving a prior dose of DPT. Persistent, inconsolable crying lasting for at least 3 hours, within 48 hours of receiving a prior dose of DPT	The events or conditions listed as precautions, although not contraindications, should be carefully reviewed. The benefits and risks of administering a specific vaccine to an individual under the circumstances should be considered. If the risks are believed to outweigh the benefits, the immunization should be withheld; if the benefits are believed to outweigh the risks (for example, during an outbreak or foreign travel), the immunization should be given. Whether and when to administer DPT to children with proven or suspected underlying neurologic disorders should be decided on an individual basis.

Immunizations for Infants, Children, Adolescents, and Adults

Vaccine	Schedule and Dosage	Age Groups	Precautions/Contraindications	Special Considerations
Live-Virus Vaccines				
Measles live-virus vaccine	1 dose SC; no booster	All infants at 15 months of age. All adults born after 1956 without documentation of live vaccine on or after 1st birthday or physician-diagnosed measles or laboratory evidence of immunity; persons born before 1957 are generally considered immune. Susceptible travelers	Known altered immunodeficiency (hematologic and solid tumors; congenital immunodeficiency; and long-term immunosuppressive therapy). Pregnancy; immunocompromised persons; history of anaphylactic reactions following egg ingestion or receipt of neomycin	Measles, mumps, rubella vaccine (MMR) is the vaccine of choice if recipients are likely to be susceptible to rubella and/or mumps as well as to measles. Persons vaccinated between 1963 and 1967 with a killed-measles vaccine, followed by live vaccine within 3 months or with a vaccine of unknown type, should be revaccinated with live-measles-virus vaccine. Measles vaccination may temporarily suppress tuberculin reactivity. If testing cannot be done the day of MMR, the test should be postponed for 4–6 weeks.
Mumps live-virus vaccine	1 dose SC; no booster	All infants at 15 months of age. All adults, particularly males, believed to be susceptible can be vaccinated. Most adults can be considered immune	Known altered immunodeficiency (hematologic and solid tumors; congenital immunodeficiency; and long-term immunosuppressive therapy). Pregnancy; immunocompromised persons; history of anaphylactic reaction following egg ingestion or receipt of neomycin	MMR is the vaccine of choice of recipients who are likely to be susceptible to measles and rubella as well as to mumps.

SC—subcutaneous (under the skin).   ID—intradermal (into the skin).   IM—intramuscular.   I.U.—international unit.

Immunizations for Infants, Children, Adolescents, and Adults

Vaccine	Schedule and Dosage	Age Groups	Precautions/Contraindications	Special Considerations
Live-Virus Vaccines (cont.)				
Rubella live-virus vaccine	1 dose SC; no booster	All infants at 15 months of age. Indicated for adults, both male and female, lacking documentation of live vaccine on or after 1st birthday or laboratory evidence of immunity, particularly women of childbearing age and young adults who work or congregate in places such as hospitals, colleges, and the military. Susceptible travelers	Known altered immunodeficiency (hematologic and solid tumors; congenital immunodeficiency; and long-term immunosuppressive therapy). Pregnancy; immunocompromised persons; history of anaphylactic reaction following receipt of neomycin	Women pregnant when vaccinated or who become pregnant within 3 months of vaccination should be counseled on the theoretical risks to the fetus. The risk of rubella-vaccine-associated malformations in these women is so small as to be negligible. MMR is vaccine of choice of recipients who are likely to be susceptible to measles or mumps as well as to rubella.
Smallpox vaccine (vaccinia virus)	None for the general civilian population	There are no indications for the use of smallpox vaccine in the general civilian population.	There are no indications for the use of smallpox vaccine in the general civilian population.	Laboratory workers involved with orthopox virus or in the production and testing of smallpox vaccines should receive regular smallpox vaccinations.

SC—subcutaneous (under the skin).   ID—intradermal (into the skin).   IM—intramuscular.   I.U.—international unit.

Immunizations for Infants, Children, Adolescents, and Adults

Vaccine	Schedule and Dosage	Age Groups	Precautions/Contraindications	Special Considerations
Live-Virus Vaccines (cont.)				
Yellow fever live, attenuated virus (17D strain)	1 dose SC 6 days to 10 years before travel; booster every 10 years	Selected persons traveling or living in areas where yellow fever infection exists	Although specific information is not available concerning adverse effects on the developing fetus, it is prudent on theoretical grounds to avoid vaccinating pregnant women unless the individual must travel to areas where the risk of yellow fever is high. Immunocompromised persons; history of hypersensitivity to egg ingestion	Some countries require a valid International Certification of Vaccination showing receipt of vaccine. If the only reason to vaccinate a pregnant woman is an international requirement, efforts should be made to obtain a waiver letter.
Live-Virus and Inactivated-Virus Vaccines				
Polio vaccines: killed-poliovirus vaccine (IPV); live-poliovirus vaccine (OPV)	IPV preferred for primary vaccination; 3 doses SC 4 weeks apart; a 4th dose 6–12 months after 3rd; for adults with a completed primary series and for whom a booster is indicated, either OPV or IPV can be given. If immediate protection is needed, OPV is recommended.	Infants from 2 months to 15 months old, then again between ages 4 and 6. Persons traveling to areas where wild poliovirus is epidemic or endemic and certain health-care personnel	Although there is no convincing evidence documenting adverse effects of either OPV or IPV on the pregnant woman or developing fetus, it is prudent on theoretical grounds to avoid vaccinating pregnant women. However, if immediate protection against poliomyelitis is needed, OPV is recommended. OPV should not be given to immunocompromised individuals or to persons with known or possibly immunocompromised family members; IPV is recommended in such situations.	Although a protective immune response to IPV in the immunocompromised individual cannot be assured, the vaccine is safe and some protection may result from its administration. There is a theoretical risk that the administration of multiple live-virus vaccines (OPV and MMR) within 30 days of one another if not given on the same day will result in a suboptimal immune response.

SC—subcutaneous (under the skin).   ID—intradermal (into the skin).   IM—intramuscular.   I.U.—international unit.

Immunizations for Infants, Children, Adolescents, and Adults

Vaccine	Schedule and Dosage	Age Groups	Precautions/Contraindications	Special Considerations
Inactivated-Virus Vaccines				
Hepatitis B (HB) inactivated-virus vaccine	2 doses IM 4 weeks apart; 3rd dose 5 months after 2nd; need for boosters unknown	Adults at increased risk of occupational, environmental, social, or family exposure	Data are not available on the safety of the vaccine for the developing fetus. Because the vaccine contains only noninfectious hepatitis B surface antigen particles, the risk should be negligible. Pregnancy should not be considered a vaccine contraindication if the woman is otherwise eligible.	The vaccine produces neither therapeutic nor adverse effects on HBV-infected persons. Pre-vaccination serologic screening for susceptibility before vaccination may or may not be cost-effective depending on costs of vaccination and testing and on the prevalence of immune individuals in the group.
Influenza vaccine (inactivated whole-virus and split-virus) vaccine	Annual vaccination with current vaccine. Either whole- or split-virus vaccine may be used.	Adults with high-risk conditions, residents of nursing homes or other chronic care facilities, medical care personnel, healthy persons over 65	Although no evidence exists of maternal or fetal risk when vaccine is given in pregnancy because of an underlying high-risk condition in a pregnant woman, waiting until the 2nd or 3rd trimester, if possible, is reasonable. History of anaphylactic hypersensitivity to egg ingestion	

SC—subcutaneous (under the skin).   ID—intradermal (into the skin).   IM—intramuscular.   I.U.—international unit.

Immunizations for Infants, Children, Adolescents, and Adults

Vaccine	Schedule and Dosage	Age Groups	Precautions/Contraindications	Special Considerations
Inactivated-Virus Vaccines (cont.) Human diploid cell rabies vaccine (HDCV) (inactivated, whole-virion and subvirion)	Preexposure prophylaxis: 2 doses 1 week apart; 3rd dose 3 weeks after 2nd; if exposure continues, booster doses every 2 years, or an antibody titer determined and a booster dose given if titer inadequate. All postexposure treatment should begin with immediate cleansing of the wound with soap and water. (1) Persons who have (a) previously received postexposure prophylaxis with HDCV, (b) received recommended IM preexposure series of HDCV, (c) received recommended ID preexposure series of HDCV in the U.S., or (d) have a previously documented rabies antibody titer considered adequate: 2 doses HDCV, 1 ml IM, 1 each on days 1 and 3. (2) Persons not previously immunized as above: HRIG 20 I.U./kg body weight, half infiltrated at bite site if possible, remainder IM; and 5 doses HDCV, 1 ml IM, 1 each on days 1, 3, 7, 14, 28	Veterinarians, animal handlers, certain laboratory workers, and persons living in or visiting countries for longer than 1 month where rabies is a constant threat	If there is substantial risk of exposure to rabies, preexposure vaccination may be indicated during pregnancy. Corticosteroids and immunosuppressive agents can interfere with the development of active immunity. History of anaphylactic or Type III hypersensitivity reaction to previous dose of HDCV	Complete preexposure prophylaxis does not eliminate the need for additional therapy with rabies vaccine after a rabies exposure. The Food and Drug Administration has not approved the ID use of HDCV. Recommendations for the ID use of HDCV are currently being discussed. ("Rabies Prevention—United States, 1984," *MMWR*, vol. 33 [1984] 393–402, 407–8.) The decision for postexposure use of HDCV depends on the species of biting animal, the circumstances of biting incident, and the type of exposure (i.e., bite, saliva contamination of wound, etc.). The type of and schedule for postexposure prophylaxis depends upon the person's previous rabies vaccination status, or the result of previous or current serologic test for rabies antibody. For postexposure prophylaxis, HDCV should always be administered IM, *not* ID.

SC—subcutaneous (under the skin).   ID—intradermal (into the skin).   IM—intramuscular.   I.U.—international unit.

Immunizations for Infants, Children, Adolescents, and Adults

Vaccine	Schedule and Dosage	Age Groups	Precautions/Contraindications	Special Considerations
Inactivated-Bacteria Vaccines				
Cholera vaccine	Two .5 ml doses SC or IM or two .2 ml doses ID 1 week to 1 month apart; booster doses .5 ml IM or .2 ml ID every 6 months	Travelers to countries requiring evidence of cholera vaccination for entry	No specific information on vaccine safety during pregnancy. Use in pregnancy should reflect actual increased risk. Persons who have had severe local or systemic reactions to a previous dose	1 dose generally satisfies International Health Regulations. Some countries may require evidence of a complete primary series or a booster dose given within months before arrival. Vaccination should not be considered as an alternative to continued careful selection of foods and water.
Meningococcal polysaccharide vaccines (bivalent A and C and tetravalent A, C, W135, and Y)	1 dose in volume and by route specified by manufacturer; need for boosters unknown	Travelers visiting areas of a country that are recognized as having epidemic meningococcal disease	Pregnancy, unless there is substantial risk of infection	

SC—subcutaneous (under the skin).   ID—intradermal (into the skin).   IM—intramuscular.   I.U.—international unit.

Immunizations for Infants, Children, Adolescents, and Adults

Vaccine	Schedule and Dosage	Age Groups	Precautions/Contraindications	Special Considerations
Inactivated-Bacteria Vaccines (cont.)				
Plague vaccine	3 IM doses; 1st dose 1 ml; 2nd dose .2 ml 1 month later; 3rd dose .2 ml 5 months after 2nd; booster doses .2 ml at 1–2- year intervals if exposure continues	Selected travelers to countries reporting cases, for whom avoidance of rodents and fleas is impossible; all laboratory and field personnel working with *Yersinia pestis* organisms possibly resistant to antimicrobials, those engaged in *Y. pestis* aerosol experiments or in field operations in areas with enzootic plague where regular exposure to potentially infected wild rodents, rabbits, or their fleas cannot be prevented	Pregnancy, unless there is substantial and unavoidable risk of exposure; persons with known hypersensitivity to any of the vaccine constituents (see manufacturer's label); patients who have had severe local or systemic reactions to a previous dose	Prophylactic antibiotics may be recommended for definite exposure whether or not the exposed person has been vaccinated.

SC—subcutaneous (under the skin).   ID—intradermal (into the skin).   IM—intramuscular.   I.U.—international unit.

Immunizations for Infants, Children, Adolescents, and Adults

Vaccine	Schedule and Dosage	Age Groups	Precautions/Contraindications	Special Considerations
Inactivated-Bacteria Vaccines (cont.)				
Pneumococcal polysaccharide vaccine (23 valent)	1 dose, booster not recommended	Adults who are at increased risk of pneumococcal disease and its complications because of underlying health conditions; older adults, especially those age 65 and over, who are healthy	The safety of vaccine in pregnant women has not been evaluated; it should not be given during pregnancy unless the risk of infection is high. Previous recipients of any type of pneumococcal polysaccharide vaccine should not receive another dose of vaccine.	
Typhoid vaccine	Two .5 ml doses SC 4 or more weeks apart; booster .5 ml SC or .1 ml ID every 3 years if exposure continues	Travelers to areas where there is a recognized risk of exposure to typhoid	Severe local or systemic reaction to a previous dose. Acetone killed and dried vaccines should not be given ID.	Vaccination should not be considered as an alternative to continued careful selection of foods and water.
Hemophilus influenzae type b (Hib)	Several doses should be administered until immunity has been established.	All infants beginning at 2 months of age	Since Hib vaccines have been available for only a short period of time, there are few reported side effects and/or long-term effects.	

SC—subcutaneous (under the skin).   ID—intradermal (into the skin).   IM—intramuscular.   I.U.—international unit.

Immunizations for Infants, Children, Adolescents, and Adults

Vaccine	Schedule and Dosage	Age Groups	Precautions/Contraindications	Special Considerations
Live-Bacteria Vaccine				
BCG	1 ID or SC dose	Prolonged close contact with untreated or ineffectively treated active tuberculosis patients; groups with excessive rates of new infection in which other control measures have not been successful	Pregnancy, unless there is unavoidable exposure to infective tuberculosis; immunocompromised patients	In the United States tuberculosis control efforts are directed toward early identification, treatment of cases and preventive therapy with isoniazid.
Immune Globulins				
Immune globulin (IG)	Hepatitis A prophylaxis: Preexposure: 1 IM dose of .02 ml/kg for anticipated risk of 2–3 months; IM dose of .06 ml/kg for anticipated risk of 5 months; repeat appropriate dose at above intervals if exposure continues. Postexposure: 1 IM dose of .02 ml/kg given within 2 weeks of exposure Measles prophylaxis: .25 ml/kg IM (maximum 15 ml) given within 6 days after exposure	Hepatitis A prophylaxis: household and sexual contacts of persons with hepatitis A; travelers to high-risk areas outside tourist routes; staff, attendees, and parents of diapered attendees in day care center outbreaks Measles prophylaxis: exposed susceptible contacts of measles cases	Measles prophylaxis: IG should *not* be used to control measles.	Hepatitis A prophylaxis: For travelers IG is not an alternative to continued careful selection of foods and water. Frequent travelers should be tested for hepatitis antibody. Measles prophylaxis: IG given within 6 days after exposure can prevent or modify measles. Recipients of IG for measles prophylaxis should receive live-measles vaccine 3 months later.

SC—subcutaneous (under the skin).   ID—intradermal (into the skin).   IM—intramuscular.   I.U.—international unit.

Immunizations for Infants, Children, Adolescents, and Adults

Vaccine	Schedule and Dosage	Age Groups	Precautions/Contraindications	Special Considerations
Immune Globulins (cont.)				
Hepatitis B immune globulin (HBIG)	.06 ml/kg IM as soon as possible after exposure followed by a 2nd dose 1 month later except when HB vaccine is given	Following percutaneous or mucous membrane exposure to blood known to be positive for hepatitis B surface antigen (HBsAG); following sexual exposure to or a bite from a person with acute HBV or an HBV carrier		IG (.06 ml/kg) may be used if HBIG is not available.
Tetanus immune globulin (TIG)	250 units IM	Part of management of nonclean, nonminor wound in a person with unknown tetanus toxoid status, with less than 2 previous doses, or with 2 previous doses and a wound more than 24 hours old		

SC—subcutaneous (under the skin).   ID—intradermal (into the skin).   IM—intramuscular.   I.U.—international unit.

Immunizations for Infants, Children, Adolescents, and Adults

Vaccine	Schedule and Dosage	Age Groups	Precautions/Contraindications	Special Considerations
Immune Globulins (cont.)				
Rabies immune globulin, human (HRIG)	20 I.U./kg, up to half infiltrated around wound, remainder IM	Part of management of rabies exposure in persons lacking a history of recommended preexposure or postexposure prophylaxis with HDCV		Although preferable to be given with the 1st dose of vaccine, can be given up to the 8th day after the 1st dose of vaccine
Varicella-zoster immune globulin (VZIG)	Persons who weigh up to 50 kg (110 lbs.): 125 units/10 kg IM; persons who weigh more than 50 kg: 625 units	Immunocompromised patients known or likely to be susceptible with close and prolonged exposure to a household contact case or to an infectious hospital staff member or hospital roommate		

SC—subcutaneous (under the skin).   ID—intradermal (into the skin).   IM—intramuscular.   I.U.—international unit.

Physical Disabilities

Physical disabilities, which limit or destroy the body's ability to accomplish certain physical functions, result from birth defects, heredity, illness, and injuries.

Some physical disabilities can be overcome through operations, physical therapy, or the use of specialized medical equipment such as wheelchairs, artificial limbs, and hearing aids (see section 7, "Medical Equipment"). The negative effects of some disabilities have been mitigated by construction of such public facilities as wheelchair ramps and elevators.

In recent years, with the help of scientific research and social support organizations, physically disabled people have learned to cope with or even overcome their handicaps and, thus, enjoy activities, such as working and schooling, that were not available to earlier victims of disabilities. With the signing into law of the Americans with Disabilities Act in July 1990, many previously closed avenues of employment, transportation, public accommodation, and communication were opened to those with physical disabilities.

TYPES OF PHYSICAL DISABILITIES

The causes associated with *blindness and impaired vision* include birth defects, disease, aging, injury, medication, allergies, poor circulation, and pollution.

Cataracts and glaucoma, the two leading causes of blindness in the U.S., can be treated with surgery. Diabetic retinopathy—damage to the retina caused by circulatory problems—is a common complication of diabetes and another leading cause of blindness, but it can be treated effectively when diagnosed early. Another cause of vision loss is retinitis, or inflammation of the retina; it can occur as a complication of disease or a result of heredity.

Retinitis pigmentosa, an inherited condition, results in the degeneration of the retina, severely limiting vision until only a narrow field of vision remains. Often called tunnel vision, because the field of vision narrows, it results in greatly decreased peripheral vision. There is no effective treatment; however, newer optic devices have been employed that widen the field of vision. Although they are somewhat effective, they carry a rather prohibitive price tag of around $2,000 for the unit.

Cerebral palsy is a neuromuscular disorder resulting from damage to the brain during its development before or after birth. Victims exhibit spastic movements of the arms and legs, speech impairments, and jerky movements of the torso and head. Treatment includes medication to reduce spasticity, physical and speech therapy, and sometimes family support therapy. The last is important because victims, while not impaired intellectually, may develop emotional problems.

Various types of equipment have been designed to meet the needs of individuals affected by neuromuscular disorders, including wheelchairs, walkers, and special gripping tools.

Deafness and hearing loss result from disease, exposure to loud noises, injury, circulation problems, tumors, use of certain drugs, and, in rare cases, heredity. Deafness can also occur in infants whose mothers took drugs or had German measles during the pregnancy. Gradual loss of hearing also occurs naturally as a result of aging.

Those suffering from hearing loss can understand words if a speaker stands close and speaks loudly and clearly. Types of impairments include presbycusis, conduction deafness, and central deafness. Presbycusis occurs when changes in the inner ear lead to a difficulty in understanding speech and sensitivity to loud noises. Conduction deafness results from blockage or poor mechanical movement in the outer or middle ear. Central deafness is caused by damage to the nerve centers in the brain and results in poor understanding of speech.

Hearing impairments can be treated with hearing aids, medication, flushing of the ear, and, in some cases, surgery. A surgical procedure called stapedectomy is recommended for people suffering from deafness caused by otosclerosis, in which the stapes, a sound-conducting bone of the inner ear, becomes immobilized and incapable of amplifying sound. The stapes is replaced by a Teflon or wire substitute that restores the vibration of the tiny bones of the inner ear. The operation is 98 percent successful.

Many telecommunications devices, especially a form of teletype, can be modified to help the deaf communicate effectively.

Multiple sclerosis (MS) is a chronic degenerative disease of the central nervous system and brain that strikes women twice as often as men. First symptoms include difficulty in movement, eye disorders, speech slurring, tremors, difficulty walking, and mood changes. Onset usually occurs between the ages of 20 and 40. The cause is unknown, but scientists suspect an allergy or virus might cause the body to attack its own tissue.

MS attacks and subsides, allowing the body time to heal between attacks. Succeeding attacks usually grow more severe. Heat, physical exertion, trauma, and other illnesses can sometimes trigger new attacks of MS. Rest and steroids are prescribed to control attacks, but most treatments are aimed at management of symptoms and at rehabilitation. Canes can be used to relieve a weary or weak leg. A plastic foot-drop orthosis (a splint inside the shoe) offers support for weak feet that won't bend. Knee braces, crutches, and wheelchairs can be recommended in severe cases.

Muscular dystrophy (MD), a hereditary, incurable, and very often fatal disease, causes the muscles to wither and waste away, sometimes resulting in the complete loss of muscle strength. An estimated 250,000 Americans have MD, about two-thirds of them children.

MD usually affects voluntary muscles, those over which we have conscious control. The disease causes muscle cells and fibers to die, rendering the muscle incapable of contracting and moving a joint.

MD is actually a group of nine types of disorders ranging in severity and age of onset. The most severe type, Duchenne's dystrophy, occurs only in males, usually starts by the age of 5, leads to complete paralysis, and is fatal. At the other end of the range is distal dystrophy, which does not cause paralysis or death. The other types of MD are Becker's (late onset, slow progression), facioscapulohumeral (atrophy of the muscles of the face, shoulder girdle, and arm), limb-girdle (weakness in the shoulder or pelvic girdle), myotonic (atrophy of the muscles of the face and neck), and congenital (present at birth).

In 1991 researchers discovered that the drug prednisone appears to slow down—but not stop or reverse—the weakening of the muscles caused by Duchenne's dystrophy. But because of the drug's side effects, including weight loss, high blood pressure, and softening of bone tissue, few doctors prescribe prednisone.

Exercise helps MD patients strengthen their remaining muscle fiber and their unaffected muscles, but does not slow or stop the advance of the disease. Improved facilities, especially elevators and ramps, and better equipment (such as powered wheelchairs) enable many MD patients to continue attending school and working.

Strokes kill about 200,000 people a year in the U.S. and leave another 300,000 with some form of disability or paralysis. Strokes result from ischemia, or the sudden interruption in blood flow to the brain. Causes include high blood pressure, stress, hardening of the arteries, smoking, obesity, diabetes, and the use of some oral contraceptives. Prevention involves the treatment or relief of those factors. Aspirin is given to inhibit formation of blood clots; blood-clotting drugs may be prescribed.

Paralysis caused by a stroke often occurs on one side of the body. Slurred speech, double vision, drooping eyelids, loss of vision in one eye, and an enlarged pupil in one eye also result from strokes, and often persist. Rehabilitation, involving physical therapy and sometimes speech, occupational, and nutritional therapy, is most effective when begun as soon as possible after a stroke. Passive therapy may be necessary; a therapist moves paralyzed limbs to maintain their potential for motion. The goal is for the patient to regain as much function as possible in damaged areas.

Women's Health

For all women, regular gynecological exams and cancer tests are vital. Some problems arise with the onset of menstruation, others not until the beginning of sexual activity, and still others immediately pre- and postmenopausally.

THE PELVIC EXAM

During the first part of the pelvic exam, the external genitals are checked for lumps, sores, inflammation, and hormone status. The labia (vaginal lips) are separated to check the urinary and vaginal openings. A woman who has given birth may be asked to cough or bear down—this allows the doctor to check for any relaxation in the supporting tissues of the vagina.

A speculum is then placed inside the vagina and opened. When opened, the speculum holds open the vaginal walls and allows the doctor to see the vagina and cervix and to check for inflammation, infection, scars, or other abnormalities. A Pap test is performed at this time; it is the scraping of a few cells from the cervix to examine them for cancer.

The doctor then performs a bimanual pelvic exam by placing two fingers in the vagina and the other hand on the abdomen to check the size, shape, and general health of the uterus and ovaries. Oftentimes the doctor will then place a finger in the rectum to check the rectum and surrounding structures.

PAP SMEAR

The Pap smear is named for Dr. George Papanicolaou, who developed this method of cancer screening. Random cells from the cervix and vagina are smeared onto a glass slide and examined under a microscope. False-negative results are possible when abnormal cells are present but not scraped off during the procedure. False-positives are possible when suspicious cells are found that represent infection rather than cancer. Abnormal Pap smears must be confirmed with a repeat smear.

Pap smear results can be divided into these categories:

Class I. Normal smear. Repeat at intervals suggested by your doctor.

Class II. "Atypical" cells indicative of inflammatory changes, but no evidence of cancerous changes. Any infection should be treated and the Pap smear should be repeated in 6 to 12 months.

Class III. "Suspicious" cells present indicating dysplasia and sometimes "carcinoma in situ" (surface cancer). Inflammation, if present, should be treated and the Pap smear repeated after the next menstrual period.

Class IV. Positive. Cells strongly suggest cancer. A biopsy is always taken to confirm or rule out cancer.

Class V. Positive. Cancer cells present. Following biopsy, surgery or other treatment is carried out immediately.

In 1988 a new method of classifying pap smears, known as the Bethesda System, was developed by the National Cancer Institute at a workshop in Bethesda, Maryland. According to an interlaboratory comparison by the College of American Pathologists, the system has been generally well received by professional societies and in laboratory practice. Its elements are:

1. A statement of whether the specimen is adequate for diagnosis.
2. A general categorization of the diagnosis as "normal" or "other." The latter category can include anything from a bacterial or viral infection to cell abnormalities.
3. A descriptive diagnosis detailing the findings under "other." (When the older terminology is used, dysplasia and carcinoma in situ may be combined as cervical intraepithelial neoplasia [CIN], with a subscript indicating degree of severity.)

The newer system separates all degrees of dysplasia (and CIN) into two categories:

a. Low-grade squamous intraepithelial lesions (includes mild dysplasia as well as CIN 1).
b. High-grade squamous intraepithelial lesions (includes moderate dysplasia, CIN 2, severe dysplasia, carcinoma in situ, and CIN 3).

What Is Involved in Diagnosis and Treatment?

These days, most doctors follow a clearly abnormal or suspicious Pap smear with a cervical biopsy. They remove bits of tissue from the cervix, using a magnifying instrument called a colposcope that allows the doctor to view the lesions that need to be sampled. (Don't agree to a "blind" or random biopsy. Their inaccuracy makes them worthless.)

A biopsy can take from 5 to 20 minutes. Since the cervix has few nerve endings, the procedure causes little pain and is done without anesthesia. During the biopsy, bits of tissue about the size of half a grain of rice are removed, using an instrument that resembles a paper punch.

During the colposcopy, your gynecologist should also scrape cells from the cervical canal, a procedure called endocervical curettage. Both the biopsy and curettage tissue samples are sent to a pathologist for microscopic examination. Both colposcopic-directed biopsy and endocervical curettage are considered to be highly accurate ways of diagnosing cervical cancer.

If your biopsy confirms cell changes that you and your doctor decide require treatment, you may have several choices.

Most forms of dysplasia on the surface of the cervix are removed in a simple, in-office procedure that usually requires no anesthesia. The lesions are destroyed by freezing in a procedure called cryosurgery or vaporized with a carbon dioxide laser. Some doctors burn lesions with a cauterizing probe, but since this older treatment can hurt and is more likely to cause the cervical canal to constrict with scar tissue, it's less frequently used nowadays.

If your abnormal cells extend into the cervical canal, your doctor should suggest a cone biopsy (or conization), a surgical procedure in which a cone-shaped piece of tissue is removed from the center of the cervix. Since it is surgery and involves general anesthesia and a hospital stay, it is usually reserved for cases in which invasive cancer needs to be ruled out.

Cone biopsies can interfere with a woman's fertility and with her ability to carry a child to term. You can get more than one conization, but most doctors don't like to do more than two. (They'll recommend a hysterectomy.) If you do have a "cone," you should be followed closely enough in the future so that if abnormal cells return, they are detected early enough to be removed by cryosurgery or laser.

In select cases, conization can be used instead of hysterectomy as a treatment for very early invasive cancer, called microinvasive cancer. To be eligible for this treatment:

- Your cancer should not have penetrated more than 3 mm into the tissue of the uterus. (Some doctors will do conizations up to 5 mm penetration, but this carries more risk that the cancer has spread.)
- The cone should remove all the cancer, not just part of it.
- The edges of the cone should show that the cancer has not spread into the blood vessels.

Simple hysterectomy is still the "treatment of choice" for microinvasive cancer. That's because, even though a fairly large number of women have been treated by conization for this condition, no large, long-term study has followed them to see if the procedure really does cure their cancer.

GYNECOLOGICAL PROBLEMS AND TREATMENTS

Below is a brief discussion of the common gynecological problems and treatments. See "Gynecology and Obstetrics" in section 3, "Healing Arts," for a more detailed look at these and others.

Prolapse of the uterus. The dropping of the uterus into the vagina due to weakening of muscles during childbirth. This can often cause discomfort. Weakness of the bladder often happens at the same time, leading to inability to hold urine, especially during the stress of coughing, sneezing, or moving of bowels. Minor cases can be controlled by insertion of a pessary, a device similar to a diaphragm that helps hold the uterus in place. Uterine resuspension is a surgery performed to reposition the prolapsed uterus.

Cystitis and urethritis. Frequent and painful urination. This often means bacterial infection. A urine culture can determine the cause. This is treated with antibiotics. The problem can often be relieved by wearing cotton underwear and by wiping from front to back after a bowel movement.

Infected Bartholin's glands. Glands on either side of the vaginal opening may become blocked. This is extremely painful. The treatment is heat, antibiotics, and cutting into the pus to drain it.

Vaginitis. Inflammation of the vagina that produces severe itching and burning of the vulva. The most common kinds of vaginitis are caused by the infectious agents Herpes Simplex Type II, Trichomonas vaginalis, and Monilia or Candida albicans. This is a great nuisance and some women are very vulnerable to it. This is treated with antifungal creams or suppositories. Again, cotton underwear, along with keeping the area dry, can help ward off this infection.

Pelvic inflammatory disease (PID). IUDS are often associated with serious pelvic infections. The condition itself is bacterial and is often secondary to gonorrhea or chlamydia. Treatment is antibiotics or, in some cases, a combination of antibiotics and surgery.

Toxic shock syndrome. Illness during menstruation characterized by fever, severe diarrhea, aching, and a rash. This can lead to death. It may be brought on by use of super tampons and is believed to be caused by staph bacteria. When using tampons, change them frequently, never leaving them in for more than 4 hours.

Endometriosis. Disease in which tissue from the lining of the uterus implants outside the uterus, usually on the ovaries. This occurs most often in women 20 to 35 years of age. It can cause painful periods and pain during intercourse and can lead to infertility. Hormonal treatments are often useful. Conservative surgery to remove the endometrial implants may be needed.

Ovarian cysts. Not painful unless they twist or hemorrhage into the abdominal cavity. These are usually removed surgically.

Cancer of the cervix. Most common cancer of the reproductive tract. Symptoms may be regular bleeding, bleeding after intercourse, pain, and weight loss. If detected early, the cure rate of preinvasive cancer is almost 100 percent.

Cancer of the uterus. About three-fourths of cases of cancer of the lining of the uterus are found in women past the menopause. Primary symptom is bleeding. Treatment is removal of the uterus, fallopian tubes, and ovaries. Radiotherapy may follow. Outlook is favorable.

Cancer of the ovary. Fourth leading cause of death from cancer among women. Sixty percent of malignant tumors occur in women aged 40 to 60, 20 percent in women under 40, and the remainder in women over 60. Treatment consists of drug therapy, X-ray therapy, or surgery.

BREAST CANCER

A woman's risk of breast cancer normally begins in her late 20s and steadily increases throughout the remainder of her life. A family history of the disease is the most significant predictor. The highest incidence occurs among women with two or more close maternal relatives who have had breast cancer. A strong family history of this disease also points to the possible early development of breast cancer. Other risk factors include obesity, lack of pregnancies, pregnancy late in life, and an unusually long menstrual life. The mammogram is the number-one method of detecting breast cancer.

Breast cancers start predominantly in the cells lining the ducts inside the breast. The cancer can spread in three ways: local extension, lymphatics, and blood vessels. In local extension, the cancer cells break through the membranes surrounding the ducts and attack the connective and supportive tissue of the breast. Lymphatic spreading refers to the invasion of cancer cells into the lymph nodes. The nodes most often affected are the underarm (axillary) lymph nodes. The nodes above the clavicle bone can also be affected. In some cases the cancer can spread to nodes far away from the original cancer site. The blood vessels can be invaded by breast cancer cells. In these cases, cancers can spread to other parts of the body.

Breast cancers are classified by stages I, II, or III. Stage I cancers are the least invasive, stage III the most invasive. Breast cancer treatment is determined individually. The three main types of treatment are surgery, radiation, and chemotherapy.

Total mastectomy—also called modified radical mastectomy—is the most common surgical procedure. This operation removes all breast tissue but does not disturb the underlying pectoral muscles.

Radical mastectomy, which includes the removal of the pectoral muscles, is used only if warranted by circumstances. In total mastectomy, the lymph nodes in the armpit are dissected to see if cancer has spread, but nodes are not automatically removed as they are in radical procedure. Surgery with or without removal of lymph nodes is often followed by radiation treatment.

The lumpectomy is a newer surgical operation in which the tumor itself is removed along with bordering tissue that seems to be cancer-free. Comparative studies of women who have had lumpectomies plus radiotherapy and those who have had total mastectomy show approximately equal survival rates.

New research suggests that scheduling a woman's breast cancer surgery according to her menstrual cycle may increase her chances of survival. At least seven studies have shown that women who have their cancers removed during the week or so following ovulation are two to four times more likely to be alive and cancer-free ten years later than those operated on at other times.

Recent studies also suggest that sunshine may offer some protection against breast cancer. Death rates from the disease are higher (about 30 deaths per 100,000 women) in the northern United States, while they are lowest (about 20 deaths per 100,000) in the sunny South. Researchers link the association to vitamin D.

Mammogram

"Should I have a mammogram?" is a typical question. The answer is debatable. If you can feel a suspicious lump in your breast, a *diagnostic* mammogram definitely is in order. If a *screening* mammogram is recommended to detect tiny lumps, you may want to think twice, depending on your age and your risk for breast cancer.

Mammograms are X rays of the breast that can detect lumps while they are still too small to be felt by hand. Because they can find cancer at an early stage, mammograms are considered to be lifesavers, at least for some women.

If you are age 50 to 65, the benefits seem to be clear. Studies done around the world show that regular screening mammograms can cut the death rate from breast cancer by 30 percent or more in these women. Few doctors dispute those findings.

But among women aged 40 to 49 or younger, the benefit of regular screening mammograms is much less clear, and the risk of undergoing unnecessary treatment (or not getting treatment you need) because of inaccurate results is much greater.

The American Cancer Society and the National Cancer Institute (along with nine other medical organizations, four of them professional radiology groups) endorse screening mammograms at one- or two-year intervals for women aged 40 to 49. They base their recommendations primarily on the findings of two studies.

One, the Breast Cancer Detection Demonstration Project, was cosponsored by the American Cancer Society and the National Cancer Institute. It enrolled 280,000 women aged 35 to 70 to have mammographic screening for five years during the 1970s. The findings of the project suggested that, at eight years' follow-up, mammographic screening did contribute to longer survival rates for women aged 35 to 49 years with breast cancer. This study has been criticized, though, because it did not include a control group (a similar group of women who did not get mammograms to compare with the group having mammograms). Instead, it used the general population as a comparison group.

The other study, the Health Insurance Plan of Greater New York, did have two distinct groups: women having mammograms and women not having mammograms. This study included some 28,000 women who were in their 40s when the study started in 1963. After eighteen years of follow-up, this study found sixteen fewer deaths from breast cancer in those women who had mammograms than in those who did not. The problem with this finding, critics say, is that the difference in death rates between the two groups is not considered "statistically significant." That is, the difference is small enough to have occurred by chance.

To complicate matters further, more recent studies in Sweden and the Netherlands have found mammography screening beneficial only for women older than age 50.

And in some of those studies, a few women who had mammograms while in their 40s were *more* likely to have died of breast cancer than those who did not have mammograms. That finding may be a statistical fluke; it may mean that younger women's breasts are more sensitive to radiation than older women's; or it may mean that breast cancer in younger women tends to be more aggressive, so that, in some women, even early detection does not prevent death from breast cancer. Researchers still don't know the answers.

Two large professional groups, the American College of Surgeons and the American College of Physicians, have declined to recommend routine mammography screening for women aged 40 to 49. (They *do* recommend breast self-exam and a yearly exam by a doctor.) And a committee of cancer experts for the U.S. Department of Health and Human Services (which oversees the National Cancer Institute) recently issued its own recommendations. They say that the only women under age 50 for whom mammography screening may be wise are those with a family or personal history of the disease.

"We decided the potential benefit to women in this age group isn't strong enough to make general screening recommendations," says Steven Woolf, M.D., the task team's scientific adviser. "Even the most accurately done mammograms produce inaccurate results if you are dealing with someone whose risk is low enough, as it is in most women younger than age 50."

So discuss the issues with your doctor before you agree to a mammogram. Chances are your gynecologist will recommend you have a screening mammogram if you're 35 or older. If you're at risk for breast cancer because your mother or a sister developed breast cancer at a young age, you may be asked to have a mammogram as early as age 25. You may also be asked to have a mammogram before you begin hormone replacement therapy, or if you're age 35 or older and about to begin taking oral contraceptives, to make sure the hormones aren't fueling a hidden tumor.

If you have lumpy breasts, as many women do, your gynecologist may recommend a mammogram to make sure cancer isn't hidden among the benign, fluid-filled cysts. He or she may also recommend a mammogram if you detect new lumps that don't fit the normal cyclical pattern of lumpy breasts. You and your doctor may decide a mammogram is appropriate in your case.

What Do Mammograms Show?

Mammograms show the nature of a lump. If a lump is cancerous, its borders tend to be irregular or its shape poorly defined or spindle-shaped. A benign lump usually has well-defined, clear borders that are not irregular. Mammograms do not show cancer per se, so any positive mammogram needs to be confirmed by a biopsy, and many negative mammograms are also confirmed by biopsy. Screening mammograms that show a suspicious lump are usually followed up by a more extensive set of diagnostic mammograms before a biopsy is performed.

The Risk of False-Positive Results
A false-positive result, in this case, means the mammogram detects a lump that, on biopsy, proves to be nonmalignant. It means you will have an unnecessary breast biopsy. Unfortunately, the smaller a cancer, the more it may resemble a benign lump, so there is always a trade-off between finding early cancer and tolerating a certain number of benign biopsies. As mammography improves in its ability to detect even tiny specks, many doctors believe the number of biopsies done on nonmalignant lumps is increasing.

False-positive rates vary with a woman's age and with a doctor's diagnostic skill. It's been calculated that a woman who has yearly mammograms from age 40 to 50 has a 1 in 3 chance of having a false-positive result sometime during that time. A woman having yearly mammograms from age 55 to 65 has a 20 percent chance. And women younger than age 40 have very high rates of false positives.

The Risk of False-Negative Results
A false-negative result, in this case, means the mammogram shows no signs of cancer when cancer is actually present. It can mean you fail to continue to do breast self-exam, or discount lumps that do appear. It can lead to a delay in treatment. It's the reason the American College of Radiology warns doctors not to rely on mammograms alone to make a diagnosis. They should be combined with a physical examination of the breast and, if necessary, a biopsy.

Studies have shown that in 10 to 15 percent of cases of known breast cancer, the mammogram does not reveal it. In women under 50, whose breast tissue is more dense, making it harder to detect abnormalities, a mammogram is only 60 to 70 percent accurate in picking up a cancer. Mammograms are least likely to detect cancer in the small, dense breasts of young women who have never had children.

Biopsy
These days, virtually every doctor does a mammogram before he does a biopsy. The mammogram gives him information about the size, location, and possible spreading of the lump that allows him to do a more accurate biopsy. It may also reveal additional lumps.

In only a few cases can a mammogram clearly show a tumor that does not need to be biopsied. These include a tumor called a calcified fibroadenoma and two kinds of fatty tumors, lipomas and fibroadenolipomas. Mammograms that indicate cysts can often be confirmed by ultrasound or needle aspiration (see sidebar) rather than biopsy.

What Happens If You Don't Have a Mammogram?
Is your doctor willing to wait and watch for a month or so to see if the lump disappears on its own? He may, especially if you are a premenopausal woman with fibrocystic condition. But these days he may have you sign a release form that includes details of his findings and recommendations to you, and your refusal. It doesn't mean he won't still be your doctor. It means that, in a court of law, he won't be held responsible if your lump turns out to be cancer.

Other Diagnostic Tests Available
Ultrasound (which uses the echoes from sound waves to visualize lumps) can save you from an unnecessary biopsy by clearly showing your lump to be a cyst. It is 96 to 100 percent accurate at distinguishing fluid-filled cysts from solid tumors, making it better than either physical examination or mammography. It is most often used for small or deep lumps that cannot be felt by hand and are hard to pinpoint for needle aspiration. It's not a substitute for mammography, though, since it can miss small solid lumps.

Both thermography (which supposedly shows tumors as "hot spots") and transillumination (shining a bright light through the tissue of the breast) are considered unreliable at detecting lumps.

How Do I Need to Prepare for a Mammogram?
Ask your doctor to schedule your mammogram during the first week following your period, when your breasts are least tender. (During the X ray, they are briefly compressed.) Some breast screening centers also caution against wearing deodorant, since some contain minerals that can show up on the X ray.

Breast Biopsy
Your doctor may be able to do a biopsy without cutting into your breast. He can use a needle to draw out

The Risk of Developing Breast Cancer from the X-Ray Radiation

These days, most doctors agree that mammograms done at a reputable breast imaging center are relatively safe. That is, your risk of developing breast cancer as a result of being exposed to the radiation needed to make the mammogram is minimal. (It's been calculated to be comparable to the risk of getting lung cancer after smoking a quarter of a cigarette.)

Doctors do have some considerations, though. No one knows a woman's lifetime risk of developing cancer as a result of regular radiation exposure from yearly mammograms starting at age 40. It's thought that younger women's breasts are more sensitive to radiation exposure than older women's breasts, but no one really knows what that means in terms of an increased risk of radiation-induced cancer. (It's been estimated that about 1 in 25,000 women who begin mammography screening at age 40 will develop radiation-induced breast cancer sometime during her life.)

Studies have shown, too, that radiation dosages can vary widely among mammography centers, and among different kinds of breast X-ray techniques. That's why it's important to ask the radiology technician (who takes the X rays) what your radiation absorbed dose (rad) will be. Compare that figure with those below, which the National Council on Radiation Protection says provide good image quality at low dosage:

- For xeromammography (a technique where the image is produced as a positive, on paper) .8 rad per two-view exposure
- For film screen with grid (a Venetian-blind-type device that improves image quality when X-raying large breasts) .8 rad per two-view exposure
- For film screen without grid, .2 rad per two-view exposure

fluid and cells from the lump (fine-needle aspiration) or to punch holes into the lump and withdraw several cores of tissue (core-needle biopsy). He's more likely to do a needle aspiration or needle biopsy if the lump appears to be benign, is close to the surface of the skin, and can be felt by hand. It's also possible to do a needle biopsy on small lumps found deeper in the breast, but this requires more skill and special equipment to pinpoint the lump during the biopsy. Needle biopsy is relatively quick and painless. The doctor may first numb the skin where he'll insert the needle. It does not require general anesthesia.

Your doctor may want to do an "open," or excisional, biopsy, making about a 1½-inch cut in the breast, then removing the entire lump, or, if it's large, a section of the lump. This kind of biopsy is easier than needle biopsy to do accurately. It's also the choice of women who want their lump removed even if it isn't cancer. Unless the lump is large or very deep in the breast, open breast biopsy is now generally done under local anesthesia on an outpatient basis.

Open biopsy does leave a scar. Although you can negotiate with your doctor as to where he'll cut (he can hide the scar under your breast or around your nipple), most doctors prefer to cut directly over the lump. They believe that if the lump does prove to be cancerous, a direct route makes it easier to see just where the tumor has spread. Some also think it's less likely to spread cancer cells to other areas of the breast.

What Does the Biopsy Show?
The biopsy will determine, once and for all, whether or not the lump is cancer. A biopsy sample taken and read correctly is highly accurate. An open biopsy is slightly more accurate than a needle biopsy.

The Breast "Disease" That's Normal— and When It's Not

Many women's breasts become swollen, tender, and lumpy premenstrually, as hormones stimulate fluid buildup in the breasts' milk glands and ducts. These lumps are usually symmetrical and in both breasts. They feel like masses of peas, grapes, or even golf balls. Doctors used to call this condition fibrocystic "disease," a misnomer since the condition is so common it's considered normal. It's now called fibrocystic changes or condition.

When should you see a doctor about lumpy breasts? If you discover a solitary, dominant, or asymmetric lump or thickening, one that doesn't seem to fit the pattern of fibrocystic changes. (Regular breast self-exam will help you make this distinction.) In this case, you may need a mammogram, ultrasound, fine-needle aspiration (which will collapse the lump if it's a cyst), or a biopsy.

Most forms of fibrocystic condition are harmless. But two forms are thought to carry about five times the risk of developing breast cancer. They are atypical lobular hyperplasia and atypical ductal hyperplasia. (Both are an excessive growth of abnormal cells in the breast's glandular tissue.) Either of these abnormalities is found in 2 to 4 percent of the biopsies done on women with fibrocystic disease.

Only a biopsy can determine if you have either one of these conditions. If you do, your doctor will follow you more closely than usual. He may want to see you every 6 months and do a yearly mammogram. He will do further biopsies only if you develop a solitary or dominant mass. Generally, hyperplastic masses are not removed. That's because hyperplasia tends to spread throughout the breast, through the network of milk ducts, making it impossible to remove it all unless you remove the entire breast. In women with a strong family history of early breast cancer (especially a mother or sister who had premenopausal cancer in both breasts), some doctors will suggest just that. But most doctors consider prophylactic mastectomy unnecessary and, in most cases, irresponsible.

If you have one of these high-risk forms of hyperplasia, with no family history of early breast cancer, your chances of developing breast cancer are still only 1 in 5. Those are pretty good odds. If your family history is grim, your odds may go as high as 50 percent.

Any diagnosis of a precancerous condition should be based on a biopsy, not a mammogram, family history, or "guessing." And keep in mind that even when a biopsy is done, not all doctors agree what cell changes are precancerous, or even cancerous.

HORMONE REPLACEMENT THERAPY

One of the most mind-boggling health decisions a menopausal woman faces is whether or not to take supplemental hormones to replace those no longer being produced by her aging ovaries.

Hormone replacement therapy (HRT) includes estrogen, a major female hormone that has many functions, including thickening the uterine lining. It often includes progesterone (usually a synthetic mix of progestins), a hormone that counterbalances estrogen, making the uterine lining shed each month as menstrual bleeding. And HRT occasionally includes androgen, male hormones that women, too, naturally produce in small amounts, and which are thought to influence sex drive, energy levels, and mood.

Why is the decision so confusing?

- Because even among well-done studies published in prestigious medical journals, results are sometimes contradictory or hard to interpret, especially when it comes to hormone replacement therapy and heart disease or breast cancer.
- Because many questions about HRT remain unanswered, especially questions about the benefits and risks of long-term use of estrogen-progestin combinations. (Unfortunately, in the past, and especially with female hormone treatments like DES, today's "medical miracle" has backfired to become tomorrow's horror story.)
- Because even doctors sometimes have trouble separating hype from fact, especially when it comes to estrogen's alleged ability to preserve youthful good looks and ensure a sense of well-being. As the National Women's Health Network points out in its booklet *Taking Hormones and Women's Health,* some doctors continue to claim estrogen relieves depression and keeps skin "young-looking" even after a National Institutes of Health Conference in 1979 found no evidence of those effects.

And drug companies are constantly marketing their various hormone replacement products—and funding research in this area—because it means big bucks.

Despite this confusion, most gynecologists apparently think hormone replacement benefits outweigh the risks, especially for women who have had their ovaries removed. At a recent national conference on menopause, speakers' pro-hormone comments got rounds of applause from an audience of mostly doctors, points out editor Mary Ann Napoli in *HealthFacts,* a newsletter published by the Center for Medical Consumers, New York City.

And some 4-million-plus women do choose to take hormones. They either simply follow their doctor's recommendation, or, wisely, they get more information and decide that, for them, the benefits of HRT outweigh the risks, including, they hope, those risks that are still unknown.

So how can you decide if HRT is for you? Well, you can start by asking your gynecologist a few questions:

Why Do You Think I Should Have HRT?
If you are bothered by hot flashes (upper body flushing usually followed by heavy sweating) or vaginal atrophy (thinning and dryness, which can cause painful intercourse), HRT definitely can help.

Estrogen *is* FDA-approved to treat both these very uncomfortable symptoms of menopause. It controls hot flashes in about 2 weeks of use, provided the dose is adequate. Vaginal atrophy is more slowly resolved, depending on the severity of the condition. Without hormone treatment, hot flashes usually eventually lessen, but vaginal atrophy only gets worse. (If it is a woman's only menopausal symptom, vaginal atrophy is often treated with an estrogen-containing topical cream for as long as a woman remains sexually active.)

Although anecdotal evidence, and some studies, suggest estrogen therapy can help such other symptoms as urinary incontinence, vaginal infections, muscle and joint pains, mood swings, and insomnia, it is *not* FDA-approved to treat these symptoms. "But women whose hot flashes disturb their sleep do sometimes find that estrogen helps relieve symptoms of anxiety or depression," says Isaac Schiff, M.D., chief of Vincent Memorial Gynecology Service at Massachusetts General Hospital.

You may decide to try HRT to see if it helps relieve any of these symptoms, but keep in mind that you may need other, or additional, treatment.

Even if you aren't bothered by hot flashes, vaginal atrophy, or other symptoms, your gynecologist may recommend HRT. His reasons? To help prevent osteoporosis (porous, fragile bones) and heart disease, the number-one killer of women after they reach the age of menopause.

Admittedly, these both seem like good reasons to take HRT, but is the evidence of benefits strong enough to subject yourself to the possible risks of prolonged hormone treatment? That's something you'll have to decide for yourself.

Does HRT Really Prevent Osteoporosis?
Studies are clear that one component of HRT, estrogen, can help slow the rapid bone loss that occurs after menopause. Some doctors think that even just a few years of hormone therapy will help prevent osteoporosis; others believe HRT must be long-term. In fact, it's anyone's guess how long HRT must be given to avoid bone fractures. Treatment may well depend on the individual woman. It's also unclear what role progestins play in preventing osteoporosis.

What Is My Risk for Osteoporosis?

Some doctors may frighten women by telling them just how widespread osteoporosis is among older women. One in every two postmenopausal women are "diagnosed" with osteoporosis. The truth is, though, that even experts don't agree on exactly how much bone mass a woman has to lose before she should be diagnosed as having osteoporosis. And ways of measuring bone loss are notoriously inaccurate.

What really counts is not osteoporosis itself, but what it can lead to—fractures, says Joseph Melton III, M.D., of the Mayo Clinic's Department of Medical Statistics and Epidemiology. "That's where you have real numbers and can come up with real risks."

According to his statistics, a white woman's lifetime risk of a hip or wrist fracture is about 15 percent; of a spinal fracture (fracture of a vertebra), about 33 percent. (Most black women are heavier-boned, and so are less likely to break bones as they age.)

Your own risks may be much greater than this, though, if you:

- Undergo menopause, including surgical menopause (removal of the ovaries), before age 45
- Are light-skinned
- Are small-boned and thin
- Are inactive
- Are a heavy drinker or smoker

Why Can't I Just Take Calcium?

Researchers now know that extra calcium is useless in older women who are estrogen-deficient. Their bodies can't use calcium to build up bones unless estrogen is present. Women who do take estrogen, though, may reap additional bone-building benefits from a calcium-rich diet and regular exercise.

Does HRT Really Help Prevent Heart Disease?

Here evidence is less clear. It is known that one component of HRT, estrogen, raises blood levels of beneficial high-density lipoproteins (HDLs), a type of cholesterol that lowers the risk for heart disease. Naturally occurring estrogen may protect younger women from heart disease. After menopause, when estrogen levels drop, women's risk for heart disease climbs.

But there are also nagging suspicions about estrogen's role in blood clotting and strokes. Estrogen is generally not prescribed to women who've had thrombophlebitis (blood clots in the veins) or a stroke

or who are heavy smokers. Most doctors, though, think that these negative effects are related to the dosage of estrogen. "Clotting problems have been seen in women who take birth control pills containing high dosages of estrogen. But they have not been seen in women taking postmenopausal estrogen, which contains much lower dosages," Dr. Schiff says.

Most studies do show that postmenopausal women who take estrogen (without progestins) are less likely to develop heart disease than women who do not take estrogen. One often-cited study, done in 1985 by researchers at Harvard Medical School, showed that estrogen use cut in half the risk for both fatal and nonfatal heart attacks.

There is one major problem with at least some of these studies, though, contends Sadja Greenwood, M.D., author of *Menopause Naturally* (Volcano, Calif.: Volcano Press, 1989).

"The studies ignore the fact that doctors tend to suggest estrogen to their healthier patients, and to discourage the use of hormones in women who already have risk factors such as obesity, high blood pressure, chest pains, diabetes, or heavy use of tobacco or alcohol," Dr. Greenwood says. So it's possible estrogen's beneficial effects are exaggerated in these studies.

"To get around this bias, what really needs to be done is a totally randomized study, where the women who get estrogen (and those who don't) are selected entirely by chance, not by a doctor," Dr. Schiff says. Such a study has yet to be done.

To make things even more confusing, researchers now think that progestins, the often-added second component of HRT, may negate at least some of estrogen's heart-protecting effects. Progestins are known to lower good HDLs and to raise bad LDLs and triglycerides, fatty particles that tend to stick to blood vessel walls and block arteries.

Studies have yet to be done that look at the development of heart disease in women taking long-term estrogen-progestin combinations.

A National Institutes of Health study, the Postmenopausal Estrogen/Progesterone Intervention (PEPI), currently in progress, may help answer questions about the effects of estrogen-progestin combinations on the incidence of heart disease in postmenopausal women. It will be several years before results are available. Until then, it's up to you and your doctor to decide.

Heart disease is certainly more of a risk in women who undergo early menopause, either naturally or by

The "Medicalization" of Menopause

If you decide to take hormone replacement therapy, you will (and should) be closely monitored by your doctor. That means yearly visits that include:

- A full medical history
- A full physical examination
- Questions about compliance (if you've been taking the hormones as prescribed, or if not, how you've been taking them)
- A breast examination by the doctor
- A mammogram (breast X rays that can detect early cancer)
- A Pap smear (a sampling of cervical cells which is checked under a microscope for precancerous signs)
- A blood pressure check
- Blood tests to determine cholesterol and other blood fat levels
- An endometrial biopsy if you are taking estrogen without progestins (and still have a uterus)
- Possibly, an ultrasound examination of the ovaries

What all this means is that as long as you are taking HRT, you are going to be a patient. Some women may find that reassuring (and it's responsible—no doctor should give HRT without close follow-up). Other women dislike it, both personally and politically. They believe menopause is being treated as a "disease" rather than part of the natural aging process.

Is menopause so bad? A recent study by Sonja McKinlay, Ph.D., of the American Institutes for Research, Cambridge, Massachusetts, compared women undergoing natural menopause with those undergoing surgically induced menopause (removal of the ovaries). She found significant differences between the two groups.

Asked to assess their overall health, the women undergoing surgically induced menopause were one and one-half times more likely to report two or more chronic conditions such as arthritis, hypertension, diabetes, or allergic diseases. They were also the main consumers of medical services and prescription drugs. Twenty-five percent of the women undergoing surgically induced menopause used hormones, compared to 5 percent of the other menopausal women, and they used more tranquilizers and sleeping pills. Overall, they used medications at twice the rate of other women their age. They also reported 80 percent more surgery for benign breast disease than other women.

"In general, women who go through a natural menopause don't see it as a health problem. The majority go through it without going near a doctor," Dr. McKinlay says. "It's a relative minority who have symptoms severe enough that they see a health professional."

having their ovaries removed. And many doctors do prescribe HRT for these women.

But doctors seem to be reluctant to prescribe HRT to women with other major risk factors for heart disease: obesity, smoking, high blood pressure, high cholesterol, or a history of blood clotting. "There is no evidence to show that HRT is harmful in these women," Dr. Schiff says. "Some of those doctors may not know the data; others fear that if their patient is at risk for heart disease, and gets into trouble, that they will blame the hormones, and sue the doctor."

One point on which all doctors agree: Stopping smoking, losing weight, exercise, and eating low-fat foods are surer ways than HRT to cut your risk for heart disease.

What's Known About the Cancer Risks of HRT?

Doctors say that women who decline to take replacement hormones often do so because of a fear of cancer. The unknown possible risks, perhaps, scare women most.

It's clear that estrogen, taken alone, in any form, increases a woman's risk of developing cancer of the endometrium (uterine lining) from four to fifteen times. Estrogen causes the uterine lining to grow and thicken, which eventually can lead to abnormal cell growth that can become cancerous.

That's why progestins are added during therapy. Progestin allows the uterine lining to break down and be shed as menstrual fluid. The monthly shedding prevents cancer from developing. Women who take progestins run less risk of endometrial cancer than women who take no replacement hormones.

One possible problem with this treatment, though, is that doctors sometimes don't prescribe progestins for the number of days each month that is necessary to ensure complete shedding of endometrial lining, which reduces the risk of endometrial cancer to zero. In the past, it was common practice to prescribe progestins for 10 days. "Some doctors still do that, even though studies show that women need to be taking progestins 12 to 14 days," warns Robert Rebar, M.D., professor of obstetrics and gynecology at the University of Cincinnati College of Medicine.

And some doctors don't prescribe progestins at all. "Currently, only about half of menopausal women taking estrogen also take progestins," Dr. Rebar says. Women who've had hysterectomies may account for some of those, and for them, estrogen alone is safe.

Others are reluctant to continue to have periods, or develop premenstruallike symptoms from progestins, and so their doctors don't include progestins, or the women stop taking the hormone.

Any woman whose uterus is intact, who's taking estrogens alone, in any form, needs to be carefully monitored for signs of endometrial hyperplasia (cell overgrowth), a condition that can lead to endometrial cancer. Some doctors do an annual endometrial biopsy, a quick office procedure that removes a bit of tissue from the uterine lining.

Problems with both cyclic estrogen-progestin therapy, and estrogen alone, are one reason more and more doctors are experimenting with a combination of continual estrogen-progestin therapy, which may provide the benefits of both estrogen and progestins without monthly periods. The problem with this therapy, though, admits Wulf Utian, M.D., director of obstetrics and gynecology at University McDonald Women's Hospital in Cleveland, is that no one knows if it creates a risk for endometrial cancer. "Most of us think the excess risk is eliminated, but that has not yet been proven," he says. (Most doctors do not do a yearly endometrial biopsy when using this therapy.) And no one knows its effect on blood lipids and heart disease.

The risks for breast cancer are much less clear. Most researchers agree that, theoretically, both estrogen and progestins could cause breast cancer, since they stimulate the growth of cells in the breast. (And breast cancer can be induced by estrogen in laboratory animals.) But most researchers think this effect is weak in older women, whose breast tissue cells are fairly inactive.

Most of the few studies done show no connection between hormone replacement therapy (mostly estrogen) and breast cancer.

But a study by Swedish researchers, published in the August 3, 1989, *New England Journal of Medicine,* did show a connection. Women who took replacement hormones had a 10 percent greater risk of developing breast cancer than women who had not taken hormones. That's a very slight risk.

Several higher-risk groups stood out: women who took estrogen for six years or more; and women who took more potent forms of estrogen not generally used in the U.S.

More important to U.S. women, those who took estrogen-progesterone combinations for more than six years appeared to have 4.4 times the average risk of developing breast cancer. A major problem with this part of the study, though, was that there were only ten women in this group, a number much too small to provide a statistically reliable result, according to experts reviewing the study for the *Harvard Medical School Newsletter*. Their consensus: The Swedish study highlights the need for more research, especially in the area of long-term estrogen/progestin therapy.

What Other Risks Does HRT Have?

Estrogen use has been associated with an increase in gallstones and gallbladder pain. Women who use replacement estrogen are more likely to have their gallbladder removed than women who do not use estrogen. Obesity, high cholesterol, and diabetes are additional risk factors for gallbladder problems.

Replacement estrogen can cause flare-ups of some conditions that may have improved as you've gotten older. It can cause fibroid tumors or endometriosis implants to grow. It can also cause painful, lumpy breasts.

Hormone replacement treatment can be complex. Various formulations and dosages abound, in pills, wafers dissolved under the tongue, suppositories, vaginal creams, estrogen-releasing skin patches, even injections. Your doctor needs to know his or her way around this pharmaceutical maze in order to be able to prescribe what's best for you. Different dosages may be given to women just beginning menopause, perhaps still menstruating irregularly, than to older women who completed menopause years ago. Women with risk factors like diabetes or cancer need to be monitored very closely. And different dosages may be needed depending on the symptoms being treated, or the side effects a woman experiences as a result of treatment. Those are all good reasons to make sure you're seeing a doctor who knows what he or she is doing, whether it's your regular gynecologist or an endocrinologist.

Do I Have to Decide Now?

Don't think that just because your doctor suggests hormone replacement therapy at this time in your life, you need to decide right now (unless you choose to do so because your symptoms are so distressing). There is time to wait and think, talk with friends, read up on the topic, even to see if your symptoms get worse or better. And don't think that deciding one way or the other about hormone replacement therapy leaves you stuck with your decision. You can always try HRT later if you want. If you decide you don't like the effects, or the bother, you can stop. And you can start again later if you find yourself being bothered by symptoms. A study by Sonja McKinlay, Ph.D., of the American Institutes for Research, Cambridge, Massachusetts, shows that many women do just that, with no apparent ill effects. You may simply want to tell your gynecologist: "I need time to think about this."

HYSTERECTOMY

In the United States, hysterectomy (removal of the uterus) remains the second most frequently performed surgery, with 650,000 to 675,000 performed annually. That's double the rate of England and many European countries.

With such statistics, you might ask if you really need a hysterectomy. A second opinion is warranted. You should think before having a hysterectomy for these reasons:

1. Hysterectomy carries a high risk of postoperative depression and other hormone-related psychological problems, especially in women who have the surgery for other than life-threatening illness.
2. It can put a serious crimp in your sexual desire and your ability to achieve orgasm.
3. It can cause urinary tract, bowel, and back and joint problems.
4. It is major surgery with a risk of death of 1–2 per 1,000 operations performed.
5. One-quarter to one-half of women have complications of fever or hemorrhage following the operation.

Statistics show that hysterectomies are most likely to be performed for fibroid tumors, uterine prolapse, and endometriosis; however, all three conditions can be helped by less invasive means.

Hysterectomy is necessary for spreading cancer of the uterus, vagina, fallopian tubes, and ovaries, and usually for invasive cervical cancer; for severe uncontrollable infection; for severe, uncontrollable bleeding; for life-threatening blockages of the bladder or bowels by the uterus or growths on the uterus; and for some rare complications of childbirth, such as uterine rupture.

Types of Hysterectomies

Several different types of hysterectomies and related operations exist. Ask your doctor to be up front with you, stating which organs he is removing, which he isn't, and which are maybes. You might ask for this information in writing or add it to a surgical consent form.

1. A *simple hysterectomy* removes the entire uterus with the cervix and the fallopian tubes. This is also referred to as a total hysterectomy. (It does not involve removal of the ovaries.)
2. A *subtotal or partial hysterectomy* involves amputation of the uterus above the cervix. The cervix remains in place. Fewer nerves are severed during this surgery, so the bladder, bowel, and sexual functions are less likely to be impaired. But it means you still run the risk of cervical cancer.
3. *Oophorectomy* means the removal of one ovary. Bilateral oophorectomy means the removal of both ovaries.
4. A *radical hysterectomy,* reserved for invasive cancer, involves removal of the uterus, removal of the upper one-third of the vagina, and a sampling of lymph nodes in the groin. (It does not necessarily include the ovaries.)
5. A *modified or type II radical hysterectomy* is similar to a radical, but attempts to preserve enough nerve fibers to the bowel and bladder to maintain normal function. Ask your doctor about this procedure if he suggests a radical.
6. An *abdominal hysterectomy* removes the uterus through an incision in the abdomen, most often a 6-to-8-inch cut just below the pubic hairline.
7. A *vaginal hysterectomy* removes the uterus through an incision in the vagina. Although it may be cosmetically acceptable, studies show that this kind of surgery has a higher postoperative wound infection rate, and that 5 to 10 percent of women having vaginal hysterectomy require further surgery for complications.

Your doctor may say, or imply, that a hysterectomy is "indicated" or standard medical practice, but that doesn't mean it's your best choice. So you'll want to ask:

Do I *Really* Need a Hysterectomy?

That's a crucially important question. You'll want to thoroughly explore the answer before you decide whether or not a hysterectomy (removal of the uterus) is going to improve *your* quality of life. It's a question that should never be answered solely by your gynecologist (since he's the one recommending the hysterectomy!). And your second opinion should come from an independent source, preferably not the colleague recommended by your own doctor.

Can I Save My Ovaries?

In about 40 percent of hysterectomies, the ovaries are also removed. The old double standard in medicine has been: "No ovary is good enough to leave in. No testicle is bad enough to take out." Doctors contend the ovaries could become cancerous, and that ovarian cancer is a deadly and hard-to-diagnose disease. That's true, but it's also so rare that some researchers have calculated that only 1 in 700 women whose ovaries are removed would have developed ovarian cancer.

If you're 40 or older, your doctor may try to persuade you that you don't "need" your ovaries anymore, and that hormone replacement therapy will restore your blood hormone levels. In fact, researchers now know that the ovaries continue to produce an array of hormones well past menopause. They also know that hormone replacement therapy is far from perfect. Even if your doctor agrees to spare your ovaries, there's a chance the ovaries will stop producing hormones, most likely because the surgery disrupts their blood supply. Some studies show this happens to more than a third of women, and in up to half of women who have one ovary removed. This is another side effect, though, that some gynecologists will claim is still unproven.

INFERTILITY

If you are slow in conceiving, a gynecologist can provide direction that may help you conceive. For instance, he or she can help pinpoint your most fertile time of month, or determine if lubricants or other products you or your husband use (including nonprescription drugs like antihistamines and cough medicines) are thwarting the normal reproductive process. The gynecologist should also recommend a semen analysis of your mate to make sure he is fertile. This is a simple, noninvasive test that checks the number, shape, and viability of the sperm.

A gynecologist can usually also perform some basic tests that will give him enough information to de-

A *reproductive endocrinologist* is a doctor specializing in the treatment of infertility problems in women. (Urologists usually treat infertility in men.) This is the doctor who can diagnose and treat hormone problems; use drugs to stimulate ovulation; perform microsurgery to open blocked fallopian tubes; use a laser to blast away painful patches of endometriosis; remove fibroid tumors from your uterus in a way that restores or preserves your fertility; and do assisted fertility procedures (perform high-tech procedures like in vitro fertilization [IVF], gamete intrafallopian transfer [GIFT], and inseminations). These doctors are expert in the surgical techniques that minimize scar tissue formation, which is a common occurrence with any kind of abdominal surgery and which can cause pain and infertility.

termine whether or not you need to see an infertility specialist. Before you agree to any course of action, though, do make sure your gynecologist has adequate training and experience in infertility. How many couples has he treated, and for what? How many babies has he produced? If he suggests he can do a certain test or procedure, ask how many times he's done it, and his complication rate.

Besides a routine pelvic exam, a gynecologist can usually:

- Do urine and blood tests to measure levels of various hormones
- Do a postcoital test (examination of the woman's vagina and cervical mucus shortly after intercourse to determine whether the sperm are capable of penetrating the cervical mucus)
- Order a radiologist to do a hysterosalpingogram (X-ray picture of the uterus, fallopian tubes, and ovaries to check for malformations and blockage)
- Do an endometrial biopsy (extraction of a small piece of tissue from the uterus for examination to determine if a woman is ovulating)

If surgery is indicated, note this: Although all board-certified gynecologists are trained to do certain types of gynecologic surgery, most are not trained specifically in surgery for infertility problems. Be especially wary if a gynecologist recommends an operation to open blocked fallopian tubes. These delicate organs can be further damaged by poorly done surgery, so you'll want to select a surgeon highly skilled in scar-minimizing microsurgery. That's most likely to be an infertility expert, usually a gynecologist who is board-certified in reproductive endocrinology.

When Should You Seek Help for an Infertility Problem?

If you've been trying unsuccessfully to conceive for a year or more (6 months if you're age 35 or older), or if you've had pelvic inflammatory disease (PID) or painful periods (which could mean endometriosis), you may want to ask your gynecologist about possible infertility problems, or see a board-certified reproductive endocrinologist.

Studies show that, ultimately, a specific diagnosis for infertility can be made in virtually all but a small percent. Among women, the most commonly diagnosed causes of infertility are fallopian tube problems, ovulatory problems, endometriosis, and cervical problems.

In men, they are varicoceles (varicose veins in the testicles), testicular failure, semen motility or volume problems, endocrine problems, and tubal obstructions.

Studies on surgery—for instance, reconstruction of fallopian tubes (extensive surgery to remove internal blockage and constricting scar tissue) and correction of varicoceles—report varying success rates.

Couples who are not able to conceive through surgery, induced ovulation, or other hormone treatments may move on to the next step: an assisted fertility procedure. That could include artificial insemination with the husband's sperm, or donor sperm, both fairly simple procedures with good success rates. Artificial insemination by the husband, in which the husband's sperm is injected into the uterus, has varying success rates, depending on the husband's sperm count; artificial insemination by a donor is successful 57 percent of the time.

Or couples may opt for in vitro fertilization (IVF), a process that allows fertilization to take place outside a woman's body and produces what the popular press has dubbed "test-tube babies."

In this procedure, a woman is given hormones to induce ovulation, a process called a stimulation cycle. Then, with a laparoscope, a number of eggs are removed from her ovaries, called a retrieval. The eggs are mixed with her husband's sperm, not in a test tube but in a flat round dish. Once the fertilized eggs have started to grow (after the cell has divided about four times) a number of eggs are injected into the woman's uterus, where, it is hoped, at least one egg will implant and grow into a full-term baby.

Gamete intrafallopian transfer (GIFT) is a technological spin-off of in vitro fertilization. Similar to IVF

Questions to Ask a Specialist

If you and your gynecologist determine that you should be seeing a specialist, choose carefully, just as you would any doctor who may be operating on you, or recommending a course of treatment. If your gynecologist refers you to a particular doctor, make sure you know why he's recommending that doctor. If you shop for an infertility specialist yourself, make sure you have a get-acquainted visit and ask plenty of questions, including these:

• Are you a board-certified reproductive endocrinologist?

Although it doesn't guarantee competency, board certification means a doctor has met stringent training requirements and passed an exam given by the American Board of Medical Specialties. Professional affiliations, such as membership or "fellowship" in the American Fertility Society or the Society for Reproductive Technology, do *not* mean a doctor has special credentials.

• What is your training in in vitro fertilization? When and where were you trained? How many of these procedures have you done?

Do you want a doctor who has trained and studied for a few weeks, or a few years? Who just started doing the procedure last week, or five years ago? Who trained at a major medical center with a nationwide reputation in infertility, or at your local hospital? Studies show that the more of a procedure a doctor does, and the longer he does it, the better he gets at it.

• What is your success rate for my type of fertility problem?

Doctors (and clinics) tend to specialize in the types of infertility problems they treat. Some are unable to handle certain types of infertility, or won't take on many tough cases because it lowers their success rate.

• Do you have any restrictions on treatment?

Some clinics require a couple to sign up in advance for a certain number of "tries." Some allow only a certain number of tries. Some won't handle certain kinds of fertility problems or take women over a certain age. (Those restrictions improve their success rates.)

• How much is this going to cost us?

Try to get a firm figure from the doctor, or, at least, a dollar amount "per try." Treatment for infertility problems is expensive, with costs for in vitro fertilization $7,000 or more per attempt. Always check with your medical insurance carrier to see what tests and procedures are covered before you have treatment. Many insurance companies do not provide coverage for in vitro fertilization.

DES Daughters and Mothers

Any woman born in the U.S. during 1941–71, and even beyond, faces a special health risk. Her mother may have been one of the 5 million women who took the drug DES (diethylstilbestrol, a synthetic estrogen) during her pregnancy to prevent miscarriage. If that's the case, she runs a higher than normal risk for fertility problems, reproductive organ abnormalities, cervical and vaginal cell changes, and cancer. (See "Gynecology and Obstetrics" in section 3, "Healing Arts," for more information.)

in its use of ovulation-inducing drugs, egg retrieval, ultrasound examinations, and blood tests, GIFT is a process in which the retrieved eggs and treated sperm are placed directly in the fallopian tubes for fertilization to occur as it normally would, in vivo. GIFT is available only to women with at least one normal, unobstructed fallopian tube and one healthy ovary, but it may be appropriate for some male fertility problems and cervical mucus or sperm antibody problems. The procedure is used most often for couples with unexplained infertility and minimal endometriosis and therefore may result in a higher pregnancy rate due to the types of women being treated.

Because a laparoscopy or a minilaparotomy (a small incision made in the abdomen above the pubic bone) must be done to place the eggs, GIFT's chief disadvantage over modern IVF is that it is invasive.

Zygote intrafallopian transfer (called ZIFT) is a new variation of GIFT. In this process, the egg is fertilized in vitro and the embryo placed in the fallopian tube about 18 hours later. Reports warn that the procedure is too new for its success to be measured.

Because there are few enough guarantees in this field of medicine to begin with, it's especially important to be careful in your selection of a "fertility" center or specialist.

According to a recent Federal Trade Commission (FTC) investigation, some of these centers have a reputation for "inflating" their success rates for "take-home babies." They do that by presenting their statistics in a way that is different from that recommended. Clinics with lower rates will try to improve the appearance of their program by telling you the number of deliveries per egg retrieval attempt, which ups their percentage of live births. But members of government are trying to standardize infertility centers' success rates by requiring that it be calculated by using live births per stimulation cycle.

The FTC investigation also found that even when success rates were calculated the same way, there was a wide range, from 1.5 percent (live births per egg recovery) to 25.5 percent.

Glossary of Gynecologic Terms

Abdomen—the part of the body between the chest and the pelvis; the belly. The abdominal cavity contains most of the body's digestive organs, among them the stomach and intestines. Also in this cavity, which is separated from the chest by the diaphragm, are the liver, gallbladder, spleen, and kidneys.

Adhesions—scar tissue that forms after infection, surgery, or curettage that can close off the cervix, make the sides of the uterus stick together, block the fallopian tubes, or constrict other pelvic organs and cause pain. Adhesion formation is particularly common in abdominal surgery; microsurgery techniques can minimize adhesions.

Ambulatory—walk-in, same-day, or outpatient (usually referring to surgery, and distinct from inpatient or hospital care).

Amenorrhea—failure to begin menstruating by age 16. A physical exam may be necessary to determine if breast development shows that ovaries are secreting estrogen, if hymen has an opening, and if vagina and uterus are normal. Other genetic and hormonal tests may follow.

Amniocentesis—withdrawal with a long needle of fluid from the sac surrounding a fetus to test for genetic and other disorders in the fetus.

Biopsy—the removal of a portion of body tissue for microscopic examination and diagnosis. It is widely used to determine the status of growths that may be cancerous. An open biopsy is done by an incision through the skin. A needle biopsy or needle aspiration biopsy is done by injecting a needle into the area where tissue is to be taken. It's used to check breast lumps thought to be fluid-filled cysts. A punch biopsy uses a surgical instrument similar to a small paper punch to extract a plug of skin and tissue. It's used on the type of surface lesions found on the cervix, vulva, or in the vagina.

Catheterization—the passage of a flexible surgical tube into an opening. Urinary catheterization refers to passage of a tube into the bladder to allow drainage of urine. It is a common cause of bladder infections.

Cauterization—the application of a caustic substance, a hot instrument, an electric current, or other agent to destroy diseased tissue. Cauterization might be used to remove venereal warts from the cervix or vagina.

Cervical intraepithelial neoplasm (CIN)—neoplasm means "new and abnormal tissue growth," which may or may not be cancerous. Intraepithelial means "among the cells" lining the cervix. This is a relatively new term used by pathologists to replace an older and less specific term, "dysplasia," which simply means "abnormal development of cells."

Cervicitis—inflammation of the cervix. (There are several types.)

Cervix—the neck of the uterus which extends into the upper part of the vagina; a fairly common site for cancer, and the area from which a Pap smear is taken.

Cesarean section—the surgical procedure in which the uterus is cut open to deliver a baby.

Chlamydia (pronounced *klah-mid-DEE-ah*)—a strange, viruslike, sexually transmitted bacterium that can cause severe pelvic inflammatory disease.

Colposcopy—a procedure that uses a magnifying instrument to examine the surface of the cervix and vagina for lesions, and to pinpoint the areas from which tissue will be taken for biopsy.

Conization—the surgical procedure in which a cone-shaped piece of tissue is cut out of the center of the cervix; used to diagnose or rule out the presence of invasive cancer. Also known as a cone biopsy.

Cryosurgery—destruction of tissue by extreme cold. Cryosurgery often replaces cauterization today as a way to remove surface lesions.

Cul-de-sac—in gynecology, a "blind pouch" of tissue between the vagina and rectum that sometimes harbors endometriosis or tumors; it is examined by touch through the rectum.

Cyst—a noncancerous, fluid-filled cavity or sac. In fibrocystic condition of the breast or benign breast condition, the breasts have numerous cysts.

Cystitis—inflammation of the urinary bladder.

Cystocele—a condition where the bladder bulges through the vaginal wall. Also known as a cystic hernia.

Danazol—a synthetic hormone used to treat endometriosis. Derived from the male hormone testosterone, this drug stops menstruation and the hormonal peaks of ovulation. It also dissolves small endometrial implants and may shrink larger ones. Marketed in the U.S. as Danocrine.

DES (diethylstilbestrol)—a synthetic hormone prescribed to 3 to 6 million pregnant women in the U.S. between 1941 and 1971, usually to prevent miscarriage. (The drug was never proven to do this.) DES has been found to cause abnormalities of the reproductive system and, in some cases, cancer at an early age. Women who know or suspect they've been exposed to DES should have a special pelvic and vaginal exam done by a doctor experienced with DES patients.

Diagnosis—the determination of the nature of the case of a disease; the art of distinguishing one disease from another.

Dilation and curettage (D&C)—a procedure in which the opening of the cervix is stretched, and a curette (a sharp spoon-shaped instrument) is inserted and used to scrape away the uterine lining. This procedure has been mostly replaced by techniques that use a flexible plastic tube and suction.

Dysmenorrhea—painful periods; most common is the uterine cramping associated with menstruation, which is considered normal if not incapacitating. Pain that begins after years of pain-free periods is usually due to causes such as endometriosis, polyps, or fibroids. Dysmenorrhea is associated with use of the IUD as a contraceptive device.

Dysplasia—a term doctors often use to refer to possibly precancerous cells. It simply means "abnormal development of cells."

Ectopic pregnancy—development of a fertilized egg outside of the uterus, usually in the fallopian tubes. Very painful; often requires emergency surgical removal.

Endocervical curettage—a process in which tissue is scraped from the endocervix, the opening in the cervix to the uterus. This is most often done as part of a cervical biopsy, after a Pap smear shows signs of abnormalities.

Endometriosis—a painful condition in which the endometrium, the tissue lining the uterus, migrates outside the uterus and grows on organs within the abdomen.

Endometrium—the tissue lining the uterus which responds to hormone levels and is shed every month as menstrual flow.

Estrogen—a female hormone produced in the ovaries that is responsible for most feminine sex characteristics. Estrogen is used in birth control pills, to treat symptoms of menopause, and to prevent osteoporosis.

Estrogen receptor assay—a test done on breast cancer tumors and other gynecological tumors immediately upon removal to determine if, and how much, their growth is enhanced by the hormone estrogen. Women with estrogen-receptive tumors are often given estrogen-suppressing drugs.

Fallopian tubes—the tiny, muscular tubes that carry eggs from the ovaries to the body of the uterus. Scarred or blocked fallopian tubes are a common cause of infertility in women.

Fibroid tumors—solid, usually benign tumors that grow on the outside, inside, or within the wall of the uterus. (Technically known as leiomyomas or myomas.) A common reason gynecologists recommend hysterectomy, although fibroids can be treated by other means, and often don't require treatment.

Genitourinary—pertaining to the area around the genitals and urinary tract.

Gonadotrophin-releasing hormones—new drugs used in the treatment of endometriosis and infertility that inhibit ovarian function and lower estrogen levels.

Gynecologic oncologist—a gynecologist with special training in the treatment of cancer of women's reproductive organs.

Gynecologist—a medical doctor specializing in the treatment of diseases of women's reproductive organs.

Hematocrit—a measurement of the volume of red blood cells found in a certain amount of blood; used along with other factors to determine a woman's blood iron level.

Hemoglobin—the oxygen-carrying pigment found in red blood cells; used along with other factors to determine a woman's blood iron level.

Hormone replacement therapy (HRT)—the use of synthetic or naturally occurring hormones to replace those the body is no longer producing because of menopause or removal of the ovaries. HRT most often includes estrogen and progesterone, and sometimes, male hormones called androgens.

Human papillomavirus (HPV)—a large group of sexually transmitted viruses that cause all forms of venereal warts and lesions. Some types of this virus have been linked with cervical cancer.

Hysterectomy—the surgical removal of the uterus. There are a number of different kinds of hysterectomies, depending on how the operation is performed.

Hysteroscopy—a diagnostic and surgical procedure in which a thin, tubular viewing scope is inserted through the cervix into the uterus. It's used to look for internal uterine growths like polyps or fibroid tumors.

Infertility—diminished or absent capacity to produce offspring. The term does not denote complete inability to produce offspring, which is called sterility. Primary infertility is that occurring in people who have never conceived; secondary infertility occurs in people who have previously conceived.

In situ—in place; cancer that has not yet spread.

Intrauterine device (IUD)—a form of contraception in which a small plastic piece is inserted into the uterus, with withdrawal string extending through the cervix into the vagina. Currently, only two IUDs are available in the U.S. IUDs have been associated with pelvic inflammatory disease and are not recommended to women who intend to have children in the future and/or who are not in a monogamous relationship.

In vitro fertilization—the process of joining egg and sperm outside the body, in a laboratory-controlled environment, then injecting the newly fertilized egg in the mother's womb. In vitro means, literally, "in glass" or "observable in a test tube."

Laparoscopy—examination of the interior of the abdomen by means of a laparoscope, a thin metal viewing scope, which is inserted through a small incision. Laparoscopy is often done to diagnose endometriosis and other infertility problems.

Laser surgery—the process of using a laser (a concentrated beam of light which can produce a tremendous amount of heat) to cut or otherwise destroy tissue. In the hands of a well-skilled surgeon, certain lasers have the advantage of being more precise and of causing less blood loss than traditional surgery with a knife.

Mammography—the process of X-raying the breasts (mammary glands) to detect lumps or thickened tissue that could be cancerous.

Mastectomy—the surgical removal of the breast. There are several different kinds of mastectomies.

Menopause—the cessation of menstrual periods in women, usually occurring around age 50. Surgically induced menopause is caused by the removal of the ovaries.

Menstruation—the shedding through the vagina of the uterine lining, consisting of blood and tissue. Average cycle is 28 days; average length of menstrual period, 5 days.

Microinvasive cancer—cancer that has just started to invade surrounding tissue, and that may still be treated by local removal.

Microsurgery—surgical techniques that use a microscope to incise and stitch tiny structures such as the fallopian tubes; also, refined surgical techniques that minimize bleeding and scarring.

Myomectomy—the surgical removal of fibroid tumors from the uterus.

Oncology—the study of cancer, especially tumors.

Oophorectomy (pronounced *oh-for-REK-tow-me*)—the surgical removal of one ovary; also called ovariectomy. Bilateral oophorectomy indicates removal of both ovaries.

Osteoporosis—a condition in which the bones lose mass and become porous, resulting in weak bones which can fracture easily. Osteoporosis is most common in small-boned, light-skinned, sedentary women past the age of menopause.

Ovaries—olive-shaped glands connected by the fallopian tubes to the uterus which secrete estrogen, the main female hormone, and which, in fertile women, produce an egg each month.

Ovulation—the process during which the ovary produces an egg.

Ovum—the egg (cell) produced monthly in the ovaries.

Pap smear—a test in which cells are scraped from the cervix, smeared on a glass slide, and examined under a microscope for signs of cancer or infection.

Pelvic Inflammatory Disease (PID)—a serious, sexually transmitted infection of the uterus, fallopian tubes, and/or ovaries. PID can result in sterility. Symptoms of pelvic pain, fever, chills, and pus-like vaginal discharge require a doctor's immediate attention.

Pelvis—the lower portion of the trunk of the body, including the pelvic bones and those organs within the hipbones. In women, this includes the entire reproductive tract.

Pessary—a plastic or metal ring or cap used to hold a fallen (prolapsed) uterus in place.

Progesterone—a female hormone secreted by the ovaries which causes changes in the endometrium that help to ensure pregnancy. Adequate levels of progesterone after ovulation, followed by a sharp drop in both progesterone and estrogen at the end of the menstrual cycle, lead to menstruation. Progesterone is used to correct abnormal bleeding in women near menopause; with estrogen for menopausal hormone replacement therapy; and sometimes, as a treatment for premenstrual syndrome. Progestins are synthetic forms of progesterone.

Progesterone receptor assay—a test done on breast cancer tumors and other gynecological tumors immediately upon removal to determine if, and how much, their growth is enhanced by the hormone progesterone. Women with progesterone-receptive tumors are often given progesterone-suppressing drugs.

Prognosis—a forecast as to the probable outcome of a disease; the prospects for recovery from a disease as indicated by the nature and symptoms of the case. Distinct from diagnosis.

Prolapse—the falling down or sinking of an organ. In uterine prolapse, the uterus drops into the vagina. The bladder and rectum can also prolapse, sometimes bulging into the vagina. And, after a hysterectomy, the vagina can prolapse, caving in on itself.

Reproductive Endocrinology—the study of the hormone-secreting organs (the endocrine system) in the body. This includes the study of the ovaries in women, and in men the testicles.

Sacrum—the triangular bone near the bottom of the spine, usually formed by five fused spinal vertebrae that are wedged between the hipbones.

Speculum—a duck-bill-shaped instrument inserted into the vagina and locked open that allows one to view the cervix and to insert and withdraw instruments without touching the sides of the vagina.

Toxic shock syndrome—a rare disease, believed caused by staph bacteria, that causes high fever, vomiting, and sometimes death. (Five percent of all women who get toxic shock syndrome die.) In women, the disease has been associated with the use of tampons. It has been estimated that each year 6–17 of every 100,000 menstruating women and girls will get toxic shock syndrome. To minimize your risks, use the least absorbent tampon needed to meet your needs and alternate with sanitary napkins.

Tubal ligation—a process of sterilization where the fallopian tubes are tied to prevent egg and sperm from uniting.

Ultrasound—the visualization of deep structures in the body by recording the echoes of sound waves directed into the tissue. Also known as sonography, the technique is used to examine the unborn fetus and to detect fluid-filled cysts on the ovaries or in the breasts.

Urethra—the canal conveying urine from the bladder to the outside of the body. In women, the urethra is about 1 inch long.

Urinary incontinence—the inability to control the flow of urine, resulting in leaking of urine at inappropriate times.

Uterus—the hollow, muscular, pear-shaped organ in women in which a fertilized egg becomes embedded and in which the developing fetus is nourished.

Vacuum aspiration—a procedure in which suction is used to draw out fluid and tissue. A vacuum aspiration of the uterus removes the endometrial lining and other contents, and may be used as a means of terminating an early pregnancy.

Vagina—the muscular canal leading from the vulva to the cervix.

Vaginitis—infection of the vagina, caused by any number of bacteria and microorganisms. Most common are yeast infections (also called *Candida, Monilia,* or fungus), *Trichomonas vaginalis* (trich), and *Gardnerella.*

Vulva—the region of the external genitalia of a woman.

Xeromammography—a certain type of X ray of the breast that uses a photoelectric rather than film screen process. Although it provides sharper images than the film screen method, xeromammography requires more radiation, so it's not as widely used as film screen mammography.

Contraception

Contraception, also called birth control and family planning, is the practice of preventing pregnancies in order to limit the number of births.

Methods of preventing pregnancy, how they work, and possible side effects, include:

Birth control pills. Monthly series of pills taken one a day. Hormonelike ingredients prevent ovaries from releasing eggs. Advantages: Reliable and convenient to use. Periods more regular with less blood loss and cramping. Warnings: Do not use if over 35 and smoke more than fifteen cigarettes a day. Report immediately: swelling or pain in legs, chest or arms; yellowing of skin or eyes; severe headaches; severe depression; blurred or double vision.

Intrauterine device (IUD). A small plastic device inserted into uterus and allowed to remain there for months or years in order to prevent pregnancy. Affects lining of the uterus, making it difficult for pregnancy to occur. Advantages: Can be left in place from one to six years, depending on type. Eliminates need to remember birth control. Warnings: Do not use with the following: recent infection of tubes or ovaries; abnormal vaginal bleeding; history of tubal pregnancy. Copper IUD not recommended if sensitive to copper or having heat treatments. Report immediately: severe cramping; pain or bleeding during sex; unexplained fever and chills; light or missed periods.

Diaphragm. A soft rubber cup with flexible rim that is inserted into the vagina and covers cervix. Used with spermicidal cream or jelly, a diaphragm prevents sperm from entering the uterus. Must be left in place 6 to 8 hours after last intercourse. Advantages: Easy insertion. Not felt by either partner during sex. Most women have no side effects, but mild allergic reactions to rubber, cream, or jelly may occur. Report immediately: irritation; frequent bladder infections; unusual discharge; diaphragm not staying in place.

Condom (also called a prophylactic or rubber). A sheath of thin rubber or animal tissue worn on penis during intercourse. Collects semen, preventing it from entering vagina. Most effective in preventing pregnancy if used with contraceptive cream or jelly. Advantages: Easy to obtain. Allows men to take responsibility for birth control. Latex condoms protect against sexually transmitted diseases. Warning: Condoms may break during intercourse.

Coitus interruptus (also called withdrawal). A method in which the male withdraws his penis from his partner's vagina before he ejaculates. One of the oldest and simplest methods of preventing pregnancy. Advantage: no equipment. Disadvantage: a high failure rate.

Other over-the-counter methods: Foams, creams, jellies, and suppositories are liquids or solids that melt into liquids after inserted deep into the vagina before intercourse. All are spermicides, chemical substances that kill live sperm inside the vagina for the purpose of birth control. Advantage: easy to buy in drugstores and some supermarkets. Disadvantage: may cause irritation of penis or vagina.

Periodic abstinence. Abstaining from unprotected intercourse for 5 days before and 3 days after an egg is released from an ovary. Women record body temperature and check vaginal mucus daily to determine when egg is released. Advantages: No medication and little equipment needed. Acceptable to all religious groups.

Cervical cap. Thimble-shaped cup of latex rubber that fits tightly over the cervix by suction. Used with spermicidal cream or jelly, the cap prevents sperm from entering uterus. Advantages: Can be left in place up to 48 hours. Less chance of bladder infections than with diaphragm. Warnings: Not recommended for women with physical abnormalities of vagina, cervix, uterus, or with history of toxic shock syndrome. Report immediately: any itching, odor, discharge, or if cap does not stay in place; bladder infection.

Sponge. Synthetic, spongelike substance that contains spermicide. Moistened with water, sponge is then inserted into vagina and acts as barrier between uterus and sperm. Advantage: Can remain inserted up to 24 hours. Intercourse can be repeated up to 6 hours before sponge is removed. Warning: Do not use if history of toxic shock syndrome. Report immediately: any itching, odor, or discharge.

Female condom. Rubber pouch with two hoops is folded in half and inserted into the vagina. One hoop is held in place by the pubic bone, the other hangs loose. Advantage: Unlike the condom, the woman takes responsibility for birth control.

Norplant. Six matchstick-sized capsules, containing a low dose of progestin (a synthetic hormone) and no estrogen, are placed in the skin of the upper arm using a local anesthetic. Progestin is slowly released into the bloodstream. Advantages: Most effective reversible method of birth control. Capsules can remain in place for up to five years. Warnings: Can cause menstrual irregularity, spotting, breakthrough bleeding, or missed periods.

Depo-Provera. Synthetic progesterone given by injection once every 3 months. Advantages: Very effective. Unlike the pill, no need to take medication daily. However, in 1978 the Food and Drug Administration issued a warning saying that it had not been approved for contraceptive use because of potentially serious side effects; further, it has been linked with breast and uterine cancers in animals and, in humans, cervical cancer and irregular bleeding.

Cyclofem and Mesigna. Two new once-a-month injectable contraceptives recently approved for use in the United States. Uses a combination of estrogen and progestogen. Advantage: Fewer side effects than Depo-Provera.

Morning-after pill. Combination of hormones (specific birth control pills in certain dosage) given to woman within 72 hours of single act of unprotected intercourse. Prevents ovulation from occurring, or, if ovulation does occur, will change lining of uterus making it difficult for fertilized egg to attach itself. Warnings: To be used only in an emergency. Nausea a very common side effect.

Vasectomy (male sterilization). Tubes that carry sperm to mix with seminal fluid are blocked. Minor surgery takes place in doctor's office. Local anesthesia is injected into scrotum and a small cut is made to each tube (vas). Advantage: permanent method for man who is positive he wants to father no more children. Possible problems: inflammation or infection; blood clot; adhesion (skin binding to vas); fluid buildup; swelling; transient pain; recanalization (the growing together of cut ends of the vas), which may restore fertility; decreased sexual desire, which occurs in 4 cases per 1,000.

Tubal ligation (female sterilization). Surgery that blocks woman's tubes to prevent eggs from passing into the uterus. Small cut is made in lower abdomen, and through this the tubes are brought into view to be sealed. Or doctor may use laparoscope (telescopelike tool) to see tubes. A harmless gas stretches abdomen to prevent injury to other organs. Local or general anesthesia can be used. Advantage: permanent method for woman who is positive she wants no more children. Possible problems: bleeding at site of cut or inside abdomen; infection; injury to blood vessels; harm to nearby organs.

Contraception Effectiveness

Method	Number of Pregnancies per 100 Women During One Year of Use
Sterilization	less than 1
The pill	2.5
IUD	4
Condom with foam	10
Condom without foam	
unmarried women	11
married women	14
Diaphragm/cervical cap	18
Sponge	18
Foams, creams, jellies,	
suppositories	20
Withdrawal	20
Periodic abstinence	24
No method	60–80

Radon

WHAT IS RADON?

Radon, a decay product of radium, is an odorless, colorless, tasteless, nonflammable gas that does not react or combine with other chemical elements. While radon itself is relatively harmless, its breakdown products, called radon daughters, are very dangerous. Radon daughters are radioactive and cannot be detected by the human senses.

WHERE IS IT?

Radon travels through rock, soil, and water. Some types of rock and soil are more heavily concentrated with radon, however, so some areas of the United States have more difficulty with radon than others, for example, the Middle Atlantic States. Granite, phosphate, shale, and uranium are particular carriers of the radon. Levels are higher in winter than they are in summer because ventilation is usually lower in cold weather.

Radon usually travels by way of simple diffusion. As radium decays and forms radon, the gas fills tiny air pockets in soil. While radon can travel only a few yards at most, it can still reach and escape into the air, into water, and into natural gas, all sources that are accessible to and utilized by people.

One way radon can leak into a home is through tiny cracks in its foundation. When warm air rises through the house and escapes from cracks and windows in the upper levels of the house, it draws air, and possibly radon gas, up through the soil underneath the home. Radon can also travel through well water, floor cracks and joints, basement floor walls and joints, concrete basement floors, basement drains, and showers. Exposure to radon is usually through indoor air, but miners who work underground are sometimes also at risk.

RADON AND HEALTH

Radon daughters are related to a number of health difficulties. They often enter the lungs either as gases or attached to air particles. The alpha particles in radon, moving at a rate of more than 4 million feet per second, can smash past molecules in their paths. The damage caused by this bombarding of molecules can kill the body's cells, or, worse yet, alter them. Any alteration of cells by radon may lead to cancer, especially lung cancer, which may not become detectable for twenty years or more. Radon has also been linked to stomach cancer and bone cancer.

Most people are not exposed to enough radon to have it seriously harm their health; however, prolonged exposure may lead to serious health problems. Children, on the other hand, may be at higher risk than adults from indoor radon because they receive a higher dose per unit of exposure. According to the International Commission of Radiologic Protection, those aged 20 and younger who are exposed to radon appear to have a higher risk of developing lung cancer than those exposed later in life.

A resident of the United States has about a 1 in 300 chance of developing lung cancer from indoor radon. In other words, about 10 percent of people who get lung cancer develop it from exposure to radon. The National Academy of Sciences has noted that cigarette smoke acts synergistically (two things acting together) with radon gas in causing lung cancer, amplifying the effects of cigarette smoking on lung cancer rates. Obviously, smokers can reduce their risk of radon-caused lung cancer by quitting smoking.

TESTING

There are several inexpensive ($15 to $40 per test) and easy-to-use kits that can measure the level of radon present in your home. The federal Environmental Protection Agency (EPA) estimates that up to 8 million homes may have radon levels that exceed current allowable limits and that require corrective action. This means that there is about a 10 percent chance that your home contains a significant amount of radon.

FIXING HIGH LEVELS

If the test determines that your home has a radon level of 4 picocuries per liter of air or higher, the EPA recommends that you undertake corrective action. Begin by carefully examining those areas where radon is most likely to enter your home. Look for cracks, crevices, loose joints, penetrations (such as water and sewer pipes, basement drains), exposed earth, or any opening that allows the flow of radon into the home.

Applying a sealant (a silicone or rubber-based product similar to caulking material) to these areas may initially reduce the amount of radon entering your home; however, this method may not be effective in all cases. The most effective method for removing radon from homes is ventilation. Pressurizing your basement by installing an exhaust fan will improve the natural ventilation and assist in removing excess radon. Installing ventilation pipes in the soil beneath your home will also vent radon before it has an opportunity to seep through the basement floor. In addition, radon can be removed from drinking water by a filtering system. And finally, building materials that emit radon gas should be replaced or sealed.

Travel and Health

To travel outside of the United States or to travel anyplace away from home exposes one to foreign smells, tastes, and microorganisms and naturally engenders health risks. However, traveling abroad does not have to be such a risky endeavor. If the traveler is prepared sufficiently for the certain kind of trip he/she is planning and is knowledgeable of what kinds of precautionary measures he/she can take in advance, there is no reason why anyone cannot experience safe and fun travel.

PRE-TRIP PLANNING

Pre-trip planning is essential for any trip one may take, and it is worthwhile to begin planning at least 6 weeks prior to departure. This pre-trip preparation includes examinations by a family doctor or a travel

medicine specialist and research on the particular place of visit (what health risks are involved regarding climate, food, and lifestyle, what immunizations are required for that area, what special first-aid products are needed). Consultation with a doctor prior to departure ensures that one is healthy enough to travel and makes one aware of any problems or special health concerns that need attention while traveling.

A standard physical examination, however, should not exclude a consultation with a dentist as well. Satisfactory dental care may be more difficult to find than standard medical services when traveling abroad. Some basic pre-trip health precautions may include a tuberculosis test, a chest X ray, various blood tests for type and for AIDS (required for some countries), an electrocardiogram, and immunizations (depending on the country).

IMMUNIZATIONS

Immunization for specific diseases should be well thought out in advance, for some vaccines need to be in the body's system before exposure to the disease, some are given in a series of shots over a period of weeks, and some cannot be given along with others. Basic vaccinations that one should already have are tetanus, diptheria, polio, influenza, pneumococcal pneumonia, measles, mumps, and rubella (German measles). Vaccinations that are often required for international travel are yellow fever and cholera. And other vaccinations specific to a particular region or often recommended for international travel include malaria, hepatitis A and B, Japanese B encephalitis, typhoid, plague, rabies, and meningococcal meningitis. Because different countries require certain immunizations and sometimes alter them due to changing worldwide health trends, it is wise to contact the Centers for Disease Control and Prevention, a local or state health department, or a doctor in order to confirm exactly which immunizations the traveler will need for his/her trip.

WHAT TO TAKE ALONG

Particularly vexing in the pre-trip stage is the question of what essentials to take. Besides packing the appropriate types of clothing, shoes, etc., and other personal items, the traveler should consider these indispensable and essential items for a healthy trip:

Any medications (prescription or otherwise) being taken regularly should be included. Prescription drugs should be updated, be in plentiful supply, and be transported in their original container. Extra written prescriptions should be obtained from one's doctor as well as a listing of the generic equivalent or other brand names of the drug. Because brand names of drugs sometimes vary in different countries, it is beneficial to know the generic name of the drug and in what dosage to take it.

If one wears eyeglasses or contact lenses, one should know their prescription and take along an extra pair of glasses or lenses.

Other medical/pharmaceutical products that are useful to take along on a trip are sunscreens and lotions; sunglasses; insect repellent; eye and nose drops; antihistamine/decongestant medicines; travel-related medications for diarrhea prevention/treatment, motion sickness, and altitude sickness; women's sanitary supplies; contraceptives; water purification tablets; moleskin (for shoe discomfort or blisters); antifungal powder; scissors; safety pins; and tweezers. A first-aid kit consisting of bandages, antiseptic, aspirin, adhesives and gauze pads, thermometer, elastic bandage wrap, and topical antibiotics should be taken along as well.

Finally, important medical information and records, containing the traveler's medical history, should be on hand for emergencies or in case of sudden illness. The medical information, whether compiled on an identification card or on a document, should list one's Social Security number, chronic diseases or health problems if any, blood type, prescription medications, X-ray or EKG abnormalities, immunization records, allergies, medical insurance information, and name, address, and telephone number of one's physician and closest relative.

Medical Insurance and Assistance

Travel medical insurance is important to consider especially when taking trips outside of the United States. Some health insurance policies such as Medicare or Medicaid do not reimburse the traveler for any bills incurred outside of the United States. Travel health insurance offers many benefits and services ranging from paying hospital bills to reimbursement for lost baggage.

In addition to travel insurance, another helpful resource available to the traveler is the International Association for Medical Assistance to Travelers (IAMAT). Travelers may join IAMAT at no charge (donations are accepted) and can receive an annual directory of a worldwide network of English-speaking doctors, information about world health concerns, and 24-hour-a-day service. Various doctor referral services are available to the traveler through major credit card companies, such as American Express, MasterCard, and Visa.

Common Travel Ailments

Two common ailments one frequently encounters during traveling are jet lag and traveler's diarrhea (*turista*). Jet lag, or the general feeling of fatigue, disorientation, and lack of mental facility, plagues many travelers who experience changes in time zones. The effects of jet lag will eventually wear off—some experts estimate that the body needs 24 hours per time zone for readjustment to the new time zone.

There are steps, however, one can take to prepare the body for this sudden shift in time and to acclimate the system to the new time zone. When flying eastward, the body's clock is moved forward, making it more difficult for the traveler to adjust to the new time. It is wise then to book an early flight to eastern destinations so that the discrepancy in the time zones will not be so great to the body's clock. Conversely, the traveler should fly at a later time when traveling to westward destinations—the change in time zone will seem like an extended day to the body and it will be able to resynchronize to the new time zone faster. In order to ward off the effects of jet lag, one should sleep before the flight; eat light, high-protein meals before, during, and after the flight; avoid beverages containing alcohol or caffeine; and drink lots of fluids. One may also prevent jet lag by acclimating the body to the new time zone before the flight. Setting watches for the new time zone, sleeping later or waking earlier, or using light-exposure treatments are ways in which the body clock can be altered to the new time zone.

Traveler's diarrhea is a condition equally as besetting as jet lag, but it can be combated if one follows certain precautionary measures. Traveler's diarrhea produces gastrointestinal distress due to the inclusion of foreign bacteria (the organisms salmonella and shigella and bacteria *Campylobacter jejuni* and *Escherichia coli*) in the body's system. The foreign bacteria are usually found in the food and water of the new country. Places where the risk of contracting traveler's diarrhea is the greatest are Africa, Asia, Latin America, and the Middle East.

The best prevention against getting traveler's diarrhea is careful selection of what one consumes—the old adage of "If you can't boil it, cook it, or peel it, then forget it" still holds true in areas where the food quality is questionable. The traveler should avoid unsafe water or tap water, ice cubes, fruit juices diluted with tap water, raw fruits and vegetables, and food that is not cooked thoroughly. In areas of unhealthy sanitation, the traveler should drink well-known brands of bottled water, bottled wine and beer, coffee or tea (made with boiling water), carbonated water and sodas, or should boil tap water (140° to 150°F) to avoid microorganisms. In addition, one can use iodine or chlorine tablets or water filters to purify an impure water source. Finally, one can prevent traveler's diarrhea by taking various medications including bismuth subsalicylate (Pepto-Bismol), kaolin and pectin (Kaopectate), loperamide hydrochloride (Imodium), and antibiotics doxycycline (Vibramycin), norfloxacin and ciprofloxacin, and the combination of trimethoprim and sulfamethoxazole (TMP/SMX) (Bactrim DS, Cotrim DS, Septra DS).

Care should be taken, however, in the use of antibiotics as a preventive measure rather than a treatment for traveler's diarrhea. There are side effects and the use of antibiotics before exposure to foreign bacteria may eventually promote the growth of antibiotic resistant bacteria and thereby hamper the treatment of the diarrhea itself.

Listed below are useful addresses and phone numbers which travelers may consult for more information on their specific area of travel or their particular travel concern.

INFORMATION FOR TRAVEL NEEDS

Directory of Travel Health Clinics

Dr. Leonard C. Marcus
Traveler's Health and Immunization Services
148 Highland Avenue
Newton, MA 02160
Send 8 1/2 x 11 SASE.

General Travel Consultants

Centers for Disease Control and Prevention
Department of Health and Human Services
Public Inquiries
Building 1, Room B63
1600 Clifton Road N.E.
Atlanta, GA 30333
404-639-3670

Superintendent of Documents
U.S. Government Printing Office
Washington, DC 20402
202-783-3238
Re: Health Information for International Travel

International Association for Medical Assistance to Travelers (IAMAT)
417 Center Street
Lewiston, NY 14902
716-754-4883

International Health Care Service
New York Hospital—Cornell Medical Center
525 E. 68th Street
Box 210
New York, NY 10021
212-746-1601

Public Health Service
Department of Health and Human Services
200 Independent Avenue S.W., Room 716G
Washington, DC 20201
202-245-7694

World Health Organization
2 United Nations Plaza
New York, NY 10017
212-963-6001

Travel Insurance Information

Access America Inc.
Blue Cross and Blue Shield
600 Third Avenue
Box 807
New York, NY 10163
800-654-6686

Health Care Abroad
243 Church Street N.W., Suite 100D
Vienna, VA 22180
800-237-6615

International SOS Assistance Inc.
P.O. Box 11568
Philadelphia, PA 19116
215-244-1500
800-523-8930

Travel Assistance International
1133 15th Street N.W., Suite 400
Washington, DC 20005
202-347-2025
800-821-2828

TravMed
P.O. Box 10623
Baltimore, MD 21204
410-296-5225
800-732-5309

WorldCare Travel Assistance
1995 W. Commercial Boulevard
Fort Lauderdale, FL 33307-3008
800-521-4822

Travel Medical Information Services

The following groups organize medical information for travelers.

Emergicard
National Health Awareness Center
P.O. Box 3559
Abeline, TX 79604
915-698-3712

Medical Passport Foundation
P.O. Box 820
Deland, FL 32721
904-734-0639

MedicAlert Foundation
2323 N. Colorado
Turlock, CA 95380
209-668-3333
800-ID-ALERT

Phone Numbers for Medical Assistance (doctor referral)

Global Assistance Hotline (American Express card holders)
800-554-2639 in U.S.
202-554-2639 international collect

Club Assistance (Diners Club card holders)
800-356-3448 in U.S.
214-996-0904 international collect

Master Assist (Gold MasterCard holders)
800-622-7747 in U.S.
202-296-4650 international collect

Visa Assistance Center (Visa Gold card holders)
800-847-2911 in U.S.
214-669-8888 international collect

FOREIGN LANGUAGE HEALTH PHRASES

1. Do you speak English?
2. I am sick.
3. Please call a doctor./ I need a doctor.
4. Help!
5. Where is the hospital?/ pharmacy?

French
1. Parlez-vous anglais?
2. Je suis malade.
3. Appelez un docteur./ J'ai besoin d'un médecin.
4. Au secours!
5. Où est l'hôpital?/ la pharmacie?

German
1. Sprechen Sie Englisch?
2. Ich bin krank.
3. Bitte rusen einen Arzt./ Ich brauche einen Arzt.
4. Hilfe!
5. Wo ist das Krankenhaus?/ die Apotheke?

Italian
1. Parla inglese?
2. Sto male.
3. Chaimi un dottore./ Ho bisogno d'un dottore.
4. Aiuto!
5. Dove'è l'ospedale?/ una farmacia?

Spanish
1. ¿Habla usted inglés?
2. No me siento bien. Estoy enfermo.
3. ¡Por favor llame un médico./ Necesito un médico.
4. ¡Auxilio!/ ¡Ayuda!/ ¡Socorro!
5. ¿Dónde está el hospital?/ ¿la farmacia?

Japanese
1. Eigo ga wakarimasuka?
2. Kibun ga suguremasen.
3. Isha o yonde kudasai./ Sugu isha o yonde kudasai.
4. Tasukete!
5. Wa doko desuka byoin?/ kusuriya?

Health Periodicals

All prices are for a year's subscription.

Advances. $39.00. Quarterly
Institute for the Advancement of Health
423 Washington Street, 3rd Floor
San Francisco, CA 94111

Aging. $6.50. Quarterly
Superintendent of Documents
U.S. Government Printing Office
Washington, DC 20402

American Family Physician. $75.00. Monthly
American Academy of Family Physicians
8880 Ward Parkway
Kansas City, MO 64114-2797

American Fitness. $27.00. Monthly
American Fitness
15250 Ventura Boulevard, Suite 310
Sherman Oaks, CA 91403

American Health. $17.97. Monthly
American Health: Fitness of Body and Mind
P.O. Box 3015
Harlan, IA 51537-3015

American Journal of Public Health. $160.00. Monthly
American Public Health Association
1015 15th Street N.W.
Washington, DC 20005

Annual Review of Public Health. $49.00. Annual
Annual Reviews Inc.
4139 El Camino Way
Palo Alto, CA 94303-0897

Archives of Environmental Health. $97.00. Bimonthly
Heldref Publications
1319 18th Street N.W.
Washington, DC 20036-1802

BB's Health Watch. $24.95. Bimonthly
Nutritional Designs
3379 Shore Parkway
Brooklyn, NY 11235

Body Bulletin. $18.95. Monthly
Rodale Press Inc. c/o Lisa Zver
400 S. 10th Street
Emmaus, PA 18098-0099

Black Health. $10.00. Quarterly
Black Health Inc.
P.O. Box 5276, FDR Station
New York, NY 10150-5276

Changing Times. $18.00. Monthly
1729 H Street N.W.
Washington, DC 20006

Child Health Alert. $21.00. Monthly
Child Health Alert
P.O. Box 338
Newton Highlands, MA 02161

Consumer Health. $10.00. Monthly
Medical Second Opinion Inc.
156 Algonquin Parkway
Whippany, NJ 07981

Consumer Reports on Health. $24.00. Monthly
Consumer Reports
Subscription Department
P.O. Box 52148
Boulder, CO 80321-2148

Current Health 2. $6.50. Monthly
Current Health 2
Publication and Subscription Offices
Weekly Reader Corporation
4343 Equity Drive
Columbus, OH 43228

Geriatrics. $40.00. Monthly
Edgell Communications Inc.
One E. First Street
Duluth, MN 55802

Harvard Medical School Letter. $18.00. Monthly
Harvard Medical School
79 Garden Street
Cambridge, MA 02138

Health. $18.00. Monthly
Health
P.O. Box 56863
Boulder, CO 80322-6863

Health and Environment Digest. $80.00. 11 times a year
Freshwater Foundation
Box 90
2500 Shadywood Rd.
Navarre, MN 55392

Health and Fitness Magazine for Healthy, Sound Living: HF. $2.95 (single issue). Quarterly
Fell Publishers Inc.
2131 Hollywood Boulevard, Suite 304
Hollywood, FL 33020

Health and You. $10.00. Quarterly
Health Ink Publishing Group
1 Executive Drive
Moorestown, NJ 08057

Health Care and Financing Review. $24.00. Quarterly
Superintendent of Documents
U.S. Government Printing Office
Washington, DC 20402-9371

Health Confidential. $49.00. Monthly
Health Confidential
330 W. 42nd Street
New York, NY 10036

Health Facts. $21.00. Monthly.
Center for Medical Consumers
237 Thompson Street
New York, NY 10012

The Health Letter. $22.00. Semimonthly
P.O. Box 19622
Irvine, CA 92713

Health Letter. $18.00. Monthly
Public Citizen Health Research Group
2000 P Street N.W.
Washington, DC 20036

Healthline. $24.00. Monthly
Mosby-Year Inc.
11830 Westline Industrial Drive
St. Louis, MO 63146

Health News and Review. $7.95. Bimonthly
Keats Publishing Inc.
27 Pine Street
New Canaan, CT 06840

Health Safety and Education. $90.00. Monthly
Predicasts Inc.
11001 Cedar Avenue
Cleveland, OH 44106

Health Science. $25.00. Bimonthly
American Natural Hygiene Society
P.O. Box 30630
Tampa, FL 33630

Health Watch. $14.95. Bimonthly
Health Watch
P.O. Box 5321
Boulder, CO 80322-3231

Health Wise. $19.70. Monthly
Health Wise
P.O. Box 1786
Indianapolis, IN 46206

Health World. $12.00. Bimonthly
Health World
1540 Gilbreth Road
Burlingame, CA 94010

Insider's Guide to Personal Wellness. $34.95. Monthly
Insider's Guide to Personal Wellness c/o Grace Publishing
2888 Bluff Street, Suite 461
Boulder, CO 80301-9002

*Johns Hopkins Health Letter: Health
After 50*. $15.00. Monthly
The Johns Hopkins Medical Institutions
Baltimore, MD 21205

Journal of Community Health. $195.00. Bimonthly
Human Sciences Press
72 5th Avenue
New York, NY 10011-8004

Journal of Environmental Health. $45.00. Bimonthly
National Environmental Health Association
720 S. Colorado Boulevard
South Tower, Suite 970
Denver, CO 80222

Journal of Nutrition. $185.00. Monthly
Journal of Nutrition
9650 Rockville Pike
Bethesda, MD 20814

Lancet. $130.00. Weekly
Williams and Wilkins Co.
428 E. Preston Street
Baltimore, MD 21202-3993

Mayo Clinic Health Letter. $24.00. Monthly
Mayo Clinic Proceedings
Mayo Clinic
200 First Street S.W.
Rochester, MN 55905

Men's Health. $17.70. Bimonthly
Men's Health
33 Minor Street
Emmaus, PA 18098

The Milbank Quarterly. $66.00. Quarterly
Cambridge University Press
40 W. 20th Street
New York, NY 10011-4211

Mother Jones. $24.00. Bimonthly
Mother Jones
P.O. Box 58259
Boulder, CO 80322

Natural Body and Fitness. $33.50. Bimonthly
Fitness Lifestyles
P.O. Box A
New Britain, PA 18901

The New England Journal of Medicine. $96.00. Weekly
Massachusetts Medical Society
10 Shattuck Street
Boston, MA 02115-6094

The New Health Standard Journal. $18.00. Bimonthly
Burgundy Court Publishers
P.O. Box 8181
Collins, CO 80526-8003

The NIH Record. $45.00. Biweekly
Superintendent of Documents
U.S. Government Printing Office
Washington, DC 20402

Nutrition Reviews. $75.00. Monthly
Springer-Verlag New York Inc.
Journal Fulfillment Services
44 Hartz Way
Secaucus, NJ 07094

Nutrition Today. $59.00. Bimonthly
Williams and Wilkins
428 E. Preston Street
Baltimore, MD 21202

People's Medical Society Newsletter. $20.00. Bimonthly
People's Medical Society
462 Walnut Street, Lower Level
Allentown, PA 18102

The Physician and Sportsmedicine. $46.00. Monthly
Physician and Sportsmedicine
430 W. 77th Street
Minneapolis, MN 55435

Prevention. $19.97. Monthly
Rodale Press Inc.
33 E. Minor Street
Emmaus, PA 18049

Psychology Today. $17.95. 6 times a year
Psychology Today
P.O. Box 55046
Boulder, CO 80322-5046

Public Health Comments. $96.00. Monthly
Public Health Information Services Inc.
11661 Charter Oak Court
Reston, VA 22090

Public Health Reports. $12.00. Bimonthly
Superintendent of Documents
U.S. Government Printing Office
Department 36KK
Washington, DC 20402

Second Opinion. $50.00. Monthly
Coalition for the Medical Rights of Women
2945 24th Street
San Francisco, CA 94110

Shape. $35.00. Monthly
Weider Health and Fitness
21100 Erwin Street
Woodland Hills, CA 91367

Total Health. $13.00. Bimonthly
Trio Publications Co.
6001 Topanga Canyon Boulevard
Woodland Hills, CA 92367

To Your Health. $25.00. Bimonthly
Cornell Publishing and Communications
330 Garfield Avenue
Eau Claire, WI 54701

Tufts University Nutrition Letter. $18.00. Monthly
332 W. 57th Street
P.O. Box 34T
New York, NY 10019

*University of California, Berkeley,
Wellness Letter.* $20.00. Monthly
University of California at Berkeley
P.O. Box 10922
Des Moines, IA 50340

Vitality. $12.99. Monthly
Vitality Magazine
8080 N. Central, Suite 1510
Dallas, TX 75206

Whole Life. $20.00. 6 times a year
Whole Life Magazine
P.O. Box 205B
New York, NY 10159

Women and Health. $110.00. Quarterly
Haworth Press Inc.
Subscription Department
10 Alice Street
Binghamton, NY 13904-1580

Women's Sports and Fitness. $19.97. 8 times a year
Women's Sports and Fitness
P.O. Box 472
Mt. Morris, IL 61054

Women Wise. $7.00. Quarterly
Women Wise
38 S. Main Street
Concord, NH 03301

World Health. $22.00. Bimonthly
World Health
World Health Organization Distribution and Sales
Avenue Appia
1211 Geneva 27
Switzerland

Your Health and Fitness. $16.50. Bimonthly
General Learning Corporation
60 Revere Drive
Northbrook, IL 60062-1563

Health Books for Children

CARE AND HYGIENE

A Checkup with the Doctor. (gr. k-1). 1989. big bk. $19.98 (0-8123-6516-X); tiny bk. $3.00 (0-8123-6517-8) McDougall-Littell & Co.

Allen, Eleanor. *Wash and Brush Up.* (Illus.). 64p. (gr. 7 and up). 1984. $14.95 (0-7136-1639-3) Dufour Editions, Inc.

Arnold, Caroline. *Too Fat? Too Thin? Do You Have a Choice?* LC 83-23841. 112p. (gr. 5 and up). 1984. PLB $12.88 (0-688-02780-6); pap. $5.95 (0-688-02779-2) Morrow Junior Bks.

Bains, Rae. *Health and Hygiene.* Zink-White, Nancy, illus. LC 84-2627. 32p. (gr. 3-6). 1985. PLB $9.49 (0-8167-0180-6); pap. text ed. $2.95 (0-8167-0181-4) Troll Assocs.

Baldwin, Dorothy. *Health and Drugs.* (Illus.). 32p. 1987. PLB $15.93 (0-86592-292-6) Rourke Corp.

———. *Health and Exercise.* (Illus.). 32p. (gr. 3-8). 1987. PLB $15.93 (0-86592-293-4) Rourke Corp.

———. *Health and Feelings.* (Illus.). 32p. (gr. 3-8). 1987. PLB $15.93 (0-86592-290-X) Rourke Corp.

———. *Health and Food.* (Illus.). 32p. (gr. 3-8). 1987. PLB $15.93 (0-86592-294-2) Rourke Corp.

———. *Health and Friends.* (Illus.). 32p. (gr. 3-8). 1987. PLB $15.93 (0-86592-289-6) Rourke Corp.

———. *Health and Hygiene.* (Illus.). 32p. (gr. 3-8). 1987. PLB $15.93 (0-86592-291-8) Rourke Corp.

Berry, Joy. *Teach Me About Bathtime.* (Illus.). 32p. (gr. ps-2). 1987. PLB $11.93 (0-516-02132-X) Children's Press.

Bleich, Alan R. *Coping with Health Risks and Risky Behavior.* Rosen, Roger, ed. (gr. 7-12). 1990. PLB $13.95 (0-8239-1072-5) Rosen Publishing Group, Inc.

Brady, Janeen. *Standin' Tall Cleanliness.* Galloway, Neil, illus. 22p. (gr. ps-6). 1984. pap. text ed.

$1.50 activity bk. (0-944803-54-7); cassette and bk. $8.95 (0-944803-55-5) Brite International.

Brown, Laurie K., and Brown, Marc. *Dinosaurs Alive and Well! A Guide to Good Health*. (gr. ps-3). 1990. $14.95 (0-316-10998-3) Little, Brown & Co.

Cobb, Vicki. *Keeping Clean*. Hafner, Marilyn, illus. LC 88-2930. 32p. (gr. k-3). 1989. $11.95 (0-397-32312-3); PLB $11.89 (0-397-32313-1) Harper-Collins Children's Bks.

Collinson, Alan. *Choosing Health*. LC 90-25849. (Illus.). 48p. (gr. 5-8). 1991. PLB $18.60 (0-8114-2801-X) Raintree Steck-Vaughn Publishers.

Davies, Leah G. *Kelly Bear Health*. Davies, Joy D., illus. LC 89-85159. 28p. (gr. ps-3). 1989. pap. $4.50 (0-9621054-2-2) Kelly Bear Bks.

Diehl, Harold S., et al. *Health and Safety for You*. 5th ed. 1980. text ed. $29.52 (0-07-016863-6) McGraw-Hill Publishing Co.

Figtree, Dale. *Eat Smart: A Guide to Good Health for Kids*. LC 92-4550. 128p. 1992. $10.95 (0-8329-0465-1) New Win Publishing Co.

Fraser, K., and Tatchell, J. *Fitness and Health*. (Illus.). 48p. (gr. 6-10). 1987. PLB $13.96 (0-88110-234-2); pap. $6.95 (0-7460-0004-9) EDC Publishing.

Friedland, Bruce. *Childhood*. (Illus.). 112p. (gr. 7-12). 1993. $18.95 (0-7910-0036-2) Chelsea House Publishers.

Greenbaum, David, and Wasser, Edward. *My First Health and Nutrition Coloring Book: Mr. Carrots Coloring Book*. Puglisi, Lou, illus. 40p. (gr. 2). 1988. pap. $.99 (0-9621833-0-X) David J. Greenbaum.

Greenhaven Staff, ed. *How Can the Health of America's Children Be Improved?* (Illus.). 50p. (gr. 10 and up). 1991. pap. text ed. $3.45 (0-89908-278-5) Greenhaven Press, Inc.

———. *How Can Health Be Improved?* (Illus.). 50p. (gr. 10 and up). 1989. pap. text ed. $3.45 (0-89908-913-5) Greenhaven Press, Inc.

Hafford, Jeanette N. *Help Mates for Your Playmates*. (Illus.). 18p. 1986. pap. $4.22 (0-9616549-1-0) Tiny's Self Help Bks for Children.

Hayes, Marilyn. *Jumbo Health Yearbook: Grade 3*. 96p. (gr. 3). 1978. $18.00 (0-8209-0063-X) ESP, Inc.

———. *Jumbo Health Yearbook: Grade 4*. 96p. (gr. 4). 1979. $18.00 (0-8209-0064-8) ESP, Inc.

Houston, Jack. *Jumbo Health Yearbook: Grade 5*. 96p. (gr. 5). 1979. $18.00 (0-8209-0065-6) ESP, Inc.

———. *Jumbo Health Yearbook: Grade 6*. 96p. (gr. 6). 1979. $18.00 (0-8209-0066-4) ESP, Inc.

———. *Jumbo Health Yearbook: Grade 7*. 96p. (gr. 7). 1979. $18.00 (0-8209-0067-2) ESP, Inc.

———. *Jumbo Health Yearbook: Grade 8*. 96p. (gr. 8). 1979. $18.00 (0-8209-0068-0) ESP, Inc.

Jacobsen, Karen. *Health*. LC 81-6193. (Illus.) 48p. (gr. k-4). 1981. PLB $15.27 (0-516-01622-9) Children's Press.

Jones, Lorraine H., and Tsumura, Ted K. *Health and Safety for You*. 7th ed. 480p. 1987. text ed. $29.96 (0-07-065386-0) McGraw-Hill Publishing Co.

Long, Lynette. *On My Own: The Kids' Self Care Book*. Hall, Joann, illus. LC 84-463. 160p. (gr. 1-7). 1984. pap. $7.95 (0-87491-735-2) Acropolis Bks.

McDonnell, Janet. *Good Health: A Visit from Droopy*. Dunnington, Tom, illus. LC 90-1871. 32p. (gr. ps-2). 1990. PLB $19.95 (0-89565-582-9) Child's World, Inc.

Moncure, Jane B. *Healthkins Help*. Axeman, Lois, illus. LC 82-14713. 32p. (gr. ps-2). 1982. PLB $18.50 (0-89565-242-0) Child's World, Inc.

———. *Magic Monsters Learn About Health*. Endres, Helen, illus. LC 79-24240. (gr. ps-3). 1980. PLB $19.95 (0-89565-117-3) Child's World, Inc.

Neff, Fred. *Keeping Fit Handbook for Physical Conditioning and Better Health*. Reid, James, illus. LC 75-38478. 56p. (gr. 5 and up). 1977. PLB $9.95 (0-8225-1157-6) Lerner Publications.

Odor, Ruth. *What's a Body to Do?* Letwenko, Ed, illus. LC 81-17031. 112p. (gr. 2-6). 1980. PLB $19.95 (0-89565-209-9) Child's World, Inc.

Orlandi, Mario, et al. *Maintaining Good Health*. 128p. (gr. 5 and up). 1989. $18.95 (0-8160-1667-4) Facts on File, Inc.

Parker, Steve. *Catching a Cold: How You Get Ill, Suffer and Recover*. (Illus.). 32p. (gr. k-4). 1992. PLB $11.40 (0-531-14146-2) Franklin Watts, Inc.

Petty, Kate. *Going to the Doctor*. Kopper, Lisa, illus. 24p. (gr. 1-3). 1987. PLB $10.40 (0-531-17069-1) Franklin Watts, Inc.

Rayner, Claire. *The Don't Spoil Your Body Book*. (Illus.). 48p. (gr. 3 and up). 1989. pap. $4.95 (0-8120-6098-9) Barron's Educational Services, Inc.

Roettger, Doris. *Growing Up Healthy*. (gr. k-3). 1991. pap. $8.95 (0-86653-970-0) Fearon Teacher Aids.

Salter, Charles A. *Looking Good, Eating Right: A Sensible Guide to Proper Nutrition and Weight Loss for Teens*. (Illus.). 144p. (gr. 7 and up). 1991. PLB $14.90 (1-56294-047-3) Milbrook Press, Inc.

Sheehan, Angela, ed. *Encyclopedia of Health.* 14 vols. LC 89-17336. (Illus.). 900p. (gr. 4-8). 1991. PLB $299.95 (1-85435-203-2) Marshall Cavendish Corp.

Springate, Kay W. *Let's Learn about Good Health.* 64p. (gr. ps-2). 1988. wkbk. $7.95 (0-86653-438-5) Good Apple.

Stein, Sara. *The Body Book.* (Illus.). (gr. 4-7). 1992. pap. $11.95 (0-89480-805-2) Workman Publishing Co., Inc.

Ward, Brian R. *Health and Hygiene.* (Illus.). 48p. (gr. 4-12). 1988. PLB $12.40 (0-531-10561-X) Franklin Watts, Inc.

CARE AND HYGIENE: FICTION

Arrick, Fran. *What You Don't Know.* 1992. $16.00 (0-553-17471-7) Bantam Bks, Inc.

Bottner, Barbara. *Messy.* (Illus.). LC 78-50420. (gr. k-2). 1979. $6.95 (0-440-15492-3); pap. $6.46 (0-440-05493-1) Delacorte Press.

Bowling, David L., and Bowling, Patricia H. *Dirty Dingy Darryl.* Martz, John, ed. Bowling, Patricia H., illus. LC 81-83120. 24p. (gr. ps-4). 1981. $6.00 (0-939700-00-X); pap. $3.00 (0-939700-01-8) Inka Dinka Ink Children's Press.

Buchanan, J. *Taking Care of My Cold.* (Illus.). 24p. (gr. ps-8). 1990. pap. $4.95 (0-88753-197-0) Firefly Bks Ltd.

Burningham, John. *Time to Get out of the Bath, Shirley.* (Illus.). LC 76-58503. 32p. (gr. k-2). 1978. $13.95 (0-690-01378-7) HarperCollins Children's Bks.

Edwards, Frank B. and Bianchi, John. *Mortimer Mooner Stopped Taking a Bath.* (Illus.). 24p. (gr. ps-2). 1990. $14.95 (0-921285-21-3); pap. $4.95 (0-921285-20-5) Firefly Bks Ltd.

Guymon, Maurine B. *The Adventures of Micki Microbe.* Zagone, Arlene T., illus. 88p. (gr. 2-5). 1987. $15.00 (0-9618650-0-8) MoDel Publishers.

Hamsa, Bobbie. *Dirty Larry.* LC 83-10079. (Illus.). 32p. (gr. ps-2). 1983. PLB $11.93 (0-516-02040-4); pap. $2.95 (0-516-42040-2) Children's Press.

Henkes, Kevin. *Clean Enough.* (Illus.). LC 81-6386. 24p. (gr. k-3). 1982. PLB $10.98 (0-688-00829-1) Greenwillow Bks.

Hutchins, Pat. *Tidy Titch.* LC 90-38483. (Illus.). 32p. (gr. ps and up). 1991. $13.95 (0-688-09963-7); PLB $13.88 (0-688-09964-5) Greenwillow Bks.

Jacobs, Don. *Happy Exercise: An Adventure into a Fit World.* Spiedel, Sandy, illus. LC 80-23547. 48p. (gr. ps-5). 1980. pap. $4.95 (0-89037-170-9) Anderson World, Inc.

McPhail, David. *Andrew's Bath.* (Illus.). (gr. ps-3). 1984. $13.95 (0-316-56319-6) Little, Brown & Co.

Moncure, Jane B. *Caring for My Body.* McCallum, Jodie, illus. 32p. (gr. ps-2). 1990. PLB $17.25 (0-89565-668-X) Child's World, Inc.

Nelson, Ray, Jr. *The Internal Adventures of Donovan Willoughby.* LC 91-18810. (Illus.). 48p. (gr. ps-7). 1991. $12.95 (0-89802-572-9) Beautiful America Publishing Co.

Smollin, Michael. *Ernie's Bath Book.* (gr. ps-3). 1982. $3.95 (0-394-85402-0) Random House Bks for Young Readers.

Starbuck, Marnie. *The Gladimals Learn Healthy Habits.* 16p. (gr. ps-3). 1991. pap. text ed. $.75 (1-56456-227-1) William Gladden Foundation.

Wells, Rosemary. *Fritz and the Messy Fairy.* LC 90-26671. (Illus.). 32p. (gr. ps-2). 1991. $13.95 (0-8037-0981-1); PLB $13.89 (0-8037-0983-8) Dial Bks for Young Readers.

Wolcott, Patty. *The Marvelous Mud Washing Machine.* Brown, Richard, illus. LC 91-8196. 32p. (gr. ps-2). 1991. $3.50 (0-679-81926-6); PLB $6.99 (0-679-91926-0) Random House Bks for Young Readers.

DEATH

Berry, Joy. *About Death.* 48p. (gr. 3 and up). 1990. PLB $15.00 (0-516-02952-5) Children's Press.

Bisnignano, Judith. *Living with Death—Middle School.* 64p. (gr. 5-9). 1991. $7.95 (0-86653-584-5) Good Apple.

Blackburn, Lynn B. *Timothy Duck: The Story of the Death of a Friend.* Johnson, Joy, ed. Borum, Shari, illus. 24p. (gr. 1-6). 1989. pap. $3.25 (1-56123-013-8) Centering Corp.

Boulden, Jim. *Saying Goodbye.* 2nd ed. (Illus.). (gr. 1-7). 1991. pap. $3.95 (1-878076-02-7) Boulden Publishing.

Bratman, Fred. *Everything You Need to Know When a Parent Dies.* (gr. 7-12). 1992. PLB $13.95 (0-8239-1324-4) Rosen Publishing Group, Inc.

Cera, Mary J. *Living with Death—Primary.* 64p. (gr. 1-4). 1991. $7.95 (0-86653-588-8) Good Apple.

Cohn, Janice. *I Had a Friend Named Peter: Talking to Children About the Death of a Friend.* Owens,

Gail, illus. LC 86-31150. 32p. (gr. ps-2). 1987. $13.00 (0-688-06685-2) Morrow Jr Bks.

Corley, Elizabeth. *Tell Me About Death, Tell Me About Funerals.* (Illus.). 36p. (gr. 3-6). 1973. pap. text ed. $2.00 (0-686-02638-1) Grammatical Sciences.

Crouthamel, Thomas G., Sr. *It's OK.* 2nd ed. Hasty, Patti, illus. LC 86-27694. 36p. (gr. 6 and up). 1990. pap. $6.95 (0-940701-18-9) Keystone Press.

Fayerweather Street School Staff. *The Kids' Book About Death and Dying.* Rofes, Eric, ed. 119p. (gr. 5 and up). 1985. $15.95 (0-316-75390-4) Little, Brown & Co.

Gravelle, Karen, and Haskins, Charles. *Teenagers Face to Face with Bereavement.* Steltenpohl, Jane, ed. 128p. (gr. 7 and up). 1989. $12.98 (0-671-65856-5) Simon & Schuster Trade.

Greenlee, Sharon. *When Someone Dies.* Drath, Bill, illus. 40p. (gr. 1-7). 1992. $12.95 (1-56145-044-8) Peachtree Publishers, Inc.

Grollman, Earl A. *Talking About Death: A Dialogue Between Parent and Child; With Parent's Guide and Recommended Resources.* 3rd ed. Heau, Gisela, illus. LC 89-46061. 128p. (gr. k-4). 1990. $18.95 (0-8070-2364-7) Beacon Press.

Haasl, Beth, and Marrocha, Jean. *Bereavement Support Group Program for Children: Participant Workbook.* 39p. (gr. ps-8). 1990. $6.95 (1-55959-012-2) Accelerated Development, Inc.

Hammond, Janice M. *When My Mommy Died: A Child's View of Death.* (Illus.). 27p. (gr. ps-5). 1980. pap. $6.95 (0-9604690-0-1) Cranbrook Publishing.

Heegaard, Marge E. *When Someone Very Special Dies: Children Can Learn to Cope with Grief.* (Illus.). 32p. (gr. 1-6). 1988. wkbk. $4.95 (0-9620502-0-2) Woodland Press.

Hyde, Margaret O., and Hyde, Lawrence E. *Meeting Death.* 129p. (gr. 5 and up). 1989. $14.95 (0-8027-6873-3) Walker & Co.

Johnson, Joy, and Johnson, Marvin. *Tell Me, Papa: A Family Book for Children's Questions about Death and Funerals.* Borum, Shari, illus. 24p. (gr. 2-7). 1978. pap. $3.25 (1-56123-011-1) Centering Corp.

Juneau, Barbara F. *Sad, but OK—My Daddy Died Today: A Child's View of Death.* Clemens, Paul M., ed. LC 88-155937. (Illus.). 112p. (gr. 5 and up). 1988. pap. $9.95 (0-931892-19-8) Blue Dolphin Publishing, Inc.

LaVelle, Steven. *Just Passing Through.* (Illus.). 32p. (gr. k-3). 1980. pap. $3.50 (0-87516-402-1) DeVorss & Co.

LeShan, Eda. *Learning to Say Goodbye: When a Parent Dies.* Giovanopoulous, Paul, illus. LC 76-15155. 96p. (gr. 3 and up). 1976. $13.95 (0-02-756360-X) Macmillan Children's Bk Group.

McGuire, Leslie. *Death and Illness.* (Illus.). 64p. (gr. 7 and up). 1990. $15.93 (0-86593-079-1) Rourke Corp.

Nystrom, Carolyn. *What Happens When We Die?* 32p. (gr. ps-2). 1981. pap. $4.99 (0-8024-6154-9) Moody Press.

Powell, E. Sandy. *Geranium Morning: A Book About Grief.* (gr. ps-3). 1991. pap. $4.95 (0-87614-542-X) Carolrhoda Bks, Inc.

Pringle, Laurence. *Death Is Natural.* LC 90-46402. 64p. (gr. 1 and up). 1991. pap. $5.95 (0-688-10528-9) William Morrow & Co., Inc.

Raab, Robert A. *Coping with Death.* Rosen, Ruth, ed. (gr. 7-12). 1989. PLB $13.95 (0-8239-0960-3) Rosen Publishing Group, Inc.

Russell, Katherine B. *Guiding Children Through Grief: A Resource Manual of Recommended Books to Help Young Children Cope with Death, Dying and Grief.* (Illus.). 48p. (gr. ps and up). 1989. pap. $5.25 (1-56123-036-7) Centering Corp.

Stein, Sara B. *About Dying.* LC 73-15268. (Illus.). 48p. (gr. ps-8). 1984. pap. $8.95 (0-8027-7223-4) Walker & Co.

Stewart, Gail. *Death.* LC 89-31257. (Illus.). 48p. (gr. 4-5). 1989. $11.95 (0-89686-446-4) Macmillan Children's Bk Group.

Temes, Roberta. *The Empty Place: A Story for Children.* (Illus.). 50p. (gr. 1-6). 1989. $12.95 (0-8290-1345-8) Irvington Publishers.

DEATH: FICTION

Angell, Judie. *Ronnie and Rosey.* 192p. (gr. 6-9). 1979. pap. $2.95 (0-440-97491-7) Dell Publishing Co., Inc.

Auer, Martin. *The Blue Boy.* Klages, Simone, illus. LC 91-39130. 32p. (gr. 2 and up). 1992. $11.95 (0-02-707610-5) Macmillan Children's Bk Group.

Bacon, Katherine J. *Shadow and Light.* LC 86-23789. 208p. (gr. 7 and up). 1987. $14.95 (0-689-50431-4) Macmillan Children's Bk Group.

Balter, Lawrence. *A Funeral for Whiskers: Understanding Death.* Schanzer, Roy, illus. 40p. (gr. ps-3).

1991. $5.95 (0-8120-6153-5) Barron's Educational Services, Inc.

Blume, Judy. *Tiger Eyes.* 224p. (gr. 7 and up). 1982. $3.99 (0-440-98469-6) Dell Publishing Co., Inc.

Boyd, Candy D. *Forever Friends.* 192p. (gr. 5-9). 1986. pap. $4.99 (0-14-032077-6) Puffin Bks.

Brown, Margaret W. *The Dead Bird.* Charlip, Remy, illus. LC 84-43124. 48p. (gr. k-3). 1989. PLB $11.89 (0-06-020758-2) HarperCollins Children's Bks.

Bunting, Eve. *A Sudden Silence.* 107p. (gr. 7 and up). 1988. $14.95 (0-15-282058-2) Harcourt Brace Jovanovich, Inc.

Byars, Betsy. *Good-Bye, Chicken Little.* LC 78-19829. 112p. (gr. 5 and up). 1979. PLB $13.89 (0-06-020911-9) HarperCollins Children's Bks.

Cameron, Eleanor. *Beyond Silence.* LC 80-10350. 208p. (gr. 5-9). 1980. $9.95 (0-525-26463-9) Dutton Children's Bks.

Carlstrom, Nancy W. *Blow Me a Kiss, Miss Lily.* Schwartz, Amy, illus. LC 89-34505. 32p. (gr. ps-3). 1990. $13.00 (0-06-021012-5) HarperCollins Children's Bks.

Carrick, Carol. *The Accident.* Carrick, Donald, illus. LC 76-3532. 32p. (gr. ps-3). 1981. $13.45 (0-395-28774-X); pap. $4.80 (0-89919-041-3) Houghton Mifflin Co.

Chambers, Aidan. *Dance on My Grave.* LC 82-48258. 256p. (gr. 7 and up). 1983. PLB $13.89 (0-06-021254-3) HarperCollins Children's Bks.

Conley, Bruce H. *Butterflies, Grandpa and Me.* (Illus.). 25p. (gr. 4 and up). 1976. pap. $2.00 (0-685-65885-6) Thum Printing.

Conrad, Pam. *My Daniel.* LC 88-19850. 144p. (gr. 5 and up). 1991. pap. $3.95 (0-06-440309-2) HarperCollins Children's Bks.

Dabcovich, Lydia. *Mrs. Huggins and Her Hen Hannah.* (Illus.). LC 85-4406. 24p. (gr. ps-2). 1988. $12.95 (0-525-44203-0); pap. $3.95 (0-525-44368-1) Dutton Children's Bks.

Douglas, Eileen. *Rachel and the Upside Down Heart.* (Illus.). 32p. 1990. pap. $6.95 (0-8431-2734-1) Price Stern Sloan, Inc.

Engel, Diana. *Eleanor, Arthur and Claire.* (Illus.). LC 91-21781. 32p. (gr. k-3). 1992. $14.95 (0-02-733462-7) Macmillan Children's Bk Group.

Fassler, Joan. *My Grandpa Died Today.* Krantz, Stewart, illus. LC 71-147126. 32p. (gr. ps-3). 1983. $14.95 (0-87705-053-8); pap. $9.95 (0-89885-174-2) Human Sciences Press, Inc.

Gibson, Roxie C. *Hey God! What Is Death?* LC 90-70219. (Illus.). 50p. (gr. k-5). 1990. $4.95 (1-55523-329-5) Winston-Derek Publishers, Inc.

Gikow, Louise. *Muppet Kids in Good-Bye, Horace Hamster.* Brannon, Tom, illus. (gr. ps-3). 1991. pap. $1.25 (0-307-12655-2) Western Publishing Co., Inc.

Godreau, Cecile. *Call Me Jonathan for Short.* Peterson, Mary J., illus. 64p. (gr. 4-5). 1991. pap. $2.95 (0-8198-1463-6) St. Paul Bks & Media.

Grant, Cynthia D. *Phoenix Rising: or How to Survive Your Life.* 160p. (gr. 7 and up). 1991. pap. $3.50 (0-06-447060-1) HarperCollins Children's Bks.

Green, Martha G. *Grampa's in Heaven.* LC 90-71356. (Illus.). 44p. (gr. 3-8). 1991. pap. $5.95 (1-55523-399-6) Winston-Derek Publishers, Inc.

Greene, Constance C. *Beat the Turtle Drum.* 128p. (gr. 5-8). 1979. pap. $3.25 (0-440-40875-X) Dell Publishing Co., Inc.

Hammond, Janice M. *When My Dad Died: A Child's View of Death.* (Illus.). 48p. (gr. k-6). 1981. pap. $6.95 (0-9604690-3-6) Cranbrook Publishing.

Hermes, Patricia. *You Shouldn't Have to Say Good-Bye.* 128p. (gr. 4-6). 1984. pap. $2.50 (0-590-41359-7) Scholastic, Inc.

Hines, Anna G. *Remember the Butterflies.* Hines, Anna G., illus. LC 90-3536. 32p. (gr. ps-2). 1991. $12.95 (0-525-44679-6) Dutton Children's Bks.

Jewell, Nancy. *Time for Uncle Joe.* Sandin, Joan, illus. LC 79-2695. 48p. (gr. k-3). 1981. $8.95 (0-06-022843-1) HarperCollins Children's Bks.

Joosse, Barbara M. *Pieces of the Picture.* LC 88-28150. 144p. (gr. 5-7). 1991. pap. $3.50 (0-06-440310-6) HarperCollins Children's Bks.

Kroll, Virginia L. *Helen the Fish.* Mathews, Judith, ed. Weidner, Teri, illus. LC 91-17230. 32p. (gr. k-3). 1992. PLB $23.95 (0-8075-3194-4) Albert Whitman & Co.

Lanton, Sandy. *Daddy's Chair.* Haas, Shelley O., illus. LC 90-44908. 32p. (gr. k-4). 1991. $12.95 (0-929371-51-8) Kar Ben Copies, Inc.

Laufer, Judy E. *Where Did Papa Go: Looking at Death from a Young Child's Perspective.* Wingfield, Ken, Jr., illus. 32p. (gr. ps-2). 1991. pap. $9.95 (1-8811669-00-9) Little Egg Publishing Co.

Lowry, Lois. *A Summer to Die.* Olivier, Jenni, illus. (gr. 3-7). 1977. $13.45 (0-395-25338-1) Houghton Mifflin Co.

Madenski, Melissa. *Some of the Pieces.* Ray, Deborah K., illus. (gr. ps-3). 1991. $15.95 (0-316-54324-1) Little, Brown & Co.

Madler, Trudy. *Why Did Grandma Die?* LC 79-23892. (Illus.). 32p. (gr. k-6). 1980. PLB $16.67 (0-8172-1354-6) Raintree Steck-Vaughn Publishers.

Manber, David. *Zachary of the Wings.* 88p. (gr. 9-12). 1993. PLB $10.95 (1-879567-27-X) Wonder Well Publishers.

McDaniel, Lurlene. *If I Should Die Before I Wake.* 128p. (gr. 5-8). 1985. $.50 (0-87406-077-X) Willowisp Press, Inc.

———. *Six Months to Live.* 144p. (gr. 5-8). 1985. $2.95 (0-87406-007-9) Willowisp Press, Inc.

———. *Why Did She Have to Die?* 128p. (gr. 5-8). 1986. $2.50 (0-87406-071-0) Willowisp Press, Inc.

Nystrom, Carolyn. *Emma Says Goodbye.* (Illus.). 48p. (gr. 4-8). 1990. $7.99 (0-7459-1826-3) Lion Publishing Corp.

O'Toole, Donna. *Aarvy Aardvark Finds Hope: A Read-Aloud Story for People of All Ages.* McWhirter, Mary Lou, illus. 80p. (gr. ps and up). 1989. pap. $9.95 (1-878321-25-0) Rainbow Connection.

Paterson, Katherine. *Bridge to Terabithia.* Diamond, Donna, illus. LC 77-2221. (gr. 5 and up). 1977. $14.00 (0-690-01359-0) HarperCollins Children's Bks.

Pfeffer, Susan B. *About David: A Novel.* LC 80-65837. 176p. (gr. 7 and up). 1980. $11.95 (0-385-28013-0) Delacorte Press.

Ruckman, Ivy. *Who Invited the Undertaker?* LC 89-1865. 192p. (gr. 3-7). 1991. pap. $3.95 (0-06-440352-1) HarperCollins Children's Bks.

Sanford, Doris. *It Must Hurt a Lot: A Child's Book About Death.* Evans, Graci, illus. LC 86-25009. 32p. (gr. ps-5). 1985. $7.99 (0-88070-131-5) Multnomah Press.

Shott, James. *The House Across the Street.* LC 87-51498. 30p. (gr. 2-4). 1988. $6.95 (1-55523-129-2) Winston-Derek Publishers, Inc.

Steel, Danielle. *Max and Grandma and Grandpa Winky.* (gr. ps-3). 1991. $9.95 (0-385-30165-0) Doubleday & Co., Inc.

Talbert, Marc. *Dead Birds Singing.* LC 85-147. 224p. (gr. 6 and up). 1985. $13.95 (0-316-83125-5) Little, Brown & Co.

Velthuijs, Max. *Frog and the Birdsong.* (gr. ps-3). 1991. $13.95 (0-374-32467-0) Farrar Straus & Giroux Inc.

Vigna, Judith. *Saying Good-bye to Daddy.* Levine, Abby, ed. Vigna, Judith, illus. LC 90-12757. 32p. (gr. k-2). 1991 $13.95 (0-8075-7253-5) Albert Whitman & Co.

Viorst, Judith. *The Tenth Good Thing About Barney.* Blegvad, Eric, illus. LC 71-154764. 32p. (gr. k-4). 1971. $12.95 (0-689-20688-7) Macmillan Children's Bk Group.

Warburg, Sandol S. *Growing Time.* Weisgard, Leonard, illus. LC 69-14729 (gr. k-3). 1975. $13.95 (0-395-16966-6) Houghton Mifflin Co.

Westall, Robert. *The Promise.* 208p. (gr. 5 and up). 1991. $13.95 (0-590-43760-7) Scholastic, Inc.

Windsor, Patricia. *The Summer Before.* 176p. (gr. 7 and up). 1974. pap. $1.95 (0-440-98382-7) Dell Publishing Co., Inc.

Wright, Betty R. *The Cat Next Door.* Owens, Gail, illus. LC 90-29080. 32p. (gr. ps-3). 1991. $14.95 (0-8234-0896-5) Holiday House, Inc.

Wurmfeld, Hope H. *Baby Blues.* LC 92-5828. 80p. (gr. 7 and up). 1992. $14.00 (0-670-84151-X) Viking Children's Bks.

Young, Alida E. *Is My Sister Dying?* 144p. (gr. 5-8). 1991. pap. $2.95 (0-87406-541-0) Willowisp Press, Inc.

Zemach, Margot. *Jake and Honeybunch Go to Heaven.* LC 82-71752. (Illus.). 40p. (gr. 3 and up). 1982. $16.00 (0-374-33652-0) Farrar Straus & Giroux Inc.

Diet and Weight Control

Coyle, Neva, and Chapian, Marie. *Slimming Down and Growing Up.* LC 85-15028. 160p. (gr. 4-7). 1985. pap. $5.99 (0-87123-833-0) Bethany House Publishers.

Jones, Lucile. *Tony's Tummy.* Van Dolson, Bobbie J., ed. 32p. (gr. k and up). 1981. pap. $3.95. (0-8280-0039-5) Review and Herald Publishing Assn.

Kane, June K. *Coping with Diet Fads.* Rosen, Ruth, ed. (gr. 7-12). 1990. PLB $13.95 (0-8239-1005-9) Rosen Publishing Group Inc.

Landau, Elaine. *Weight: A Teenage Concern.* 160p. (gr. 7 and up). 1991. $15.00 (0-525-67335-0) Dutton Children's Bks.

Phillips, Barbara. *Don't Call Me Fatso.* Cogancherry, Helen, illus. LC 85-24341. 32p. (gr. k-6). 1980. PLB $16.67 (0-8172-1350-3) Raintree Steck-Vaughn Publishers.

Sachs, Marilyn. *The Fat Girl.* LC 83-11697. 176p. (gr. 6 and up). 1984. $13.95 (0-525-44076-3) Dutton Children's Bks.

Silverstein, Alvin, et al. *So You Think You're Fat?* LC 90-40761. 224p. (gr. 7 and up). 1991. $14.00 (0-06-021641-7): PLB $13.89 (0-06-021642-5) HarperCollins Children's Bks.

Ward, Brian R. *Diet and Nutrition.* (Illus.). 48p. (gr. 4-12). 1987. PLB $12.40 (0-531-10259-9) Franklin Watts, Inc.

Wolhart, Dayna. *Anorexia and Bulimia.* LC 88-21553. (Illus.). 48p. (gr. 5-6). 1988. $11.95 (0-89686-416-12) Macmillan Children's Bk Group.

DIET AND WEIGHT CONTROL: FICTION

Bottner, Barbara. *Dumb Old Casey Is a Fat Tree.* LC 78-19474. (Illus.). 48p. (gr. 1-4). 1979. $11.89 (0-06-020616-0) HarperCollins Children's Bks.

DeClements, Barthe. *Nothing's Fair in Fifth Grade.* 144p. (gr. 3 and up). 1990. pap. $3.50 (0-14-034443-8) Puffin Bks.

Greenberg, Jan. *The Pig-Out Blues.* LC 82-2552. 121p. (gr. 7 and up). 1982. $14.00 (0-374-35937-7) Farrar Straus & Giroux Inc.

Hargreaves, Roger. *Little Miss Plump.* (Illus.). 32p. (gr. ps-k). 1981. pap. $1.75 (0-8431-0895-9) Price Stern Sloan, Inc.

Holland, Isabelle. *Dinah and the Green Fat Kingdom.* 192p. (gr. 5 and up). 1986. pap. $1.75 (0-440-91918-5) Dell Publishing Co., Inc.

Hunt, Angela. *Cassie Perkins: Much Adored Shore.* 176p. (gr. 4-8). 1992. pap. $4.99 (0-8423-1065-7) Tyndale House Publishers.

Lipsyte, Robert. *One Fat Summer.* LC 76-49746. (gr. 7 and up). 1977. PLB $14.89 (0-06-023896-8) HarperCollins Children's Bks.

Perl, Lila. *Hey, Remember Fat Glenda?* 192p. (gr. 3-6). 1981. $14.45 (0-395-31023-7) Houghton Mifflin Co.

Ruckman, Ivy. *The Hunger Scream.* LC 83-6522. 200p. (gr. 6 and up). 1983. $14.95 (0-8027-6514-9) Walker & Co.

DISEASES

Brown, Fern G. *Hereditary Disease.* (Illus.). 96p. (gr. 4-9). 1987. PLB $10.40 (0-531-10386-2) Franklin Watts, Inc.

Eagles, Douglas A. *Nutritional Diseases.* (Illus.). (gr. 4-8). 1987. PLB $10.40 (0-531-10391-9) Franklin Watts, Inc.

Fox, Cecil H. *AIDS and HIV Diseases.* Head, J. J., ed. Botzis, Ka, illus. 16p. (gr. 10 and up). 1991. pap. text ed. $2.15 (0-89278-120-3) Carolina Biological Supply Co.

Hathaway, Joe, and Hathaway, Nancy. *How John Was Unique.* 12p. (gr. k-3). 1984. pap. text ed. $3.95 (0-918335-01-9) National Marfan Foundation.

Krementz, Jill. *How It Feels to Fight for Your Life.* (Illus.). 1989. $15.95 (0-316-50364-9) Little, Brown & Co.

Lampton, Christopher. *Epidemic.* LC 91-21413. (Illus.). 64p. (gr. 4-6). 1992. PLB $13.40 (1-56294-126-7) Millbrook Press, Inc.

Nourse, Alan E. *Lumps, Bumps, and Rashes: A Look at Kids' Diseases.* rev. ed. (Illus.). 64p. (gr. 5-8). 1990. PLB $12.40 (0-531-10865-1) Franklin Watts, Inc.

Ogden, John A. *The Medibears Guide to the Doctor's Exam: For Children and Parents.* Ogden, Ethel F., illus. (gr. k-5). 1991. $9.95 (0-8130-1082-9) University Press of Florida.

Richardson, Joy. *What Happens When You Catch a Cold?* LC 86-3730. (Illus.). 32p. (gr. 2-3). 1986. PLB $11.95 (1-55532-104-6) Gareth Stevens, Inc.

DISEASES: FICTION

Barnes, Caroline. *It's No Fun to Be Sick!* (Illus.). 32p. (gr. ps-k). 1989. (0-307-12031-7) Western Publishing Co., Inc.

Blume, Judy. *Deenie.* 144p. (gr. 7 and up). 1991. pap. $3.50 (0-440-93259-9) Dell Publishing Co., Inc.

Gehret, Jeanne. *I'm Somebody Too.* 176 p. (gr. 4-7). 1992. text ed. $16.00 (0-9625136-7-9); pap. $12.00 (0-9625136-6-0) Verbal Images Press.

Getz, David. *Thin Air.* LC 90-34137. 128p. (gr. 3-7). 1992. pap. $3.95 (0-06-440422-6) HarperCollins Children's Bks.

Gilow, Betty, and Tickle, Phyllis. *It's No Fun to Be Sick by Paula and Her Friends.* (Illus.). (gr. 2-6). 1976. $3.95 (0-918518-02-4) St. Luke's Press.

Girard, Linda W. *Alex, the Kid with AIDS.* Levine. Abby, ed. Sims, Blanche, illus. LC 89-77592. 32p. (gr. 2-5). 1991. PLB $13.95 (0-8075-0245-6) Albert Whitman & Co.

Jones, Shelley D. *When Laughing Isn't Funny.* (Illus.). 1990. $6.95 (0-533-08541-1) Vantage Press, Inc.

Laird, Elizabeth. *Loving Ben.* (gr. 5 and up). 1989. $14.95 (0-385-29810-2) Delacorte Press.

MacLachlan, Patricia. *The Sick Day.* DuBois, William P., illus. LC 78-11686. (gr. k-3). 1979. $6.95 (0-394-83876-9) Pantheon Bks.

Sinykin, Sheri. *Apart at the Seams.* 120p. (gr. 6-12). 1991. pap. $3.95 (0-89486-733-4) Hazelden Foundation.

Starkman, Neil. *Z's Gift.* Ellen, G., and Sasaki, Joy, illus. LC 88-71483. 52p. (gr. 4-6). 1988. pap. $7.00 (0-935529-08-X) Comprehensive Health Education Foundation.

COMMUNICABLE DISEASES

Diskavich, Laura, and Woods, Samuel, Jr. *Everything You Need to Know about STD.* Rosen, Ruth, ed. (gr. 7-12). 1990. PLB $13.95 (0-8239-1010-5) Rosen Publishing Group, Inc.

Donahue, Parnell, and Capellaro, Helen. *Germs Make Me Sick: A Health Handbook for Kids.* Oechsli, Kelly, illus. LC 74-15309. 96p. (gr. 4 and up). 1975. Alfred A. Knopf Bks for Young Readers.

Metos, Thomas H. *Communicable Diseases.* (Illus.). 96p. (gr. 4-9). 1987. PLB $10.40 (0-531-10380-3) Franklin Watts, Inc.

Norse, Alan E. *Sexually Transmitted Diseases.* Matthews, V., ed. (Illus.). 144p. (gr.9-12). 1992. PLB $13.90 (0-531-11065-6) Franklin Watts, Inc.

EXERCISE

Baldwin, Dorothy. *Health and Exercise.* (Illus.). 32p. (gr. 3-8). 1987. PLB $15.93 (0-86592-293-4) Rourke Corp.

Charles, Donald. *Calico Cat's Exercise Book.* LC 82-9640. (Illus.). (gr. ps-3). 1982. PLB $15.00 (0-516-03457-X) Children's Press.

Duyff, Roberta, L. *Big Bug Book of Exercise.* McKissack, Patricia, and McKissack, Frederick, eds. LC 87-61656. 24p. (gr. k-1). 1987. $14.95 (0-88335-761-5); pap. text ed. $4.95 (0-88335-771-2) Milliken Publishing Co.

Goldstein, Rebecca. *The Mind-Body Problem.* 304p. (gr. 5 and up). 1985. pap. $4.95 (0-440-35651-2) Dell Publishing Co., Inc.

Isenberg, Barbara, and Jaffe, Marjorie. *Albert the Running Bear's Exercise Book.* De Groat, Diane, illus. LC 84-7064. 64p. (gr. ps-4). 1984. Clarion Bks.; pap. $4.80 (0-89919-318-8) Houghton Mifflin Co.

Jones, Lucile. *Hop, Skip and Jump.* Van Dolson, Bobbie J., ed. 32p. (gr. k and up). 1981. pap. $3.95 (0-8280-0038-7) Review & Herald Publishing Assn.

Liptak, Karen. *Aerobics Basics.* D'Amato, Janet, illus. 48p. (gr. 3-7). 1983. $9.95 (0-13-018218-4) Prentice Hall.

Moncure, Jane B. *Healthkins Exercise!* Endres, Helen, illus. LC 82-14712. 32p. (gr. ps-2). 1982. PLB $18.50 (0-89565-241-2) Childs World, Inc.

Nardo, Don. *Exercise.* (Illus.). 112p. (gr. 6-12). 1992. $18.95 (0-7910-0017-6) Chelsea House Publishers.

Reiss, Elayne, and Friedman, Rita. *Exercise Expert.* (gr. k-1). $10.50 (0-89796-866-2) New Dimensions in Education.

Richardson, Joy. *What Happens When You Run?* LC 86-3707. (Illus.). 32p. (gr. 2-3). 1986. PLB $11.95 (1-55532-110-0) Gareth Stevens, Inc.

Schwarzenegger, Arnold, and Gaines, Charles. *Arnold's Fitness for Kids: A Guide to Health, Exercise, and Nutrition.* LC 92-28577. (gr. 1-5). 1993. $15.00 (0-385-42267-9) Doubleday & Co., Inc.

———. *Arnold's Fitness for Kids Ages Birth to Five: A Guide to Health, Exercise, and Nutrition.* LC 92-26209. (gr. ps-k). 1993. $15.00 (0-385-42266-0) Doubleday & Co., Inc.

HOSPITALS

Alsop, Peter, et al. *In the Hospital.* 64p. (gr. k-6). 1989. pap. $12.98 (1-877942-00-6) Moose School Records.

Butler, Daphne. *First Look in the Hospital.* LC 90-10245. (Illus.). 32p. (gr. 1-2). 1991. $11.95 (0-8368-0563-1) Gareth Stevens, Inc.

Carter, Sharon, and Monnig, Judith. *Coping with a Hospital Stay.* Rosen, Ruth, ed. 128p. (gr. 7 and up). 1987. PLB $13.95 (0-8239-0682-5) Rosen Publishing Group, Inc.

Coleman, William L. *My Hospital Book.* Walles, Dwight, illus. LC 81-10094. 96p. (gr. 2-7). 1981. pap. $5.99 (0-87123-354-1) Bethany House Publishers.

Elliot, Ingrid G. *Hospital Roadmap: A Book to Help Explain the Hospital Experience to Young Chil-*

dren. LC 82-80226. (Illus.). 36p. (gr. k-2). 1984. pap. $8.95 (0-9608150-0-7) Resources for Children in Hospitals.

———. *Hospital Roadmap Manual: A Curriculum Guide to Explain the Hospital Experience to Young Children.* 100p. (gr. k-2). 1986. pap. $11.95 (0-9608150-1-5) Resources for Children in Hospitals.

Going into Hospital. (Illus.). (gr. ps). $3.50 (0-7241-0849-4) Ladybird Bks, Inc.

Going to the Hospital. (Illus.). 32p. (gr. ps). 1990. $2.99 (0-517-69197-3) Outlet Bk Co., Inc.

Krall, Carlotte B., and Jim, Judith M. *Fat Dog's First Visit: A Child's View of the Hospital.* Hull, Nancy, ed. and illus. LC 87-2745. 28p. (gr. ps-3). 1987. pap. text ed. $4.00 (0-939838-23-0) Pritchett & Hull Assocs., Inc.

Livingston, Carole, and Ciliotta, Claire. *Why Am I Going to the Hospital?* Walter, Paul, illus. (gr. 1 and up). 1981. $12.00 (0-8184-0316-0) Carol Publishing Group.

Rosenstock, Judith D., and Rosenstock, Harvey A. *Your Hospital Stay . . . It'll Be Okay.* Sorg, James M., illus. 36p. (gr. 1-5). 1988. pap. $4.95 (0-9622172-0-4) D. Miller Foundation.

Sauer, Sue, et al. *Stevie Has His Heart Examined.* Goldstein, Nancy, ed. Albury, Mary, illus. (gr. ps-7). 1983. pap. text ed. $4.25 (0-937423-00-9) University of Minnesota Hospital & Clinic.

———. *Stevie Has His Heart Repaired.* Goldstein, Nancy, ed. Albury, Mary, illus. (gr. ps-7). 1979. pap. text ed. $4.25 (0-937423-01-7) University of Minnesota Hospital & Clinic.

Shepherd, Sue, et al. *Color Me Special.* Albury, Mary, illus. (gr. ps-3). 1982. pap. text ed. $4.00 (0-937423-02-5) University of Minnesota Hospital & Clinic.

Stein, Sara B. *A Hospital Story.* LC 73-15269. (Illus.). 48p. (gr. ps-8). 1984. pap. $8.95 (0-8027-7222-6) Walker & Co.

———. *A Hospital Story.* LC 73-15269. (Illus.). 48p. (gr. 1 and up). 1974. $12.95 (0-8027-6173-9) Walker & Co.

HOSPITALS: FICTION

Balter, Lawrence. *Alfred Goes to the Hospital.* Schanzer, Roz, illus. 40p. (gr. 3-7). 1990. $5.95 (0-8120-6150-0) Barron's Educational Services, Inc.

Bucknall, Caroline. *One Bear in the Hospital.* (Illus.). LC 90-2994. 32p. (gr. ps-2). 1991. $11.95 (0-8037-0847-5) Dial Bks for Young Readers.

Civardi, Anne, and Cartwright, Steven. *Going to the Hospital.* 16p. (gr. ps and up). 1987. $3.95 (0-7460-0073-1) EDC Publishing.

Coles, Allison. *Mandy and the Hospital.* Charlton, Michael, illus. 28p. (gr. ps and up). 1985. $3.95 (0-88110-269-5) EDC Publishing.

Davidson, Martine. *Maggie and the Emergency Room.* Hafner, Marilyn, illus. LC 91-31413. 32p. (gr. ps-2). 1992. PLB $5.99 (0-679-91818-3); pap. $2.25 (0-679-81818-9) Random House Bks for Young Readers.

———. *Rita Goes to the Hospital.* Jones, John, illus. LC 91-43293. 32p. (gr. ps-2). 1992. PLB $5.99 (0-679-91820-5); pap. $2.25 (0-679-81820-0) Random House Bks for Young Readers.

Hantzig, Deborah. *A Visit to the Sesame Street Hospital.* Mathieu, Joe, illus. LC 84-17852. 32p. (gr. ps-4). 1985. $5.99 (0-394-97062-4); pap. $2.25 (0-394-87062-X) Random House Bks for Young Readers.

Hogan, Paula Z., and Hogan, Kirk. *The Hospital Scares Me.* Thelen, Mary, illus. LC 79-23886. 32p. (gr. k-6). 1980. PLB $16.67 (0-8172-1351-1) Raintree Steck-Vaughn Publishers.

Howe, James. *A Night Without Stars.* LC 82-16278. 192p. (gr. 4-7). 1983. $13.95 (0-689-30957-0) Macmillan Children's Bk Group.

Keller, Holly. *The Best Present.* LC 87-38086. (Illus.). 32p. (gr. k and up). 1989. $11.95 (0-688-07319-0) Greenwillow Bks.

Rockwell, Anne. *The Emergency Room.* Rockwell, Harlow, illus. LC 84-20161. 24p. (gr. ps-2). 1985. $13.95 (0-02-777300-0) Macmillan Children's Bk Group.

Steel, Danielle. *Max's Daddy Goes to the Hospital.* Rogers, Jacqueline, illus. (gr. ps-2). 1989. $8.95 (0-385-29797-1) Delacorte Press.

PHYSICIANS

Berry, Joy W. *Teach Me About the Doctor.* Dickey, Kate, ed. (Illus.). 36p. (gr. ps). 1986. $4.98 (0-685-10723-X) Grolier, Inc.

Drescher, Joan. *Your Doctor, My Doctor.* 32p. (gr. 1-3). 1987. $10.95 (0-8027-6668-4) Walker & Co.

Rockwell, Harlow. *My Doctor.* (Illus.). LC 72-92442. 24p. (gr. ps-1). 1973. $13.95 (0-02-777480-5) Macmillan Children's Bk Group.

Rogers, Fred. *Going to the Doctor.* Judkis, Jim, illus. 32p. (gr. ps-2). 1986. $12.95 (0-399-21298-1); pap. $5.95 (0-399-21299-X) Putnam Publishing Group.

Watson, Jane W., et al. *My Friend the Doctor: A Read Together Book for Parents and Children.* Smith, Catherine B., illus. 32p. (gr. ps and up). 1987. pap. $3.50 (0-517-56485-8) Crown Bks for Young Readers.

PHYSICIANS: FICTION

Allen, Julia. *My First Doctor Visit.* Reese, Bob, illus. (gr. k-3). 1987. $7.95 (0-89868-187-1); pap. $2.95 (0-89868-188-X) ARO Publishing Co.

Cole, Joanna. *Doctor Change.* Carrick, Donald, illus. LC 86-881. 32p. (gr. ps-3). 1986. $12.95 (0-688-06135-4) Morrow Jr Bks.

Fine, Anne. *Poor Monty.* Vulliamy, Clara, illus. 32p. (gr. ps-1). 1992. $14.95 (0-395-60472-9) Houghton Mifflin Co.

Freeman, Don. *Corduroy's Busy Street and Corduroy Goes to the Doctor.* (2 bks.). Reprint of 1987 ed. McCue, Lisa, illus. (gr. ps-k). 1989. $12.95 w/cassette (0-87499-133-1) Live Oak Media.

Kuklin, Susan. *When I See My Doctor.* LC 87-25621. (Illus.). 32p. (gr. ps-k). 1988. $13.95 (0-02-751232-0) Macmillan Children's Bk Group.

Sommers, Tish. *Big Bird Goes to the Doctor.* Cooke, Tom, illus. LC 85-81562. 32p. (gr. ps-k). 1986. (0-307-12019-8) Western Publishing Co., Inc.

Steel, Danielle. *Freddie and the Doctor.* Rogers, Jacqueline, illus. 32p. (gr. 1-3). 1992. pap. 2.99 (0-440-40575-0) Dell Publishing Co., Inc.

Self-Help Clearinghouses in the U.S.

These groups can assist in a number of ways. They may be able to provide current information on your particular medical concern or condition or, in some cases, advise you of any existing local self-help groups concerned with that health or medical topic/condition.

California*	800-222-LINK (CA only)
	For verification 310-825-1799
Connecticut	203-789-7645
Illinois*	708-328-0470
	For administrative 708-328-0471
Iowa	800-383-4777 (IA only)
	515-576-5870
Kansas	800-445-0116 (KS only)
	316-689-3843
Massachusetts	413-545-2313
Michigan*	800-777-5556 (MI only)
	517-484-7373
Minnesota	612-224-1133
Missouri (Kansas City)	816-472-HELP
Missouri (St. Louis)	314-773-1399
Nebraska	402-476-9668
New Jersey	800-FOR-MASH (NJ only)
	201-625-9565
New York (Brooklyn)	718-875-1420
New York (Westchester)†	914-949-6301
North Carolina (Mecklenberg area)	704-331-9500
Ohio (Dayton area)	513-225-3004
Oregon (Portland area)	503-222-5555
Pennsylvania (Pittsburgh area)	412-261-5363
Pennsylvania (Scranton area)	717-961-1234
South Carolina (Midlands area)	803-791-9227
Tennessee (Knoxville area)	615-584-6736
Tennessee (Memphis area)	901-323-0633
Texas*	512-454-3706
Greater Washington, D.C.	703-941-LINK

*Maintains listings of additional local clearinghouses operating within that state.

†Call Westchester only for referral to local clearinghouses in upstate New York.

For national U.S. listings and directories:

American Self-Help Clearinghouse	201-625-7101
	201-625-9053 TDD
	201-625-8848 fax
National Self-Help Clearinghouse	212-642-2944

Top 300+ Toll-Free Medical, Nutritional, and General Health-Related Hotlines

The emerging consumer health movement has spawned an army of well-informed, proactive individuals who no longer limit their sources of health and medical information to their personal physicians. No longer do consumers have limited access to cutting-edge data about specific conditions, medications, or treatment options, just to name a few. A nationwide network of self-help and support groups has been formed around such interests as adoption services, organ transplants, substance abuse counseling, and women's health.

What follows are more than 300 useful and important health-related organizations that offer toll-free telephone numbers for public use. These numbers give you access to agencies and organizations that can tell you about a medical condition, answer your questions about toxic substances, test your hearing over the phone, or locate a local support group. And you don't need to leave your home to obtain any of this information. The only piece of equipment you need is your telephone!

ADOPTION

AASK America
657 Mission Street, Suite 601
San Francisco, CA 94105
800-232-2751
Provides information on how to adopt children with special needs, such as mental and physical handicaps.

Child Reach
155 Plan Way
Warwick, RI 02886
800-556-7918
Provides information on how to become a foster parent to third-world children.

Concerned United Birthparents
2000 Walker Street
Des Moines, IA 50317
800-822-2777
515-263-9558 in Iowa
Provides information on support groups designed for birthparents who gave up their child for adoption and are now seeking to come to terms with their decision. Makes referrals to support groups throughout the country.

Edna Gladney Center
2300 Hemphill Street
Ft. Worth, TX 76110
800-433-2922
800-772-2740 in Texas
8:30 A.M. to 5:00 P.M. (central time) Monday–Saturday
Provides counseling and shelter to single pregnant women who want to place their children for adoption. Free information packet available upon request.

International Children's Care
2711 N.E. 134th Street
Vancouver, WA 98686
800-422-7729
Provides information to couples or individuals who are interested in foreign adoptions. Counsels prospective parents on the adoption and immigration laws of the foreign country.

National Adoption Center
1218 Chestnut Street
Philadelphia, PA 19107
800-862-3678
215-925-0200 in Philadelphia area
Provides adoption information concerning hard-to-place children and children with special needs.

Pregnancy Counseling Services
Liberty Godparent Home
1000 Villa Road
Lynchburg, Virginia 24503
800-542-4453
804-384-3043 in Virginia
24 hours a day
Provides information on residential programs for unwed mothers and offers counseling and adoption services. Also makes referrals to other support groups and similar homes in the caller's area.

AEROBIC EXERCISE

Aerobic and Fitness Association of America
15250 Ventura Boulevard, Suite 310
Sherman Oaks, CA 91403
800-446-2322
800-445-5950
800-343-2584 in California
800-225-2322 in Canada and Mexico
8:30 A.M. to 5:00 P.M. (Pacific time) Monday–Friday
Provides basic information on aerobic exercise, certified instructors, and prevention and treatment of aerobics-related injuries.

National Dance-Exercise Instructors Training Association
1503 S. Washington Avenue, Suite 208
Minneapolis, MN 55454
800-237-6242
612-340-1306 in Minnesota
Provides information on aerobics instructors and seminars nationwide.

AIDS

AIDS Hotline
c/o American Social Health Association
P.O. Box 13827
Research Triangle Park, NC 27709
800-342-2437
800-243-7889 Hearing-impaired
24 hours a day
800-344-7432 Spanish
8:00 A.M. to 2:00 A.M. (eastern time) 7 days a week
Provides information on HIV and AIDS transmission and prevention. Answers specific questions concerning HIV and AIDS and also makes referrals for testing and counseling. Free information packet available upon request.

American Academy of Pediatrics
Pediatric AIDS Coalition
1331 Pennsylvania Avenue N.W., Suite 721-N
Washington, DC 20004
800-336-5475
202-662-7460 in District of Columbia
9:00 A.M. to 5:00 P.M. (eastern time) Monday–Friday
Provides information on AIDS education programs for adults and children in churches, schools, and other community organizations.

Clinical Trials Information Service
P.O. Box 6421
Rockville, MD 20849-6421
800-874-2572
800-243-7012 Hearing-impaired
9:00 A.M. to 7:00 P.M. (eastern time) Monday–Friday
Provides information on the status of federally and privately sponsored experimental drug trials for HIV and AIDS. Free materials available upon request.

Haitian AIDS Hotline
8037 N.E. 2nd Avenue
Miami, FL 33138
800-722-7432
8:30 A.M. to 5:00 P.M. (eastern time) Monday–Friday
Provides HIV and AIDS information specifically tailored to the Haitian population.

Multicultural Training Resource Center
1540 Market Street, Suite 320
San Francisco, CA 94102
800-545-6642 in California
Provides HIV and AIDS information specifically targeted to diverse cultural groups.

Names Project
2362 Market Street
P.O. Box 14573
San Francisco, CA 94114
415-863-5511
800-872-6263 in California
9:00 A.M. to 6:00 P.M. (Pacific time) Monday–Friday
Provides information on how to add names to the AIDS Memorial Quilt project, which commemorates those men, women, and children who have lost their lives to AIDS.

National AIDS Information Clearinghouse
P.O. Box 6003
Rockville, MD 20849-6003
800-458-5231
9:00 A.M. to 7:00 P.M. (eastern time) Monday–Friday
Provides recorded messages in English and Spanish with information on organizational and educational materials, clinical drug trials, and how to order publications.

National Association of People with AIDS
2025 I Street N.W., Suite 1118
Washington, DC 20006
800-673-8538
Provides information and referrals to local chapters of People with AIDS. Also maintains a national system of self-empowering programs for people infected with HIV or who have AIDS-related complex or AIDS.

National Native American AIDS Prevention Center
3515 Grand Avenue, Suite 100
Oakland, CA 94610
800-283-2437
510-444-2051 Oakland area
8:30 A.M. to 5:00 P.M. (Pacific time) Monday–Friday
510-444-1593 fax
Provides referrals to counseling and testing centers. Free information packet available upon request.

Project Inform
220 Market Street
San Francisco, CA 94103
800-822-7422
800-334-7422 in California
10:00 A.M. to 4:00 P.M. (Pacific time) Monday–Friday
10:00 A.M. to 1:00 P.M. (Pacific time) Saturday
Answering machine at all other times
Provides current information on treatment options for persons with HIV and AIDS, as well as information on organizations that provide the treatments. Also operates an outreach and advocacy program.

Teens Teaching AIDS Prevention
3030 Walnut Street
Kansas City, MO 64108
800-234-8336
816-561-8784 in Kansas City area
4:00 P.M. to 8:00 P.M. (central time) Monday–Friday
Answering machine at all other times
Provides information and counseling on HIV and AIDS from a teen's perspective. Makes referrals to AIDS organizations and other resources. Some literature available at a nominal charge.

ALCOHOL TREATMENT PROGRAMS

See Substance Abuse.

ALLERGIES AND ASTHMA

Allergy Information Referral Line
American Academy of Allergy and Immunology
611 E. Wells Street
Milwaukee, WI 53202
800-822-2762
414-272-6071 in Wisconsin
8:00 a.m to 5:00 p.m. (central time) Monday–Friday
Provides information on the diagnosis and treatment of
allergies and asthma and makes referrals to allergy
specialists.

American College of Allergy and Immunology
800 W. Northwest Highway, Suite 1080
Palatine, IL 60067
800-842-7777
24 hours a day, Monday–Friday
Provides information on various allergies and the treatment
options available.

Asthma and Allergy Foundation of America
1717 Massachusetts Avenue N.W., Suite 305
Washington, DC 20036
800-727-8462
202-466-7643 in District of Columbia
Provides U.S. maps showing zones where plants are likely
to cause allergic problems. Also provides educational materials on asthma and allergies.

National Jewish Asthma Center
1400 Jackson Street
Denver, CO 80206
800-222-5864
303-398-1477 in Denver
8:00 A.M. to 5:00 P.M. (mountain time) Monday–Friday
Answers questions about asthma, emphysema, chronic
bronchitis, and other respiratory diseases. Also makes referrals to doctors in caller's local area. Free information
packets available upon request.

ALZHEIMER'S DISEASE

Alzheimer's Association
919 N. Michigan Avenue, Suite 1000
Chicago, IL 60611
800-272-3900
8:30 A.M. to 5:00 P.M. (central time) Monday–Friday
Answering machine at all other times
Provides information on Alzheimer's and related disorders
and also makes referrals to local chapters of the association.

American Health Assistance Foundation
15825 Shady Grove Road, Suite 140
Rockville, MD 20850
800-437-2423
301-948-3244 in Maryland
9:00 A.M. to 5:00 P.M. (eastern time) Monday–Friday
Provides public education materials on Alzheimer's relief
programs and provides funding for such programs. Also
provides financial assistance to families in need of relief
services.

AMYOTROPHIC LATERAL SCLEROSIS (ALS) ("LOU GEHRIG'S DISEASE")

ALS Association
21021 Ventura Boulevard, Suite 321
Woodland Hills, CA 91364
800-782-4747
818-340-7500 in San Fernando Valley
8:00 A.M. to 5:00 P.M. (Pacific time) Monday–Friday
Provides education, information, and referral services to
ALS patients and their families. Also makes referrals to local chapters and support groups.

ANEMIA

Cooley's Anemia Foundation
105 E. 22nd Street, Room 911
New York, NY 10010
800-221-3571
800-522-7222 in New York State
9:00 A.M. to 5:00 P.M. (eastern time) Monday–Friday
Provides information on patient care, support groups, and
the latest research into Cooley's anemia.

National Association for Sickle Cell Disease
3345 Wilshire Boulevard, Suite 1106
Los Angeles, CA 90010-1880
800-421-8453
213-736-5455 in Los Angeles
8:30 A.M. to 5:00 P.M. (Pacific time) Monday–Friday
Provides materials, trains counselors, and offers programs
to medical professionals and the public. Also supports research, conducts public education campaigns, and provides
diagnostic screening.

ARTHRITIS

Arthritis Consulting Services
4620 N. State Road 7, Suite 206
Ft. Lauderdale, FL 33319
800-327-3027
8:30 A.M. to 4:00 P.M. (eastern time) Monday–Friday
Provides information on holistic approaches to treating
arthritis.

Arthritis Foundation Information Line
P.O. Box 19000
Atlanta, GA 30326
800-283-7800
404-872-7100 in Georgia
9:00 A.M. to 7:00 P.M. (eastern time) Monday–Friday
Provides local physician referrals and information concerning local chapters of the Arthritis Foundation. Free brochures and other literature available upon request.

BLOOD DISORDERS

National Marrow Donor Program
3433 Broadway Street N.E., Suite 400
Minneapolis, MN 55413-1762
800-654-1247
8:00 A.M. to 5:00 P.M. (central time) Monday–Friday
Answering machine at all other times
Maintains a registry of bone marrow donors and also provides information on how interested individuals can become active in the registry program.

BURN CARE

Phoenix Society
National Organization for Burn Survivors
11 Rust Hill Road
Levittown, PA 19056
800-888-2876
215-946-BURN
Provides information on the self-help services available to burn victims and their families. Helps burn victims deal with their trauma and provides the psychological support they need to return to normal lives and interests. Distributes information on burns and trauma and their treatment.

Shriners Hospital Referral Line
2900 Rocky Point Drive
Tampa, FL 33607-1435
800-237-5055
800-282-9161 in Florida
8:00 A.M. to 5:00 P.M. (eastern time) Monday–Friday
Provides information about burn treatment programs available at Shriners hospitals.

CANCER

American Association of Oral and Maxillofacial Surgeons
9700 Bryn Mawr Avenue
Rosemont, IL 60018
800-467-5268
8:30 A.M. to 5:00 P.M. (central time) Monday–Friday
Answering machine at all other times
Provides information on oral cancer and makes referrals to oral surgeons in the caller's area.

American Cancer Society
1599 Clifton Road N.E.
Atlanta, GA 30329
800-227-2345
8:30 A.M. to 4:30 P.M. (eastern time) Monday–Friday
Provides general information on the society's programs and services and makes referrals to local chapters. Also answers questions about cancer, including prevention, diagnosis, treatment, and rehabilitation.

American Institute for Cancer Research
Nutrition Hotline
1759 R Street N.W.
Washington, DC 20009
800-843-8114
202-328-7744 in District of Columbia
9:00 A.M. to 9:00 P.M. (eastern time) Monday–Thursday
9:00 A.M. to 5:00 P.M. (eastern time) Friday
Answering machine at all other times
Provides information on the role of diet and nutrition in cancer prevention and how nutrition may be used to assist a cancer treatment program. Also responds to specific requests.

American International Hospital Cancer Program
1321 Shiloh Boulevard
Zion, IL 60099-2646
800-FOR-HELP
Provides information on cancer treatment programs available at the hospital.

American Medical Center
Cancer Information and Counseling Line
1600 Pierce Street
Denver, CO 80214
800-525-3777
303-233-6501 in Denver area
8:30 A.M. to 4:45 P.M. (mountain time) Monday–Friday
Provides the latest information on cancer prevention, detection, and treatment methods. Also offers counseling and makes referrals to support groups.

Breast Cancer Hotline
Physicians Committee for Responsible Medicine
P.O. Box 6322
Washington, DC 20015
800-875-4837
9:00 A.M. to 5:00 P.M. (eastern time) Monday–Friday
Answering machine at all other times
Provides information on the link between diet and breast cancer. Caller may leave name and address and receive a free packet of information.

Candlelighters Childhood Cancer Foundation
7910 Woodmont Avenue, Suite 460
Bethesda, MD 20814
800-366-2223
24 hours a day
Provides information and services, such as a 24-hour crisis line and transportation, to families of childhood cancer patients. Serves as a clearinghouse and liaison between parents and medical professionals. Established Ronald McDonald houses where family members of patients may stay while the patient undergoes treatment.

National Cancer Institute
Cancer Information Service
9000 Rockville Pike, Suite 414
Bethesda, MD 20892
800-422-6237
800-638-6070 in Alaska
800-524-1234 in Hawaii
9:00 A.M. to 10:00 P.M. (eastern time) Monday–Friday
Provides information on various types of cancers and the latest treatments available for those cancers. Free information is available in both English and Spanish.

Y-Me Breast Cancer Support Program
18220 Harwood Avenue
Homewood, IL 60430
800-221-2141
708-799-8228 in Illinois
Provides information and support to women undergoing treatment for breast cancer. Also provides information on prostheses after breast surgery.

CEREBRAL PALSY

United Cerebral Palsy Association
7 Penn Plaza, Suite 804
New York, NY 10001
800-872-1827
212-268-6655 in New York City area
9:00 A.M. to 5:00 P.M. (eastern time) Monday–Friday
Provides information on the diagnosis and treatment of cerebral palsy and works to establish local programs that help people with the disease move into mainstream society.

CHILDREN'S SERVICES

American Academy of Pediatrics
P.O. Box 927
141 N.W. Point Boulevard
Elk Grove, IL 60007
800-433-9016
800-421-0589 in Illinois
Provides information on pediatric care and the role of the pediatrician.

American Association for Protecting Children
Division of American Humane Association
63 Inverness Drive E.
Englewood, CO 80112
800-227-5242
303-792-9900 in Colorado
8:30 A.M. to 5:00 P.M. (mountain time) Monday–Friday
Answering machine at all other times
Provides services to professionals who work in the child-protection field and conducts research and program evaluations of child welfare agencies. List of books and other publications available upon request.

Boys Town Hotline
Father Flanagan's Boys Town
Boys Town, NE 68010
800-448-3000
Provides assistance to runaway and homeless children regardless of race, color, or creed.

Child Find
P.O. Box 277
New Paltz, NY 12561
800-426-5678
914-255-1848 in New York
Operates an international locator service for missing children and maintains a registry of missing children.

Children's Defense Fund
122 C Street N.W., Suite 400
Washington, DC 20001
800-CDF-1200
202-628-8787 in District of Columbia
Provides information on the expanding field of children's rights as recognized by law and is involved in social and educational programs affecting children. Free information available upon request.

Children's Wish Foundation
7840 Roswell Road, Suite 301
Atlanta, GA 30350
800-323-9474
404-393-9474 in Georgia
Provides information on programs that seek to grant a dying child his or her final wish. Works with organizations and individuals who want to become Wish Foundation supporters.

Covenant House
460 W. 41st Street
New York, NY 10036
800-999-9999
Provides 24-hour assistance to runaways and homeless youth. Also provides temporary shelter until the child's situation at home can be resolved.

Feingold Association of the United States
P.O. Box 6550
Alexandria, VA 22306
800-321-3287
24 hours a day
Provides information on the Feingold Program, which uses diet to treat children with learning and behavioral problems. Also makes referrals to local support groups. Free information available upon request.

"Just Say No" Kids Club International
2101 Webster Street, Suite 1300
Oakland, CA 94612
800-258-2766
510-939-6666
Provides information on drug prevention programs for children and on how to start a "Just Say No" chapter.

Kevin Collins Foundation for Missing Children
P.O. Box 590473
San Francisco, CA 94159
800-272-0012
Provides counseling and education to the families of missing or abducted children and helps them through the ordeal.

Kidsrights
10100 Park Cedar Drive
Charlotte, NC 28210
800-892-5437
Provides information to parents and other interested individuals on how to establish programs that work to combat teen suicide.

Missing Children Awareness Foundation
13094 95th Street N.
Largo, FL 34643
800-741-7233
Provides assistance and referrals to parents of missing children.

Missing Children Help Center
410 Ware Boulevard, Suite 400
Tampa, FL 33619
800-872-5437
Provides assistance to parents of missing children by publicizing the children's photographs in newspapers, brochures, and flyers.

National Association for the Education of Young Children
1834 Connecticut Avenue N.W.
Washington, DC 20009
800-424-2460
Provides information and referrals to accredited child care programs.

National Child Watch Campaign
P.O. Box 1368
Jackson, MI 49204
800-222-1464
Provides information on child safety and how to establish a child watch program to protect children from being kidnapped. Also provides counseling and support services to parents whose child has been kidnapped or is missing.

National Hotline for Missing and Exploited Children
2101 Wilson Boulevard, Suite 550
Arlington, VA 22201
800-843-5678
7:30 A.M. to 11:00 P.M. (eastern time) Monday–Friday
10:00 A.M. to 6:00 P.M. (eastern time) Saturday
Operates a hotline for reporting sightings of missing children and children exploited by crime, prostitution, and pornography. Provides technical assistance to legal authorities in the hunt for missing or kidnapped children.

National Information Clearinghouse for Infants with Disabilities and Life-Threatening Conditions
University of South Carolina
Benson Building, 1st Floor
Columbia, SC 29208
800-922-9234 Voice- and hearing-impaired
800-922-1107 Voice- and hearing-impaired in South Carolina
9:00 A.M. to 5:00 P.M. (eastern time) Monday–Friday
Answering machine at all other times
Provides information to families with children who have rare or life-threatening conditions. Also offers referrals to professional and community services in the caller's area. Offers special services to Vietnam veterans and their families.

National Resource Center on Child Sexual Abuse
107 Lincoln Street
Huntsville, AL 35801
800-543-7006
Provides resources to agencies dealing with children who have been sexually abused. Also provides bibliographies and articles on the sexual abuse of children.

National Runaway Hotline
Office of the Governor
P.O. Box 12428
Austin, TX 78711
800-231-6946
800-392-3352 in Texas
Provides assistance to runaway children by making referrals to shelters and other agencies. Also delivers messages to the families of runaway children.

National Runaway Switchboard
3080 N. Lincoln
Chicago, IL 60657
800-621-4000
Provides counseling and referral to runaway youths 18 years of age and younger.

Operation Lookout National Center for Missing Youth
P.O. Box 231
Mt. Lake Terrace, WA 98043
800-782-7335
Provides assistance in locating missing children.

Parent Help Line
Nashua Brookside Hospital
11 Northwest Boulevard
Nashua, NH 03063
800-543-6381
Provides referrals to organizations that can aid parents in obtaining treatment and counseling for troubled kids.

Shriners Hospital Referral Line
2900 Rocky Point Drive
Tampa, FL 33607-1435
800-237-5055
800-282-9161 in Florida
8:00 A.M. to 5:00 P.M. (eastern time) Monday–Friday
Provides information about children's services available at Shriners hospitals.

Teen Crisis Hotline
498 S. Spring Street
Crestview, FL 32536
800-262-8336 in Florida
Provides information and referrals to teenagers facing crises in their lives.

Toughlove International
P.O. Box 1069
Doylestown, PA 18901
800-333-1069
215-348-7090 in Pennsylvania
Serves as a support group for parents of children with behavioral problems. Makes referrals in both the United States and Canada.

Vanished Children's Alliance
1407 Parkmoor Avenue, Suite 200
San Jose, CA 95126
800-826-4743
408-971-4822
24 hours a day
Provides information on missing and recovered children.

Youth Crisis Hotline
10225 Ulmerton Road, Suite 4-A
Largo, FL 34641
800-442-4673
Provides information on child abuse and serves as an advocacy group for abused children.

CLEFT PALATE

American Cleft Palate Educational Foundation
1218 Grandview Avenue
Pittsburgh, PA 15211
800-24-CLEFT
800-242-5338
800-232-5338 in Pennsylvania
Assists parents by providing information about feeding, dental care, and local professional and support groups. Free information available upon request.

CORNELIA DE LANGE SYNDROME (CDLS)

Cornelia de Lange Foundation
60 Dyer Avenue
Collinsville, CT 06022
800-223-8355
800-753-2357 in Canada
9:00 A.M. to 4:30 P.M. (eastern time) Monday–Friday
Answering machine at all other times
Provides general information on the birth defects caused by CDLS. Operates a support system for parents and makes referrals to local chapters. Free information available upon request.

DENTAL CARE

American Academy of Cosmetic Dentistry
2711 Marshall Court
Madison, WI 53705
800-543-9220
Provides information on cosmetic dentistry and referrals to practitioners in the caller's area.

American Association of Orthodontists
460 N. Lindbergh Boulevard
St. Louis, MO 63141
800-222-9969
Provides information on orthodontic treatments and referrals to orthodontists in the caller's area.

Environmental Dental Association
9974 Scripps Ranch Boulevard, Suite 36
San Diego, CA 92131
800-388-8124
Provides information on alternatives to mercury fillings and how to locate dentists who do not use mercury fillings.

DIABETES MELLITUS

American Diabetes Association
1660 Duke Street
Alexandria, VA 22314
800-232-3472
703-549-1500
8:30 A.M. to 5:00 P.M. (eastern time) Monday–Friday
Provides general information on the diagnosis and
treatment of diabetes. Information packets available
upon request.

Diabetes Center, Inc.
P.O. Box 47945
Minneapolis, MN 55447
800-848-2793
Provides information on diabetic supplies, including pre-
scription medications.

Juvenile Diabetes Foundation
432 Park Avenue S.
New York, NY 10016
800-223-1138
212-889-7575
Provides information on the latest research into the cause
and prevention of juvenile diabetes. Also provides grants
to support ongoing research.

DIGESTIVE DISEASES

Crohn's and Colitis Foundation
444 Park Avenue S.
New York, NY 10018
800-343-3637
9:00 A.M. to 5:00 P.M. (eastern time) Monday–Friday
Provides information on digestive diseases and their diagnosis and treatment. Also makes referrals to support groups
and local chapters of the organization. Free literature available upon request.

DOMESTIC VIOLENCE

Hit Home Youth Crisis Line
Youth Development International
P.O. Box 178408
San Diego, CA 92177-8408
800-448-4663
619-292-5683
Provides counseling and referrals on child abuse, run-
aways, suicide, molestation, and pregnancy.

National Child Abuse Hotline
ChildHelp USA
P.O. Box 630
Hollywood, CA 90028
800-422-4453
24 hours a day
Provides 24-hour crisis counseling and intervention for any
abuse-related situation. Also offers information and referral
service that includes national, regional, or local organizations, agencies, and groups. Free literature available upon
request.

National Council on Child Abuse and Family Violence
1155 Connecticut Avenue N.W., Suite 300
Washington, DC 20036
800-222-2000
202-429-6695 in District of Columbia
7:30 A.M. to 4:30 P.M. (eastern time) Monday–Friday
Provides referrals to local community services and support
groups. Free information packet available upon request.

Parents Anonymous/Abusive Parents
520 S. Lafayette Park Place, Suite 316
Los Angeles, CA 90057
800-421-0353
800-352-0386 in California
8:30 A.M. to 5:00 P.M. (Pacific time) Monday–Friday
Answering machine at all other times
Provides information on the prevention and treatment of
child abuse. Also makes referrals to self-help groups and
local chapters for parents involved in abusive situations.

DOWN SYNDROME

National Down Syndrome Congress
1800 Dempster Street
Park Ridge, IL 60068
800-232-6372
9:00 A.M. to 5:00 P.M. (central time) Monday–Friday
Provides information and referrals for families concerning
Down syndrome. Publishes a newsletter and sponsors an
annual convention.

National Down Syndrome Society
666 Broadway
New York, NY 10012
800-221-4602
9:00 A.M. to 5:00 P.M. (eastern time) Monday–Friday
Answering machine at all other times
Provides free information packets on Down syndrome and
makes referrals to local support groups in caller's area.
Publications available for a small fee.

DRINKING WATER

GEO/Resource Consultant, Inc.
1555 Wilson Boulevard, Suite 500
Arlington, VA 22209
800-426-4791
8:00 A.M. to 5:00 P.M. (eastern time) Monday–Friday
Provides information on drinking water standards that must
be met by community and municipal water supplies.

DRUG TREATMENT PROGRAMS

See Substance Abuse.

DYSLEXIA

Orton Dyslexia Society
Chester Building, Suite 382
8600 LaSalle Road
Baltimore, MD 21286-2044
800-222-3123
410-296-0232 in Baltimore
9:00 A.M. to 5:00 P.M. (eastern time) Monday–Friday
Provides information on support networks and resources
for people with dyslexia.

EATING DISORDERS

FIT-AHL
Food Addiction Hotline
2000 Commerce Street
Melbourne, FL 32904
800-872-0088
Provides information on eating disorders and makes referrals to local services. Information packets available upon
request.

Take Off Pounds Sensibly (TOPS)
4575 S. 5th Street
Milwaukee, WI 53207
800-932-8677
Provides information on sensible dieting methods. Also
makes referrals to local chapters of TOPS.

EMERGENCY MEDICAL COMMUNICATION SYSTEMS

American Medical Alert Corporation
3265 Lawson Boulevard
Oceanside, NY 11572
800-645-3244
Provides information on telecommunications devices that
are used by people with life-threatening conditions or, in
the case of accidents, that can be used to summon help in
emergency situations.

Lifeline Systems
1 Arsenal Marketplace
Watertown, MA 02172
800-451-0525
617-923-4141 in Alaska, Hawaii, and Massachusetts
Provides information on communications systems that link
elderly and handicapped persons directly to hospitals.

ENDOMETRIOSIS

Endometriosis Association
8585 N. 76th Place
Milwaukee, WI 53223
800-992-3636
800-426-2363 in Canada
24 hours a day
Provides free information on endometriosis.

EPILEPSY

Epilepsy Foundation of America
4351 Garden City Drive
Landover, MD 20785
800-332-1000
9:00 A.M. to 6:00 P.M. (eastern time) Monday–Friday
Provides information on the diagnosis and treatment of
epilepsy and makes referrals to doctors in caller's area.
Also operates a discount pharmacy available to members.

HANDICAPPED SERVICES

American Paralysis Association
500 Morris Avenue
Springfield, NJ 07081
800-225-0292
800-526-3456 in New Jersey
8:30 A.M. to 5:00 P.M. (eastern time) Monday–Friday
Provides information on the treatment of spinal cord injuries and makes referrals to local support groups. Free information packet available upon request.

AT&T National Special Needs Center
2001 Route 46, Suite 310
Parsippany, NJ 07054
800-233-1222
800-833-3232 Hearing-impaired
8:30 A.M. to 7:00 P.M. (eastern time) Monday–Friday
Provides information on special equipment available to
people with hearing, speech, vision, or motion impairment.

Devereux Foundation
19 S. Waterloo Road
Devon, PA 19333
800-345-1292 ext. 3109
8:45 A.M. to 9:00 P.M. (eastern time) Monday–Friday
Provides information on treatment programs for children,
adolescents, and adults with psychiatric, emotional, neurological, and developmental handicaps.

Institute of Logopedics
2400 Jardine Drive
Wichita, KS 67219
800-835-1043
800-937-4644 (includes Canada)
8:00 A.M. to 5:00 P.M. (central time) Monday–Friday
Provides information on residential programs for children
with multiple disabilities.

Job Accommodation Network
809 Allen Hall
P.O. Box 6123
West Virginia University
Morgantown, WV 26506-6123
800-526-7234
800-526-4698 in West Virginia
Provides information to employers and the public on how
to accommodate the disabled in the workplace.

National Association of Rehabilitation Facilities
P.O. Box 17675
Washington, DC 20041
800-368-3513
8:30 A.M. to 5:30 P.M. (eastern time) Monday–Friday
Answering machine at all other times
Provides the names and locations of rehabilitation facili-
ties. Also makes referrals to local support groups.

National Center for Youth with Disabilities
University of Minnesota Box 721
420 Delaware Street N.E.
Minneapolis, MN 55455
800-333-6293
612-624-3939 Hearing-impaired
7:45 A.M. to 4:30 P.M. (central time) Monday–Friday
Provides free information to assist parents, educators, care-
givers, advocates, and others in helping children and youth
with disabilities become fully participating members of
society.

**National Clearinghouse on Postsecondary Education
for Individuals with Disabilities**
One Dupont Circle, Suite 800
Washington, DC 20036-1193
800-544-3284
202-939-9320 in District of Columbia
Provides information for disabled individuals on job opportunities following graduation from high school.

National Easter Seal Society
70 E. Lake Street
Chicago, IL 60601
800-221-6827
8:30 A.M. to 5:00 P.M. (central time) Monday–Friday
Provides information on therapy, counseling, and educational programs for the disabled. Also makes referrals to
community-based programs operated by the Easter Seal
Society.

**National Information Center for Children and
Youth with Disabilities**
7926 Jones Branch Drive
McLean, VA 22102
800-999-5599
703-893-6061 in Virginia
Provides information on programs for handicapped children and youth.

National Organization on Disability
910 16th Street N.W., Suite 600
Washington, DC 20006
800-248-2253
Provides information on how to improve living conditions
for disabled individuals.

National Rehabilitation Information Center
8455 Colesville Road, Suite 935
Silver Spring, MD 20910-3319
800-346-2742
8:00 A.M. to 6:00 P.M. (eastern time) Monday–Friday
Provides information on research, resources, and products
for the disabled.

National Tour Association
Handicapped Travel Division
546 E. Main Street
Lexington, KY 40508
800-682-8886
Provides information to travelers who require special accommodations because of handicaps or other limitations.
Provides a list of travel operators who have booked accommodations for handicapped individuals.

Pathways Awareness Foundation
123 N. Wacker Drive
Chicago, IL 60606
800-955-2445
9:00 A.M. to 5:00 P.M. (central time) Monday–Friday
Provides information on the detection of disabilities in early childhood.

Tele-Consumer Hotline
1910 K Street N.W., Suite 610
Washington, DC 20006
800-332-1124
Assists the disabled in locating communications equipment
that can be adapted to their individual needs.

HANSON'S DISEASE (LEPROSY)

American Leprosy Missions
One American Leprosy Mission Way
Greenville, SC 29601
800-543-3131
8:00 A.M. to 5:00 P.M. (eastern time) Monday–Friday
Provides information on the diagnosis and treatment of
Hanson's disease and makes referrals to treatment pro-
grams. Free information packet available upon request.

HEADACHE

National Headache Foundation
5252 N. Western Avenue
Chicago, IL 60625
800-843-2256
9:00 A.M. to 5:00 P.M. (central time) Monday–Friday
Provides general information on the diagnosis and treatment of headaches. Also makes referrals to local support and mutual aid groups.

New England Headache Treatment Program
778 Longridge Road
Stamford, CT 06902
800-245-0088
203-968-1799 in Connecticut
9:00 A.M. to 4:00 P.M. (eastern time) Monday–Friday
Provides general information on headaches and treatment programs available at Greenwich Hospital in Greenwich, Connecticut. Free information available upon request.

HEAD INJURY

National Head Injury Foundation
1776 Massachusetts Avenue N.W., Suite 100
Washington, DC 20036
800-444-6443
202-296-6443 in District of Columbia
9:00 A.M. to 5:00 P.M. (eastern time) Monday–Friday
Provides information on the treatment of head injuries and makes referrals to local support groups.

HEALTH INFORMATION

American Institute for Preventive Medicine
30445 Northwestern Highway
Farmington Hills, MI 48075
800-345-2476
313-539-1800 in Michigan
8:30 A.M. to 5:30 P.M. (eastern time) Monday–Friday
Provides information on programs designed for lifestyle improvement, such as stress reduction, weight control, smoking cessation, and health education. Free information available upon request.

American Medical Radio News
515 N. State Street
Chicago, IL 60610
800-448-9384
Provides a recorded message on a current health topic or feature story in medicine.

American Osteopathic Association
142 E. Ontario Street
Chicago, IL 60611
800-621-1773
312-280-5800
8:30 A.M. to 4:30 P.M. (central time) Monday–Friday
Provides information on osteopathic medicine and makes referrals to local osteopathic physicians and medical centers.

American Trauma Society
8903 Presidential Parkway, Suite 512
Upper Marlboro, MD 20772-2656
800-556-7890
301-420-4189
9:00 A.M. to 5:00 P.M. (eastern time) Monday–Friday
Provides information on injury prevention and trauma care. Free information available upon request.

California Self-Help Center
UCLA Psychology Department
405 Hilgard Avenue
Los Angeles, CA 90024
800-222-5465 in California
Provides consumer information on a variety of health topics and makes referrals to local, regional, and national organizations.

Center for Self Help
Riverwood Center
P.O. Box 547
Benton Harbor, MI 49022-0547
800-336-0341 in Michigan
Provides information on self-help resources available in the caller's area.

Consumer Health Information Resource Institute
3521 Broadway
Kansas City, MO 64111
800-821-6671
816-753-8850
9:00 A.M. to 5:00 P.M. (central time) Monday–Friday
Provides referrals to local, regional, and national organizations and also maintains a patient education library. Suggests sources of health information on various conditions, procedures, and medications.

Doctor Referral Service of Mt. Sinai Medical Center
One Gustave L. Levy Place
P.O. Box 1083
New York, NY 10029-6575
800-637-4624
8:30 A.M. to 6:00 P.M. (eastern time) Monday–Friday
Provides referrals to physicians located in the New York City area who are affiliated with Mt. Sinai Medical Center.

Health Information Network International
4213 Montgomery Drive
Santa Rosa, CA 95405
800-743-6996
707-539-3966
9:00 A.M. to 5:00 P.M. (Pacific time) Monday–Friday
Provides consumers with the latest research and information on natural health substances, medical conditions, and treatment alternatives.

Joseph and Rose Kennedy Institute of Ethics
National Reference Center for Bioethics Literature
Georgetown University
Washington, DC 20057
800-633-3849
202-687-3885
Provides information to medical professionals and the public on the topic of medical bioethics.

National Health Information Center
U.S. Department of Health and Human Services
Office of Disease Prevention and Health Promotion
P.O. Box 1133
Washington, DC 20013
800-336-4797
301-565-4167 in Maryland
9:00 A.M. to 5:00 P.M. (eastern time) Monday–Friday
Provides information to consumers and professionals on a variety of health-related topics. Also makes referrals to national organizations. Free literature available upon request.

National Library of Medicine
8600 Rockville Pike, 4th Floor
Bethesda, MD 20894
800-638-8480
Provides computer access to medical literature and information-retrieval systems. Also searches current medical literature on a variety of topics.

New Jersey Self-Help Clearinghouse
St. Clares–Riverside Hospital
Denville, NJ 07834
201-625-7101
201-625-9053 Hearing-impaired
800-367-6274 in New Jersey
Provides information to consumers on self-help groups and other organizations. Produces materials on how to establish a self-help group. Also publishes a directory of self-help and mutual aid organizations.

Office of Minority Health
Resource Center
1010 Wayne Avenue, Suite 300
Silver Spring, MD 20910
800-444-6472
9:00 A.M. to 5:00 P.M. (eastern time) Monday–Friday
Provides information to minority groups on health topics that are of special interest to them. Free information packet available upon request. English- and Spanish-language personnel available to callers.

People's Medical Society
462 Walnut Street, Lower Level
Allentown, PA 18102
800-624-8773
610-770-1670
8:30 A.M. to 5:00 P.M. (eastern time) Monday–Friday
Answering machine at all other times
Provides information on how to become a better-informed medical consumer. Also publishes consumer-oriented medical information on topics ranging from pediatrics to Medicare. Free membership information and publication list available upon request.

Total Health Foundation
P.O. Box 5
Yakima, WA 98907
800-348-0120
24 hours a day
Provides information on a variety of medical topics.

HEARING IMPAIRMENTS

American Speech-Language-Hearing Association Helpline
10801 Rockville Pike
Rockville, MD 20852
301-897-8682
800-638-8255 Voice- and hearing-impaired
800-897-8682 in Alaska, Hawaii, and Maryland
8:30 A.M. to 4:30 P.M. (eastern time) Monday–Friday
Provides general information on speech, language, and hearing problems and makes referrals to professionals. Free information packet available upon request.

Better Hearing Institute
P.O. Box 1840
Washington, DC 20013
703-642-0580
800-424-8576 in Virginia
9:00 A.M. to 5:00 P.M. (eastern time) Monday–Friday
Provides information on deafness and other types of hearing problems.

Captioned Films for the Deaf
5000 Park Street N.
St. Petersburg, FL 33709
800-237-6213
813-545-8781
Provides information on films that are available with captioning for the hearing-impaired.

Deafness Research Foundation
9 E. 38th Street, 7th Floor
New York, NY 10016-0003
800-535-3323 Voice- and hearing-impaired
212-684-6556 in New York City
9:00 A.M. to 5:00 P.M. (eastern time) Monday–Friday
Provides information on hearing problems and makes referrals to local physicians. Also provides information on how to select a hearing aid and detect hearing problems in children. Free materials available upon request.

Delta Society
P.O. Box 1080
Renton, WA 98057-1080
800-869-6898
206-226-7357
Provides information on how to obtain hearing dogs for the deaf.

Hearing Aid Hotline
20361 Middlebelt Road
Livonia, MI 48152
800-521-5247
313-478-2610
Provides information on hearing loss and hearing aids. Also makes referrals to hearing-aid specialists.

Hearing Information Center
P.O. Box 1880
Media, PA 19063
800-622-3277
Provides hearing screening over the phone and also answers general questions about hearing.

Hear Now
4001 S. Magnolia Way, Suite 100
Denver, CO 80237
800-648-4327 Voice- and hearing-impaired
303-758-4919 in Colorado
8:30 A.M. to 4:00 P.M. (mountain time) Monday–Friday
Answering machine at all other times
Provides information on hearing aids and ear implants. Also sponsors a national hearing-aid bank and makes referrals to local organizations and agencies.

National Captioning Institute
5203 Leesburg Pike
Falls Church, VA 22041
800-533-9673
703-998-2443
Provides captioning services for television programs and films.

Sensor Hearing Aids
300 S. Chester Road
Swarthmore, PA 19081
800-622-3277
215-544-2700
9:00 A.M. to 5:00 P.M. (eastern time) Monday–Friday
Provides free information on hearing loss and hearing aids. Also makes referrals to audiologists in caller's area.

TRIPOD Grapevine
2901 N. Keystone Street
Burbank, CA 91504
800-352-8888 Voice- and hearing-impaired
800 287-4763 Voice- and hearing-impaired in California
9:00 A.M. to 5:00 P.M. (Pacific time) Monday–Friday
Provides information and services to parents who are raising a hearing-impaired child.

HEART DISEASE

American Heart Association
7272 Greenville Avenue
Dallas, TX 75231
800-242-8721
Provides information on coronary conditions and makes referrals to local support groups.

HOSPICE

Children's Hospice International
900 N. Washington Street, Suite 700
Alexandria, VA 22314
800-242-4453
703-684-0330 in Virginia
8:30 A.M. to 5:30 P.M. (eastern time) Monday–Friday
Answering machine at all other times
Provides information on hospice programs especially designed for children with life-threatening conditions or who are terminally ill.

Hospice Education Institute
5 Essex Square
P.O. Box 713
Essex, CT 06246
800-544-2213
203-767-1620 in Alaska and Connecticut
9:00 A.M. to 4:30 P.M. (eastern time) Monday–Friday
Provides information and counseling on death and dying and the role of the hospice. Also makes referrals to local agencies and publishes a directory of hospices.

National Hospice Organization
1901 N. Moore Street, Suite 901
Arlington, VA 22209
800-658-8898
8:30 A.M. to 5:30 P.M. (eastern time) Monday–Friday
Provides information on hospice programs available in the caller's area.

HOSPITAL CARE

Hill-Burton Hospital Program
Division of Facilities Compliance
Parklawn Building, Room 11-25
5600 Fishers Lane
Rockville, MD 20857
800-638-0742
800-492-0359 in Maryland
9:30 A.M. to 5:30 P.M. (eastern time) Monday–Friday
Answering machine at all other times
Provides information on hospitals that are participating in the Hill-Burton Free Care Program in the caller's area. Free information packet available upon request.

HUNTINGTON'S DISEASE

Huntington's Disease Society of America
140 W. 22nd Street, 6th Floor
New York, NY 10011-2420
800-345-4372
212-242-1968 in New York
9:00 A.M. to 5:00 P.M. (eastern time) Monday–Friday
Provides information and referrals to individuals with
Huntington's disease and their families. Also offers crisis
intervention and makes referrals to support groups. Free information available upon request.

INCONTINENCE

Simon Foundation for Continence
P.O. Box 815
Wilmette, IL 60091
800-237-4666
708-864-3913 in Illinois
9:00 A.M. to 6:00 P.M. (central time) 7 days a week
Provides information on incontinence. Also makes referrals to specialists in the field and support groups in the
caller's area.

INSURANCE

Alternative Health Insurance Services
P.O. Box 9178
Calabasas, CA 91372-9178
800-331-2713
818-509-5742 in Los Angeles
Provides information on insurance plans that cover alternative health care practitioners.

Communicating for Seniors
P.O. Box 677
Fergus Falls, MN 56538
800-432-3276
8:00 A.M. to 4:30 P.M. (central time) Monday–Friday
Provides information on insurance matters to the elderly,
especially in the area of Medicare supplemental insurance.
Free information available upon request.

Coop-America
2100 M Street N.W., Suite 403
Washington, DC 20037
800-424-2667
202-872-5200 in District of Columbia
Provides information on worker-owned and cooperatively
structured health insurance plans that provide coverage for
conventional as well as alternative practitioners.

National Insurance Consumer Helpline
American Council of Life Insurance
Health Insurance Association of America
Insurance Information Institute
1001 Pennsylvania Avenue N.W.
Washington, DC 20004
800-942-4242
Provides general information on how to choose an agent or
broker and an insurance company. Also provides information on the following types of insurance: health, long-term
care, disability, Medicare supplemental, and major medical. Does not provide information on specific policies or
companies.

KIDNEY DISEASES

American Association of Kidney Patients
111 S. Parker Street, Suite 405
Tampa, FL 33606
800-749-2257
813-251-0725 in Tampa area
9:00 A.M. to 5:00 P.M. (eastern time) Monday–Friday
Provides information to kidney patients and their families
on coping with kidney disease.

American Kidney Fund
6110 Executive Boulevard, Suite 1010
Rockville, MD 20852
800-638-8299
800-492-8361 in Maryland
8:00 A.M. to 5:00 P.M. (eastern time) Monday–Friday
Provides information on kidney diseases and organ donor
programs. Also offers financial assistance to kidney patients. Public education materials available upon request.

National Kidney Foundation
30 E. 33rd Street
New York, NY 10016
800-622-9010
8:30 A.M. to 5:30 P.M. (eastern time) Monday–Friday
Provides information on research into kidney and urinary
tract diseases, organ donations, and transplant programs.
Also provides materials for public education programs.

National Medical Care Patient Travel Service
Reservoir Place
1601 Trapelo Road
Waltham, MA 02154
800-634-6254
Provides information to dialysis patients on how to arrange
for dialysis at a National Medical Center dialysis facility
while on vacation.

LIVER DISEASES

American Liver Foundation
1425 Pompton Avenue
Cedar Grove, NJ 07009
800-223-0179
201-857-2626 in New Jersey
8:30 A.M. to 4:30 P.M. (eastern time) Monday–Friday
Provides information and assistance to children and adults with liver diseases. Also makes referrals to specialists and support groups.

LUNG DISEASES

Cystic Fibrosis Foundation
6931 Arlington Road
Bethesda, MD 20814
800-344-4823
301-951-4422
8:30 A.M. to 5:30 P.M. (eastern time) Monday–Friday
Provides information on cystic fibrosis and makes referrals to hospital treatment centers and local support groups. Free information available upon request.

LUPUS

Lupus Foundation of America
4 Research Place, Suite 180
Rockville, MD 20850-3226
800-558-0121
301-670-9292 in Maryland
24 hours a day
Provides free information concerning books written by doctors and patients who have lupus and refers callers to local chapters of the Lupus Foundation.

Terri Gotthelf Lupus Research Institute
3 Duke Place
South Norwalk, CT 06854
800-825-8787
203-852-0120
9:00 A.M. to 7:30 P.M. (eastern time) Monday–Friday
Provides information on medical centers that conduct research into the cause and treatment of lupus. Also provides general information on lupus to patients and their families. Free information available upon request.

MEDIC ALERT

Medic Alert Foundation International
2323 N. Colorado Avenue
Turlock, CA 95380
800-432-5378
800-468-1020 in California
209-668-3333 in Alaska and Hawaii
24 hours a day
Provides information on how to register with Medic Alert and obtain an emergency identification bracelet. Also maintains a record of the patient's medical record that can be retrieved in an emergency. Free registration form and catalog available upon request.

MEDICARE/MEDICAID

Inspector General's Hotline
U.S. Department of Health and Human Services
P.O. Box 17303
Baltimore, MD 21203-7303
800-368-5779
800-638-3986 in Maryland
Handles complaints from recipients relating to overcharges and possible fraud and waste of funds in the Medicare and Medicaid programs.

Medicare Information Hotline
U.S. Department of Health and Human Services
Health Care Financing Administration
Washington, DC 20201
800-888-1770 Recorded message
800-888-1998 To request written material or ask questions
8:00 A.M. to midnight (eastern time) 7 days a week
Provides general information on the Medicare program and responds to specific questions concerning Medicare coverage.

Medicare Medigap Insurance Fraud Line
U.S. Department of Health and Human Services
Health Care Financing Administration
Washington, DC 20201
800-638-6833
Provides information on the new Medicare supplemental, or Medigap, policies and also receives complaints from beneficiaries concerning instances of Medigap fraud and abuse.

MEN'S HEALTH

Impotence Foundation
800-221-5517
9:00 A.M. to 5:00 P.M. (Pacific time) Monday–Friday
Provides information on the treatment of impotence.

Impotence Information Center
P.O. Box 9
Minneapolis, MN 55440
800-843-4315
8:00 A.M. to 5:30 P.M. (central time) Monday–Friday
Answering machine at all other times
Provides free information on the causes and treatments of
impotence, but does not provide on-line counseling. Also
provides the names and addresses of urologists in the
caller's area.

Star Center
27211 Lahser Road, Suite 208
Southfield, MI 48034
800-835-7667
313-357-1314 in Michigan
24 hours a day
Provides general information on impotency and makes referrals to practitioners in the caller's area.

Us Too (Prostate Cancer)
American Foundation for Urologic Disease, Inc.
300 W. Pratt Street, Suite 401
Baltimore, MD 21201
800-828-7866
Provides information on the latest developments in the diagnosis and treatment of prostate cancer. Also makes referrals to local chapters of Us Too.

MENTAL HEALTH

American Board of Professional Psychology
2100 E. Broadway, Suite 313
Columbia, MO 65201-6082
800-255-7792
Provides information on psychologists who have met the
standards required for certification.

American Mental Health Counselors Association
5999 Stevenson Avenue
Alexandria, VA 22304
800-326-2642
703-823-9800
8:30 A.M. to 4:30 P.M. (eastern time) Monday–Friday
Provides information on professionals in the counseling
field and makes local referrals.

American Mental Health Fund
1021 Price Street
Alexandria, VA 22314
800-433-5959
703-684-2201 in Virginia
24 hours a day
Provides general information on mental illness. Callers
may request packets of information that include the location and telephone numbers for local chapters.

Camelback Helpline
7575 E. Earl Drive
Scottsdale, AZ 85251
800-253-1334
24 hours a day
Provides information on such subjects as mental health,
eating disorders, and substance dependency. Makes referrals to treatment centers nationwide. Free information
available upon request.

National Alliance for the Mentally Ill
2101 Wilson Boulevard, Suite 302
Arlington, VA 22201
800-950-6264
9:00 A.M. to 5:00 P.M. (eastern time) Monday–Friday
Answering machine at all other times
Provides information on local chapters, advocacy, and support groups for the mentally ill. Free literature available
upon request.

National Foundation for Depressive Illness
P.O. Box 2257
New York, NY 10116
800-248-4344
24 hours a day
Provides general information on depression and directs the
caller to other organizations that can provide additional information on specific conditions and physician referrals.

National Mental Health Association
1021 Prince Street
Alexandria, VA 22314-2971
800-969-6642
703-684-7722 in Virginia
9:00 A.M. to 6:00 P.M. (eastern time) Monday–Friday
Provides information on mental health and mental illnesses. Also makes referrals to local support groups, mental
health centers, self-help clearinghouses, and other organizations. Free packet of information available upon request.

MENTAL RETARDATION

American Association on Mental Retardation
1719 Kalorma Road N.W.
Washington, DC 20009
800-424-3688
202-387-1968 in District of Columbia
9:00 A.M. to 5:00 P.M. (eastern time) Monday–Friday
Provides general information on mental retardation and
makes referrals to practitioners. Free information packet on
the association's services and publications available upon
request.

MULTIPLE SCLEROSIS (MS)

National Multiple Sclerosis Society
733 3rd Avenue
New York, NY 10017-3288
800-624-8236
212-986-3240 in New York
24 hours a day
Provides general information on multiple sclerosis and makes referrals to local groups. Free information packet lists MS centers, board-certified neurologists, and updates on the latest research into the causes and treatments of MS.

MYASTHENIA GRAVIS (MG)

Myasthenia Gravis Foundation
53 W. Jackson Boulevard, Suite 660
Chicago, IL 60604
800-541-5454
8:00 A.M. to 5:00 P.M. (central time) Monday–Friday
Provides information on the diagnosis and treatment of MG and also makes referrals to local support groups.

NEUROFIBROMATOSIS

National Neurofibromatosis Foundation
141 5th Avenue, Suite 7-S
New York, NY 10010
800-323-7938
212-460-8980 in New York
9:00 A.M. to 5:00 P.M. (eastern time) Monday–Friday
Provides information and assistance to neurofibromatosis patients and their families. Free information packet available upon request.

NUTRITION INFORMATION

Akpharma Foods, Inc.
P.O. Box 111
Pleasantville, NJ 08232-0111
800-257-8650
9:00 A.M. to 5:00 P.M. (eastern time) Monday–Friday
Provides information on a product that helps people digest beans and vegetable fiber. Free information and sample of the product available upon request.

American Dietetic Association
Consumer Nutrition Hotline
216 W. Jackson Boulevard, Suite 800
Chicago, IL 60606
800-366-1655
10:00 A.M. to 5:00 P.M. (central time) Monday–Friday
Recorded messages 24 hours a day
Provides general information on nutrition, including cholesterol, weight control, and healthy snacks. Also makes referrals to nutritional counselors in the caller's area. Provides special service for teenagers.

American Institute for Cancer Research
AICR Nutrition Hotline
1759 R Street N.W.
Washington, DC 20009
800-843-8114
202-328-7744 in District of Columbia
9:00 A.M. to 9:00 P.M. (eastern time) Monday–Thursday
9:00 A.M. to 5:00 P.M. (eastern time) Friday
Answering machine at all other times
Provides information on the relationship between diet and nutrition and cancer. Callers may ask specific questions about cancer and diet.

Beech-Nut Nutrition, Inc.
Checkerboard Square
Consumer Affairs, 1-B
St. Louis, MO 63164
800-523-6633
800-492-2384 in Pennsylvania
9:00 A.M. to 8:00 P.M. (eastern time) Monday–Friday
Provides information on nutritional content of baby food and answers food-related questions.

Gerber Hotline
Consumer Relations Gerber Products
445 State Street
Fremont, MI 49413
800-443-7237
Provides information on infant nutrition and specific baby care topics.

HCF Foundation
High Carbohydrate Fiber
University of Kentucky
800 Rose Street
Lexington, KY 40536
800-727-4423
Provides information on the role of fiber in the diet as it relates to cholesterol, diabetes, and blood sugar levels. Callers may leave specific questions on voice-mail system.

International Olive Oil Council
P.O. Box 2506
Stuart, FL 34995-2506
800-232-6548
9:00 A.M. to 5:00 P.M. (eastern time) Monday–Friday
Provides information on the nutritional and fat content of olive oil. Free information available upon request.

Lactaid, Inc.
McNeil Consumer Affairs
P.O. Box 85
Camp Hill Road
Ft. Washington, PA 19034
800-522-8243
9:00 A.M. to 5:00 P.M. (eastern time) Monday–Friday
Provides information on Lactaid and lactose intolerance. Free information and samples available upon request.

Meat and Poultry Hotline
U.S. Department of Agriculture
Room 1165 S, FSIS
Washington, DC 20250
800-535-4555
202-720-3333 in District of Columbia
10:00 A.M. to 4:00 P.M. (eastern time) Monday–Friday
Provides information on the proper handling and storage of meat and poultry products. Free information available upon request.

Molly McButter Information Hotline
800-622-3274
9:00 A.M. to 5:00 P.M. (eastern time) Monday–Friday
Provides information on the fat and calorie content of foods. Callers may ask questions of registered dietitians.

Mrs. Dash Sodium Information Hotline
800-622-3274
9:00 A.M. to 5:00 P.M. (eastern time) Monday–Friday
Provides low-sodium recipes and information on the sodium content of foods for people on sodium-restricted diets. Free information available upon request.

ORGAN DONOR PROGRAMS

The Living Bank
P.O. Box 6725
Houston, TX 77265
800-528-2971
713-528-2971 in Texas
24 hours a day
Operates a registry and referral program for people wishing to donate their vital organs or bodies to research.

National Marrow Donor Program
3433 Broadway Street N.E., Suite 400
Minneapolis, MN 55413
800-654-1247
8:00 A.M. to 5:00 P.M. (central time) Monday–Friday
Answering machine at all other times
Provides information on how to become a bone marrow donor. Also maintains a national registry of volunteers. Free information available upon request.

Organ Donor Hotline
United Network for Organ Sharing
1100 Boulders Parkway, Suite 500
P.O. Box 13770
Richmond, VA 23225-8770
800-243-6667
804-330-8500
9:00 A.M. to 5:00 P.M. (eastern time) Monday–Friday
Provides information on organ donor programs and transplants. Also provides organ donor cards upon request.

ORPHAN DRUGS AND RARE DISEASES

Friends of Karen
P.O. Box 217
Croton Falls, NY 10519
800-637-2774
9:00 A.M. to 5:00 P.M. (eastern time) Monday–Friday
Provides information on financial support that may be available to families with children who have life-threatening or rare diseases. Also provides information on support groups to aid the families. Free information available upon request.

National Information Center for Orphan Drugs and Rare Diseases
P.O. Box 1133
Washington, DC 20013
800-336-4797
202-429-9091 in District of Columbia
9:00 A.M. to 5:00 P.M. (eastern time) Monday–Friday
Provides information on how to locate a source for orphan drugs. (Orphan drugs, for which there is only a small market, are used to treat rare illnesses.)

National Information Clearinghouse for Infants with Disabilities and Life-Threatening Conditions
University of South Carolina
Benson Building, 1st Floor
Columbia, SC 29208
800-922-9234 Voice- and hearing-impaired
800-922-1107 Voice- and hearing-impaired in South Carolina
9:00 A.M. to 5:00 P.M. (eastern time) Monday–Friday
Answering machine at all other times
Provides information to families with children who have rare or life-threatening conditions. Also makes referrals to professional and community services in the caller's area. Offers special services to Vietnam veterans and their families.

National Organization for Rare Disorders
P.O. Box 8923
New Fairfield, CT 06812-1783
800-447-6673
9:00 A.M. to 5:00 P.M. (eastern time) Monday–Friday
Answering machine at all other times
Provides information on how individuals may apply for the drug cost-sharing program that the pharmaceutical industry sponsors to help consumers pay the cost of medications. Free information available upon request.

OSTEOPOROSIS

National Osteoporosis Foundation
2100 M Street N.W., Suite 602-B
Washington, DC 20037
800-223-9994
Provides information on osteoporosis, including a publication answering basic questions about the condition. Free information packet available upon request.

PARALYSIS AND SPINAL CORD INJURY

APA Spinal Cord Injury Hotline
2201 Argonne Drive
Baltimore, MD 21218
800-526-3456
8:30 A.M. to 5:30 P.M. (eastern time) Monday–Friday
Answering machine at all other times
Provides information on spinal cord injuries and referrals
to local organizations, agencies, and treatment centers.

American Paralysis Association
Montebello Hospital
500 Morris Avenue
Springfield, NJ 07081
800-225-0292
201-379-2690 in New Jersey
8:30 A.M. to 5:00 p.m (eastern time) Monday–Friday
Provides information on research into treatment of spinal
cord injuries and prospects for recovery. Free information
available upon request.

National Spinal Cord Injury Association
600 W. Cummings Park, Suite 2000
Woburn, MA 01801
800-962-9629
617-935-2722 in Massachusetts
9:00 A.M. to 5:00 P.M. (eastern time) Monday–Friday
Provides information for patients and their families on services available from organizations, agencies, and local
support groups. Free information packet available upon
request.

PARENTING

A Way Out
7 Innis Avenue
New Paltz, NY 12561
800-292-9688
914-255-1907
Provides 24-hour-a-day assistance to parents who are considering abducting their children or who already have taken
their children.

Father Advocacy Information Referral
140-B Sandune Drive
Pittsburgh, PA 15239
800-722-3247
Provides assistance with visitation rights and custody for
divorced fathers.

Foster Parents Plan
155 Plan Way
Warwick, RI 02886
800-556-7918
Provides information on becoming a foster parent.

**National Association for Parents of the
Visually Impaired**
P.O. Box 317
Watertown, MA 02272-0317
800-562-6265
608-362-4945 in Wisconsin
9:00 a.m to 5:00 P.M. (central time) Monday–Friday
Provides general information and counseling to families
with visually impaired children.

Parents Anonymous/Abusive Parents
520 S. Lafayette Park Place, Suite 316
Los Angeles, CA 90057
800-421-0353
800-352-0386 in California
Provides assistance and counseling to parents who have
been involved in child abuse or abusive situations.

Parents Without Partners
8807 Colesville Road
Silver Spring, MD 20910
800-637-7974
301-588-9354 in Maryland
Provides information on area support groups for single
parents.

Technical Assistance to Parent Programs Network
Federation for Children with Special Needs
95 Berkeley Street, Suite 104
Boston, MA 02116
800-331-0688 in Massachusetts
9:00 A.M. to 5:00 P.M. (eastern time) Monday–Friday
Provides information to parents with children who have
special needs because of developmental disabilities. Also
provides information on special education laws, and provides training and workshops for parents of children with
special needs. Makes referrals to a national network of support groups.

Toughlove, Inc.
P.O. Box 1069
Doylestown, PA 18901
800-333-1069
215-348-7090 in Pennsylvania
Provides information on psychological treatment programs
for children with behavioral problems.

PARKINSON'S DISEASE

American Parkinson's Disease Association
60 Bay Street, Suite 401
Staten Island, NY 18901
800-223-2732 in New York
9:00 A.M. to 5:00 P.M. (eastern time) Monday–Friday
Answering machine at all other times
Provides brochures and sends information on medicines
used to treat Parkinson's. Also offers counseling services
and makes referrals to treatment centers.

National Parkinson's Foundation
1501 N.W. 9th Avenue
Miami, FL 33136
800-327-4545
800-433-7022 in Florida
305-547-6666 in Miami area
8:00 A.M. to 5:00 P.M. (eastern time) Monday–Friday
Provides information on Parkinson's disease and makes referrals to physicians.

Parkinson's Disease Foundation
William Black Medical Research Building
650 W. 168th Street
New York, NY 10032
800-457-6676
9:00 A.M. to 5:00 P.M. (eastern time) Monday–Friday
Provides information on patient care and rehabilitation, including lists of self-help groups and of clinics where treatment is available. Publishes newsletter four times a year. Clinical specialists available to answer questions.

Parkinson's Education Program
3900 Birch Street, Suite 105
Newport Beach, CA 92660
800-344-7872
714-640-0218 in California
24 hours a day
Provides written materials, including newsletters and other publications and definitions of key terms. Also makes referrals to support groups. Caller may leave name and address to receive materials.

PESTICIDES

National Pesticides Information Clearinghouse
National Pesticides Telecommunications Network
Texas Tech University
Health Science Center/Department of
Preventative Medicine
Lubbock, TX 79430
800-858-7378
800-292-7664 in Texas
24 hours a day
Provides information to the public and the medical profession on the hazards of pesticides.

PHYSICIAN CREDENTIALING

ABMS Certification Line
American Board of Medical Specialties
180 Allen Road, Suite 302
Atlanta, GA 30328
800-776-2378
9:00 A.M. to 6:00 P.M. (eastern time) Monday–Friday
Provides information on the certification status of physicians, including their specialty and year certified. Caller should have physician's name and location ready before calling.

PREGNANCY SERVICES

Abortion Hotline
National Abortion Federation
1436 U Street N.W.
Washington, DC 20009
800-772-9100
202-667-5881 in District of Columbia
9:30 A.M. to 5:30 P.M. (eastern time) Monday–Friday
Provides information on services available at clinics in the caller's area. Also provides information on state laws applicable to abortion services.

American Academy of Husband-Coached Childbirth
P.O. Box 5224
Sherman Oaks, CA 91413-5224
800-422-4784
818-788-6662 in Sherman Oaks area
24 hours a day
Provides information on the Bradley method of childbirth and makes referrals to local instructors. Free information, including directory of instructors, available upon request.

American Society for Psychoprophylaxis in Obstetrics/Lamaze
1101 Connecticut Avenue N.W., Suite 700
Washington, DC 20036
800-368-4404
202-857-1128 in District of Columbia
9:00 A.M. to 5:00 P.M. (eastern time) Monday–Friday
Provides information on the Lamaze technique and makes referrals to local centers.

Be Healthy, Inc.: Positive Pregnancy and Parenting Fitness
51 Saltrock Road
Baltic, CT 06330
800-433-5523
203-822-8573 in Connecticut
9:00 A.M. to 5:00 P.M. (eastern time) Monday–Friday
Answering machine at all other times
Provides information on pregnancy and parenting, including audio and visual aids. Free packet of information available upon request.

Bethany Christian Services
901 Eastern Avenue N.E.
Grand Rapids, MI 49503
800-238-4269
9:00 A.M. to 5:00 P.M. (eastern time) Monday–Friday
Provides pregnancy testing, counseling services, and adoption services to pregnant women.

Birthright
686 N. Broad Street
Woodbury, NJ 08096
800-848-5683
609-848-1818 in New Jersey
8:00 A.M. to 3:00 P.M. (eastern time) Monday–Friday
Provides confidential pregnancy counseling to girls who are homeless because of their pregnancy. Also provides maternity and baby clothes and support services, such as medical and financial referrals.

Edna Gladney Center Pregnancy Hotline
2300 Hemphill
Ft. Worth, TX 76110
800-452-3639
817-926-3304 in Texas
9:00 A.M. to 5:00 P.M. (central time) Monday–Saturday
Provides information on all the options of pregnancy, especially adoption. Residential services are provided to women who are considering placing their babies for adoption.

International Childbirth Education Association
P.O. Box 20048
Minneapolis, MN 55420
800-624-4934
Provides information on pregnancy, childbirth, and other related infant health needs. Also operates a book center. Free information and catalog available upon request.

La Leche League International
P.O. Box 1209
9616 Minneapolis Avenue
Franklin Park, IL 60131-8209
800-525-3243
9:00 A.M. to 3:00 P.M. (central time) Monday–Friday
Provides information on breast-feeding.

Planned Parenthood Federation
810 7th Avenue
New York, NY 10019
800-829-7732
212-541-7800 in New York
8:30 A.M. to 5:00 P.M. (eastern time) Monday–Friday
Provides information on family planning matters, including the use of contraceptives. Makes referrals to Planned Parenthood clinics in the caller's area.

PREMENSTRUAL SYNDROME

PMS Access
P.O. Box 9326
Madison, WI 53715
800-222-4767
608-257-8682 in Wisconsin
9:00 A.M. to 5:00 P.M. (central time) Monday–Friday
Provides information on all aspects of PMS. Makes referrals to physicians and clinics in the caller's area. Free information packet available upon request.

PRODUCT SAFETY

U.S. Consumer Product Safety Commission
5401 Westbard Avenue
Bethesda, MD 20207
800-638-CPSC
800-638-8270 Hearing-impaired
800-492-8104 Hearing-impaired in Maryland
9:00 A.M. to 5:00 P.M. (eastern time) Monday–Friday
Provides information on how to report complaints of injuries caused by consumer products.

RETINITIS PIGMENTOSA (RP)

National Retinitis Pigmentosa Foundation
1401 Mt. Royal Avenue, 4th Floor
Baltimore, MD 21217
800-683-5555
410-225-9400 in Maryland
8:30 A.M. to 5:00 P.M. (eastern time) Monday–Friday
Answering machine at all other times
Provides information on the latest developments in the treatment of RP and answers questions.

Retinitis Pigmentosa International Fighting Blindness
P.O. Box 900
Woodland Hills, CA 91367
800-344-4877
Provides information on RP and reports on research into the diagnosis and treatment of this condition.

REYE'S SYNDROME

National Reye's Syndrome Foundation
426 N. Lewis
P.O. Box 829
Bryan, OH 43506
800-233-7393
800-231-7393 in Ohio
24 hours a day
Provides information on symptoms of Reye's syndrome and on treatment and support networks.

SENIOR CITIZENS' SERVICES

Alcohol Rehabilitation for the Elderly
Hopedale Medical Complex
P.O. Box 267
Hopedale, IL 61747
800-354-7089
800-344-0824 in Illinois
24 hours a day
Provides information and also makes referrals to treatment programs for people aged 50 and older.

Life Extension Foundation
2835 Hollywood Boulevard
P.O. Box 229120
Hollywood, FL 33022
800-327-6110
Provides information on anti-aging research.

National Council on the Aging, Inc.
409 3rd Street S.W.
Washington, DC 20024
800-424-9046
202-479-1200 in District of Columbia
9:00 A.M. to 5:00 P.M. (eastern time) Monday–Friday
Provides general information on the subject of aging. Also serves as a clearinghouse for other organizations that provide programs to the elderly. Free information packet available upon request.

National Eye Care Project Hotline
P.O. Box 429098
San Francisco, CA 94142
800-222-3937
8:00 A.M. to 4:00 P.M. (Pacific time) Monday–Friday
Provides information on a program designed for senior citizens aged 65 or older who are considered economically disadvantaged. Income and resources test for eligibility. Makes referrals to medical professionals in the caller's area.

SEXUALLY TRANSMITTED DISEASES

STD National Hotline
American Social Health Association
P.O. Box 13827
Research Triangle Park, NC 27709
800-227-8922
919-361-8400 in North Carolina
8:00 A.M. to 11:00 P.M. (eastern time) Monday–Friday
Provides free and confidential information on sexually transmitted diseases. Also provides referrals for diagnosis and treatment.

SKIN DISORDERS

American Society for Dermatological Surgery
930 N. Meacham Road
Schaumburg, Il 60173
800-441-2737
9:00 A.M. to 5:00 P.M. (central time) Monday–Friday
Provides information on surgical procedures related to skin damage from the sun, disease, or aging. List of specialists in the caller's area available upon request.

United Scleroderma Foundation
P.O. Box 350
Watsonville, CA 95077
800-722-4673
8:00 A.M. to 5:00 P.M. (Pacific time) Monday–Friday
Provides information on scleroderma and other related skin diseases. Makes referrals to local support groups and treatment centers.

SLEEP DISORDERS

American Narcolepsy Association
P.O. Box 26230
San Carlos, CA 94126
800-222-6085
24 hours a day
Provides information on narcolepsy and makes local referrals.

Better Sleep Council
P.O. Box 13
Washington, DC 20044
800-827-5337
Provides guidelines to better sleeping.

SOCIAL SECURITY

National Association of Social Security Claimants Representatives
6 Prospect Street
Midland Park, NJ 07432
800-431-2804
914-735-8812 in New York (call collect)
Provides the names of attorneys who specialize in Social Security cases.

Social Security Administration
Social Security Hotline
U.S. Department of Health and Human Services
6401 Security Boulevard
Baltimore, MD 21235
800-234-5772
7:00 A.M. to 7:00 P.M. (eastern time) Monday–Friday
Answering machine at all other times
Provides information on Social Security claims and general information concerning eligibility for the program.

SPASMODIC TORTICOLLIS

National Spasmodic Torticollis Association, Inc.
P.O. Box 476
Elm Grove, WI 53122-0476
800-487-8385
24 hours a day
Provides referrals to physicians and support groups. Free information packet available upon request.

Speech Impairments

American Speech-Language-Hearing Association Helpline
1081 Rockville Pike
Rockville, MD 20852
800-638-8255
8:30 A.M. to 4:30 P.M. (eastern time) Monday–Friday
Provides information on speech, hearing, and language problems. Makes referrals to professionals in the field of speech therapy. Free information available upon request.

AT&T Special Needs Center
2001 Route 46, 3rd Floor
Parsippany, NJ 07054
800-833-3232
Provides information on purchasing or renting special equipment and services for speech- and hearing-impaired individuals.

Institute of Logopedics
2400 Jardine Drive
Wichita, KS 67219
800-835-1043 (includes Canada)
8:00 A.M. to 5:00 P.M. (central time) Monday–Friday
Provides information on services offered by the institute's outpatient audiology department.

National Center for Stuttering
200 E. 33rd Street, Suite 17-C
New York, NY 10016
800-221-2483
9:00 A.M. to 5:00 P.M. (eastern time) Monday–Friday
Provides information on methods used to treat stuttering in children and adults. Free information available upon request.

Spina Bifida

Spina Bifida Association of America
4590 MacArthur Boulevard N.W., Suite 250
Washington, DC 20007
800-621-3141
301-770-7222 in Maryland
9:00 a.m to 5:00 P.M. (eastern time) Monday–Friday
Answering machine at all other times
Provides free information on the birth defect spina bifida. Also makes referrals to local chapters.

Sports Medicine

International Institute of Sports Science and Medicine
Center for Hip and Knee Surgery
1199 Hadley Road
Mooresville, IN 46158
800-237-7678 in Indiana
Provides information on surgical procedures to repair hip and knee injuries.

Stroke

Courage Stroke Network
3915 Golden Valley Road
Golden Valley, MN 55422
800-553-6321
612-588-0811 in Minnesota
8:00 A.M. to 4:00 P.M. (central time) Monday–Friday
Provides consultation, information, public education, and referrals to local support groups.

National Stroke Association
300 E. Hampden Avenue, Suite 240
Englewood, CO 80110-2654
800-787-6537
8:00 A.M. to 5:00 P.M. (central time) Monday–Friday
Provides information on support networks for stroke victims and their families. Also serves as a clearinghouse of information on stroke, including referrals to local support groups.

Substance Abuse: Drugs and Alcohol

Al-Anon Family Groups Headquarters
P.O. Box 862, Midtown Station
New York, NY 10018
800-356-9996
800-245-4656 in New York
800-443-4525 in Canada
9:00 A.M. to 5:00 P.M. (eastern time) Monday–Friday
Provides information on twelve-step recovery programs for alcoholics and their families. Free information available upon request.

Alcohol and Drug Referral Helpline
Highland Ridge Hospital
4578 S. Highland Drive
Salt Lake City, UT 84117
800-821-4357
24 hours a day
Provides information on alcohol and drug abuse and also makes referrals to local support programs.

Alcohol Helpline
Adcare Hospital of Worcester
107 Lincoln Street
Worcester, MA 01605
800-252-6465
24 hours a day
Provides basic information on alcohol treatment programs and makes referrals to local treatment facilities.

Alcoholism and Drug Addiction Treatment Center

Scripps-Memorial Hospital
9904 Genesee Avenue
La Jolla, CA 92037
800-382-4357 California
619-457-4123
Provides information on substance-abuse programs and makes referrals to treatment services for adults and adolescents.

American Council on Alcoholism

5024 Campbell Boulevard, Suite H
Baltimore, MD 21236
800-527-5344
410-931-9393 in Baltimore area
9:00 A.M. to 5:00 P.M. (eastern time) Monday–Friday
Answering machine at all other times
Provides information on alcoholism prevention programs for adults and children. Also provides counseling and referrals to treatment programs.

ASAP Treatment Hotline

31129 Via Colinas, Suite 701
Westlake Village, CA 91362
800-367-2727
Provides telephone counseling to callers and information on alcohol and drug rehabilitation programs.

BABES World, Inc.

Beginning Alcohol and Addiction Basic Education Studies
17330 Northland Park Court
Southfield, MI 48075
800-542-2237
Provides information on alcohol and drug prevention programs designed for children.

Cocaine Anonymous

3740 Overland Avenue, Suite G
Los Angeles, CA 90034
800-347-8998
310-559-5833 in Los Angeles area
Provides information on cocaine addiction and rehabilitation programs.

Cottage Program International

57 W. South Temple Street, Suite 420
Salt Lake City, UT 84101
800-752-6100
24 hours a day
Provides information on substance abuse programs aimed at the family. Also makes referrals to local organizations and support groups.

Drug Abuse Information and Treatment Referral Line

National Institute on Drug Abuse
11426 Rockville Pike, Suite 410
Rockville, MD 20852
800-662-4357
800-662-9832 Spanish
800-228-0427 Hearing-impaired
9:00 A.M. to 3:00 A.M. (eastern time) Monday–Friday
Noon to 3:00 A.M. (eastern time) Saturday and Sunday
Provides counseling and referral services to callers. Also provides general information on substance abuse and addiction.

Drug Abuse Resistance Education (DARE)

P.O. Box 2090
Los Angeles, CA 90051-0090
800-223-3273
Provides information on programs that teach people how to avoid using drugs and other harmful substances.

Families Anonymous

P.O. Box 528
Van Nuys, CA 91408
800-736-9805
818-989-7841
Provides information for families with children who have substance abuse or behavioral problems. Also provides counseling for family members and friends.

Family Talk About Drinking

Anheuser-Busch Company
Department of Consumer Awareness and Education
One Busch Place
St. Louis, MO 63118
800-359-8255
Provides information to families on how to discuss alcohol use with young children and teenagers. Callers may request information booklets by leaving name and address on voice-mail system.

Hazelton Foundation

15251 Pleasant Valley Road
P.O. Box 11
Center City, MN 55102
800-328-9000
800-262-5010 in Minnesota
7:00 A.M. to 6:00 P.M. (central time) Monday–Friday
Answering machine at all other times
Provides information on substance abuse treatment and rehabilitation programs and on publications for sale. Operates rehabilitation center and also makes referrals to other organizations and resources. Free information available upon request.

Johnson Institute

7205 Ohms Lane
Minneapolis, MN 55439-2159
800-231-5165
800-247-0484 in Minnesota
Provides educational materials and information on community substance abuse prevention programs.

Mothers Against Drunk Drivers (MADD)
511 E. John Carpenter Freeway, Suite 700
Irving, TX 75062
800-438-6233
24 hours a day
Provides information on programs designed to prevent
drunk driving.

**National Clearinghouse for Alcohol and
Drug Information**
6000 Executive Boulevard, Suite 402
Rockville, MD 20852
800-729-6686
Provides information and referrals to callers with questions
about alcohol and drug treatment programs.

National Cocaine Hotline
P.O. Box 100
Summit, NJ 07901-0100
800-262-2463
Provides information and referrals to drug treatment and
rehabilitation programs. Also answers specific questions on
drug abuse.

**National Council on Alcoholism and Drug
Dependence, Inc.**
Hopeline
12 W. 21st Street
New York, NY 10010
800-622-2255
212-206-6770 in New York City area
24 hours a day
Provides referrals to local organizations and support
groups. Callers may obtain the location of the nearest affili-
ate office by entering their zip code on the voice-mail system. Free information available upon request.

National Federation of Parents for a Drug-Free Youth
8730 Georgia Avenue, Suite 200
Silver Spring, MD 20910
800-554-5437
Provides information on programs designed to help parents
and children prevent drug abuse. Also makes referrals to
support groups.

**National Parents Resources Institute for
Drug Education**
50 Hurt Plaza, Suite 210
Atlanta, GA 30303
800-677-7433
404-577-4500 in Atlanta area
Provides information on starting community drug education programs for young people.

New Life (Women for Sobriety)
P.O. Box 618
Quakertown, PA 18951
800-333-1606
215-536-8026
Provides help and assistance to women alcoholics.

Pride Institute
14400 Martin Drive
Eden Prairie, MN 55344
800-547-7433
24 hours a day
Provides information for persons addicted to alcohol or
drugs. Also makes referrals to treatment centers.

Target Resource Center
P.O. Box 20626
Kansas City, MO 64195
800-366-6667
8:00 A.M. to 4:30 P.M. (central time) Monday–Friday
Provides information on substance abuse avoidance programs designed for preschool and school-age children,
kindergarten through high school. Free catalog available
upon request.

SUDDEN INFANT DEATH SYNDROME (SIDS)

American Sudden Infant Death Syndrome Institute
275 Carpenter Drive
Atlanta, GA 30328
800-232-7437
800-847-7437 in Georgia
8:00 A.M. to 5:00 P.M. (eastern time) Monday–Friday
Answering machine at all other times
Provides information on research into the cause of SIDS
and also provides counseling and referral services.

Sudden Infant Death Syndrome Alliance
10500 Little Patuxent Parkway, Suite 420
Columbia, MD 21044
800-221-7437
8:00 A.M. to 5:00 P.M. (eastern time) Monday–Friday
Answering machine at all other times
Provides information to parents of young infants and also
offers counseling and support services to parents who have
lost a child to SIDS.

SURGERY SERVICES

American Academy of Cosmetic Surgery
401 N. Michigan Avenue
Chicago, IL 60611
800-221-9808
8:00 A.M. to 5:00 P.M. (central time) Monday–Friday
Provides information on cosmetic surgery and also makes
referrals to physician members of the academy in the
caller's area.

American Academy of Facial Plastic and Reconstructive Surgeons
1110 Vermont Avenue N.W., Suite 220
Washington, DC 20005
800-332-3223
800-532-3223 in Canada
202-842-4500 in District of Columbia
24 hours a day
Provides general information on plastic surgery. Callers may request lists of surgeons in their areas.

American Association of Oral and Maxillofacial Surgeons
9700 Bryn Mawr Avenue
Rosemont, IL 60018
800-467-5268
8:30 A.M. to 5:00 P.M. (central time) Monday–Friday
Answering machine at all other times
Provides information and referrals to oral surgeons.

American Plastic Surgery Information
6707 First Avenue S.
St. Petersburg, FL 33707
800-522-2222 in Florida
Provides information on plastic and reconstructive surgery and makes referrals in caller's area.

American Society of Plastic and Reconstructive Surgeons
444 E. Algonquin Road
Arlington Heights, IL 60005
800-635-0635
8:30 A.M. to 4:30 P.M. (central time) Monday–Friday
Provides information on surgical procedures and makes referrals to specialists within specified geographical areas. Also verifies credentials of plastic surgeons.

Plastic and Aesthetic Surgery Center
217 E. Chestnut Street
Louisville, KY 40202
800-327-3613
800-633-8923 in Kentucky
24 hours a day
Provides information about various plastic surgery procedures, including cost estimates. Also makes local referrals.

TOURETTE SYNDROME

Tourette Syndrome Association
42-40 Bell Boulevard
Bayside, NY 11361
800-237-0717
8:30 A.M. to 4:30 P.M. (eastern time) Monday–Friday
Answering machine at all other times
Provides information on the syndrome to patients and their families. Also makes referrals to local chapters in the caller's area.

TOXIC SUBSTANCES

Asbestos Technical Information Service
P.O. Box 12194
Research Triangle Park, NC 27709
800-334-8571
9:00 A.M. to 5:00 P.M. (eastern time) Monday–Friday
Provides information about different types of asbestos and proper removal and disposal procedures. Also provides information on home tests for asbestos.

Chemical Manufacturers Association
2501 M Street N.W.
Washington, DC 20037
800-262-8200
202-887-1315 in District of Columbia
9:00 A.M. to 6:00 P.M. (eastern time) Monday–Friday
Answering machine at all other times
Provides general information on the safe handling of chemicals. Makes referrals to the manufacturers of specific chemical products who are responsible for providing more detailed information on the proper use and safety of the product. Each company provides a fact sheet on the specific effects of exposure to the chemical.

Emergency Planning and Community Right-to-Know Information Hotline
U.S. Environmental Protection Agency
401 M Street N.W.
Washington, DC 20460
800-535-0202
202-479-2449 in District of Columbia
Provides information on chemicals used in the community and the workplace.

Environmental Defense Fund Hotline
1616 P Street N.W.
Washington, DC 20036
800-225-5333
202-387-3500 in District of Columbia
Provides information to the public on the issue of environmental protection, including ways in which individuals can help keep the environment clean.

National Center for Toxicological Research
NCTR Drive
Highway 365 N.
County Road 3
Jefferson, AR 72079-9502
800-638-3321
Provides information on the effects of toxic substances on the environment.

TUBEROUS SCLEROSIS

National Tuberous Sclerosis Association
8000 Corporate Drive, Suite 120
Landover, MD 20785
800-225-6872
301-459-9888 in Maryland
9:00 A.M. to 5:00 P.M. (eastern time) Monday–Friday
Answering machine at all other times
Provides referrals to local representatives of the association
and also provides information on parent-to-parent support
networks. Free packet of materials available upon request.

VIETNAM VETERANS

Agent Orange Veteran Payment Program
P.O. Box 110
Hartford, CT 06104
800-225-4712
800-922-9234 Birth defect information line
8:00 A.M. to 6:00 P.M. (eastern time) Monday–Friday
Provides counseling and assistance to Vietnam veterans
who are involved in the class action lawsuit against the
manufacturers of the defoliant Agent Orange. Also provides information and counseling to families with children
who have disabilities that may be linked to Agent Orange.

Vietnam Veterans Agent Orange Victims, Inc.
P.O. Box 2465
Darien, CT 06820-0465
800-521-0198
9:00 A.M. to 4:00 P.M. (eastern time) Monday–Friday
Provides medical and legal advice, information, and counseling to veterans who were exposed to the defoliant Agent
Orange. Has established a children's fund to aid families
whose children may be suffering from birth defects and developmental disabilities linked to Agent Orange.

VISION IMPAIRMENTS

See also Retinitis Pigmentosa.

American Council of the Blind
1155 Vermont Avenue N.W., Suite 720
Washington, DC 20005
800-424-8666
202-467-5081 in District of Columbia
3:00 P.M. to 5:30 P.M. (eastern time) Monday–Friday
Provides information and referrals to clinics, organizations,
and government agencies that provide services to the blind.

American Foundation for the Blind
15 W. 16th Street
New York, NY 10011
800-232-5463
8:30 A.M. to 4:30 P.M. (eastern time) Monday–Friday
Provides answers to questions concerning vision loss and
blindness. Free information available upon request.

AT&T National Special Needs Center
2001 Route 46, 3rd Floor
Parsippany, NJ 07054
800-833-3232
Provides information on equipment that can be adapted to
meet the needs of the visually impaired.

Audio Reader
P.O. Box 847
Lawrence, KS 66044
800-772-8898 in Kansas
Provides information on reading services available to the
visually impaired.

Blind Children's Center
4120 Marathon Street
Los Angeles, CA 90029-0159
800-222-3566
800-222-3567 in California
Provides information on blindness and makes referrals to
local organizations and support groups.

Books on Tape
P.O. Box 7900
Newport Beach, CA 92658-7900
800-626-3333
Provides information on talking books that may be rented
or purchased.

Guide Dog Foundation for the Blind
371 E. Jericho Turnpike
Smithtown, NY 11787
800-548-4337
9:00 A.M. to 5:00 P.M. (eastern time) Monday–Friday
Provides information on guide dogs and refers callers to local organizations.

International Orthokeratology Society
1575 W. Big Beaver Road
Troy, MI 48084
800-626-7846
8:00 A.M. to 5:00 P.M. (eastern time) Monday–Friday
10:00 A.M. to 2:00 P.M. (eastern time) Saturday
Answering machine at all other times
Provides information on the use of contact lenses to correct
astigmatism and myopia. Makes referrals in caller's local
area. Free brochure and other information available upon
request.

Job Opportunities for the Blind
National Federation of the Blind
1800 Johnson Street
Baltimore, MD 21230
800-638-7518
8:00 A.M. to 5:00 P.M. (eastern time) Monday–Friday
Provides career counseling, job listings, and referrals to the
visually impaired who are seeking employment.

Library of Congress
National Service for the Blind and Physically Handicapped
1291 Taylor Street N.W.
Washington, DC 20542
800-424-8567
202-794-8650 in District of Columbia
Provides information on libraries that offer talking books and books in braille.

National Society to Prevent Blindness
National Center for Sight
500 E. Remington Road
Schaumburg, IL 60173
800-221-3004
9:00 A.M. to 4:00 P.M. (central time) Monday–Friday
Provides literature on specific vision problems and conditions. Also produces educational materials and offers professional education programs.

WOMEN'S HEALTH

Breast Implant Information Service
Food and Drug Administration
P.O. Box 1802
Rockville, MD 20704-1802
800-532-4440
800-688-6167 Hearing-impaired
9:00 A.M. to 7:00 P.M. (eastern time) Monday–Friday
Answering machine at all other times
Provides information on the status of clinical studies being conducted on the safety of silicone gel-filled breast implants. Free packet of information available upon request.

Johnson & Johnson, Inc.
Personal Products Consumer Response Center
New Brunswick, NJ 08901
800-526-3967
Provides information on a wide range of women's health concerns, including toxic shock syndrome.

Women's Sports Foundation
342 Madison Avenue, Suite 728
New York, NY 10173
800-227-3988
9:00 A.M. to 5:00 P.M. (eastern time) Monday–Friday
Provides information on women and sports, physical fitness, and sports medicine.

State Agencies on Aging

These agencies, established under the Older Americans Act, coordinate many of the services and programs offered to older Americans. They also assist Area Agencies on Aging and other affiliated agencies to implement these programs at the local level.

Alabama
Commission on Aging
136 Catoma Street
Montgomery, AL 36130
205-242-5743
800-243-5463 (in AL)

Alaska
State Agency on Aging
Older Alaskans Commission
P.O. Box C
Juneau, AK 99811-0209
907-465-3250

Arizona
State Agency on Aging
Aging and Adult Administration
1400 W. Washington Street, 950A
Phoenix, AZ 85007
602-542-4446

Arkansas
State Agency on Aging
Office of Aging and Adult Services
Department of Human Services
P.O. Box 1437
Little Rock, AR 72203-1437
501-682-2441
800-482-8049 (in AR)

California
Department of Aging
1600 K Street
Sacramento, CA 95814
916-322-5290
800-231-4024 (in CA)

Colorado
State Agency on Aging
Department of Social Services
1575 Sherman Street
Denver, CO 80203-1714
303-866-5700

Connecticut
Department on Aging
175 Main Street
Hartford, CT 06106
203-566-3238
800-443-9946 (in CT)

Delaware
Division of Aging
Department of Health and Social Services
1901 N. DuPont Highway
New Castle, DE 19720
302-421-6791
800-223-9074 (in DE)

District Of Columbia
State Office on Aging
1424 K Street N.W., 2nd Floor
Washington, DC 20005
202-724-5623

Florida
State Agency on Aging
Aging and Adult Services
1321 Winewood Boulevard, Room 323
Tallahassee, FL 32399-0700
904-488-8922

Georgia
Office of Aging
878 Peachtree Street N.E., Suite 632
Atlanta, GA 30309
404-894-5333

Hawaii
Executive Office on Aging
335 Merchant Street, Room 241
Honolulu, HI 96813
808-548-2593
800-468-4644 (in HI)

Idaho
State Office on Aging
Statehouse, Room 108
Boise, ID 83720
208-334-3833

Illinois
Department on Aging
421 E. Capitol Avenue
Springfield, IL 62701
217-785-2870
800-252-8966 (in IL)

Indiana
State Agency on Aging
Aging/In-Home Care Services Division
Department of Human Services
P.O. Box 7083
Indianapolis, IN 46207-7083
317-232-7020
800-622-4972 (in IN)

Iowa
State Agency on Aging
Department of Elder Affairs
914 Grand Avenue, Suite 236
Des Moines, IA 50319
515-281-5187
800-532-3213 (in IA)

Kansas
Department on Aging
Docking State Office Building, Room 122 South
915 S.W. Harrison Street
Topeka, KS 66612-1500
913-296-4986
800-432-3535 (in KS)

Kentucky
Division for Aging Services
Department for Social Services
275 E. Main Street, 6th Floor West
Frankfort, KY 40621
502-564-6930
800-372-2991 (in KY)

Louisiana
State Agency on Aging
Governor's Office of Elder Affairs
P.O. Box 80374
Baton Rouge, LA 70898
504-925-1700

Maine
State Agency on Aging
Bureau of Elder and Adult Services
35 Anthony Avenue
Statehouse Station 11
Augusta, ME 04333-0011
207-626-5335

Maryland
Office on Aging
301 W. Preston Street, 10th Floor
Baltimore, MD 21201
410-225-1100
800-243-3425 (in MD)

Massachusetts
State Agency on Aging
Executive Office of Elder Affairs
38 Chauncy Street
Boston, MA 02111
617-727-7750
800-882-2003 (in MA)

Michigan
State Agency on Aging
Office of Services to the Aging
P.O. Box 30026
Lansing, MI 48909
517-373-8230

Minnesota
Board on Aging
444 Lafayette Road
St. Paul, MN 55155-3843
612-296-2544
800-652-9747 (in MN)

Mississippi
State Agency on Aging
Division of Aging and Adult Services
421 W. Pascagoula Street
Jackson, MS 39203
601-949-2070
800-345-6347 (in MS)

Missouri
Division of Aging
P.O. Box 1337
Jefferson City, MO 65102
314-751-8535
800-392-0210 (in MO)

Montana
State Agency on Aging
Governor's Office
State Capitol
Helena, MT 59620
406-444-4204
800-332-2272 (in MT)

Nebraska
Department on Aging
State Office Building
P.O. Box 95044
Lincoln, NE 68509
402-471-2306

Nevada
Division for Aging Services
Department of Human Resources
340 N. 11th Street
Las Vegas, NV 89158
702-486-3545

New Hampshire
Division of Elderly and Adult Services
6 Hazen Drive
Concord, NH 03301
603-271-4680
800-351-1888 (in NH)

New Jersey
Division on Aging
Department of Community Affairs
101 S. Broad Street, CN-807
Trenton, NJ 08625
609-292-4833
800-792-8820 (in NJ)

New Mexico
State Agency on Aging
224 E. Palace Avenue, 4th Floor
Santa Fe, NM 87501
505-827-7640
800-432-2080 (in NM)

New York
State Agency on Aging
Agency Building 2
Empire State Plaza
Albany, NY 12223
518-474-5731
800-342-9871 (in NY)

North Carolina
Division of Aging
Department of Human Resources
Caller Box Number 2953
693 Palmer Drive
Raleigh, NC 27626-0531
919-733-3983
800-662-7030 (in NC)

North Dakota
State Agency on Aging
Department of Human Services
600 E. Boulevard
Bismarck, ND 58505
701-224-2310
800-472-2622 (in ND)

Ohio
Department of Aging
50 W. Broad Street, 9th Floor
Columbus, OH 43266-0501
614-466-5500
800-282-1206 (in OH)

Oklahoma
State Agency on Aging
Special Unit on Aging
P.O. Box 25352
Oklahoma City, OK 73125
405-521-2281

Oregon
State Agency on Aging
Department of Human Resources
313 Public Service Building
Salem, OR 97310
503-378-4728
800-232-3020 (in OR)

Pennsylvania
Department of Aging
231 State Street
Harrisburg, PA 17101
717-783-1549

Puerto Rico
State Agency on Aging
Office of Elder Affairs
Call Box 563
Old San Juan Station, PR 00902
809-721-4560

Rhode Island
State Agency on Aging
Department of Elderly Affairs
160 Pine Street
Providence, RI 02903
401-277-2880
800-322-2880 (in RI)

South Carolina
Commission on Aging
400 Arbor Lake Drive, Suite B-500
Columbia, SC 29223
803-735-0210
800-868-9095 (in SC)

South Dakota
State Agency on Aging
Office of Adult Services And Aging
700 Governor's Drive
Pierre, SD 57501
605-773-3656

Tennessee
Commission on Aging
706 Church Street, Suite 201
Nashville, TN 37243-0860
615-741-2056

Texas
Department on Aging
P.O. Box 12786
Capitol Station
Austin, TX 78711
512-444-2727
800-252-9240 (in TX)

Utah
State Agency on Aging
Division of Aging and Adult Services
P.O. Box 45500
Salt Lake City, UT 84145-0500
801-538-3910

Vermont
State Agency on Aging
Department of Aging and Disabilities
103 S. Main Street
Waterbury, VT 05671-2301
802-241-2400

Virgin Islands
State Agency on Aging
Department of Human Services
Barbel Plaza S.
Charlotte Amalie
St. Thomas, VI 00802
809-774-0930

Virginia
Department for the Aging
700 E. Franklin Street, 10th Floor
Richmond, VA 23219
804-225-2271
800-552-4464 (in VA)

Washington
State Agency on Aging
Aging and Adult Services Administration
OB-44A
Olympia, WA 98504
206-493-2509
800-422-3263 (in WA)

West Virginia
Commission on Aging
State Capitol
Charleston, WV 25305
304-558-3317

Wisconsin
Bureau on Aging
P.O. Box 7851
Madison, WI 53707
608-266-2536

Wyoming
Division on Aging
139 Hathaway Building
Cheyenne, WY 82002-0480
307-777-7986
800-442-2766 (in WY)

Healthiest States

Every year since 1989 Northwestern National Life Insurance Company has issued a report on the healthiness of the population of each state. The ranking is based on a holistic view of health outlined by the World Health Organization, which defines health as "a state of complete physical, mental, and social well-being and not merely the absence of diseases or infirmity."

Below is the overall ranking of each state, representing a broad range of issues that affect a population's health. Following that are seven different rankings: five based on components that reflect the lifestyle of a population and its impact on health—prevalence of smoking, motor vehicle deaths, violent crime, risk for heart disease, and high school graduation—and two concerning access, or the measure of the availability of health care to the population of a state.

OVERALL STATE HEALTH RANKINGS

(from healthiest to least healthy)

Rank	State
1	Minnesota
2	New Hampshire
3	Hawaii
3	Connecticut
5	Utah
6	Vermont
6	Kansas
8	Massachusetts
9	Iowa
9	Colorado
11	Wisconsin
11	Nebraska
13	Virginia
14	Maine
15	New Jersey
16	Maryland
16	Ohio
18	North Dakota
18	Rhode Island
18	Pennsylvania
21	Washington
22	Indiana
23	Delaware
24	California
25	Michigan
26	Montana
26	Oregon
26	Arizona
29	Missouri
29	Oklahoma
31	Texas
31	Idaho
33	Illinois
33	South Dakota
35	Wyoming
36	New York
37	North Carolina
38	Georgia
38	Kentucky
40	Tennessee
40	Florida
42	Nevada
43	Alabama
43	Alaska
43	Arkansas
46	South Carolina
46	New Mexico
48	West Virginia
49	Louisiana
50	Mississippi

STATES RANKED BY HIGH SCHOOL GRADUATION

(from highest percent graduating to lowest)

Rank	State
1	Minnesota
1	North Dakota
1	Nebraska
1	Iowa
5	Montana
6	South Dakota
7	Wisconsin
8	New Jersey
8	Wyoming
10	Kansas
10	Vermont
12	Idaho
12	Massachusetts
14	Maine
14	Utah
16	Connecticut
16	Pennsylvania
18	Illinois
18	West Virginia
18	Nevada
21	Arkansas
22	New Hampshire
22	Hawaii
24	Oklahoma
24	Indiana
26	Colorado
26	Washington
28	Virginia
28	Maryland
30	Missouri
30	Arizona
30	Alaska
30	Ohio
30	Rhode Island
35	Oregon
36	Kentucky
36	Michigan
36	New Mexico
39	North Carolina
39	Delaware
41	Tennessee
41	California
43	Texas
44	Alabama
45	New York
45	Georgia
47	Mississippi
48	Florida
48	South Carolina
50	Louisiana

STATES RANKED BY MOTOR VEHICLE DEATHS

(from fewest deaths per 100,000 miles to highest)

Rank	State
1	Massachusetts
2	Connecticut
2	Rhode Island
4	New Hampshire
5	New Jersey
5	Virginia
7	California
7	Minnesota
7	North Dakota
7	Washington
7	Wisconsin
12	Hawaii
12	Michigan
12	Ohio
15	Illinois
15	Indiana
15	Kansas
15	Maryland
15	New York
15	Vermont
21	Maine
21	Oregon
21	Pennsylvania
21	Utah
25	Colorado
25	Georgia
25	Iowa
25	Oklahoma
29	Missouri
29	Nebraska
29	Texas
29	Wyoming
33	Delaware
33	Florida
35	Montana
36	Alabama
36	Arizona
36	Idaho
36	Kentucky
36	Nevada
36	South Carolina
36	South Dakota
43	Louisiana
43	Mississippi
43	North Carolina
43	Tennessee
47	West Virginia
48	Alaska
48	Arkansas
50	New Mexico

STATES RANKED BY PREVALENCE OF SMOKING

(from lowest percent of population to highest)

Rank	State
1	Utah
2	Montana
3	California
4	North Dakota
5	Idaho
6	Kansas
6	South Dakota
6	Arizona
9	Hawaii
10	Colorado
10	Minnesota
12	Vermont
13	Iowa
13	New Jersey
13	Oregon
16	Maryland
16	New Hampshire
18	Connecticut
18	Washington
18	New Mexico
21	Alabama
22	Arkansas
22	New York
24	Virginia
24	Nebraska
26	Texas
27	Delaware
28	Massachusetts
28	Florida
28	Pennsylvania
31	Georgia
31	Mississippi
33	Illinois
33	Wyoming
35	Wisconsin
36	Louisiana
36	South Carolina
38	Alaska
39	Rhode Island
40	Ohio
40	Missouri
42	Oklahoma
42	Indiana
42	West Virginia
45	Tennessee
46	Maine
47	North Carolina
48	Nevada
49	Michigan
49	Kentucky

STATES RANKED BY RISK FOR HEART DISEASE

(from lowest to highest risk)

Rank	State
1	Colorado
2	Massachusetts
3	Utah
4	New Mexico
4	New Hampshire
6	Arizona
6	Virginia
6	Washington
6	Vermont
6	Montana
11	Illinois
12	Oregon
12	California
12	Hawaii
15	Minnesota
16	Texas
16	Idaho
18	Louisiana
19	South Dakota
19	North Dakota
19	Georgia
22	Nebraska
23	Connecticut
24	Rhode Island
24	Wisconsin
24	New York
27	Maryland
27	Missouri
29	Ohio
30	Oklahoma
31	Maine
31	Delaware
31	Pennsylvania
31	Iowa
35	Florida
35	North Carolina
37	Alabama
37	Tennessee
39	Alaska
39	Arkansas
39	Kansas
39	Nevada
39	New Jersey
39	Wyoming
45	Kentucky
46	Michigan
47	South Carolina
48	Indiana
49	West Virginia
50	Mississippi

STATES RANKED BY VIOLENT CRIME

(from lowest number of offenses per 100,000 population to highest)

Rank	State
1	North Dakota
1	Vermont
1	New Hampshire
1	Maine
1	Montana
1	South Dakota
7	West Virginia
8	Hawaii
9	Wisconsin
10	Utah
10	Idaho
12	Iowa
13	Wyoming
14	Minnesota
15	Nebraska
16	Virginia
17	Mississippi
18	Kentucky
19	Pennsylvania
20	Rhode Island
21	Kansas
22	Indiana
22	Oregon
24	Washington
25	Connecticut
26	Colorado
26	Ohio
28	Oklahoma
29	Arkansas
30	Alaska
31	New Jersey
32	North Carolina
33	Arizona
34	Nevada
35	Delaware
36	Tennessee
37	Massachusetts
37	Georgia
39	Missouri
40	Michigan
41	New Mexico
42	Texas
42	Alabama
44	Louisiana
45	Maryland
46	South Carolina
47	Illinois
48	California
49	New York
50	Florida

STATES RANKED BY ACCESS TO PRIMARY CARE

(from highest percent of
population to lowest)

Rank	State
1	Connecticut
2	Hawaii
3	New Hampshire
4	Kansas
5	Minnesota
6	Delaware
6	Maryland
8	New Jersey
9	Colorado
10	Pennsylvania
11	Vermont
12	Massachusetts
13	Maine
14	Virginia
15	Florida
16	California
17	Arizona
18	Indiana
19	Ohio
20	New York
21	Nevada
22	Iowa
23	Oregon
24	Texas
25	Michigan
25	Utah
27	Oklahoma
28	Washington
29	Wisconsin
30	Missouri
31	Tennessee
32	Nebraska
33	Rhode Island
34	Kentucky
35	North Carolina
36	Illinois
37	Georgia
38	Arkansas
38	Alaska
38	Montana
41	Alabama
42	South Carolina
43	Louisiana
44	West Virginia
45	Wyoming
46	Idaho
47	New Mexico
47	South Dakota
47	Mississippi
47	North Dakota

STATES RANKED BY ADEQUACY OF PRENATAL CARE

(from highest percent of population
receiving to lowest)

Rank	State
1	New Hampshire
2	Massachusetts
2	Iowa
2	Rhode Island
5	Connecticut
6	Maryland
7	Maine
8	Kansas
9	Wisconsin
10	Michigan
10	Nebraska
10	Utah
13	Ohio
13	Delaware
15	Minnesota
15	Virginia
17	New Jersey
18	Missouri
19	Kentucky
19	Wyoming
21	Alaska
21	North Carolina
21	Pennsylvania
21	Indiana
25	Washington
25	Colorado
27	Oregon
27	Tennessee
29	South Dakota
30	Mississippi
31	Illinois
32	Idaho
32	Vermont
32	Louisiana
35	Montana
35	West Virginia
35	Florida
35	Georgia
39	Alabama
40	North Dakota
41	Nevada
42	Oklahoma
43	Arkansas
43	California
45	New York
46	Arizona
46	Texas
48	South Carolina
49	Hawaii
50	New Mexico

Source: The NWNL State Health Rankings, 1993 edition. Northwestern National Life Insurance Company, 20 Washington Avenue S., Minneapolis, MN 55401.

10. Consumer Protection: Your Legal and Medical Rights

INTRODUCTION

When we cross the threshold of a hospital, when a family member is being kept alive by artificial means, or when an injury occurs because of a physician's negligence, we are not without rights. In fact, under no circumstances does a consumer yield or give up his rights by merely seeking medical attention.

Most consumers are unaware of their medical rights. A hospital stay can often have the feeling of being held in custody, when a person reads the forms and documents presented upon admission. Even gaining access to your medical record frequently involves hassles or denials.

In this section, your legal and medical rights as a health care consumer are reviewed. You will learn how to file a complaint against a doctor or medical facility in your state. You will acquire a better understanding of the legal concept of "informed consent," without which a medical practitioner or facility cannot proceed with treatment. Even dying comes with rights, which you will find reviewed.

Knowing your medical rights is an important part of your overall health care. By being cognizant of your rights, you will be in a better position to be more active in your own health care decision-making.

Your Medical Rights: Do You Really Know Them?

We're always talking about demanding our rights—but do we really know what our rights are? Do you know for sure which legal actions are under your control and which are beyond it? Do you know what you are empowered to do when it comes to your medical care, and especially the care when you are critically ill and perhaps even too ill to make decisions?

Test your knowledge of such things and see what your R.Q.—your Rights Quotient—really is. Take this quiz and see. It could mean the difference between first-class and low-class treatment, and it could help avoid family disruptions and heartbreak.

The questions and answers are based on current law, advice from People's Medical Society's legal advisers, and in part on information from two sources sponsored by the American Civil Liberties Union:

The Rights of the Critically Ill, by John A. Robertson (New York: Bantam Books, 1983), and *The Rights of Hospital Patients,* by George J. Annas (Carbondale, Ill.: Southern Illinois University Press, 1989).

1. There is a legal right to health care in the United States. True or False?
2. A doctor can lie to a patient about the seriousness of an illness if the doctor thinks it will spare the patient anxiety and grief. True or False?
3. A patient can override objections by the family and can demand to be told the nature of his or her illness. True or False?
4. A patient has the legal right to keep his or her illness a secret from the family. True or False?
5. The family has the legal right to stop treatment of a competent, critically ill family member, even if the patient wants it continued. True or False?
6. A cancer patient has a right to have his or her doctor prescribe or administer laetrile. True or False?
7. A competent adult can refuse medical care that could keep him or her alive. True or False?
8. A patient can sue a doctor who treats him or her against his or her will, in order to keep him or her alive. True or False?
9. A patient can be thrown out of a hospital if he or she can't pay. True or False?
10. A doctor can (a) refuse to treat a patient who can't pay; (b) stop treating a patient who can't pay. True or False?
11. If, in an emergency situation, a person is brought to a hospital that does not have an emergency room the hospital has the obligation to take in and care for the person anyway. True or False?
12. A hospital can prevent a patient from leaving. True or False?
13. A doctor must refer a patient to a specialist or seek a consultation if the patient requests it. True or False?
14. A doctor can refuse to continue to see a patient without first obtaining the services of another doctor for the patient. True or False?
15. A hospital patient has the right to refuse to be examined by medical students, interns, or residents. True or False?

Check your answers against the ones below.

1. False. Neither the Constitution nor the Declaration of Independence guarantees this right. There is no legal right to demand medical care.

2. False. A doctor is obligated, under all circumstances, to tell a patient his diagnosis and prognosis. If the doctor fails to do so, he can be sued for malpractice. If the patient has specifically expressed a desire to know his diagnosis and prognosis, and the doctor does not tell him, it can be construed as a breach of contract. And, if the doctor keeps back information that ultimately obstructs crucial medical, financial, or personal decisions on the part of the patient, then the doctor could be held liable for the damages that result. There are two instances when the doctor is off the legal hook: if the patient has specifically expressed a desire not to know, and if the doctor reasonably believes that bad news could do real harm to the patient (known as "therapeutic privilege").

3. True. If the patient is competent, the family has no right to have information relevant to the person's medical condition withheld from him.

4. True. A patient can ask that his condition be kept secret, and the doctor has to go along.

5. False. If the ill person is (and this is important) competent and also has the money to pay for treatments, the family has no legal power to stop it. The doctor's duty is to the ill person, not to family members. In terminal cases, the law is fuzzier. The patient has the right to treatment that will prolong life even a few days, but this right might not extend to include continued maximum treatment if he or she is in a comatose or unconscious state.

6. False. Even in states where laetrile is legal, doctors aren't obligated to use it. Writes Robertson: "Since laetrile has not been shown to be effective, a doctor who refuses to prescribe it would not be violating his duty to provide the patient with effective medical care. If the patient objects, [he or she] is free to terminate the relationship and seek care elsewhere."

7. True. According to some rulings, rejection of lifesaving treatment is protected by the constitutional guarantee of right of privacy. There would

have to be some pretty good reason for interfering with this right.

8. True. Despite a doctor's seeming good intentions or ethical concerns, he can be sued for battery, false imprisonment, or lack of informed consent. The doctor could even end up being responsible for the cost of the care. A patient can also get a court order, if necessary, to force a doctor to stop treatment on penalty of contempt of court.

9. False. Once a person has been admitted and needs continued care, the hospital probably can't discharge him. The hospital could have the person transferred to another hospital, but only if the patient were in stable enough condition to be moved. If the patient is discharged because he can't pay, and then gets worse or incurs further damage, he could sue, claiming abandonment.

10. (a) True. (b) False. Writes Robertson: "Although not obligated to begin treatment, once this is undertaken, [the doctor] is obligated to continue as long as the patient will benefit or [until] the patient withdraws." Otherwise, abandonment can be claimed, and a civil suit could follow. However, if the doctor has made it clear at the start of treatment that ability to pay is a condition of continuing care, he can cut off treatment.

11. False. In most states there is no legal obligation to do so, and a severely injured person could, within the law, be turned away. Some states have laws requiring hospitals to have emergency rooms. In these places, and in all situations where a hospital has an emergency room, that emergency room cannot turn away a person brought to it in an emergency state.

12. False. If the person is of sound mind, he can leave at any time, and the hospital can't do a thing about it—or risk a suit for false imprisonment. And this applies even if the person hasn't paid his bill, or the bill of his child. A person may be asked to sign a "discharge against medical advice" form, but there is no legal obligation for the person to do so in order to leave the hospital.

13. True. This is not a law, but good practice. It is also a portion of the American Medical Association's Principles of Medical Ethics. And, if the doctor refuses a patient's request for a referral or consultation, and it turns out that the doctor's reassurance

of proper treatment was wrong, a negligence suit is probably the patient's next (and successful) step.

14. False. The only way a doctor-patient relationship ends is if (a) both parties agree to its end, (b) if it is ended by the patient, (c) if the doctor is no longer needed, or (d) if the doctor withdraws from the case after having given reasonable notice. Otherwise, a case for abandonment can be made by the patient.

15. True. Writes Annas: "All patients have a right to refuse to be examined by anyone in the hospital setting." In addition, fraud can be claimed if consent for an examination was given when a medical student was introduced as "doctor" to the patient, and the patient believed him to be a doctor.

A Patient's Bill of Rights

Hospitals that belong to the American Hospital Association (AHA) often post or will give you a copy of AHA's Patient's Bill of Rights when you are hospitalized. Bear in mind, though, that hospitals are not bound by the document. In fact, many hospital employees are not even aware of this document or have given it much thought if they are.

To obtain these rights may require some action to ensure that they are not honored more in the breach than in the observance. It is important to see these twelve points as a bill of rights for *consumers,* which implies activism, rather than a bill of rights for patients, which implies passivity.

A Patient's Bill of Rights

The American Hospital Association presents "A Patient's Bill of Rights" with the expectation that observance of these rights will contribute to more effective patient care and greater satisfaction for the patient, his physician, and the hospital organization. Further, the association presents these rights in the expectation that they will be supported by the hospital on behalf of its patients as an integral part of the healing process. It is recognized that a personal relationship between the physician and the patient is essential for the provision of proper medical care.

The traditional physician-patient relationship takes on a new dimension when care is rendered within an organizational structure. Legal precedent has established that the institution itself also has a responsibility to the patient. It is in recognition of these factors that these rights are affirmed.

1. The patient has the right to considerate and respectful care.

2. The patient has the right to obtain from his physician complete current information concerning his diagnosis, treatment and prognosis in terms the patient can be reasonably expected to understand. When it is not medically advisable to give such information to the patient, the information should be made available to an appropriate person in his behalf. He has the right to know, by name, the physician responsible for coordinating his care.

3. The patient has the right to receive from his physician information necessary to give informed consent prior to the start of any procedure and/or treatment. Except in emergencies, such information for informed consent should include, but not necessarily be limited to, the specific procedure and/or treatment, the medically significant risks involved, and the probable duration of incapacitation. Where medically significant alternatives for care or treatment exist, or when the patient requests information concerning medical alterna-

continued on next page

tives, the patient has the right to such information. The patient also has the right to know the name of the person responsible for the procedures and/or treatment.

4. The patient has the right to refuse treatment to the extent permitted by law and to be informed of the medical consequences of his action.

5. The patient has the right to every consideration of his privacy concerning his own medical-care program. Case discussion, consultation, examination, and treatment are confidential and should be conducted discreetly. Those not directly involved in his care must have the permission of the patient to be present.

6. The patient has the right to expect that all communications and records pertaining to his care should be treated as confidential.

7. The patient has the right to expect that within its capacity a hospital must make reasonable response to the request of a patient for services. The hospital must provide evaluation, service and/or referral as indicated by the urgency of the case. When medically permissible, a patient may be transferred to another facility only after he has received complete information and explanation concerning the needs for and alternatives to such a transfer. The institution to which the patient is to be transferred must first have accepted the patient for transfer.

8. The patient has the right to obtain information as to any relationship of his hospital to other health-care and educational institutions insofar as his care is concerned. The patient has the right to obtain information as to the existence of any professional relationship among individuals, by name, who are treating him.

9. The patient has the right to be advised if the hospital proposes to engage in or perform human experimentation affecting his care or treatment. The patient has the right to refuse to participate in such research projects.

10. The patient has the right to expect reasonable continuity of care. He has the right to know in advance what appointment times and physicians are available and where. The patient has the right to expect that the hospital will provide a mechanism whereby he is informed by his physician or a delegate of the physician of the patient's continuing health-care requirements following discharge.

11. The patient has the right to examine and receive an explanation of his bill, regardless of source of payment.

12. The patient has the right to know what hospital rules and regulations apply to his conduct as a patient.

No catalog of rights can guarantee for the patient the kind of treatment he has the right to expect. A hospital has many functions to perform, including the prevention and treatment of disease, the education of both health professionals and patients, and the conduct of clinical research. All these activities must be conducted with an overriding concern for the patient, and, above all, the recognition of his dignity as a human being. Success in achieving this recognition ensures success in the defense of the rights of the patient.

A Pregnant Patient's
Bill of Rights and Responsibilities

Rights

1. The Pregnant Patient has the right, prior to the administration of any drug or procedure, to be informed by the health professional caring for her of any potential direct or indirect effects, risks or hazards to herself or her unborn or newborn infant which may result from the use of a drug or procedure prescribed for or administered to her during pregnancy, labor, birth, or lactation.

2. The Pregnant Patient has the right, prior to the proposed therapy, to be informed, not only of the benefits, risks, and hazards of the proposed therapy but also of known alternative therapy, such as available childbirth education classes which could help to prepare the Pregnant Patient physically and mentally to cope with the discomfort or stress of pregnancy and the experience of childbirth, thereby reducing or eliminating her need for drugs and obstetric intervention. She should be offered such information early in her pregnancy in order that she may make a reasoned decision.

3. The Pregnant Patient has the right, prior to the administration of any drug, to be informed by the health professional who is prescribing or administering the drug to her that any drug which she receives during pregnancy, labor and birth, no matter how or when the drug is taken or administered, may adversely affect her unborn baby, directly or indirectly, and that there is no drug or chemical which has been proven safe for the unborn child.

4. The Pregnant Patient has the right, if cesarean section is anticipated, to be informed prior to the administration of any drug, and preferably prior to her hospitalization, that minimizing her and, in turn, her baby's intake of nonessential preoperative medicine will benefit her baby.

5. The Pregnant Patient has the right, prior to the administration of a drug or procedure, to be informed of the areas of uncertainty if there is NO properly controlled follow-up research which has established the safety of the drug or procedure with regard to its direct and/or indirect effects on the physiological, mental and neurological development of the child exposed, via the mother, to the drug or procedure during pregnancy, labor, birth, or lactation (this would apply to virtually all drugs and the vast majority of obstetric procedures).

6. The Pregnant Patient has the right, prior to the administration of any drug, to be informed of the brand name and generic name of the drug in order that she may advise the health professional of any past adverse reaction to the drug.

7. The Pregnant Patient has the right to determine for herself, without pressure from the attendant, whether she will accept the risks inherent in the proposed therapy or refuse a drug or procedure.

8. The Pregnant Patient has the right to know the name and qualifications of the individual administering a medication or procedure to her during labor or birth.

9. The Pregnant Patient has the right to be informed, prior to the administration of any pro-

continued on next page

cedure, whether that procedure is being administered to her for her or her baby's benefit (medically indicated) or as an elective procedure (for convenience, teaching purposes, or research).

10. The Pregnant Patient has the right to be accompanied during the stress of labor and birth by someone she cares for, and to whom she looks for emotional comfort and encouragement.

11. The Pregnant Patient has the right after appropriate medical consultation to choose a position for labor and for birth which is least stressful to her baby and to herself.

12. The Obstetric Patient has the right to have her baby cared for at her bedside if the baby is normal, and to feed her baby according to her baby's needs rather than according to the hospital regimen.

13. The Obstetric Patient has the right to be informed in writing of the name of the person who actually delivered her baby and the professional qualifications of that person. This information should also be on the birth certificate.

14. The Obstetric Patient has the right to be informed if there is any known or indicated aspect of her baby's care or condition which may cause her or her baby later difficulty or problems.

15. The Obstetric Patient has the right to have her and her baby's hospital medical records complete, accurate and legible and to have their records, including nursing notes, and to receive a copy upon payment of a reasonable fee and without incurring the expense of retaining an attorney.

16. The Obstetric Patient, both during and after her hospital stay, has the right to have access to her complete hospital medical records, including nursing notes, and to receive a copy upon payment of a reasonable fee and without incurring the expense of retaining an attorney.

Responsibilities

1. The Pregnant Patient is responsible for learning about the physical and psychological process of labor, birth, and postpartum recovery. The better informed expectant parents are, the better they will be able to participate in decisions concerning the planning of their care.

2. The Pregnant Patient is responsible for learning what comprises good prenatal and intranatal care and for making an effort to obtain the best care possible.

3. Expectant parents are responsible for knowing about those hospital policies and regulations which will affect their birth and postpartum experience.

4. The Pregnant Patient is responsible for arranging for a companion or support person (husband, mother, sister, friend, etc.) who will share in her plans for birth and who will accompany her during her labor and birth experience.

5. The Pregnant Patient is responsible for making her preferences known clearly to the health professional involved in her case in a courteous and cooperative manner and for making mutually agreed upon arrangements regarding maternity care alternatives with her physician or hospital in advance of labor.

6. Expectant parents are responsible for listening to their chosen physician or midwife with an open mind, just as they expect him or her to listen openly to them.

7. Once they have agreed to a course of health care, expectant parents are responsible, to the best of their ability, for seeing that the program is carried out in consultation with others with whom they have made the agreement.

8. The Pregnant Patient is responsible for obtaining information in advance regarding the approximate cost of her obstetric and hospital care.

9. The Pregnant Patient who intends to change her physician or hospital is responsible for notifying all concerned, well in advance of the birth if possible, and for informing both of her reasons for changing.

10. In all their interactions with medical and nursing personnel, the expectant parents should behave toward those caring for them with the same respect and consideration they themselves would like.

11. During the mother's hospital stay, the mother is responsible for learning about her and her baby's continuing care after discharge from the hospital.

12. After birth, the parents should put into writing constructive comments and feelings of satisfaction and/or dissatisfaction with the care (nursing, medical, and personal) they received. Good service to families in the future will be facilitated by those parents who take the time and responsibility to write letters expressing their feelings about the maternity care they received.

Source: International Childbirth Education Association, P.O. Box 20048, Minneapolis, MN 55420.

Informed Consent

Informed consent is, simply, the idea that you have the right to available information about your condition and about the benefits and risks of procedures the doctors want to perform on you. Then you can make an informed decision about what is done to your body and your life before you give the go-ahead or refusal.

Unfortunately, the definition in theory is the only simple thing about informed consent. In practice, it is a complex, controversial boiling pot.

Why? Many physicians and their trade organizations believe that informed consent is a nonworkable idea that obstructs quality care. Patients and consumer groups feel that informed consent is an important tool in establishing autonomy and creating a true doctor-patient partnership, one in which physicians are willing to explain and patients are able to understand and decide.

Some doctors believe that medicine is too complicated for unschooled nonphysicians to understand, but medical consumers think that doctors ought to try to simplify medical information to make it accessible to the general public. The consumers also point out

that, since doctors do not get paid to talk but to perform procedures, doctors may consider taking time to discuss potential risks and options a loss of time and money. And more than a few doctors believe that, if they explain things accurately, you might decide not to have the test, procedure, or operation.

Many doctors also contend that patients really don't want to know everything about their conditions and upcoming procedures. They say that the fear created in a patient by hearing all the things that could go wrong is detrimental to the patient's well-being. The facts, though, paint a different picture. A survey undertaken by the President's Commission for the Study of Ethical Problems in Medicine and Biomedical and Behavioral Research found that 96 percent of patients said they wanted to know everything. That number included 85 percent who said they would even want to hear the most "dismal facts," even if one of those facts was imminent death.

Furthermore, a goodly number of studies has shown that people who are told all the possible negatives (as well as positives) ahead of time make much better postoperative adjustments to stress and pain. Psychologist Irving Janis calls this phenomenon "emotional inoculation," in which patients can prepare themselves and even rehearse recovery scenarios.

Resentment at having anything impede professional autonomy, and possibly an uncertainty about the effectiveness and safety of the procedures they are recommending, are two more reasons why doctors don't like informed consent. And they have been successful in lobbying legislators to see their side of things. Less than half the states in this country have informed consent laws on the books to protect patients.

Let's look at informed consent as it affects you directly during a hospital stay.

THE CONSENT FORM AT THE ADMISSIONS DESK

As a new patient one of the first papers you'll receive from the admissions person is a consent form. It is not exactly an informed consent situation, because although you are doing a lot of consenting, they are not doing any informing, largely because of the type of consent form it is. This is a "blanket consent form," and by signing it you are in essence saying, "Do with me as you will. I am giving up all rights to make decisions, to say no, or to sue you if you do me harm."

If that prospect does not bother you, then sign the form. On the other hand, you should know that it is within your rights to withhold your signature on such a document. Bear in mind, though, that it is almost certain that, if you refuse to sign this consent form, you will not be admitted to the hospital. You can try, but expect a rebuff. Instead, sign the form—but only after you have added to or modified it to your liking. Write on the form that you are signing it only because you would not be admitted otherwise, and that you have no intention of giving up any of the rights the form is forcing you to give up.

If there are any items to which you take specific and strong objection, note those. If the admissions person says you can't add statements to the form, ask to see her superior or a hospital administrator, if need be. How will hospital administrators and doctors react to these changes? It will vary, and some might try to convince you that you should sign the form as originally written. Most, however, will accede to your wishes. They realize that standard consent forms frequently deny patients their rights and, fearful of lawsuits or other complaints, will grudgingly allow you to make certain changes.

Once you are admitted to the hospital, it is up to your doctor, surgeon, anesthesiologist, or whoever else will be operating or performing a procedure on you to explain what is going to be done and why. He or she must tell you what you can expect before, during, and after, and about alternative forms of treat-

Standard Release Form

A frequently asked question by consumers regarding informed consent and the forms involved is: *Is the standard release form I am forced to sign when I enter the hospital binding?*

It depends on what the release says. If it's a release against negligence on the hospital's part, it doesn't really matter if you sign it. It's unenforceable. Generally, such forms have been held to be against public policy.

Some hospitals have created another type of release form, one in which you waive your right to file a lawsuit in common court and agree to arbitration as a resolution for malpractice. Again, these releases have been held to be unenforceable because they're considered "contracts of adhesion"—the hospital has such tremendous bargaining advantage that you're placed in an unequal position.

The hospital might also ask you to sign a consent form for a specific procedure. Don't sign a blanket consent, allowing them to do anything they feel is necessary. Consent only to the procedure that you've been informed about and agree is necessary.

If you refuse to sign a blanket consent form, the surgeon may refuse to operate. He has that option in some instances. He doesn't have that option, however, if any delay in the operation might result in negative consequences—if you have a ruptured appendix, for example.

ment, even ones that are more hazardous than those recommended. And because you will undergo a number of specific procedures, you should be given a consent form for each procedure. However, most of the time you will not. Instead, the hospital expects the blanket release to "cover" everything during your hospitalization.

If you are so disposed, you can demand a consent form for each procedure proposed. Remember: A consent form should say what the hospital intends to do, what is involved, what the risks are, and what, if any, are the alternatives.

If you have not been informed to your satisfaction and/or are more than a bit unsure about giving your consent to your doctor's game plan, don't sign any form. Ask for more information. Ask about survival rates and statistical proofs of the effectiveness and safety of the procedure. (A lot of this territory should have already been covered during office visits and previous discussions.) If you are really doubtful, ask for printed materials that provide support for the route your doctor wants to take.

Make sure that the procedure described in the form is the same one that your doctor described to you. If it seems that the form grants permission for other procedures that you weren't aware of, don't sign the form until the point is clarified.

Remember, too, that these forms aren't set in stone. In fact the form is provided by the hospital. It is not the law. The form is a contract that's subject to revision, and you have the right to revise it. And you also have the right to say no to anything proposed.

CONSENT FORM FOR A SPECIFIC PROCEDURE

The consent form reproduced here is similar to ones used in most hospitals, give or take a few phrases and clauses. A form of this sort is a specific consent form—that is, it indicates that by your signature you have agreed to the performance of a specific procedure in a specific way for which you have received adequate informational background. A different form should be completed before every procedure that you believe requires a consent contract.

It might be a bit too picky to ask for risk-versus-benefit statistics and a consent form before having a urinalysis or blood test performed. But exercising your right of informed consent before undergoing a stress test, ultrasound, perhaps even some X rays, or

similar "minor" procedures is justified if you want or need such assurances.

Be sure that all the clauses are true and represent your beliefs before you sign the form. Be careful. The forms are filled with booby traps. If you need to alter, amend, or revise the form to fit your situation, then do so. For example, in the form shown, you might possibly require more space to set forth your reservations than the extremely generous and expansive two lines afforded you in number 3. Or you might not go along with number 4, which, in effect, makes a mockery of the form and the entire informed consent process. You might not want your operation to be that day's surgical show, so number 6 would be something you couldn't agree to. Some forms have patients consenting to allow film and video taping of their operations. You might not want that. Let them know they are refused permission to do so. One way of interpreting number 7 is that it leaves the door wide open for cover-ups by destroying evidence of botched surgeries. You might not agree to that. Say so, in writing.

The Importance of Your Medical Record

The medical chart is a mystery to most of us. Just the way the doctor handles it—cradling it as he/she strides into the room, scribbling in it, rustling its pages, snapping it shut at the end of the session—is enough to pique the curiosity of even the least inquisitive among us. What's in it and why are its secrets so closely guarded?

The medical chart is one of the most important aspects of good care. Aside from a history of your ailments, the chart is a repository for all the information regarding where you've been medically and where you're going. In it are housed your complaints, your questions, your doctor's notes on your visits and your health, laboratory results, X-ray reports, medications you take or have taken, descriptions of procedures, other doctors' findings, and any communications among doctors about you. A thorough, well-organized, and accurate chart is the best documentation around for where your medical dollars are going.

Unfortunately, many doctors are reluctant to share your medical record with you, claiming that you might not understand their notes or that you might be frightened away from a "needed" procedure. Hospi-

Consent to Operation or Other Special Procedure

PATIENT _____ AGE_____

DATE _____ TIME _____ a.m./p.m.

CONSENT OBTAINED AT _____ (i.e., physician's office, hospital, etc.)

1. I authorize the performance upon _____ (myself or name of patient) of the following operation or procedure _____ _____(state nature and extent of operation) to be performed at The Hospital under the direction of Dr. _____ and/or such associates and assistants as may be selected by him/her.

2. The nature and purpose of the operation, referred to in Paragraph 1 hereof and the possible alternative methods of treatment have been explained to me by Dr. _____ and to my complete satisfaction. No guarantee or assurance has been given by anyone as to the results that may be obtained.

3. I acknowledge that I have been afforded the opportunity to ask any questions with respect to the operation and any risks or complications thereto and to set forth, in the space provided below, any limitations or restrictions with respect to this consent (If none, write "none."):

   _____

   _____

4. I consent to the performance of operations, procedures, and treatment in addition to or different from those now contemplated as described above, whether or not arising from presently unforeseen conditions, which the above-named doctor or his/her associates or assistants may in his/her or their judgment consider necessary or advisable in my present illness.

5. I understand that anesthesia shall be administered during this operation under the direction of the responsible physician.

6. For the purpose of advancing medical education, I consent to the admittance of observers to the operating room.

7. I consent to the disposal by hospital authorities of any tissues or parts that may be removed.

I CERTIFY THAT I HAVE READ AND FULLY UNDERSTAND THE ABOVE CONSENT, THAT THE EXPLANATIONS THEREIN REFERRED TO WERE MADE, THAT ALL BLANKS OR STATEMENTS REQUIRING INSERTION OR COMPLETION WERE FILLED IN, AND THAT INAPPLICABLE PARAGRAPHS, IF ANY, WERE STRICKEN BEFORE I SIGNED.

Signature of Patient _____

Signature of Witness _____

(Witness to signature only)

When a patient is a minor or incompetent to give consent:

Signature of person authorized to consent for patient _____

Relationship to patient _____

The foregoing consent was signed in my presence, and in my opinion the person did so freely with full knowledge and understanding.

Signature of Physician _____

Signature of Witness _____

(Witness to signature only)

continued on next page

Also mark down items that aren't on the form that you think must be on it before you will give your consent. For example, an important condition you might wish to add is that you will not consent to the operation unless it is performed by your surgeon. You do not consent to a colleague, resident, or intern doing the operation for the first time while your surgeon acts as a teacher/observer.

Don't be rushed into signing the form. Give it a few good thinks, and certainly enough time to tailor it to your specific situation. Sometimes you can understand your medical condition and treatment options just fine; it is the consent form you can't make heads or tails of. If that is the case, request that somebody from the administrator's office or the hospital's legal department clarify the form or parts of it for you. And get that explanation down on tape, too.

Two final points: Everything mentioned in this section applies equally if you are granting consent for procedures to be performed on a child who is too young to understand or give an informed consent, or on an incompetent patient. In an emergency, when there is no time for lengthy discussion, consent is implied and assumed by doctors and the law as a given.

Informed consent is not and should not be a piece of paper, but an ongoing process, a partnership of information-sharing and trust between doctor and patient.

---

tals also hedge at releasing records even though the American Hospital Association Patient's Bill of Rights gives you the right to see information on your record. (Hospitals, however, are not required to observe the bill, so many do not.) Unfortunately, too, few consumers work up the courage to ask to read their chart or get a copy.

The irony of all this is that more people than you think see your record—and not just those who need to see it, the doctors and nurses involved in your health care, but other prying eyes as well: health and life insurance carriers, employers, company medical examiners, and others with legitimate access. Aside from the matter of privacy, another problem with this arrangement—other people know what's in your record, but you don't—is that too often the record is inaccurate—in fact, largely flawed. "At the very time information machines are improving and records are becoming more important, the information transferred is getting worse," writes John F. Burnum, M.D., in the *Annals of Internal Medicine.* Consequently, inaccuracies and problems "follow you around" for life and become the basis for denial of coverage or benefits or even outright harassment.

Protect yourself *and* your investment in your health by knowing what's in your record so that you can correct any misinformation when necessary. As a

better informed consumer you stand a much better chance of getting the most for your medical dollar.

Do you have the legal right to see your medical record? Yes and no. You see, the answer depends upon where you live and your state's law governing access to medical records. The reality is that, for the most part, you cannot see the records directly related to your health and well-being unless state laws give you the thumbs-up. What can you do?

ACCESSING YOUR MEDICAL RECORDS

State Laws
Requesting and receiving copies of your medical records from doctors, dentists, chiropractors, hospitals, or mental health facilities should be a relatively easy process, yet most consumers find it a struggle. Since laws governing access to medical records are enacted at the state level, what has emerged is a patchwork of confusing laws, court decisions, and health department regulations that makes the process anything but clear and easy.

Only twenty-four states have some form of legislation that permits you direct access to your medical records. These states are:

Alaska	Minnesota
Arkansas	Montana
California	Nevada
Colorado	New Hampshire
Connecticut	New Jersey
Florida	New York
Georgia	Oklahoma
Hawaii	South Dakota
Indiana	Virginia
Louisiana	Washington
Maryland	West Virginia
Michigan	Wisconsin

Physicians in Maine, Massachusetts, and Texas have the option of providing you with a summary of your records if they choose not to release your entire record. If you did not find your state listed here, then there are no regulations governing consumer access to copies of medical records.

Don't despair! Even if your state has no regulation covering your direct access to your medical records, there is nothing to preclude your asking a practitioner or facility for copies of your records. In fact, we encourage you to do so.

As with any administrative request, knowing the formalities and going about the request in the proper way help guarantee the best outcome. We recommend you use the following procedure.

1. Contact the practitioner or facility that has your records and ask about the general procedures for releasing records. Take notes on what is said and ask additional questions if the process seems confusing. If your state is one of those with access laws, let the contact person at the office or the facility know that you know your rights of access. Some office managers and other clerical personnel often claim that it is illegal for you to have copies of your records. When this happens, ask what specific state law prohibits access. Remember, *there is no state where it is illegal to obtain copies of your medical record.*

2. Always put your request in writing. This documents your efforts and is proof that you are working through normal channels. Include your name, address, patient identification number (if known), and the specific entry or file that you want. Indicate your willingness to pay reasonable copying fees (we consider unreasonable anything over 50 cents a page).

3. If your initial request is denied by the office manager or records administrator, ask her to put the denial in writing. Also ask her to cite the reasons you are being denied access to your records—for example, state law, health department regulation, or office policy. Then ask her to cite the statute number or specific regulation.

4. Learn about any appeals process that permits you to resubmit your request for specific parts of your record.

5. Contact the hospital patient representative if you are having problems obtaining hospital records. You may wish to consider asking a physician-ally to request copies of your records.

6. When all else fails, contact a lawyer familiar with your state's laws. You may be able to obtain a court order from a magistrate or civil court judge if you can show good cause for needing your medical records.

Federal Laws

Access to your medical records from federal hospitals—including military, Veterans Administration, and prison hospitals—is covered under the federal Privacy Act and the Freedom of Information Act. A person still in active duty must write to the hospital at his or her post or at the previous duty station. Retirees and anyone else no longer in active duty must write the National Archives Record Center, 9700 Page, St. Louis, MO 63132. Be sure to include your military identification number, branch of service, and dates of service.

Medical Information Bureau

You may never have heard of the Medical Information Bureau (MIB), but it has heard of you. In fact, it probably knows more about you and your health than you can imagine. How is this possible? you ask. If you have ever completed an insurance company application form, you know that these companies want to know a lot about your present and past medical history. And most people comply and answer the many detailed questions. The chances are excellent that the information you provided on the application found its way to the MIB.

Because insurance companies rely upon the information stored at the MIB to determine whether or not they will insure you, it is very important that your file is accurate. Unfortunately, your right to inspect your file is limited to all nonmedical information, the names of insurance companies that reported information to the MIB, and the names of insurance companies that received a copy of the information in your file within the last 6 months preceding your request.

The MIB discloses medical information to physicians. Ask your physician to assist you in obtaining the medical information contained in your file. Write to the MIB and ask for a copy of the form "Request for Disclosure of MIB Record Information": Medical Information Bureau, P.O. Box 105, Essex Station, Boston, MA 02112; 617-329-4500.

Death and Dying Issues

Death is the cessation of life processes of the body as well as an inevitable outcome of life. Over the years, though, as advances in technology have made it possible to prolong lives and maintain heartbeat and breathing functions even in the face of serious illnesses, the definition of death has come under some scrutiny.

REDEFINING DEATH

Death used to be simple. If you stopped breathing, your heart stopped, and your pupils dilated, you were dead. Not so today. No longer is the traditional heart-and-lungs concept of death applicable in every case. So, if you are concerned about the issue known as *dying with dignity,* it is important to understand how the medical and legal worlds are redefining what once was the most certain thing in life—death.

The changes in the definition of death have come about, according to the *Medico-Legal Journal,* thanks to what it calls the "revolution in intensive care technology, which now enables artificial ventilation and circulation, feeding by the intravenous route, and the elimination of waste products of metabolism by dialysis machines to be resorted to on bodies whose brains have been irreversibly destroyed." Organ transplantation also changed the accepted definition of death because, for an organ to be of the utmost benefit to the recipient, it must be removed at the earliest possible moment after circulation stops.

As a result, the definition of death has been broadened to include the irreversible loss of all brain function—brain death. In a landmark report in 1968, the Ad Hoc Committee of the Harvard Medical School to Examine the Definition of Brain Death laid down four characteristics of a permanently nonfunctioning brain:

1. Unreceptivity and unresponsivity (total unawareness to externally applied stimuli)
2. No movement or breathing (1 hour's observation of spontaneous muscular movements, breathing, or response to stimuli). If the person is on a respirator, absence of breathing must be established by 3 minutes off the machine.
3. No reflexes present (fixed and dilated pupils, no eye movement or blinking, no contraction of muscles due to stimulation)
4. Flat electroencephalogram (EEG) after 10 minutes of recording

These tests, the report said, are to be done twice, 24 hours apart.

Either through laws or court decisions, most states recognize the concept of brain death, but have left the final determination to the doctor. The wording of most of the statutes conforms to what's called the Uniform Determination of Death Act: "An individual who has sustained either (1) irreversible cessation of circulatory and respiratory functions, or (2) irreversible cessation of all functions of the entire brain, including the brain stem, is dead. A determination must be made in accordance with accepted medical standards."

What about the states where there is no legislation? Generally, decisions on what constitutes death in those states are left up to physicians' own definitions. *Your state bar association can tell you what applies where you reside.*

Unfortunately, even a legal definition of brain death does not completely eliminate the uncertainty surrounding this issue. Be aware that the criteria for determining brain death may vary slightly from hospital to hospital. So you may want to call your community hospitals—first try the office of the chief of the medical staff, then go on to the hospital administrators, if necessary—to find out what "standards" they use to determine brain death. (Remember, the criteria should always include total lack of movement, inability to breathe without a respirator, total unresponsiveness to stimuli, and total absence of reflexes.)

But even with recognized and legislated definitions of brain death and established criteria for determining it, there's uncertainty among some bioethicists, philosophers, and physicians who question whether brain death refers to the entire brain, including the brain stem, or just cerebral death, which is partial death of the brain. An article in the magazine *Omni* some years back referred to a burgeoning movement to modify the concept of brain death to include people in what's called a persistent vegetative state (PVS), a number estimated to be around 10,000 in this country.

In PVS, only part of the brain is destroyed; the main stem is intact, so the person is capable of reflex functions such as breathing and sleeping, but incapable of thought or even awareness of his or her environment. PVS, often called cognitive death, can last for years, with absolutely no hope for improvement.

But the cognitive death idea has many opponents, in both the medical and the lay worlds: those who ask, "Where will it all end—experiments on these people?" and those who simply believe the long-term unconscious may someday "wake up." So the debate is liable to go on for years or even decades to come.

These are matters, too, you may want to discuss with your physician, and perhaps a lawyer knowledgeable in right-to-die issues, so that any advance directives you write encompass all the points about which you believe strongly. Any of the organizations concerned with death (which are listed later in this section) should be able to help you as well.

ADVANCE DIRECTIVES: THE PATIENT'S RIGHT TO DECIDE

All adult individuals in hospitals, nursing homes, and other health care settings have certain rights. For example, you have a right to confidentiality of your personal and medical records and to know what treatment you will receive.

You also have another right. You have the right to fill out a paper known as an advance directive. The paper says in advance what kind of treatment you want or do not want under special, serious medical conditions—conditions that would prevent you from telling your doctor how you want to be treated. For example, if you were taken to a hospital in a coma, would you want the hospital's medical staff to know your specific wishes about decisions affecting your treatment?

A relatively new federal law (see box) requires most hospitals, nursing facilities, hospices, home health care programs, and health maintenance organizations to give you information about advance directives and your legal choices in making decisions about medical care. Remember, in general an advance directive allows you to state your choices for health care or to name someone to make those choices for you, if you become unable to make decisions about your medical treatment. In short, an advance directive

The Patient Self-Determination Act

The Patient Self-Determination Act, a federal law that went into effect December 1991, requires workers at all federally funded institutions—hospitals, health maintenance organizations, hospices, skilled nursing facilities, or facilities accepting Medicare or Medicaid customers—to inform patients of their right to establish an advance directive. Advance directives are written documents that, in the case of a serious illness, either clarify an individual's wishes for health care or name a person to make health care decisions for that individual if he or she becomes unable to do so.

No state agency presides over advance directives. So in most instances the federally funded health care institution will be able to fully explain your state's provision for advance directives. There is one notable exception, according to the organization Choice in Dying: Institutions with their own ethical or moral code may impose their own restrictions on your treatment. Usually these institutions will inform you of their policies when you are admitted.

can enable you to make decisions about your future medical treatment. You can say yes to treatment you want, or say no to treatment you don't want.

Living Will

A living will is a document that lists an individual's preferences concerning life support, other life-sustaining procedures or "heroic" measures, and instructions about therapies one wishes to have or not have.

It is generally agreed that the individual has the right to decide whether he or she wants to be subjected to futile measures that may prolong an otherwise inevitable outcome. The individual can decide whether or not to be put on a respirator or dialysis machine, be resuscitated, or be nourished intravenously. Specifically, a person can refuse to receive CPR (cardiopulmonary resuscitation) by placing a DNR (Do Not Resuscitate) order in his or her advance directive.

A living will, which can be revoked at any time, can be drafted by the individual or can be obtained from state agencies or Choice in Dying. If you decide to write or sign a living will, it is a good idea that your lawyer, physician, and family are notified of and understand your wishes. It is beneficial to check the living will legislation of your particular state, because laws and stipulations vary from state to state (all states have living will legislation except Massachusetts, Michigan, and New York).

Durable Power of Attorney for Health Care

A durable power of attorney is a document that names a legal agent or proxy (DPA) who will carry out your desired method of treatment or who will make those decisions for you at the time of death or when you become incompetent. Even though your desired methods of treatment can be spelled out in a durable power of attorney, it is a good idea to have both a living will and a durable power of attorney. The document must be signed, dated, and witnessed and can be canceled (in writing) at any time.

The most critical issue is deciding who is the appropriate decision-maker. Most experts recommend that you consider these factors: Who would you trust with life-and-death decisions? Who knows you best—your attitudes and values? Who would respect your wishes? Most people appoint spouses or close family members—good choices because they know you well—but if they are beneficiaries of your estate there may be a conflict of interest.

The best strategy, some say, is to have both a living will and a durable power of attorney. A living will is only about the final moments of life. Considered more flexible than a living will, a durable power of attorney can be drafted to include the authority to make decisions about several areas of medical treatment, not just the termination of life support—on behalf of people not capable of making their own decisions, such as after a serious accident, a permanent loss of consciousness, or an incapacitating illness.

As with any advance directive, you should keep the directive in a safe place and the family, physician, designated proxy, and lawyer should be notified of your instructions and directions and should hold a copy of the document. Again, because states differ in advance directive legislation in terms of definition and limitations, it is worthwhile to know your state's policy concerning advance directives (all states and the District of Columbia have DPA legislation). You may also now obtain information on advance directives from certain federally funded health care facilities and other organizations because of the passage in 1991 of the Patient Self-Determination Act.

For further information concerning advance directives, the specific laws of your state, legal advice concerning death, or the registration of living wills, you can contact Choice in Dying, 200 Varick Street, Suite 1001, New York, NY 10014; 212-366-5540.

HOSPICE CARE

Hospices were developed solely to assist dying patients—typically cancer patients who have exhausted the various forms of curative treatment—and to help them live their remaining weeks or months as free of symptoms and as much in control as possible. Deliberately created as alternatives to traditional long-term institutions, hospices provide palliative care (care intended to comfort and to ease pain) to patients and their families, and also provide bereavement counseling for the families following the patient's death. In short, a hospice is an alternative facility to hospital and nursing home care that can offer to the patient personalized care, attention, emotional support, and relief from pain.

For people who do not wish to receive further aggressive treatment for a terminal illness, or for whom only palliative care can be provided, a hospice offers an opportunity for the patient and family to help each other during the dying process.

DNR Orders

In hospitals and nursing homes across the country, DNR stands for the order "Do Not Resuscitate." It means that, should respiration or heartbeat fail, cardiopulmonary resuscitative measures (CPR) will not be started or carried out. A DNR order means that the patient will not be given brief emergency CPR, nor will the patient be placed on long-term mechanical life-support equipment. Knowing about DNR orders—when, how, and by whom they're issued, and how they work—is an important step in gaining more control over the circumstances of your death.

Historically, in the absence of laws and guidelines, such decisions as when to turn to technology and when to let nature take over have been left to the medical team. For years, only medical and nursing personnel knew whether a person was designated DNR, because doctors believed that it was "inappropriate" to discuss the matter with the patient. An outcome of this secrecy was that there was tacit agreement among the hospital staff to engage in "slow codes" (have the resuscitation team purposely move slowly) or "show codes" (have the team feign a resuscitation effort, for the family's sake). However the DNR status was indicated—a purple dot on the patient's chart, as one New York hospital did, or any other esoteric symbol—doctors, nurses, technicians, and all the other members of the health care team knew what to do and not to do.

An important nationwide survey of DNR orders in intensive care units, reported in the *Journal of the American Medical Association* some years back, found that 75 percent of the time the ICU or attending physicians initiated the DNR orders, and only 8 percent of the time the family did so. In this thirteen-hospital study of more than 7,000 admissions, only 1 patient gave the word, and only 1 patient had a living will that stipulated no resuscitation.

For the most part, this scenario is changing, and for a variety of reasons, not the least of which is the movement toward greater patient autonomy—and doctors' fear of lawsuits by patients or their families. The bottom line here is that it's important that you find out what your hospital's specific DNR policy is.

A few questions then arise: Should you routinely upon admission to the hospital discuss your wishes for resuscitation? At what point in the course of your illness/hospitalization can the decision about resuscitation best be made? What can you do if your decision about resuscitation changes over time? Clearly, timing is essential. According to a study reported in the *Journal of the American Medical Association*, DNR orders are written at a time when most patients are not capable of participating in the decision, although the majority of the people in the survey were considered competent when they were admitted. On the other hand, if a person is critically ill when admitted to the hospital, there's not always enough time to discuss resuscitation.

What can you do to avoid such a devil-and-the-deep-blue-sea predicament?

• Talk to your physician about the appropriateness of a Do Not Resuscitate order—before it's needed, and even before admission to the hospital, if possible. Ask specifically about your illness and the probable consequences of refusing resuscitation. Force the issue, if you must, to ensure that your physician knows what aggressive and expensive medical care would be undesirable to you.

- Discuss the matter with your family so that they'll know your wishes and be able to act confidently in your behalf if necessary.
- Document your wishes concerning emergency resuscitation, and have your physician make this a part of your medical record.
- Remember, too, a DNR order is not an irrevocable decision. If the outcome of another day in the hospital or another hospital stay causes you to have second

thoughts, just speak up—and document your decision, of course. Any major improvement in your condition also would nullify the DNR order.

The important thing is to avoid the potential complications that can arise—conflicts between family members, conflicts between your family and the hospital and doctors, and the need for determination by outside parties such as the hospital ethics committee or legal counsel. We echo the finding of the President's Commission for the Study of Ethical Problems in Medicine: "Decision-making about life-sustaining care is rarely improved by resort to courts."

Model for DNR Orders

Here are some of the still-relevant guidelines issued by the 1983 President's Commission for the Study of Ethical Problems in Medicine. Use these recommendations to determine how your hospital's policy stacks up:

"A competent and informed patient or an incompetent patient's surrogate is entitled to decide with the attending physician that an order against resuscitation should be written in the chart. When cardiac arrest is likely, a patient (or a surrogate) should usually be informed and offered the chance specifically to decide for or against resuscitation.

"Physicians have a duty to assess for each hospitalized patient whether resuscitation is likely, on balance, to benefit the patient, to fail to benefit, or to have uncertain effect.

"When a patient will not benefit . . . a decision not to resuscitate, with the consent of the patient or surrogate, is justified.

"When a physician's assessment conflicts with a competent patient's decision, further discussion and consultation are appropriate; ultimately, the physician must follow the patient's decision or transfer responsibility for that patient to another physician.

"When a physician's assessment conflicts with that of an incompetent patient's surrogate, further discussion, consultation, review by an institutional committee and, if necessary, judicial review should be sought.

"[DNR policies] should require that orders not to resuscitate be in written form and . . . delineate who has the authority both to write such orders and to stop a resuscitation effort in progress."

Most states have their own living will forms, each somewhat different. It may be possible, however, to complete and sign a standard living will form available in your own community, draw up your own form, or simply write a statement of your preferences for treatment. Below is a sample living will declaration. This is just a sample and not to be taken as necessarily the correct or legally binding form for your needs. Be sure to check the requirement of the statute in your state.

Sample Living Will Declaration

Declaration made this _____ day of _____, 19_____, I, _____, being of sound mind, willfully and voluntarily make known my desire that my dying shall not be artificially prolonged under the circumstances set forth below, and do declare:

If at any time I should have an incurable injury, disease or illness certified to be a terminal condition by two physicians who have personally examined me, one of whom shall be my attending physician, and the physicians have determined that my death will occur whether or not life-sustaining procedures are utilized and where the application of life-sustaining procedures would serve only to artificially prolong the dying process, I direct that such procedures be withheld or withdrawn, and that I be permitted to die naturally with only the administration of medication or the performance of any medical procedure deemed necessary to provide me with comfort care.

In the absence of my ability to give directions regarding the use of such life-sustaining procedures, it is my intention that this declaration shall be honored by my family and physician(s) as the final expression of my legal right to refuse medical or surgical treatment and accept the consequences from such refusal.

I understand the full import of this declaration and I am emotionally and mentally competent to make this declaration.

Signed _____

Address _____

The declarant has been personally known to me and I believe him/her to be of sound mind.

Witness _____

Witness _____

Source: **President's Commission for the Study of Ethical Problems in Medicine and Behavioral Research, "Deciding to Forego Life-Sustaining Treatment" (Washington, D.C.: U.S. Government Printing Office), pp. 314–15.**

Next to the feeling of abandonment, the fear of excessive pain is a primary concern of a dying person. At a hospice, whose treatment goals include pain control through use of drug therapy or other treatments (biofeedback, relaxation therapy) and relief from other unpleasant symptoms, a dying patient can be assured that he or she will be taken care of and, most of all, will be made as comfortable as possible.

Hospice care can be performed in a hospice facility (a freestanding facility or one associated with a hospital or nursing home) or can be done at home, where a primary caregiver (usually a family member) works with the hospice team to tend to the patient. Unlike hospital care, the active contributions and support of family members are welcomed and, in fact, are an integral part of the hospice care system. A hospice team, consisting of the primary caregiver, a physician, a nurse, social workers, counselors and therapists, clergy members, and volunteers, gives the dying patient palliative care and provides emotional support and assistance to the family.

AUTOPSIES

When an individual dies, it is an event that is full of difficult emotions, responsibilities, and concerns with which the surviving spouse and family must cope. Besides securing a death certificate, making funeral arrangements, or settling the terms of a will, the family can decide whether or not to have an autopsy performed on the deceased.

An autopsy, an external and internal examination of the body, is performed by a pathologist, medical examiner, or coroner and reveals the cause of death. Internal organs are examined and weighed and tissue samples are collected for further laboratory study. Contrary to popular belief, an autopsy does not disfigure or distort the body of the deceased in any way. Because autopsies are relatively costly procedures, however, they are not usually recommended for every death.

An autopsy is usually performed when the cause of death is unknown, when the identity of the body is unknown, when the deceased was a victim of a homi-cide or a suicide, when there is a certain amount of unanswered questions concerning the death, and when there are organs to be donated for transplants. An autopsy can also be done if a genetic disorder was suspected in the deceased so that the family can be notified of the risk of the disorder. Finally, autopsies offer medical personnel a chance for research (if AIDS or other diseases undergoing current research are involved) and an opportunity to discover the efficacy and quality of medical care and treatment.

RESOURCES FOR DEATH AND DYING ISSUES

Elisabeth Kubler-Ross Center
South Route 616
Head Waters, VA 24442
703-396-3441

National Hemlock Society
P.O. Box 11830
Eugene, OR 97440
503-342-5748

National Hospice Organization
1901 N. Moore Street. Suite 901
Arlington, VA 22209
703-243-5900

Choice in Dying, Inc.
200 Varick Street, Suite 1001
New York, NY 10014
212-366-5540

The Controversial Issue of Nourishment

Perhaps more than any other life-sustaining treatment, questions on the subject of withholding or withdrawing artificial feeding have moved into the forefront of right-to-die issues. Perhaps, too, because of the symbolic significance of nourishment in the minds of many people, sustenance (food and water) appears to be more difficult to discontinue than any other treatment—whether in a person who is expected to die in a relatively short time, or a comatose person whose death may not occur for months or years.

Amidst all the controversy surrounding the issue, however, many authorities see an emerging legal trend. Courts in at least fifteen states have ruled that patients have the same right to refuse feeding tubes as to refuse any other medical treatment—a growing consensus that counts among its supporters the American Medical Association. In 1986 the American Medical Association's Council on Ethical and Judicial Affairs issued a major opinion stating that it is ethically permissible for doctors to withhold all life-prolonging treatment, including artificial nutrition and hydration, from permanently unconscious or dying patients. And in a precedent-setting ruling in 1987, the New Jersey Supreme Court affirmed a lower court decision (the Jobes case) that had been the first ruling to support removal of life-extending, artificial feeding and hydration from a patient not diagnosed as terminally ill.

Generally, competent patients have the right to refuse this treatment—and the right is not limited to comatose or terminally ill patients. For incompetent patients, artificial feeding, as with other treatments, can be stopped in accordance with the patient's previously expressed wishes.

In examining your options regarding this emotionally charged issue and your right to refuse treatments, here are some pointers:

- Document your wishes about artificial feeding (as well as other life-sustaining treatments), and be as specific as you can.

- Know your state's living will law (if it has one)—in this case, what it says and doesn't say about artificial feeding. Even in states with such laws on the books, not all of those laws specifically mention artificial feeding, and the language in some of the laws actually restricts.

- Know the common feeding and hydration treatments available should you not be able to eat in the usual way, and discuss these with your physician. What are the goals of these feedings—to prolong life, deliver calories, or provide comfort? The difficulty comes in determining whether the burdens of feeding are worth the benefits—especially since these treatments are invasive, can be painful, and sometimes are harmful to both unconscious and conscious patients.

Before it merged with another like-minded group and became Concern for Dying, the Society for the Right to Die detailed the following potential complications and side effects of the common feeding and hydration treatments. (See the glossary of life-support procedures for actual descriptions of each.) While these complications do not necessarily occur in a majority of the cases, you need to know them so that your discussions with your doctor can be productive.

Nasogastric tube: This intervention causes discomfort for the average person who also runs the risk of food aspiration, pneumonia, vomiting, injuries to tissue, and bleeding into the stomach. (Others have documented additional risk of sinus and lung infections.)

Intravenous feeding: The risks include phlebitis, hematoma, infection, blood clots, and embolism.

Gastrostomy tube: The risks are those usually associated with the use of anesthesia, as well as infection and peritonitis.

Parenteral hyperalimentation: The risks include perforation of the lung causing collapse, blood poisoning, and massive bleeding.

Be certain that you know your physician's feelings on withholding/withdrawing artificial feeding. You even may want to familiarize yourself with area hospitals' and nursing homes' policies. According to a 1988 report in the journal *Medical Staff Counselor,* no matter how unfounded the fears may be, some health care providers are still worried about the legal liability for honoring patient preferences—even when these preferences are completely documented in the medical record. Furthermore, there's always the chance that your doctor will prove unwilling, for reasons of conscience, to participate in the rejection of artificial feeding. It's far better to know these things in advance than to haggle over the issue from a hospital bed or subject your family to the conflicts that may arise.

Glossary of Life-Support Procedures

To help you make treatment decisions or to decide which specific instructions to add to your advance directive, a glossary of relevant terms is important. It should help you learn the meaning and the treatment implications of the most commonly used of today's life-support measures. Be aware, however, that slightly different terms might be used at some facilities. Your personal physician should be able to answer any questions about the precise life-support terminology used in your community hospitals.

CPR/cardiopulmonary resuscitation—an attempt to restore heartbeat (cardio) and breathing (pulmonary) in someone whose heart has stopped—i.e., suffered a cardiac arrest. This involves mouth-to-mouth breathing and closed chest compression of the heart. In a hospital setting it may also include intravenous medications, electrical shock to stimulate the heart, and intubation (an endotracheal tube is inserted into the trachea [windpipe] via the mouth to provide an airway) and ventilatory support (use of a respirator).

Code/No Code—"Code" means to institute CPR and call the cardiac-arrest team to make every effort to resuscitate someone whose heart has stopped. "No Code" means that no attempts will be made to resuscitate.

IV/intravenous—solutions that are given to patients through their veins. A needle or catheter is inserted into the vein and the solution administered through clear plastic tubing connected to the needle. An IV has many uses: to provide a route through which medications can be administered and to provide a source of hydration for a patient.

Respirator/Ventilator—a machine that assists a patient to breathe by providing artificial respiration. A respirator may be necessary after a patient has suffered a cardiac arrest and has been resuscitated.

Gastrostomy tube (G.T.), Jejunostomy tube (J.T.)—a gastrostomy is an operation to create an opening through the skin into the stomach. A jejunostomy is similar, but the opening is into a part of the small intestine called the jejunum. A G.T. or J.T. is a rubber tube or catheter inserted into the stomach or jejunum and sutured in place. The tube enables patients to be given blenderized or pureed food or special caloric supplements.

N.G. tube/nasogastric tube—a pliable plastic or rubber tube inserted through the nose into the stomach. N.G. tubes have many uses. After certain surgical procedures, a patient may have an N.G. tube connected to suctioning equipment to keep the stomach empty of secretions. An N.G. tube can be used to feed a patient who is unable to swallow and for whom T.P.N. (see below) would not be medically appropriate. An N.G. tube also can be used to decompress the stomach and reduce pain and discomfort in a patient who has a bowel obstruction.

T.P.N./total parenteral nutrition—special intravenous solutions which contain vitamins, minerals, and calories to provide nourishment for a patient. T.P.N. is used when the patient is unable to eat any food or sufficient food to maintain a good nutritional state.

Tracheostomy—opening into the trachea (windpipe) through the neck so that a tube can be inserted to provide a passageway for air. A tracheostomy may be necessary if a patient will require mechanical ventilatory support for a protracted period of time. A tracheostomy also provides a passageway for suctioning if the lungs have copious secretions which the patient is unable to bring up because of a weak cough or an inability to cough.

Reprinted by permission of Choice in Dying, 200 Varick Street, New York, NY 10014; 800-989-WILL.

Medical Malpractice

The Mosby Medical Encyclopedia (New York: Plume, 1992) describes malpractice as

> a professional mistake that is a direct cause of injury or harm to a patient. It may result from a lack of professional knowledge, experience, or skill that can be expected in others in the profession. It may also result from a failure to use reasonable care or judgment in applying professional knowledge, experience, or skill.

This is a fairly straightforward definition for a very complex, very controversial issue that is getting more so all the time.

Four standards of care, according to the *Columbia University College of Physicians and Surgeons Complete Home Medical Guide* (New York: Crown, 1989), constitute a doctor's legal obligations toward his or her patients; any one of these obligations, if violated, can be grounds for a lawsuit.

1. The doctor must obtain the patient's informed consent before treatment. This means that a patient must understand the risks involved in a procedure before consenting to it; it does *not* mean that a doctor must detail every remote possibility, nor that he must get a signed consent form every time he treats a patient. A signed consent form, however, is required by law before surgery or an invasive diagnostic test is done. If informed consent is not obtained properly—if, for example, a patient is asked to agree to "any or all" procedures, or the consent is obtained when the patient is sedated just prior to surgery—the doctor is technically open to a charge of assault and battery,

2. In treating a patient, the doctor must use reasonable skill and care in accordance with accepted medical practice, and within the limits of his competence. The key words here are "reasonable" and "accepted." Both are extremely difficult to define, and it has proven to be extremely difficult to establish in court that this standard has been violated, except in cases of extreme negligence.

3. A doctor must adequately supervise those aspects of a patient's care that he or she delegates to others. Doctors customarily delegate to nurses and other health-care personnel; this is acceptable legally as long as the doctor assumes responsibility for those who are helping. (Under certain circumstances, hospital nurses and aides, although not in the doctor's employ, are considered to be under the doctor's supervision.

4. A patient, once accepted by a doctor, cannot be abandoned by the doctor. A doctor is not under any obligation to accept a patient, but once treatment has begun, he or she must continue to care for that patient until treatment is no longer needed, or until the patient voluntarily leaves the doctor, or until the doctor has properly notified the patient that he or she is no longer responsible for the patient's care.

BACKGROUND

Of the forces reshaping contemporary medicine, certainly none is more powerful than the current malpractice crisis. From state legislatures to the halls of Congress, issues surrounding escalating malpractice premiums and an allegedly lawsuit-conscious public are hotly debated.

While the debate rages on into the 1990s, its origins are in the 1970s and 1980s, when the first of several so-called malpractice crises occurred. They were brought on when liability insurance companies raised the cost of insurance and doctors felt the impact of steep premium increases. Insurance companies justified the premium increases on the grounds that they were incurring exorbitant costs to prepare and defend doctors and also to pay out millions of dollars in jury awards. Doctors, feeling themselves under pressure to act, joined with insurance companies to lobby state lawmakers to change their tort laws (a tort is a wrongful act) to make it more difficult for injured patients to bring malpractice suits.

TORT REFORM LEGISLATION

Major components of tort reform legislation generally include: limits on awards for noneconomic damages (pain and suffering); limits on attorney's fees (for example, limiting an attorney's fee to 33 percent of the first $100,000 and 20 percent on any amount above that); reducing the statute of limitations to two years (the time period in which legal action must be taken); periodic payment of awards (stretching payments over a period of years as opposed to a lump-sum payment); inclusion of a collateral source rule (reducing a monetary award by the amount of any other payment a plaintiff may receive from a source other than the defendant); and the imposition of penalties for groundless lawsuits.

Supporters of tort reform legislation claim that these changes would put an end to the malpractice crisis and enable doctors to once again practice medicine free from the threat of unwarranted legal action. To gain the support of doctors, insurance companies also held out the promise of lower insurance premiums, thereby reducing a doctor's cost of doing business. Tort reform legislation was enacted in several states; however, this action did not necessarily result in lower malpractice premiums as promised. To put this issue in proper perspective, it's necessary to examine the factors and sides in the malpractice debate.

THE DOCTOR'S VIEW

It is generally agreed that doctors tend to view every patient as a potential lawsuit. As a result of this perception, doctor alter their normal practice patterns and engage in what is called *defensive medicine*. Defensive medicine is the ordering of a battery of diagnostic tests and procedures just to guard against missing something that could lead to a lawsuit.

Aside from the added cost to our already burgeoning medical expenses—estimated to reach $1 trillion sometime in 1995—defensive medicine also exposes patients to additional dangers. In the midst of over- and unnecessary testing, some abnormality, however insignificant, is bound to surface and be seen, or misidentified as indicative of some disease or illness. And, of course, this can lead to unnecessary treatment of a nonexistent condition, not to mention the risks associated with invasive and other procedures.

Doctors believe the only way to prevent what they consider inappropriate lawsuits is to limit the patient's ability to collect damages for pain and suffering (also called noneconomic damages) and enact other laws aimed at discouraging litigation. The assumption here, on the part of some doctors, is that patients file lawsuits against doctors hoping to "strike it rich," much like a lottery. Some states, such as California, Colorado, Kansas and Utah, limit the award

for pain and suffering to a maximum of $250,000. Further, as a result of tort reform, plaintiffs and attorneys are subject to penalties if they bring a lawsuit with little merit to the courts in Mississippi and South Carolina. This can have a chilling effect on the ability of a injured patient to find an attorney to handle his/her case. While such an approach to malpractice reform has been applauded in medical circles, it has generally been viewed with dismay among consumer groups.

THE CONSUMER'S VIEW

Medical malpractice from the consumer viewpoint, not surprisingly, is quite different. Rather than harboring get-rich-quick motives, as doctors sometime may believe, consumers see unconcerned, uncaring, and unqualified doctors as the primary reasons for malpractice. A look at the myths promulgated by the medical profession and the contradicting evidence will show just how dichotomous the positions—doctor and consumer—can be in the debate over medical malpractice.

Myth number one alleges that consumers are ready to sue a doctor or hospital at the drop of a hat. In fact, according to a Harvard University study of hospital discharge records in New York State, just the opposite is true. A review of more than 30,000 medical records revealed that about 4 percent of all hospitalized patients experience some form of adverse occurrence. Yet fewer than 50 of the patients whose records were reviewed filed a malpractice claim. When the researchers applied these figures to statewide hospitalizations they determined that some 5,000 patients received serious and disabling injuries as a result of hospitalization. However, a review of malpractice claims revealed only slightly more than 3,500 patients had filed suit.

Another study, conducted by the Pennsylvania State University College of Medicine, reported that only one patient in 65 injured by a health care worker ever filed a lawsuit.

The second myth, that malpractice victims always win their day in court, was dispelled when a study, published in the *Annals of Internal Medicine,* found that doctors win 76 percent of the time—which means that plaintiffs prevail in only 24 percent of the cases. This study also revealed that the overwhelming majority of these court cases are truly warranted:

continued on page 576

Malpractice—What Is Most Likely to Happen and Where Is Malpractice Most Likely to Occur?

Diagnostic Issues Cited Most Frequently Among Claims Reported by Insured Doctors

The following discussion and accompanying tables are taken from the St. Paul Fire & Marine Insurance Company's 1993 "Physicians and Surgeons Update," an annual report to its policyholders. Located in St. Paul, Minnesota, St. Paul Fire & Marine is the largest private malpractice insurer in the United States, with more than 30,000 physician policyholders.

The major categories of claims reported for physicians and surgeons insured by St. Paul during 1991 and 1992 showed little change from the kinds of claims reported in previous years. Claims involving failure to diagnose, improper treatment and surgery accounted for nearly 81 percent of all claims reported. The number of claims reported also remains very close to those reported in the previous year's report "Physicians and Surgeons Update."

The surgery category accounted for nearly 27 percent of all claims, as opposed to 26 percent last year. Most allegations in the surgery category were in the area of postoperative complications, with 990 claims. Some of the most frequently reported postoperative complications were cardiopulmonary arrest, strokes, nerve injuries during back surgery, hypotensive episodes, blindness and other sensory deficits, and poor results—patients not satisfied with the outcome of surgery.

Costly Categories

The costliest category was Improper Treatment—Birth-Related, with an average cost per claim of $171,526. Within that category several claims were made in the areas of fail-

ure to monitor high-risk patients, injuries due to the use of forceps, use of tocolytic terbutaline and oxytocins [drugs used to suppress premature labor], delays in cesarean sections, shoulder dystocia and delays in the treatment and diagnosing of diseases and conditions of the newborn (such as hypoglycemia and monitoring intravenous fluids).

Six of the top 10 most costly claims were in the Failure to Diagnose category, continuing the trend of recent years. The costliest allegation in this category was Failure to Diagnose Myocardial Infarction, with an average cost per claim of $134,799.

The second most costly was Failure to Diagnose Pregnancy Problems. There were several failure-to-diagnose ectopic pregnancies. Other allegations included failure to diagnose the following: uterine rupture; genetic conditions; and preeclampsia. Cesarean-section timing and placenta previa were also included. The average cost per claim was $130,788.

Failure to Diagnose Circulatory Problems was another costly claim category, with claims being made for failure to diagnose compartment syndrome, pulmonary embolism, aneurysms, amputation (as a result of circulatory problems), stroke/brain/head injury, and testicular torsion.

Location

There was a nearly 5 percent jump from last year in claims being made for incidents taking place in a physician's office or clinic.

continued on next page

Major Allegation Groups by Frequency

Group	Number	Percent of Total Claims	Percent of Total Incurred Cost
Failure to Diagnose	2,097	28.2	38.5
Improper Treatment	1,930	26.0	28.0
Surgery	1,972	26.6	23.3
Anesthesia	258	3.5	2.9
Other	1,164	15.7	7.3
Total	**7,421**	**100.0**	**100.0**

Failure to Diagnose

Top Five Allegations	Number of Claims
Failure to Diagnose Cancer	545
Failure to Diagnose Fracture/Dislocation	201
Failure to Diagnose Abdominal Problems	185
Failure to Diagnose Myocardial Infarction	176
Failure to Diagnose Infection	164

Improper Treatment

Top Five Allegations	Number of Claims
Improper Treatment—Birth-Related	404
Improper Treatment—Drug Side Effect	200
Improper Treatment—Infection	198
Improper Treatment—Fracture/Dislocation	150
Improper Treatment—Drug Incorrect	117

Surgery

Top Five Allegations	Number of Claims
Surgery—Postoperative Complications	990
Surgery—Inadvertent Act	345
Surgery—Inappropriate Procedure	179
Surgery—Postoperative Death	113
Surgery—Delay/Complications	95

Top 10 Allegations by Cost

Allegation	Number of Claims	Average Cost
Improper Treatment— Birth-Related	404	171,526
Failure to Diagnose— Myocardial Infarction	176	134,799
Failure to Diagnose— Pregnancy Problems	104	130,788
Failure to Diagnose— Circulatory Problems	146	130,220
Failure to Diagnose— Hemorrhage	54	118,679
Failure to Diagnose— Infection	164	108,712
Failure to Diagnose— Cancer	545	108,670
Surgery—Postoperative Death	113	86,290
Surgery— Delay/Complications	95	84,577
Improper Treatment— Drug Overdose	63	80,637

Top 10 Allegations by Frequency

Allegation	Number of Claims	Average Cost
Surgery—Postoperative Complications	990	66,451
Failure to Diagnose— Cancer	545	108,670
Improper Treatment— Birth-Related	404	171,526
Surgery— Inadvertent Act	345	74,065
Failure to Diagnose— Fracture/Dislocation	201	69,400
Improper Treatment— Drug Side Effect	200	66,987
Improper Treatment— Infection	198	60,105
Failure to Diagnose— Abdominal Problems/ Other	185	78,110
Failure to Diagnose— Myocardial Infarction	176	134,799

All Allegations by Location

Location & Allegation	Number of Claims	Percent of Total
Physician's Office/Clinic	3,033	40.9
Hospital		
Surgery	1,821	24.5
Patient Care Area	715	9.7
Emergency Room	677	9.1
Labor/Delivery/Nursery	462	6.2
Other	407	5.5
Outpatient Surgery	245	3.3
Surgicenter	15	0.2
Other	46	0.6
Total Hospital	**4,327**	**58.3**
Total Nonhospital	**3,094**	**41.7**
Total All Claims	**7,421**	**100.0**

Most of the cases were tried after the doctor's own insurance company had reviewed the facts and determined that the care provided was questionable.

The final malpractice myth is the "million dollar payday" for plaintiffs who file suits. Once again, reality paints an entirely different picture. According to an organization that tracks malpractice awards, the latest figures reveal the average award, in a case involving a doctor, is around $420,000. While this may appear to be a sizeable award, it should be remembered that at least one-third of this settlement goes to cover the cost of attorney's fees. Limitations on attorney's fees, now in effect in more than 20 states, make it difficult for some plaintiffs to retain adequate legal counsel. The rationale for limiting attorney's fees is to guarantee that plaintiffs receive the majority of the award, and not have it consumed by legal fees.

IF YOU DECIDE TO SUE . . .

You may decide to file a malpractice suit if your injuries are severe and you have a strong desire to get satisfaction from a clearly inadequate doctor or institution. This is a matter for you and a good, qualified malpractice attorney to go over.

Your case had better be strong, your evidence solid, and your resolve firm, because a malpractice case can take years from first to last. That is why many cases end in out-of-court settlements.

Perhaps your injuries are not quite so severe, or your attorney doesn't see much optimism for a court ruling in your favor, but you feel strongly that there was negligence. You could meet with the doctor and hospital representatives to air your grievances. Frankly, the specter of a lawsuit is often as effective as the real thing, and doctors and hospitals will often make amends based on their fear of legal action.

ARBITRATION AN OPTION

Arbitration is an option. Several states sanction arbitration as an alternative dispute-resolving forum for medical malpractice claims.

A patient who signs an arbitration agreement before treatment gives up his right to a jury trial if there is a later claim of malpractice and a lawsuit. Instead, the case is presented to a theoretically neutral panel consisting of one arbitrator chosen by the patient, one chosen by the doctor, and one disinterested arbitrator.

The panel decides all questions of fault and sets an award. This decision generally cannot be appealed in a court of law.

Doctors believe that arbitration benefits them by reducing the time and expense of a court case and avoiding excessive monetary awards to patients by sympathetic juries. Some patients choose arbitration because it can be less costly and speedier than a full-blown trial. Patients seriously injured by their physicians' incompetence may need money for immediate treatment. This may cause them to want their cases to be heard by an arbitration panel rather than wait (perhaps years) until the matter comes before a judge and jury in court.

Although arbitration might ultimately benefit many, you cannot be coerced into signing an arbitration agreement. In no state can a patient be forced to choose between signing the arbitration agreement or forgoing medical care. If you can prove that the contract was unfair or that you were coerced into signing without knowing the risks, alternatives, and disadvantages of arbitration, a court can invalidate the agreement. In some states a patient is allowed to revoke or rescind the agreement within 30 or 60 days after signing.

Arbitration is something to think about and discuss with advisers, legal and otherwise.

HOW TO SELECT A MALPRACTICE ATTORNEY

How do you find a good medical malpractice lawyer? Once you've found him or her, what can you expect?

It's vitally important to understand the process. A competent lawyer can be invaluable in your fight to preserve your rights as a health care consumer. He or she can make the difference between winning and losing a case, between a large and small settlement, between allowing an incompetent physician to get off scot-free or be punished.

Let's say you have been the victim of what you suspect is medical malpractice. What's the first thing you should do?

Resources

In virtually every major city, there are hundreds of personal injury lawyers. Very few of them specialize solely in medical malpractice. They'll probably also handle everything from workmen's compensation to product liability cases.

Begin your search for a lawyer the same way you would for a doctor. Find someone you know who can refer you to a personal injury lawyer. Ideally, the person will have worked with that lawyer in a medical malpractice situation and will recommend him.

If you have no luck with that route, there are a number of reference books in law libraries that might help you. Bar associations usually have referral lists, though they often don't screen those lists carefully. The Martindale-Hubbell legal directory and *Markham's Negligence Counsel* are two other references.

In these directories, you'll find all sorts of credentials: education, speeches, publications, memberships. Though it's difficult to evaluate some of the credentials, pay attention to whether the attorney belongs to prestigious trial societies, such as the American College of Trial Lawyers, the International Academy of Trial Lawyers, and the International Society of Barristers. It is especially noteworthy if a lawyer is a fellow of one of these groups; a fellow has over fifteen years of experience and has been thoroughly screened by colleagues and judges.

You should also look to see if a lawyer is a member of his state trial lawyers' association and the Association of Trial Lawyers of America. Also see if he is a present or past officer of these organizations.

Finally, note the articles and speeches listed in the directories. It's possible that an attorney has written or spoken on a subject relevant to your case. If, for instance, an attorney has published an article on medical negligence, he is probably qualified to help you.

Initial Meeting

Schedule appointments with the lawyer or lawyers who seem best suited to your needs. When you meet with them, you'll want to ask some key questions, including:

- What sorts of medical malpractice cases have they handled? How much experience do they have, and what were the outcomes of some of the cases?
- Who will actually try the case? Many successful personal injury attorneys have staffs, and they frequently divide responsibility for a case among staffers. That's fine, providing the staff is competent and the attorney you hired is involved in the case, especially in the courtroom.

- You should also determine whether you feel comfortable with the lawyer. This is more important than it might seem. Some lawyers communicate frequently and well with their clients; others do not. Some are autocratic; others are down-to-earth. Your relationship with the attorney might last years. The more you trust and like the attorney, the better that relationship will be.
- Is your lawyer competent to handle your type of case? In most instances, he'll be able to if he's an experienced medical malpractice attorney. If you want to sue a hospital because of a particular surgical error, you don't need an attorney who's handled the exact type of case. The only exception might be if yours is a drug case: for example, a pharmaceutical company that marketed a drug with harmful effects they didn't warn the public about. Usually, there are one or two attorneys who have done the exhaustive research necessary to litigate these cases, and it might be wise to contact them.

Fees

The standard contingency-fee contract calls for an attorney to receive one-third of all monies awarded to a client. However, that percentage can vary from attorney to attorney. In medical malpractice cases, the percentage is often as high as 40 or 45 percent because of the extensive amount of time and outside costs such cases require. You might also live in a state that provides for graduated percentages based on award amounts. In Illinois, for instance, lawyers are allowed 33 percent of the first $150,000, 25 percent over $150,000, and 20 percent over $1 million. (If you see this in your contract with a lawyer, don't automatically assume you have a chance of gaining a million bucks; the amounts are inserted because of the law rather than because of the lawyer's expectations.)

According to the attorney's code of professional responsibility and the laws of every state, clients are responsible for costs. Those costs can be high, easily topping $10,000 in many cases. They entail a variety of expenses, including expert testimony, filing fees, reprints of records, and reporting of depositions.

What are you to do if you don't have the thousands of dollars required? Here are some options.

Suggest to a lawyer that he advance you the money to pay for costs and subtract that "advance" from the final settlement or judgment. This is a fairly common practice, and many lawyers will suggest it to clients. What happens if you lose the case and there is no settlement? Though lawyers aren't legally permitted to absorb the costs, many will offer verbal assurances, such as "I've never sued a client for costs" or something to that effect. In most instances, it's not an empty promise. From a purely practical standpoint, attorneys recognize that they're not going to collect from a penniless client.

Another option is to put a clause in your contract with the lawyer that limits costs. If, for instance, you have some available cash, you might want to insert a clause that stipulates that any costs over a certain amount ($7,500, for instance) will be deducted from the lawyer's fee. Again, this is an accepted practice that many lawyers will agree to.

A third option involves marginal cases—ones the attorney is reluctant to take on. If you believe your case has merit, you might persuade him to review the case by offering an advance ($2,500 is a typical amount). That will enable him to spend sufficient time to determine whether you have a chance of winning and will also limit your costs.

What to Bring with You

Don't arrive in your attorney's office empty-handed. The more information your attorney has and the faster he gets it, the better chances for a favorable resolution of the case.

Here's what you should bring:

- All records available to you: medical history, hospital and office visits
- A written chronology of events that led up to your problem. Dates, times, places, and people involved should be clearly listed.
- Copies of relevant prescriptions
- Bills received from doctors, hospitals, and other health care facilities

Putting a Case Together

Cases are won or lost based on a lawyer's preparation. You should expect and demand that your lawyer leave no stone unturned. His ability to prepare a case thoroughly will have a tremendous impact on the outcome.

Let's look at depositions. These pretrial examinations of experts and potential witnesses are extraordinarily important. If your lawyer is able to obtain the right information in a deposition, he'll have a powerful weapon to use in court.

For instance, a man was pushed into a door after an argument with a store owner. The police came, and the man told them he was hurt, that he couldn't move his arms or legs. The police threw him into a patrol wagon. In the hospital, doctors told the man that as a result of his injuries, he would be a quadriplegic.

The man decided to sue the city, claiming his condition was the result of mishandling by the police. The defense's neurosurgeon maintained in his deposition that the man's injuries were an irreversible result of the fall into the door, that the man had suffered a burst fracture. During the deposition, the lawyer questioned the doctor about the nature of a burst fracture, eliciting the response that a burst fracture is "a rare, highly unstable fracture."

During the trial, the lawyer questioned the neurosurgeon again, pulling out a medical textbook the doctor had referred to in the deposition as the "bible."

"Doctor," the lawyer said, "you maintained a burst fracture is rare and uncommon, correct?"

"Yes," the doctor replied.

"But, Doctor," the lawyer continued, "isn't it true that this is a common fracture known by other names?"

"Absolutely not true," the doctor insisted.

"Well, Doctor, I refer you to page 52 of your bible, which states that a burst fracture is also known as a vertical compression fracture. It says that it's not at all uncommon; that when a burst fracture occurs, the lateral ligaments of the neck are seldom interrupted or damaged, so that if a person is treated properly, he won't have as much damage."

Because of the deposition in which he referred to the text as his bible, the lawyer sounded foolish to the neurosurgeon when he took issue with the statement in the text.

The man received a verdict from the jury against the city.

Many cases hinge on a lawyer's aggressiveness. Your lawyer should act quickly to get the information he needs. He shouldn't be intimidated by close-mouthed health care professionals, and he should take what they say with more than a few grains of salt.

Here's a fascinating case that illustrates the point.

A mother took her 6-month-old child to the hospital because she was spitting up blood. The bleeding was stopped but a new problem developed: The child's right hand was turning blue.

The attending physician noticed the circulation problem and noted on the chart that he wasn't sure what was going on; he questioned on the chart whether he should call in a vascular surgeon. A full 6 hours later, he did so.

Shortly thereafter, the doctor called the mother and told her a blood clot had developed and they'd have to operate; there was a chance the child might lose her arm.

Subsequently, the mother received an anonymous phone call, the caller saying, "I was in the operating room and the butchers cut a vein, and that's why your child will lose an arm; they're covering it up."

The mother tape-recorded the phone call and brought it with her to the lawyer. The mother then received another anonymous phone call, the voice saying that a bottle that had been assumed to be a glucose solution had been mislabeled, and a corroding drug was mistakenly injected into the baby's arm, resulting in the circulation problem.

Subsequently, the child's arm was amputated.

Once the amputation was performed, the lawyer acted quickly. He had the mother sign a letter messengered to the hospital's department of legal affairs. The letter requested that the amputated arm be sent to an independent pathologist for examination.

At first, the hospital refused. The lawyer then sent another letter, threatening the hospital with a lawsuit for punitive damages if they didn't turn over the arm.

The letter worked. The report of the pathologist who examined the arm for the lawyer, combined with the delay in contacting the vascular specialist, provided substantial evidence of negligence. The lawyer won a substantial settlement for the client.

Fire or Ice

Many people believe that a lawyer's courtroom oratory can sway a jury.

This happens rarely, especially in medical malpractice cases. Years ago, spellbinding courtroom oratory had more of an impact on decisions. A great deal of information was privileged, and our system was, out of necessity, a battle of wits between opposing attorneys.

Today, each side knows generally what the other is going to do before the trial begins. It's like a play that's been well rehearsed. The jury is an audience, and they will decide based on how well each "actor" has prepared for his or her role. Jurors, too, are far more sophisticated than they used to be. Study after study demonstrates that juries usually reach decisions based on the evidence they hear and not on a lawyer's histrionics.

Therefore, don't choose a lawyer because he has a mesmerizing manner or a commanding baritone. Don't make your choice because he has received favorable publicity about his courtroom antics. It's all sizzle. Far better to have a dull, mousy lawyer who prepares his cases well than a flamboyant showman who misses crucial details.

Settlements

In many medical malpractice suits, defendants wish to settle out of court. At some point during the legal process, you might be confronted with a settlement decision.

It's a tough, tricky one.

If the situation arises, here are some things you should consider.

First, remember it's your decision, not your lawyer's, the defendant's, or the judge's (though the judge can decide about a settlement if a minor is involved). A settlement can't be imposed upon you.

Second, before making that decision, be sure you have all the facts. Just as you wouldn't agree to an operation without all the facts, neither should you agree to a settlement without sufficient information. The informed consent principle is applicable here as well.

To ensure that you are fully informed, ask the following questions as soon as a lawyer proposes a settlement:

- What, if any, limitations does the state law impose on the amount of money that is recoverable? (In recent years, in response to medical lobbies, many state legislatures have passed damage limits in medical malpractice cases.)
- Is there a likelihood that more money might be offered?
- Is it likely that additional money will be offered before, or during, the trial?
- How long will the settlement offer be on the table? In many instances, the offer will change or be withdrawn depending on what develops as the case evolves.
- If you reject the settlement, what are your chances for losing the case and receiving nothing?

Be wary of hospital administrators overeager to settle. You might find that they'll contact you before you have contacted a lawyer. They'll usher you into their plush conference room, apologize profusely for your loss, and pull out a check with a number of zeros that has your name on it. They'll tell you this is a neat, clean way of settling the case and you won't have to pay attorney fees. Before letting you have the check, they'll insist you sign a form releasing the hospital of all liability for negligence and stating that you won't sue them.

Don't fall victim to this ploy. When hospitals make these offers, they almost always offer less than they should. They're counting on your naïveté.

If you do sign the release and accept the money, however, you might still be able to file a suit. In a number of instances, the courts have set aside these releases when they've determined that the hospital paid the victim an unfairly small amount.

The Jury Finds . . .

During your initial interview with a lawyer, you might be tempted to ask him what your case is worth, what a jury might give you.

Your lawyer shouldn't tell you. If he quotes a specific amount—if he says you're looking at seven figures—don't believe him. Until he spends the necessary time poring over documents and interviewing experts and witnesses, he cannot give you even an educated guess. The amount you're likely to receive is directly related to the strength of your legal case, the extent of your injuries, and your ultimate damages, and that's something a lawyer can't possibly know at the outset.

On the other hand, you are entitled to know what your lawyer thinks about your case. Is his initial impression positive or negative? Does he believe damages are extensive? What are those damages as defined by the law, and what does the law allow you to recover?

Let's say the client comes to a lawyer with a claim for the wrongful death of a spouse. He should tell him that wrongful death involves a pecuniary loss, that the next of kin may recover for loss of services, and that an economist may be called in to estimate what the value of those services are. He should explain that in most states, juries are instructed not to award anything for grief or emotional suffering in wrongful death cases. They are, however, generally allowed to give awards for loss of society and companionship.

At the very least, ask your lawyer for his impressions of your case. He might be able to tell you something like, "If we can prove that the hospital ignored your warning that you were allergic to the medication, then we've got a strong case"; or, "If the nurse is willing to testify that the doctor was drunk in the operating room, we can expect a sizable award from the jury."

Time Frame

Don't expect to resolve your case quickly. The fastest resolutions usually take at least a year. Some cases drag on for five years. Only if both parties agree to a settlement in the early stages of a case—a rare occurrence—do medical malpractice cases end in less than a year.

Why does it take so long? A number of reasons. For one thing, the extent of a plaintiff's injuries often aren't known immediately; it can take months until someone's condition stabilizes and the damages (both physical and financial) can be assessed. Another problem is that most medical malpractice cases—especially ones involving serious injuries—are complicated. It takes time for both sides to compile evidence, interview experts, etc. Finally, conflicting schedules must be reconciled before a trial date is set—schedules of defendants, plaintiffs, witnesses, lawyers, and judges.

Some cases reach the courts faster than others. Generally, because of volume, cases in large cities go more slowly than those in smaller communities; federal courts often work faster than metropolitan state courts; smaller claims move through the system faster than larger claims.

Incompetent Lawyers

It's not only physicians who are incompetent. What happens if you suspect your lawyer is negligent?

You have every right to discharge your lawyer. If you're considering this action, think hard and long before doing so. Changing lawyers in the middle of a case can be costly and counterproductive.

Many clients feel their lawyers are incompetent because months pass with seemingly little activity; or because their lawyers don't return phone calls quickly; or because they find themselves dealing with an associate of the original lawyer they hired.

Try to resolve miscommunication with your lawyer before dismissing him. Many times, he's unaware that there's a communication problem, and if you inform him of the problem, more often than not he'll correct it.

If, however, you're certain that your attorney is incompetent, fire him and look for a new attorney. Your former lawyer might insist on being paid for work to date. If you have proof that he was truly incompetent, he should receive little, if anything. The law provides that attorneys in contingency fee cases should be paid for efforts that have reasonably contributed to the successful conclusion of a case. Your new lawyer will help you resolve any fee problems.

Filing a Complaint Letter Against a Doctor or Medical Facility in Your State

As a medical consumer, you may find yourself in a situation in which you feel that you have been wronged. When this happens, it is within your rights to file a formal complaint against the offending medical practitioner, hospital, health care facility, or insurance company. But keep in mind that you are starting an administrative review process when you file a formal complaint. You should be willing and prepared to see it through to the end. To file a complaint, follow the steps outlined here.

1. Select the proper source from ones given elsewhere in this book. For state licensing boards for doctors and dentists see Section 3: Healing Arts. For state licensing boards for hospitals and nursing homes see Section 4: Settings. For complaints involving insurance companies see the State Insurance Department in Section 8: Insurance.
2. Put your complaint in writing. See sample complaint letter.
3. Include the name of the offending party.
4. Describe the nature of the complaint.
5. Tell where the incident occurred.
6. Give the date and time it occurred.
7. Include statements from witnesses, if any.
8. Include copies of bills and other pertinent items.
9. Be willing and able to provide additional documentation if requested.
10. For your own protection, consider retaining legal counsel.

The information presented here is not legal advice.

Sample Complaint Letter

Dear [Commissioner/Secretary/Director]:

I am writing to you to file a formal complaint against [name of person, institution, or organization] arising from an incident in which I believe I was wronged. I am requesting that a full administrative review process be initiated so that I may be given a full and complete hearing. I am prepared to provide the documentation to support my complaint and to cooperate fully with the investigating officer assigned to my case.

I will briefly describe what happened and why I believe I am justified in filing this complaint. [See steps 4, 5, 6, and 7 above.]

I will be awaiting your reply and will complete any additional forms if necessary. Your assistance in this matter is appreciated.

11. Government Resources

INTRODUCTION

Government, both federal and state, is an integral part of your overall health. States regulate doctors, hospitals, health insurance, and a host of other health-related entities. States also determine eligibility for Medicaid, a wealth of social services, training for handicapped individuals, and much more.

The federal government is also a major participant. Medicare is administered by the federal government. The federal government legislates, regulates, and oversees food and drug laws. It also runs health services for veterans and the military.

Government is also an information source. If you need to find out about a doctor's license, your state government has the information. If you have a concern about how a loved one is being treated in a nursing home, you should consult your state's nursing home ombudsman.

But finding these valuable resources and knowing what they do are often a problem. Government health-related services and functions, at both the federal and state levels, are in literally hundreds of departments, offices, and bureaus.

In this section, you will find a complete directory of all the important health-related government entities at the federal level and in each state.

State Attorneys General

The attorney general is the chief prosecutor and law enforcement officer of the state, and represents the state in all legal matters. The state attorney general's office may be contacted concerning state health regulations as they pertain to a consumer's medical and legal rights, especially in the area of possible fraud.

Alabama
Attorney General
11 S. Union Street
Montgomery, AL 36130
205-242-7300

Alaska
Attorney General
Department of Law
120 4th Street
Juneau, AK 99801
907-465-3600

Arizona
Attorney General
1275 W. Washington
Phoenix, AZ 85007
602-542-4266

Arkansas
Attorney General
323 Center, Suite 200
Little Rock, AR 72201
501-682-2007

California
Attorney General
Department of Justice
1515 K Street, Law Library
Sacramento, CA 95814
916-324-5437

Colorado
Attorney General
Department of Law
110 16th Street, 10th Floor
Denver, CO 80202
303-620-4500

Connecticut
Attorney General
55 Elm Street
Hartford, CT 06106
203-566-2026

Delaware
Attorney General
Carvel State Office Building
820 N. French Street
Wilmington, DE 19801
302-571-2500

District of Columbia
Attorney General
Corporation Counsel
Office of the Corporation Counsel
1350 Pennsylvania Avenue N.W., Room 329
Washington, DC 20004
202-727-6248

Florida
Attorney General
Department of Legal Affairs
The Capitol
Tallahassee, FL 32399
904-487-1963

Georgia
Attorney General
State Law Department
132 State Judicial Building
Atlanta, GA 30334
404-656-4585

Hawaii
Attorney General
425 Queen Street
Honolulu, HI 96813
808-586-1282

Idaho
Attorney General
State Capitol
Boise, ID 83720
208-334-2424

Illinois
Attorney General
500 S. 2nd Street
Springfield, IL 62706
217-782-1090

Indiana
Attorney General
219 Statehouse
Indianapolis, IN 46204
317-232-6201

Iowa
Attorney General
Hoover State Office Building
Des Moines, IA 50319
515-281-8373

Kansas
Attorney General
301 W. 10th, Judicial Center
Topeka, KS 66612
913-296-2215

Kentucky
Attorney General
State Capitol, Room 116
Frankfort, KY 40601
502-564-7600

Louisiana
Attorney General
Department of Justice
P.O. Box 94005
Baton Rouge, LA 70804
504-342-7013

Maine
Attorney General
Statehouse Station 6
Augusta, ME 04333
207-289-3661

Maryland
Attorney General
200 St. Paul Place
Baltimore, MD 21202
410-576-6300

Massachusetts
Attorney General
One Ashburton Place
Boston, MA 02108
617-727-3688

Michigan
Attorney General
525 W. Ottawa, Law Building
Lansing, MI 48913
517-373-1110

Minnesota
Attorney General
102 State Capitol
St. Paul, MN 55155
612-297-4272

Missouri
Attorney General
Supreme Court Building
P.O. Box 899
Jefferson City, MO 65102
314-751-3221

Montana
Attorney General
Department of Justice
215 N. Sanders Street
Helena, MT 59620
406-444-2026

Nebraska
Attorney General
State Capitol, Room 2115
P.O. Box 94906
Lincoln, NE 68509
402-471-2682

Nevada
Attorney General
Heroes Memorial Building
Capitol Complex
Carson City, NV 89710
702-687-4170

New Hampshire
Attorney General
Statehouse Annex, Room 208
25 Capitol Street
Concord, NH 03301
603-271-3658

New Jersey
Attorney General
Department of Law and Public Safety
Hughes Justice Complex, CN-081
Trenton, NJ 08625
609-292-8740

New Mexico
Attorney General
Bataan Memorial Building
P.O. Box 1508
Santa Fe, NM 87501
505-827-6000

New York
Attorney General
Department of Law
State Capitol
Albany, NY 12224
518-474-7330

North Carolina
Attorney General
Department of Justice
2 E. Morgan Street
Raleigh, NC 27601
919-733-3377

North Dakota
Attorney General
State Capitol, 1st Floor
600 E. Boulevard
Bismarck, ND 58505
701-224-2210

Ohio
Attorney General
30 E. Broad Street, 17th Floor
Columbus, OH 43266
614-466-3376

Oklahoma
Attorney General
112 State Capitol
Oklahoma City, OK 73105
405-521-3921

Oregon
Attorney General
Department of Justice
100 State Office Building
Salem, OR 97310
503-378-6002

Pennsylvania
Attorney General
Strawberry Square, 16th Floor
Harrisburg, PA 17120
717-787-3391

Puerto Rico
Attorney General
Department of Justice
P.O. Box 192
San Juan, PR 00904
809-721-2924

Rhode Island
Attorney General
72 Pine Street
Providence, RI 02903
401-274-4400

South Carolina
Attorney General
Dennis Building
P.O. Box 11549
Columbia, SC 29211
803-734-3970

South Dakota
Attorney General
State Capitol, 1st Floor
Pierre, SD 57501
605-773-3215

Tennessee
Attorney General
450 James Robertson Parkway
Nashville, TN 37243
615-741-6474

Texas
Attorney General
Capitol Station
P.O. Box 12548
Austin, TX 78711
512-463-2100

Utah
Attorney General
236 State Capitol
Salt Lake City, UT 84114
801-538-1326

Vermont
Attorney General
Pavilion Office Building
109 State Street
Montpelier, VT 05602
802-828-3171

Virgin Islands
Attorney General
Department of Justice
Gers Building, 2nd Floor
St. Thomas, VI 00802
809-774-5666

Virginia
Attorney General
101 N. 8th Street, 5th Floor
Richmond, VA 23219
804-786-2071

Washington
Attorney General
Highway-Licenses Building
Mail Stop PB-71
Olympia, WA 98504
206-753-2550

West Virginia
Attorney General
Department of Justice
Building 1, Room E-26
State Capitol Complex
Charleston, WV 25305
304-558-2021

Wisconsin
Attorney General
Department of Justice
114 E. State Capitol
P.O. Box 7857
Madison, WI 53707
608-266-1221

Wyoming
Attorney General
State Capitol
Cheyenne, WY 82002
307-777-7810

State Child Welfare Offices

These agencies coordinate the delivery of services to children and youth designed to protect them from abuse, exploitation, and neglect. Foster care programs for abused, neglected, and runaway children are also managed by these offices.

Alabama
Child Welfare
Bureau of Family and Children's Services
64 N. Union Street
Montgomery, AL 36130
205-242-9500

Alaska
Child Welfare
Family and Youth Services Division
Health and Social Services Department
P.O. Box H
Juneau, AK 99811
907-465-3170

Arizona
Child Welfare
Children, Youth and Families
Department of Economic Security
1717 W. Jefferson
Phoenix, AZ 85007
602-542-3981

Arkansas
Child Welfare
Department of Human Services
Children and Family Services
P.O. Box 1437
Little Rock, AR 72203
501-682-8770

California
Child Welfare
Office of Child Abuse Prevention
Department of Social Services
744 P Street, MS 9-100
Sacramento, CA 95814
916-323-2888

Colorado
Child Welfare
Family and Children's Services Division
Department of Social Services
1575 Sherman Street, 2nd Floor
Denver, CO 80203
303-866-3672

Connecticut
Child Welfare
Children and Youth Services Department
170 Sigourney Street
Hartford, CT 06105
203-566-3536

Delaware
Child Welfare
Department of Services for Children, Youth
and Their Families
1825 Faulkland Road
Wilmington, DE 19805
302-633-2500

District of Columbia
Child Welfare
Family Services Administration
Department of Human Services
First and I Street S.W., Room 215
Washington, DC 20024
202-727-5947

Florida
Child Welfare
Children and Families
Health and Rehabilitative Services Department
1317 Winewood, Building 8, 3rd Floor
Tallahassee, FL 32399
904-488-8762

Georgia
Child Welfare
Family and Children Services
Department of Human Resources
878 Peachtree Street, 4th Floor
Atlanta, GA 30309
404-894-6386

Hawaii
Child Welfare
Child and Protective Services
Department of Human Services
810 Richards Street, Suite 400
Honolulu, HI 96813
808-548-6123

Idaho
Child Welfare
Family and Children Services
Department of Health and Welfare
450 W. State Street
Boise, ID 83720
208-334-5700

Illinois
Child Welfare
Children and Family Services Department
406 E. Monroe Street
Springfield, IL 62701
217-785-2509

Indiana
Child Welfare
Division of Children and Families
Family and Social Services Administration
302 W. Washington
IGC-S, E-414
Indianapolis, IN 46204
317-233-4451

Iowa
Child Welfare
Adult, Children and Family Services
Department of Human Services
Hoover State Office Building
Des Moines, IA 50319
515-281-5521

Kansas
Child Welfare
Youth Services
Social and Rehabilitations Services Department
Smith-Wilson Building
300 S.W. Oakley
Topeka, KS 66606
913-296-3284

Kentucky
Child Welfare
Division of Family Services
Department for Social Services
275 E. Main Street
Frankfort, KY 40601
502-564-6852

Louisiana
Child Welfare
Office of Community Services
Department of Social Services
P.O. Box 44367
Baton Rouge, LA 70804
504-342-4000

Maine
Child Welfare
Child and Family Services
Department of Human Services
Statehouse Station 11
Augusta, ME 04333
207-289-5060

Maryland
Child Welfare
Child Welfare Services Office
Department of Human Resources
300 W. Preston Street
Baltimore, MD 21201
410-333-0208

Massachusetts
Child Welfare
Department of Social Services
150 Causeway Street
Boston, MA 02114
617-727-0900

Michigan
Child Welfare
Office of Children and Youth Services
Department of Social Services
300 S. Capitol
P.O. Box 30037
Lansing, MI 48909
517-373-4506

Minnesota
Child Welfare
Community Social Services Division
Department of Human Services
658 Cedar Street, 4th Floor
St. Paul, MN 55155
612-297-2673

Mississippi
Child Welfare
Division of Family and Children's Services
P.O. Box 352
Jackson, MS 39205
601-354-6661

Missouri
Child Welfare
Children's Services
Division of Family Services
Broadway Building, Box 88
Jefferson City, MO 65103
314-751-2882

Montana
Child Welfare
Department of Family Services
48 N. Last Chance Gulch
Helena, MT 59601
406-444-5902

Nebraska
Child Welfare
Division of Human Services
Department of Social Services
P.O. Box 95026
Lincoln, NE 68509
402-471-9308

Nevada
Child Welfare
Children and Family Services
Human Resources
505 E. King Street
Carson City, NV 89710
702-687-4400

New Hampshire
Child Welfare
Children and Youth Services
Department of Health and Welfare
Hazen Drive
Concord, NH 03301
603-271-4451

New Jersey
Child Welfare
Division of Economic Assistance
Department of Human Services
Quakerbridge Road, CN-716
Trenton, NJ 08625
609-588-2361

New Mexico
Child Welfare
Children's Bureau
Social Services Division
Human Services Department
P.O. Box 2348
Santa Fe, NM 87504
505-827-8439

New York
Child Welfare
Department of Social Services
40 N. Pearl Street
Albany, NY 12243
518-474-9475

North Carolina
Child Welfare
Division of Social Services
Department of Human Resources
325 N. Salisbury Street
Raleigh, NC 27603
919-733-3055

North Dakota
Child Welfare
Children and Family Services
Department of Human Services
State Capitol, Judicial Wing
600 E. Boulevard
Bismarck, ND 58505
701-224-4811

Ohio
Child Welfare
Family and Children's Services Division
Department of Human Services
51 N. High Street, 3rd Floor
Columbus, OH 43266
614-466-8783

Oklahoma
Child Welfare
Secretary of Health and Human Services
Department of Human Services
P.O. Box 25352
Oklahoma City, OK 73125
405-521-2778

Oregon
Child Welfare
Children's Services Division
Department of Human Resources
198 Commercial Street S.E.
Salem, OR 97310
503-378-4374

Pennsylvania
Child Welfare
Children, Youth and Families
Department of Public Welfare
P.O. Box 2675
Harrisburg, PA 17105
717-787-4756

Puerto Rico
Child Welfare
Fernández Juncos Station
P.O. Box 3349
Santurce, PR 00904
809-725-0753

Rhode Island
Child Welfare
Department of Children and Families
610 Mt. Pleasant Avenue
Providence, RI 02908
401-861-6000

South Carolina
Child Welfare
Children and Family Services Division
Department of Social Services
P.O. Box 1520
Columbia, SC 29202
803-734-5670

South Dakota
Child Welfare
Child Protection Services Division
Department of Social Services
Kneip Building
Pierre, SD 57501
605-773-3227

Tennessee
Child Welfare
Child Support Director
Department of Human Services
111 7th Avenue N.
Nashville, TN 37243
615-741-1820

Texas
Child Welfare
Department of Human Services
P.O. Box 149030
Austin, TX 78714
512-450-3080

Utah
Child Welfare
Division of Family Services
Department of Human Services
120 North 200 West, 4th Floor
Salt Lake City, UT 84103
801-538-4004

Vermont
Child Welfare
Division of Social Services
Social and Rehabilitation Services Department
103 S. Main Street
Osgood Building
Waterbury, VT 05671
802-241-2131

Virginia
Child Welfare
Department of Social Services
8007 Discovery Drive
Richmond, VA 23229
804-662-9236

Washington
Child Welfare
Children and Family Services
Social and Health Services Department
Office Building #2
Mail Stop OB-41
Olympia, WA 98504
206-586-8654

West Virginia
Child Welfare
Social Services Bureau
Division of Human Services
1900 Washington E.
Building 6
Charleston, WV 25305
304-558-7980

Wisconsin
Child Welfare
Children, Youth and Families
Health and Social Services Department
P.O. Box 7851
Madison, WI 53707
608-266-6946

Wyoming
Child Welfare
Division of Youth Services
Department of Family Services
Hathaway Building, 3rd Floor
Cheyenne, WY 82002
307-777-6095

State Community Affairs Offices

These agencies provide support services to communities to help them deliver essential public services to residents. Local communities may apply to the state government for grants to implement programs such as water and sewer improvement, public housing, and economic development.

Alabama
Community Affairs
Department of Economic and Community Affairs
3465 Norman Bridge Road
Montgomery, AL 36105
205-242-8672

Alaska
Community Affairs
Department of Community and Regional Affairs
P.O. Box B
Juneau, AK 99811
907-465-4700

Arizona
Community Affairs
Department of Commerce
3800 N. Central Avenue
Phoenix, AZ 85012
602-280-1306

Arkansas
Community Affairs
Department of Human Services
P.O. Box 1437, Slot 316
Little Rock, AR 72203
501-682-8650

California
Community Affairs
Division of Community Affairs
Housing and Community Development Department
1800 3rd Street
Sacramento, CA 95814
916-322-1560

Colorado
Community Affairs
Division of Local Government
Department of Local Affairs
1313 Sherman Street, #521
Denver, CO 80203
303-866-2156

Connecticut
Community Affairs
Office of Policy and Management
80 Washington Street
Hartford, CT 06106
203-566-2367

District of Columbia
Community Affairs
Office of the Mayor
2000 14th Street N.W., 3rd Floor
Washington, DC 20009
202-939-8750

Florida
Community Affairs
2740 Centerview Drive
Tallahassee, FL 32399
904-488-8466

Georgia
Community Affairs
Equitable Building, Suite 1200
100 Peachtree Street
Atlanta, GA 30303
404-656-3836

Hawaii
Community Affairs
Department of Business, Economic Development
and Tourism
P.O. Box 2359
Honolulu, HI 96804
808-548-3034

Idaho
Community Affairs
Division of Community Development
Department of Commerce
700 W. State Street
Boise, ID 83720
208-334-2470

Illinois
Community Affairs
Department of Commerce and Community Affairs
620 E. Adams Street, 3rd Floor
Springfield, IL 62701
217-785-1032

Indiana
Community Affairs
Community Development Division
Department of Commerce
One North Capitol
Indianapolis, IN 46204
317-232-8917

Iowa
Community Affairs
Community and Rural Development Division
Department of Economic Development
200 E. Grand
Des Moines, IA 50309
515-242-4728

Kansas
Community Affairs
Community Development Division
Department of Commerce
400 S.W. 8th, 5th Floor
Topeka, KS 66603
913-296-3485

Kentucky
Community Affairs
Department of Local Government
1024 Capitol Centre
Frankfort, KY 40601
502-564-2382

Louisiana
Community Affairs
Development Office
P.O. Box 94185
Baton Rouge, LA 70804
504-342-5359

Maine
Community Affairs
Division of Community Services
Executive Department
Statehouse Station 73
Augusta, ME 04333
207-289-3771

Maryland
Community Affairs
Community Services Administration
Department of Human Resources
311 W. Saratoga Street
Baltimore, MD 21201
410-333-0053

Massachusetts
Community Affairs
Executive Office of Communities and Development
100 Cambridge Street, Room 1404
Boston, MA 02202
617-727-7765

Michigan
Community Affairs
Community Assistance Services
525 W. Ottawa, 5th Floor
P.O. Box 30225
Lansing, MI 48909
517-335-2105

Minnesota
Community Affairs
Community Development Division
Department of Trade and Economic Development
150 E. Kellogg Boulevard, Room 900
St. Paul, MN 55101
612-296-5005

Mississippi
Community Affairs
Community Services
Department of Economic and Community Development
P.O. Box 849
Jackson, MS 39205
601-359-3449

Missouri
Community Affairs
Economic Development Program
Department of Economic Development
Truman Building, Box 118
Jefferson City, MO 65102
314-751-2133

Montana
Community Affairs
Local Government Assistance Division
Department of Commerce
Cogswell Building
Helena, MT 59620
406-444-3757

Nebraska
Community Affairs
Division of Community Development
Department of Economic Development
P.O. Box 94666
Lincoln, NE 68509
402-471-3111

Nevada
Community Affairs
Nevada Office of Community Services
Office of the Governor
400 W. King, Suite 400
Carson City, NV 89710
702-687-4913

New Hampshire
Community Affairs
Office of State Planning
2 ½ Beacon Street
Concord, NH 03301
603-271-2155

New Jersey
Community Affairs
101 S. Broad Street, CN-800
Trenton, NJ 08625
609-292-6420

New Mexico
Community Affairs
Economic Development Division
Department of Economic Development
1100 St. Francis Drive
Santa Fe, NM 87503
505-827-0300

New York
Community Affairs
Department of State
162 Washington Avenue
Albany, NY 12231
518-474-4750

North Carolina
Community Affairs
Department of Economic and Community Development
1307 Glenwood
P.O. Box 27687
Raleigh, NC 27605
919-733-2850

North Dakota
Community Affairs
Office of Management and Budget
State Capitol, 14th Floor
600 E. Boulevard
Bismarck, ND 58505
701-224-2094

Ohio
Community Affairs
Division of Community Development
Department of Development
30 E. Broad Street
Columbus, OH 43266
614-466-5863

Oklahoma
Community Affairs
Department of Commerce
6601 Broadway Extension
Oklahoma City, OK 73116
405-843-9770

Oregon
Community Affairs
Department of Housing and Community Services
1600 State Street, Suite 100
Salem, OR 97310
503-373-1614

Pennsylvania
Community Affairs
Department of Community Affairs
317 Forum Building
Harrisburg, PA 17120
717-787-7160

Puerto Rico
Community Affairs
Municipal Services Administration
P.O. Box 70167
San Juan, PR 00936
809-753-9151

Rhode Island
Community Affairs
Governor's Office of Housing, Energy and
Intergovernmental Relations
Statehouse, Room 111
Providence, RI 02903
401-277-2850

South Carolina
Community Affairs
Office of the Governor
P.O. Box 11369
Columbia, SC 29211
803-734-0434

South Dakota
Community Affairs
Governor's Office of Economic Development
Capitol Lake Plaza
Pierre, SD 57501
605-773-5032

Tennessee
Community Affairs
Department of Economic and Community Development
320 6th Avenue N.
Nashville, TN 37243
615-741-1888

Texas
Community Affairs
Texas Department of Community Affairs
P.O. Box 13166
Austin, TX 78711
512-475-3800

Utah
Community Affairs
Division of Business and Economic Development
Community and Economic Development Department
324 S. State Street, Suite 300
Salt Lake City, UT 84111
801-538-8820

Vermont
Community Affairs
Housing and Community Affairs Department
Agency of Development and Community Affairs
109 State Street
Montpelier, VT 05602
802-828-3217

Virgin Islands
Community Affairs
Department of Human Services
Barbel Plaza S.
St. Thomas, VI 00802
809-774-1166

Virginia
Community Affairs
Housing and Community Development Department
205 N. 4th Street
Richmond, VA 23219
804-786-1575

Washington
Community Affairs
Department of Community Development
9th and Columbia Building
Mail Stop GH-51
Olympia, WA 98504
206-586-8966

West Virginia
Community Affairs
Governor's Office of Community and
Industrial Development
State Capitol, Room 146
Charleston, WV 25305
304-558-4010

Wisconsin
Community Affairs
Division of Economic Development
Department of Development
P.O. Box 7970
Madison, WI 53707
608-266-3203

Wyoming
Community Affairs
Division of Economic and Community Development
Department of Commerce
122 W. 25th Street, 2W
Cheyenne, WY 82002
307-777-5948

State Consumer Protection Offices

These offices investigate and help to resolve complaints made by consumers against businesses. All complaints involving services, products, or charges should be made to these offices. If your complaint involves a business in another state, your complaint should be directed to that state's consumer protection office.

Alabama
Alabama Consumer Protection Division
Office of Attorney General
11 S. Union Street
Montgomery, AL 36130
205-242 7334

Alaska
The Consumer Protection Section in the Office of the Attorney General has been closed. Consumers with complaints are being referred to the Better Business Bureau, small claims court, and private attorneys.

Arizona

Arizona Consumer Protection Office
Office of the Attorney General
1275 W. Washington St., Room 259
Phoenix, AZ 85007
602-542-3702
602-542-5763

Arkansas

Arkansas Consumer Protection Division
Office of Attorney General
200 Tower Building
323 Center Street
Little Rock, AR 72201
501-682-2341
800-482-8982 (in AR)

California

California Consumer Protection Office
Department of Consumer Affairs
400 R Street, Suite 1040
Sacramento, CA 95814
916-445-0660 Complaint assistance
916-445-1254 Consumer information
800-344-9940 (in CA)

Colorado

Colorado Consumer Protection Unit
Office of Attorney General
110 16th Street, 10th Floor
Denver, CO 80202
303-620-4500

Connecticut

Connecticut Consumer Protection Office
Department of Consumer Protection
State Office Building
165 Capitol Avenue
Hartford, CT 06106
203-566-4999
800-842-2649 (in CT)

District of Columbia

District of Columbia Consumer Protection Office
Department of Consumer and Regulatory Affairs
614 H Street N.W.
Washington, DC 20001
202-727-7000

Florida

Florida Consumer Protection Office
Department of Agriculture and Consumer Services
Division of Consumer Services
218 Mayo Building
Tallahassee, FL 32399
904-488-2226
800-342-2176 TDD in FL
800-327-3382 Information and education
800-321-5366 Lemon Law

Georgia

Georgia Consumer Protection Office
Governor's Office of Consumer Affairs
2 Martin Luther King Jr. Drive S.E.
Plaza Level, East Tower
Atlanta, GA 30334
404-651-8600
404-656-3790
800-869-1123 (in GA)

Hawaii

Hawaii Office of Consumer Protection
Department of Commerce and Consumer Affairs
828 Fort Street Mall, Suite 600B
P.O. Box 3767
Honolulu, HI 96812-3767
808-586-2630

Idaho

Idaho Consumer Protection Unit
Deputy Attorney General
Office of the Attorney General
Statehouse, Room 113A
Boise, ID 83720-1000
208-334-2424
800-432-3545 (in ID)

Illinois

Illinois Consumer Protection Office
Governor's Office of Citizens Assistance
222 S. College
Springfield, IL 62706
217-782-0244
800-642-3112 (in IL)

Indiana

Indiana Consumer Protection Division
Chief Counsel and Director
Office of Attorney General
219 Statehouse
Indianapolis, IN 46204
317-232-6330
800-382-5516 (in IN)

Iowa

Iowa Consumer Protection Division
Assistant Attorney General
Office of Attorney General
1300 E. Walnut Street, 2nd Floor
Des Moines, IA 50319
515-281-5926

Kansas

Kansas Consumer Protection Division
Deputy Attorney General
Office of Attorney General
301 W. 10th
Kansas Judicial Center
Topeka, KS 66612-1597
913-296-3751
800-432-2310 (in KS)

Kentucky

Kentucky Consumer Protection Division
Office of Attorney General
209 St. Clair Street
Frankfort, KY 40601-1875
502-564-2200
800-432-9257 (in KY)

Louisiana

Louisiana Consumer Protection Section
Office of Attorney General
State Capitol Building
P.O. Box 94005
Baton Rouge, LA 70804-9005
504-342-7373

Maine

Maine Consumer Protection Office
Superintendent
Bureau of Consumer Credit Protection
Statehouse Station 35
Augusta, ME 04333-0035
207-582-8718
800-332-8529 (in ME)

Maryland

Maryland Consumer Protection Division
Office of Attorney General
200 St. Paul Place
Baltimore, MD 21202-2021
410-528-8662
410-576-6372 TDD in Baltimore area
410-565-0451 TDD in District of Columbia area
800-969-5766 (in MD)

Massachusetts

Massachusetts Consumer Protection Office
Department of Attorney General
131 Tremont Street
Boston, MA 02111
617-727-8400

Michigan

Michigan Consumer Protection Division
Assistant in Charge
Office of Attorney General
P.O. Box 30213
Lansing, MI 48909
517-373-1140

Minnesota

Minnesota Consumer Protection Office
Office of Consumer Services
Office of Attorney General
117 University Avenue
St Paul, MN 55155
612-296-2331

Mississippi

Mississippi Consumer Protection Office
Special Assistant Attorney General
Chief, Consumer Protection Division
Office of Attorney General
P.O. Box 22947
Jackson, MS 39225-2947
601-354-6018

Missouri

Missouri Consumer Protection Office
Office of Attorney General
Consumer Complaints or Problems
P.O. Box 899
Jefferson City, MO 65102
314-751-3321
800-392-8222 (in MO)

Montana

Montana Consumer Protection Office
Consumer Affairs Unit
Department of Commerce
1424 9th Avenue
Helena, MT 59620
406-444-4312

Nebraska

Nebraska Consumer Protection Division
Assistant Attorney General
Department of Justice
2115 State Capitol
P.O. Box 98920
Lincoln, NE 68509
402-471-2682

Nevada

Nevada Consumer Protection Office
Commissioner of Consumer Affairs
Department of Commerce
State Mail Room Complex
Las Vegas, NV 89158
702-486-7355
800-992-0900 (in NV)

New Hampshire

New Hampshire Consumer Protection and
Antitrust Bureau
Office of Attorney General
Statehouse Annex
Concord, NH 03301
603-271-3641

New Jersey

New Jersey Consumer Protection Office
Division of Consumer Affairs
P.O. Box 45027
Newark, NJ 07101
201-648-4010

New Mexico

New Mexico Consumer Protection Divsion
Office of Attorney General
P.O. Drawer 1508
Santa Fe, NM 87504
505-827-6060
800-432-2070 (in NM)

New York

New York Consumer Protection Office
Chairperson and Executive Director
New York State Consumer Protection Board
99 Washington Avenue
Albany, NY 12210-2891
518-474-8583

North Carolina

North Carolina Consumer Protection Section
Special Deputy Attorney General
Office of Attorney General
Raney Building
P.O. Box 629
Raleigh, NC 27602
919-733-7741

North Dakota

North Dakota Consumer Protection Office
Office of Attorney General
600 E. Boulevard
Bismarck, ND 58505
701-224-2210
800-472-2600 (in ND)

Ohio

Ohio Consumer Protection Office
Consumer Frauds and Crimes Section
Office of Attorney General
30 E. Broad Street
State Office Tower, 25th Floor
Columbus, OH 43266-0410
614-466-4986 Complaints
614-466-1393 TDD
800-282-0515 (in OH)

Oklahoma

Oklahoma Consumer Protection Office
Assistant Attorney General
Office of Attorney General
420 W. Main, Suite 550
Oklahoma City, OK 73102
405-521-4274

Oregon

Oregon Consumer Protection Office
Financial Fraud Section
Department of Justice
Justice Building
Salem, OR 97310
503-378-4320

Pennsylvania

Pennsylvania Consumer Protection Office
Bureau of Consumer Protection
Office of Attorney General
Strawberry Square, 14th Floor
Harrisburg, PA 17120
717-787-9707
800-441-2555 (in PA)

Puerto Rico

Puerto Rico Consumer Protection Office
Department of Consumer Affairs–DACO
P.O. Box 41059, Minnillas Station
Santurce, PR 00940
809-721-0940

Rhode Island

Rhode Island Consumer Protection Division
Department of Attorney General
72 Pine Street
Providence, RI 02903
401-277-2104
401-274-4400 ext. 354 Voice/TDD
800-852-7776 (in RI)

South Carolina

South Carolina Consumer Protection Office
Assistant Attorney General
Consumer Fraud and Antitrust Section
Office of Attorney General
P.O. Box 11549
Columbia, SC 29211
803-734-3970

South Dakota

South Dakota Consumer Protection Office
Division of Consumer Affairs
Office of Attorney General
500 E. Capitol
State Capitol Building
Pierre, SD 57501-5070
605-773-4400

Tennessee

Tennessee Consumer Protection Office
Antitrust and Consumer Protection Division
Office of Attorney General
450 James Robertson Parkway
Nashville, TN 37243-0485
615-741-2672

Texas

Texas Consumer Protection Division
Assistant Attorney General and Chief
Office of Attorney General
P.O. Box 12548
Austin, TX 78711
512-463-2070

Utah

Utah Division of Consumer Protection
Department of Commerce
160 East 300 South
P.O. Box 45802
Salt Lake City, UT 84145-0802
801-530-6601

Vermont

Vermont Consumer Protection Office
Assistant Attorney General and Chief
Public Protection Division
Office of Attorney General
109 State Street
Montpelier, VT 05609-1001
802-828-3171

Virgin Islands

Virgin Islands Consumer Protection Office
Department of Licensing and Consumer Affairs
Property and Procurement Building
Subbase #1, Room 205
St. Thomas, VI 00802
809-774-3130

Virginia

Virginia Consumer Protection Office
Antitrust and Consumer Litigation Section
Office of Attorney General
Supreme Court Building
101 N. 8th Street
Richmond, VA 23219
804-786-2116
800-451-1525 (in VA)

Washington

Washington Consumer Protection Office
Consumer and Business
Fair Practices Division
Office of the Attorney General
111 Olympia Avenue N.E.
Olympia, WA 98501
206-753-6210

West Virginia

West Virginia Consumer Protection Division
Office of Attorney General
812 Quarrier Street, 6th Floor
Charleston, WV 25301
304-558-8986
800-368-8808 (in WV)

Wisconsin

Wisconsin Consumer Protection Office
Division of Trade and Consumer Protection
Department of Agriculture, Trade and
Consumer Protection
801 W. Badger Road
P.O. Box 8911
Madison, WI 53708
608-266-9836
800-422-7128 (in WI)

Wyoming

Wyoming Consumer Protection Office
Office of Attorney General
123 State Capitol Building
Cheyenne, WY 82002
307-777-7874

State Developmental Disabilities Offices

These agencies are responsible for coordinating the delivery of services to children and adults with developmental disabilities, including special education classes, career counseling, and medical care. They also assist community agencies involved in providing support services to the developmentally disabled and their families.

Alabama

Developmental Disabilities
Department of Mental Health and Mental Retardation
200 Interstate Park Drive
P.O. Box 3710
Montgomery, AL 36193-5001
205-271-9295

Alaska

Developmental Disabilities
Division of Mental Health and Developmental Disabilities
Department of Health and Social Services
Alaska Office Building, Room 214
P.O. Box 110620
Juneau, AK 99811
907-465-3370

Arizona

Developmental Disabilities
Department of Economic Security
1841 W. Buchanan Street
P.O. Box 6123
Phoenix, AZ 85007
602-258-0419

Arkansas

Developmental Disabilities
Department of Human Services
Donaghey Plaza N., 5th Floor
7th and Main Streets
P.O. Box 1437, Slot 2500
Little Rock, AR 72203-1437
501-682-8662

California

Developmental Disabilities
Department of Developmental Services
Health and Welfare Agency
Gregory Bateson Building, 2nd Floor N.W.
1600 9th Street
Sacramento, CA 95814
916-323-3131

Colorado

Developmental Disabilities
Department of Institutions
3824 W. Princeton Circle
Denver, CO 80236
303-762-4550

Connecticut

Developmental Disabilities
Department of Mental Retardation
90 Pitkin Street
East Hartford, CT 06108
203-528-7141

Delaware

Developmental Disabilities
Division of Mental Retardation
Department of Health and Social Services
Robbins Building
802 Silverlake Road
Dover, DE 19901
302-736-4386

District of Columbia

Developmental Disabilities
Commission on Social Services
Department of Human Services
Bundy Building
429 O Street N.W.
Washington, DC 20001
202-673-7657

Florida

Developmental Disabilities
Developmental Services
Department of Health and Rehabilitative Services
Building V, Room 215
1311 Winewood Boulevard
Tallahassee, FL 32399-0700
904-488-4257

Georgia

Developmental Disabilities
Division of Mental Health, Mental Retardation
and Substance Abuse
Department of Human Services
878 Peachtree Street, Suite 306
Atlanta, GA 30309
404-894-6313

Hawaii

Developmental Disabilities
Community Services for the Developmentally
Disabled Branch
Developmental Disabilities Division
Department of Health
741-A Sunset Avenue, Room 208
Honolulu, HI 96816
808-732-0935

Idaho

Developmental Disabilities
State Council on Developmental Disabilities
Towers Building
450 W. State Street
Boise, ID 83720
208-334-5509

Illinois

Developmental Disabilities
Department of Mental Health and
Developmental Disabilities
William G. Stratton Office Building
401 S. Spring Street
Springfield, IL 62706
217-782-7179

Indiana

Developmental Disabilities
Division on Developmental Disabilities
Department of Mental Health
117 E. Washington Street
Indianapolis, IN 46204
317-232-7836

Iowa

Developmental Disabilities
Division of Mental Health, Retardation and
Developmental Disabilities
Department of Human Services
Hoover State Office Building, 5th Floor
1300 E. Walnut Street
Des Moines, IA 50319
515-281-6003

Kansas

Developmental Disabilities
Mental Health and Retardation Services
Department of Social and Rehabilitation Services
Docking State Office Building, 5th Floor
915 Harrison Street
Topeka, KS 66612
913-296-2608

Kentucky

Developmental Disabilities
Division of Mental Retardation
Department of Mental Health and Mental
Retardation Services
Human Resources Cabinet
Health Services Building
275 E. Main Street
Frankfort, KY 40621
502-564-7700

Louisiana

Developmental Disabilities
Office of Mental Retardation and
Developmental Disabilities
Department of Health and Human Services
Schwing Building, Room 305
721 Government Street
Baton Rouge, LA 70802
504-342-6811

Maine

Developmental Disabilities
Department of Mental Health and Mental Retardation
Nash Building
102 Sewall Street
Statehouse Station 40
Augusta, ME 04333
207-289-4213

Maryland

Developmental Disabilities
Department of Health and Mental Hygiene
Herbert R. O'Conor State Office Building, Room 422C
201 W. Preston Street
Baltimore, MD 21201
410-225-5600

Massachusetts

Developmental Disabilities
Executive Office of Human Services
Department of Mental Retardation
Hoffman Building
160 N. Washington Street
Boston, MA 02114
617-727-5608

Michigan

Developmental Disabilities
Department of Mental Health
Lewis Cass Building, 5th Floor
320 S. Walnut Street
Lansing, MI 48913
517-373-3500

Minnesota

Developmental Disabilities
Department of Human Resources
444 Lafayette Road
St. Paul, MN 55155-3825
612-296-1898

Mississippi

Developmental Disabilities
Bureau of Mental Retardation
Department of Mental Health
1101 Robert E. Lee Building
239 N. Lamar Street
Jackson, MS 39201
601-359-1288

Missouri

Developmental Disabilities
Division of Mental Retardation and Developmental
Disabilities
Department of Mental Health
1915 Southridge Drive
P.O. Box 687
Jefferson City, MO 65102
314-751-4054

Montana

Developmental Disabilities
Department of Social and Rehabilitation Services
SRS Building, Room 202
111 Sanders Street
P.O. Box 4210
Helena, MT 59604
406-444-2995

Nebraska

Developmental Disabilities
Office of Mental Retardation
Department of Public Institutions
W. Van Dorn and Folsom Streets
P.O. Box 94728
Lincoln, NE 68509
402-471-2851 ext. 5110

Nevada

Developmental Disabilities
Division of Mental Hygiene and Mental Retardation
Department of Human Resources
Kinkead Building, Room 403
505 E. King Street
Carson City, NV 89710
702-885-5943

New Hampshire

Developmental Disabilities
Division of Mental Health and Developmental Services
Department of Health and Human Services
State Office Park S.
105 Pleasant Street
Concord, NH 03301-6523
603-271-5007

New Jersey

Developmental Disabilities
Department of Human Services
Capitol Place One
222 S. Warren Street, CN-700
Trenton, NJ 08625
609-292-3742

New Mexico

Developmental Disabilities
Behavioral Health Services Division
Health and Environmental Department
Harold Runnels Building
1190 St. Francis Drive
Santa Fe, NM 87501
505-827-2573

New York

Developmental Disabilities
Mental Retardation and Developmental Disabilities Office
44 Holland Avenue
Albany, NY 12229
518-473-1997

North Carolina

Developmental Disabilities
Office of the Secretary
Department of Human Resources
1508 Western Boulevard
Raleigh, NC 27606
919-733-6566

North Dakota

Developmental Disabilities
Department of Human Services
State Capitol Annex
Bismarck, ND 58505
701-224-2768

Ohio

Developmental Disabilities
Department of Mental Retardation and
Developmental Disabilities
State Office Tower, Room 1280
30 E. Broad Street
Columbus, OH 43266-0415
614-466-5214

Oklahoma

Developmental Disabilities
Services for the Mentally Retarded and
Developmentally Disabled
Department of Human Services
Will Rogers Memorial Office Building, Room 303
2401 N. Lincoln Boulevard
Oklahoma City, OK 73125
405-521-3617

Oregon

Developmental Disabilities
Mental Health Division
Department of Human Resources
2575 Bittern Street N.E.
Salem, OR 97310
503-378-2429

Pennsylvania

Developmental Disabilities
Office of Mental Retardation
Department of Public Welfare
Health and Welfare Building, Room 302
Forster Street and Commonwealth Avenue
Harrisburg, PA 17120
717-787-3700

Puerto Rico

Developmental Disabilities
Vocational Rehabilitation Services
Department of Social Services
P.O. Box 1118
Santurce, PR 00919
809-725-1792

Rhode Island

Developmental Disabilities
Division of Retardation and Developmental Disabilities
Department of Mental Health, Retardation, and Hospitals
Aime J. Forand Building
600 New London Avenue
Cranston, RI 02920
401-464-3231

South Carolina

Developmental Disabilities
Department of Mental Retardation
2712 Middleburg Drive
P.O. Box 4706
Columbia, SC 29240
803-737-6444

South Dakota

Developmental Disabilities
Department of Social Services
Richard F. Kneip Building
700 Governor's Drive
Pierre, SD 57501
605-773-3438

Tennessee

Developmental Disabilities
Mental Retardation Services Division
Department of Mental Health and Mental Retardation
Doctors Building, 3rd Floor
706 Church Street
Nashville, TN 37219
615-741-3803

Texas

Developmental Disabilities
Department of Mental Retardation Services
Department of Mental Health and Retardation
909 W. 45th Street
P.O. Box 12668, Capitol Station
Austin, TX 78711
512-465-4521

Utah

Developmental Disabilities
Division of Services to the Handicapped
Department of Social Services
Social Services Building, Room 234
120 North 200 West
P.O. Box 45500
Salt Lake City, UT 84103
801-538-4200

Vermont

Developmental Disabilities
Agency of Human Services
Waterbury Office Complex
103 S. Main Street
Waterbury, VT 05676
802-241-2612

Virgin Islands

Developmental Disabilities
Special Services Section
Disabilities and Rehabilitation Services
Department of Human Services
Barbel Plaza S.
St. Thomas, VI 00802
809-774-4775

Virginia

Developmental Disabilities
Department of Mental Health, Mental Retardation
and Substance Abuse
James Madison Building
109 Governor Street
P.O. Box 1797
Richmond, VA 23214
804-786-5313

Washington

Developmental Disabilities
Department of Social and Health Services
Mail Stop OB-42C
Olympia, WA 98504
206-753-0541

Wisconsin

Developmental Disabilities
Division of Community Services
Department of Health and Social Services
Wilson Street State Office Building
One W. Wilson Street
P.O. Box 7851
Madison, WI 53707
608-266-9329

Wyoming

Developmental Disabilities
Division of Community Programs
Department of Health and Social Services
Hathaway Building, Room 354
2300 Capitol Avenue
Cheyenne, WY 82002-0710
307-777-7115

State Food and Drug Offices

These agencies are responsible for the purity, quality and safety of foods and drugs sold in their state. They are also responsible for inspecting agricultural and animal products brought into their state to determine if these products conform to state standards.

Alabama

Food and Drugs
Department of Agriculture and Industries
Richard Beard Building
1445 Federal Drive
P.O. Box 3336
Montgomery, AL 36193
205-242-2656

Alaska

Food and Drugs
Division of Environmental Health
Department of Environmental Conservation
3232 Channel Drive
P.O. Box 0
Juneau, AK 99811-1800
907-465-2696

Arizona

Food and Drugs
Department of Health Services
1740 W. Adams Street
Phoenix, AZ 85007
602-255-1181

Arkansas

Food and Drugs
Food and Dairy Products Section
Division of Sanitation Services
Department of Health
State Health Building
4815 W. Markham Street
Little Rock, AR 72205-3867
501-661-2171

California

Food and Drugs
Department of Food and Agriculture
1220 N Street
Sacramento, CA 95814
916-445-7126

Colorado

Food and Drugs
Consumer Protection Division
Department of Health
4210 E. 11th Avenue
Denver, CO 80220
303-320-8333

Connecticut

Food and Drugs
Food Division
Department of Consumer Protection
165 Capitol Avenue, Room 167
Hartford, CT 06106
203-566-3388

Delaware

Food and Drugs
Division of Standards and Inspections
Department of Agriculture
2320 S. DuPont Highway
Dover, DE 19901
302-739-4811

District of Columbia

Food and Drugs
Food Protection Branch
Department of Consumer and Regulatory Affairs
614 H Street N.W., Room 616
Washington, DC 20001
202-727-7250

Florida

Food and Drugs
Food Laboratory
Agriculture and Consumer Services
3125 Conner Boulevard
Tallahassee, FL 32399
904-488-0670

Georgia

Food and Drugs
Environmental Health Section
Department of Human Resources
878 Peachtree Street N.E.
Atlanta, GA 30309
404-894-6644

Hawaii

Food and Drugs
Environmental Health Administration
Department of Health
1250 Punchbowl Street
Honolulu, HI 96813
808-548-4139

Idaho

Food and Drugs
Food Program Compliance Officer
Food Section
Bureau of Health
Department of Health and Welfare
450 W. State Street
Boise, ID 83720
208-334-5938

Illinois

Food and Drugs
Department of Public Health
535 W. Jefferson Street
Springfield, IL 62761
217-782-4977

Indiana

Food and Drugs
Bureau of Consumer Protection
State Board of Health
Health Building, Room 136
1330 W. Michigan Street
Indianapolis, IN 46206
317-633-0313

Iowa

Food and Drugs
Program Manager
Inspections Division
Department of Inspections and Appeals
Lucas State Office Building, 3rd Floor
E. 12th and Walnut Streets
Des Moines, IA 50319
515-281-6538

Kansas

Food and Drugs
Bureau of Environmental Health Services
Department of Health and Environment
109 S.W. 9th, Suite 604
Topeka, KS 66620
913-296-0189

Kentucky

Food and Drugs
Division of Food Distribution
Department of Agriculture
Capitol Plaza Tower
Frankfort, KY 40601
502-564-4387

Louisiana

Food and Drugs
Department of Health and Hospitals
325 Loyola Avenue
New Orleans, LA 70112
504-568-5050

Maine

Food and Drugs
Department of Agriculture, Food and Rural Resources
Statehouse Station 28
Augusta, ME 04333
207-289-3871

Maryland

Food and Drugs
Food Protection and Community Health
Department of Health and Mental Hygiene
4201 Patterson Avenue
Baltimore, MD 21201
410-764-3579

Massachusetts

Food and Drugs
Division of Food and Drugs
Department of Public Health
305 South Street
Jamaica Plain, MA 02130
617-727-3163

Michigan

Food and Drugs
Food Division
Department of Agriculture
Ottawa Building N.
611 W. Ottawa Street
Lansing, MI 48909
517-373-1060

Minnesota

Food and Drugs
Food Inspection Division
Department of Agriculture
90 W. Plato Boulevard
St. Paul, MN 55107
612-296-2627

Mississippi

Food and Drugs
Division of Sanitation
Department of Public Health
P.O. Box 1700
Jackson, MS 39215-1700
601-960-7690

Missouri

Food and Drugs
Bureau of Community Sanitation
Department of Health
1730 E. Elm
P.O. Box 570
Jefferson City, MO 65102-0570
314-751-6095

Montana

Food and Drugs
Food and Consumer Safety Bureau
Health and Environmental Sciences
W. F. Cogswell Building, Room A104
Helena, MT 59620
406-444-2408

Nebraska

Food and Drugs
Food Division Manager
Bureau of Dairies and Foods
Department of Agriculture
State Office Building
301 Centennial Mall S.
P.O. Box 95064
Lincoln, NE 68509
402-471-2341

Nevada

Food and Drugs
Regulatory Health Services Bureau
Department of Human Resources
Kinkead Building, Room 201
505 E. King Street
Carson City, NV 89710
702-687-4475

New Hampshire

Food and Drugs
Bureau of Environmental Health
Department of Health and Welfare
Health and Human Services Building
6 Hazen Drive
Concord, NH 03301
603-271-4587

New Jersey

Food and Drugs
Division of Regulatory Services
Department of Agriculture
John Fitch Plaza, CN-330
Trenton, NJ 08625
609-292-5575

New Mexico

Food and Drugs
Department of Agriculture
New Mexico State University
Department 3189
P.O. Box 30005
Las Cruces, NM 87504-0968
505-646-3007

New York

Food and Drugs
Department of Agriculture and Markets
Capital Plaza
One Winners Circle
Albany, NY 12235
518-457-4188

North Carolina

Food and Drugs
Food and Drug Protection Division
Department of Agriculture
Constable Laboratory
4000 Reedy Creek Road
Raleigh, NC 27607
919-733-7366

North Dakota

Food and Drugs
Consolidated Laboratories
Department of Health
2635 E. Main Street
P.O. Box 937
Bismarck, ND 58502-0937
701-221-6140

Ohio

Food and Drugs
Division of Food, Dairies and Drugs
Department of Agriculture
Building 1
8995 E. Main Street
Reynoldsburg, OH 43068
614-866-6361

Oklahoma

Food and Drugs
Food Protection Service
Department of Health
1000 N.E. 10th Street, Room 355
P.O. Box 53551
Oklahoma City, OK 73152
405-271-5243

Oregon

Food and Drugs
Food and Dairy Division
Department of Agriculture
Agriculture Building
635 Capitol Street N.E.
Salem, OR 97310-0110
503-378-3790

Pennsylvania

Food and Drugs
Bureau of Food and Chemistry
Department of Agriculture
2301 N. Cameron Street, Room 112
Harrisburg, PA 17110
717-787-6416

Rhode Island

Food and Drugs
Food Protection and Sanitation
Department of Health
Cannon Building, Room 304
75 Davis Street
Providence, RI 02908
401-277-2833

South Carolina

Food and Drugs
Division of Food Protection
Department of Health and Environmental Control
Robert Mills Building, Room 0-131
2600 Bull Street
Columbia, SC 29201
803-734-5088

South Dakota

Food and Drugs
Department of Health
Joe Foss Building
523 E. Capitol Avenue
Pierre, SD 57501
605-773-3361

Tennessee

Food and Drugs
Quality Standards Dairy
Department of Agriculture
Ellington Agricultural Center
Nashville, TN 37204
615-360-0150

Texas

Food and Drugs
Bureau of Consumer Health Protection
Division of Food and Drugs
Department of Health
1100 W. 49th Street
Austin, TX 78756
512-458-7248

Utah

Food and Drugs
Bureau of Food and Consumer Services
Department of Agriculture
William Spry Building
350 N. Redwood Road
Salt Lake City, UT 84116
801-538-7150

Vermont

Food and Drugs
Division of Environmental Health
Department of Health
60 Main Street
Burlington, VT 05402
802-863-7221

Virgin Islands

Food and Drugs
Department of Health
St. Thomas Hospital
St. Thomas, VI 00802
809-774-0117

Virginia

Food and Drugs
Dairy and Foods Division
Department of Agriculture and Consumer Services
Washington Building, Capitol Square
1100 Bank Street
Richmond, VA 23209
804-786-8899

Washington

Food and Drugs
Food Safety and Animal Health Division
Department of Agriculture
2627 B Parkmont Lane S.W.
Mail Stop JT-16
Olympia, WA 98502
206-753-5043

West Virginia

Food and Drugs
Public Health Sanitation
Office of Environmental Health Services
Department of Health
State Office Building 3, Room 507
1800 Washington Street E.
Charleston, WV 25305
304-558-2981

Wisconsin

Food and Drugs
Food Division
Department of Agriculture, Trade and
Consumer Protection
801 W. Badger Road
P.O. Box 8911
Madison, WI 53708
608-266-7240

Wyoming

Food and Drugs
Food and Drug Section
Department of Agriculture
Smith Building
2219 Carey Avenue
Cheyenne, WY 82002
307-777-6587

State Governors' Offices

The governor is the chief executive officer of the state and is responsible for submitting legislation to the legislature, preparing the state budget and managing all state departments and programs.

Alabama
Alabama Governor
State Capitol
600 Dexter Avenue
Montgomery, AL 36130
205-242-7100

Alaska
Alaska Governor
P.O. Box 11001
Juneau, AK 99811-0001
907-465-3500

Arizona
Arizona Governor
Statehouse
Phoenix, AZ 85007
602-542-4331

Arkansas
Arkansas Governor
State Capitol
Little Rock, AR 72201
501-682-2345

California
California Governor
State Capitol
Sacramento, CA 95814
916-445-2841

Colorado
Colorado Governor
136 State Capitol
Denver, CO 80203
303-866-2471

Connecticut
Connecticut Governor
State Capitol
Hartford, CT 06106
203-566-4840

Delaware
Delaware Governor
Tatnall Building
William Penn Street
Dover, DE 19901
302-739-4101

Florida
Florida Governor
State Capitol
Tallahassee, FL 32399-0001
904-488-2272

Georgia
Georgia Governor
203 State Capitol
Atlanta, GA 30334
404-656-1776

Hawaii
Hawaii Governor
State Capitol
Honolulu, HI 96813
808-586-0034

Idaho
Idaho Governor
Statehouse
Boise, ID 83720
208-334-2100

Illinois
Illinois Governor
State Capitol
Springfield, IL 62706
217-782-6830

Indiana
Indiana Governor
206 Statehouse
Indianapolis, IN 46204
317-232-4567

Iowa
Iowa Governor
State Capitol
Des Moines, IA 50319
515-281-5211

Kansas
Kansas Governor
State Capitol
Topeka, KS 66612-1590
913-296-3232

Kentucky
Kentucky Governor
State Capitol
Frankfort, KY 40601
502-564-2611

Louisiana
Louisiana Governor
State Capitol
P.O. Box 94004
Baton Rouge, LA 70804
504-342-7015

Maine
Maine Governor
Statehouse Station 1
Augusta, ME 04333
207-289-3531

Maryland
Maryland Governor
Statehouse
Annapolis, MD 21401
410-974-3901

Massachusetts
Massachusetts Governor
Statehouse, Room 360
Boston, MA 02133
617-727-9173

Michigan
Michigan Governor
State Capitol
P.O. Box 30013
Lansing, MI 48909
517-373-3400

Minnesota
Minnesota Governor
130 State Capitol
St. Paul, MN 55155
612-296-3391

Mississippi
Mississippi Governor
P.O. Box 139
Jackson, MS 39205
601-359-3100

Missouri
Missouri Governor
P.O. Box 720
Jefferson City, MO 65102
314-751-3222

Montana
Montana Governor
State Capitol
Helena, MT 59620
406-444-3111

Nebraska
Nebraska Governor
State Capitol
P.O. Box 94848
Lincoln, NE 68509
402-471-2244

Nevada
Nevada Governor
State Capitol
Carson City, NV 89710
702-687-5670

New Hampshire
New Hampshire Governor
State of New Hampshire
Office of Governor
Concord, NH 03301-4990
603-271-2121

New Jersey
New Jersey Governor
Statehouse, CN-001
Trenton, NJ 08625
609-292-6000

New Mexico
New Mexico Governor
State Capitol
Santa Fe, NM 87503
505-827-3000

New York
New York Governor
State Capitol
Albany, NY 12224
518-474-8390

North Carolina
North Carolina Governor
State Capitol
Raleigh, NC 27603
919-733-4240

North Dakota
North Dakota Governor
State Capitol
600 E. Boulevard Avenue
Bismarck, ND 58505
701-224-2200

Ohio
Ohio Governor
77 S. High Street, 30th Floor
Columbus, OH 43266-0601
614-466-3555

Oklahoma
Oklahoma Governor
State Capitol
Oklahoma City, OK 73105
405-521-2342

Oregon
Oregon Governor
245 State Capitol
Salem, OR 97310
503-378-3100

Pennsylvania
Pennsylvania Governor
245 E. Capitol Building
Harrisburg, PA 17120
717-787-2500

Puerto Rico
Puerto Rico Office of the Governor
La Fortaleza
San Juan, PR 00901
809-724-2100

Rhode Island
Rhode Island Governor
Statehouse
Providence, RI 02903
401-277-2080

South Carolina
South Carolina Governor
P.O. Box 11369
Columbia, SC 29211
803-734-9818

South Dakota
South Dakota Governor
State Capitol
Pierre, SD 57501
605-773-3212

Tennessee
Tennessee Governor
State Capitol
Nashville, TN 37243-0001
615-741-2001

Texas
Texas Governor
P.O. Box 12428
Capitol Station
Austin, TX 78711
512-463-2000

Utah
Utah Governor
210 State Capitol
Salt Lake City, UT 84114
801-538-1000

Vermont
Vermont Governor
Pavilion Office Building
Montpelier, VT 05609
802-828-3333

Virgin Islands
Virgin Islands Office of the Governor
Government House
Charlotte Amalie
St. Thomas, VI 00801
809-774-0001

Virginia
Virginia Governor
State Capitol
Richmond, VA 23219
804-786-2211

Washington
Washington Governor
Legislative Building
Olympia, WA 98504
206-753-6780

West Virginia
West Virginia Governor
State Capitol
Charleston, WV 25305
304-558-2000

Wisconsin
Wisconsin Governor
115 East Washington Avenue
Madison, WI 53702
608-266-1212

Wyoming
Wyoming Governor
State Capitol
Cheyenne, WY 82002
307-777-7434

State Health Departments

State health departments are responsible for administering public health programs and policies within the states they serve. Write or telephone your state's health department to learn more about specific programs available in your community.

Alabama

Alabama Department of Public Health
State Office Building
501 Dexter Avenue
Mail to: 434 Monroe Street
Montgomery, AL 36130-1701
205-242-5095

Alaska

Alaska Department of Health and Social Services
Alaska Office Building, Room 503
350 Main Street
Pouch H-06
Juneau, AK 99811-0610
907-465-3030

Arizona

Arizona Department of Health Services
1740 W. Adams Street
Phoenix, AZ 85007
602-542-1024

Arkansas

Arkansas Department of Health
State Health Building
4815 W. Markham Street
Little Rock, AR 72205-3867
501-661-2112

California

California Department of Health Services
714 P Street, Room 1253
Sacramento, CA 95814
916-445-1248

Colorado

Colorado Department of Health
4210 E. 11th Avenue
Denver, CO 80220
303-331-4602

Connecticut

Connecticut Department of Health Services
150 Washington Street
Hartford, CT 06106
203-566-2038

Delaware

Delaware Division of Public Health
Department of Health and Social Services
Jesse Cooper Building
P.O. Box 637
Dover, DE 19901
302-736-4701

District of Columbia

District of Columbia Department of Human Services
Commission of Public Health
1660 L Street N.W., 12th Floor
Washington, DC 20036
202-673-7700

Florida

Florida Health Program Office
Department of Health and Rehabilitative Services
Building I, Room 115
1323 Winewood Boulevard
Tallahassee, FL 32399-0700
904-488-4115

Georgia

Georgia Division of Public Health
Department of Human Resources
878 Peachtree Street N.E., Suite 201
Atlanta, GA 30309
404-894-7505

Hawaii

Hawaii Department of Health
Kinau Hale
1250 Punchbowl Street
P.O. Box 3378
Honolulu, HI 96801
808-548-6505

Idaho

Idaho Bureau of Preventive Medicine
Division of Health
Department of Health and Welfare
Towers Building, 4th Floor
450 W. State Street
Boise, ID 83720
208-334-5930

Illinois

Illinois Department of Public Health
535 W. Jefferson Street
Springfield, IL 62761
217-782-4977

Indiana

Indiana State Board of Health
1330 W. Michigan Street
P.O. Box 1964
Indianapolis, IN 46206-1964
317-633-8400

Iowa

Iowa Department of Public Health
Lucas State Office Building
E. 12th and Walnut Streets
Des Moines, IA 50319
515-281-5605

Kansas

Kansas Division of Health
Department of Health and Environment
Forbes Field, Building 740
Topeka, KS 66620
913-296-1500

Kentucky

Kentucky Department for Health Services
Cabinet for Human Resources
Health Services Building, 1st Floor
275 E. Main Street
Frankfort, KY 40621
502-564-3970

Louisiana

Louisiana Department of Hospitals
Department of Health and Human Resources
Office of Public Health Services
325 Loyola Avenue
P.O. Box 60630
New Orleans, LA 70160
504-568-5052

Maine

Maine Bureau of Health
Department of Human Services
157 Capitol Street
Statehouse Station 11
Augusta, ME 04333
207-289-3201

Maryland

Maryland Department of Health and Mental Hygiene
Herbert R. O'Conor State Office Building
201 W. Preston Street
Baltimore, MD 21201
410-225-6500

Massachusetts

Massachusetts Department of Public Health
150 Tremont Street
Boston, MA 02111
617-727-0201

Michigan

Michigan Department of Public Health
Baker-Olin West Building
3423 N. Logan Street
P.O. Box 30195
Lansing, MI 48909
517-335-8000

Minnesota

Minnesota Department of Health
717 Delaware Street S.E.
P.O. Box 9441
Minneapolis, MN 55440
612-623-5460

Mississippi

Mississippi Department of Health
2423 N. State Street
P.O. Box 1700
Jackson, MS 39215-1700
601-960-7400

Missouri

Missouri Department of Health
P.O. Box 570
Jefferson City, MO 65102
314-751-6001

Montana

Montana Department of Health and
Environmental Sciences
Cogswell Building, Room C108
Helena, MT 59620
406-444-2544

Nebraska

Nebraska Department of Health
State Office Building
301 Centennial Mall S.
P.O. Box 95007
Lincoln, NE 68509
402-471-2133

Nevada

Nevada Health Division
Department of Human Resources
Kinkead Building
505 E. King Street
Carson City, NV 89710
702-885-4740

New Hampshire

New Hampshire Division of Public Health Services
Department of Health and Human Services
Health and Welfare Services Building
6 Hazen Drive
Concord, NH 03301-6527
603-271-4501

New Jersey

New Jersey Department of Health
Health and Agriculture Building
John Fitch Plaza, CN-360
Trenton, NJ 08625
609-292-7837

New Mexico
New Mexico Division of Public Health
Health and Environment Department
Harold Runnels Building
1190 St. Francis Drive
Santa Fe, NM 87503
505-827-0020

New York
New York Department of Health
Corning Tower, Room 1408
Empire State Plaza
Albany, NY 12237
518-474-2011

North Carolina
North Carolina Department of Environmental Health
and Natural Resources
Office of the State Health Director
Archdale Building
512 N. Salisbury Street
P.O. Box 27687
Raleigh, NC 27611
919-733-3446

North Dakota
North Dakota Department of Health
State Capitol
600 E. Boulevard Avenue
Bismarck, ND 58505-0200
701-224-2372

Ohio
Ohio Department of Health
246 N. High Street
Columbus, OH 43226-0588
614-466-3543

Oklahoma
Oklahoma Department of Health
1000 N.E. 10th Street
P.O. Box 53551
Oklahoma City, OK 73152
405-271-4200

Oregon
Oregon Health Division
Department of Human Resources
State Office Building, Room 811
1400 S.W. 5th Avenue
P.O. Box 231
Portland, OR 97207
503-229-5032

Pennsylvania
Pennsylvania Department of Health
Health and Welfare Building, Room 802
Commonwealth Avenue and Forster Street
P.O. Box 90
Harrisburg, PA 17108
717-787-6436

Puerto Rico
Puerto Rico Department of Health
Call Box 70184
San Juan, PR 00936
809-250-7227

Rhode Island
Rhode Island Department of Health
Cannon Building, Room 401
3 Capitol Hill
Providence, RI 02908
401-277-2231

South Carolina
South Carolina Department of Health and
Environmental Control
2600 Bull Street
Columbia, SC 29201
803-734-4880

South Dakota
South Dakota Department of Health
Joe Foss Building
523 E. Capitol Avenue
Pierre, SD 57501
605-773-3361

Tennessee
Tennessee Department of Health and Environment
Cordell Hull Building, Room 344
Nashville, TN 37219
615-741-3111

Texas
Texas Department of Health
1100 W. 49th Street
Austin, TX 78756-3199
512-458-7375

Utah
Utah Department of Health
288 North 1460 West
Salt Lake City, UT 84116-0700
801-538-6101

Vermont

Vermont Department of Health
Agency of Human Services
60 Main Street
P.O. Box 70
Burlington, VT 05402
802-863-7280

Virgin Islands

Virgin Islands Department of Heatlh
St. Thomas Hospital
Charlotte Amalie
St. Thomas, VI 00802
809-774-0117

Virginia

Virginia Department of Health
James Madison Building
109 Governor Street
Richmond, VA 23219
804-786-3561

Washington

Washington Division of Health
Department of Health
1112 S. Quince Street
Mail Stop ET-21
Olympia, WA 98504
206-753-5871

West Virginia

West Virginia Department of Health
State Office Building 3, Room 206
1800 Washington Street E.
Charleston, WV 25305
304-558-2971

Wisconsin

Wisconsin Division of Health
Department of Health and Social Services
One W. Wilson Street
P.O. Box 309
Madison, WI 53701-0309
608-266-7568

Wyoming

Wyoming Department of Health and Social Services
Hathaway Building
2300 Capitol Avenue
Cheyenne, WY 82002-0710
307-777-7656

State Mental Health and Mental Retardation Offices

These agencies are responsible for planning the delivery of mental health services to children and adults who are mentally ill or mentally retarded. They also assist community agencies involved in providing support services to the mentally ill or mentally retarded and their families.

Alabama

Mental Health Office
Mental Retardation Division
Department of Mental Health
P.O. Box 3710
Montgomery, AL 36193
205-271-9209

Alaska

Mental Health Office
Mental Health and Developmental Disabilities Division
P.O. Box H
Juneau, AK 99811
907-465-3370

Arizona

Mental Health Office
Developmental Disabilities Division
Department of Economic Security
1717 W. Jefferson
Phoenix, AZ 85007
602-542-5775

Arkansas

Mental Health Office
Division of Mental Health
Department of Human Services
4313 W. Markham
Little Rock, AR 72205
501-686-9165

California

Mental Health Office
Department of Mental Health
1600 9th Street
Sacramento, CA 95814
916-323-8173

Colorado

Mental Health Office
Developmental Disabilities Division
Department of Institutions
3824 W. Princeton Circle
Denver, CO 80236
303-762-4560

Connecticut
Mental Health Office
Department of Mental Retardation
90 Pitkin Street
East Hartford, CT 06108
203-725-3860

Delaware
Mental Health Office
Division of Alcoholism, Drug Abuse and Mental Health
1901 N. DuPont Highway
New Castle, DE 19720
302-421-6107

District of Columbia
Mental Health Office
Mental Health Service
Department of Human Services
A Building, Room 107
2100 Martin Luther King Jr. Avenue S.E.
Washington, DC 20032
202-373-7166

Florida
Mental Health Office
Alcohol, Drug Abuse and Mental Health
1317 Winewood
Building 6, Room 183
Tallahassee, FL 32399
904-488-8304

Georgia
Mental Health Office
Mental Health, Mental Retardation and Substance Abuse
878 Peachtree Street N.E.
Atlanta, GA 30309
404-894-6300

Hawaii
Mental Health Office
Waimano Training School and Hospital
Department of Health
Pearl City, HI 96782
808-456-6255

Idaho
Mental Health Office
Division of Community Rehabilitation
Department of Health and Welfare
450 W. State Street
Boise, ID 83720
208-334-5528

Illinois
Mental Health Office
Department of Mental Health and
Developmental Disabilities
401 Stratton Building
Springfield, IL 62706
217-782-2243

Indiana
Mental Health Office
Division of Mental Health and Addictions
402 W. Washington Street
Indianapolis, IN 46204
317-232-7844

Iowa
Mental Health Office
Department of Human Services
Hoover State Office Building
Des Moines, IA 50319
515-281-6360

Kansas
Mental Health Office
Mental Health and Retardation
Social and Rehabilitation Services Department
Docking Office Building, 5th Floor
Topeka, KS 66612
913-296-3774

Kentucky
Mental Health Office
Mental Health and Retardation Services Department
275 E. Main Street
Frankfort, KY 40601
502-564-4527

Louisiana
Mental Health Office
Office of Human Services
Department of Health and Hospitals
P.O. Box 2790, Bin 18
Baton Rouge, LA 70821
504-342-6717

Maine
Mental Health Office
Department of Mental Health and Mental Retardation
Statehouse Station 40
Augusta, ME 04333
207-289-4223

Maryland
Mental Health Office
Developmental Disabilities Administration
Department of Health and Mental Hygiene
201 W. Preston Street, 4th Floor
Baltimore, MD 21201
410-225-5600

Massachusetts
Mental Health Office
Department of Mental Retardation
160 N. Washington Street
Boston, MA 02114
617-727-5608

Michigan
Mental Health Office
Department of Mental Health
300 S. Walnut, 6th Floor
P.O. Box 30037
Lansing, MI 48962
517-373-3500

Minnesota
Mental Health Office
Mental Health Bureau
Department of Human Services
658 Cedar Street
St. Paul, MN 55155
612-296-2710

Mississippi
Mental Health Office
Department of Mental Health
1101 Robert E. Lee Building
Jackson, MS 39201
601-359-1288

Missouri
Mental Health Office
Department of Mental Health
1915 Southridge
P.O. Box 687
Jefferson City, MO 65102
314-751-3070

Montana
Mental Health Office
Mental Health Division
Department of Institutions
1539 11th Avenue
Helena, MT 59620
406-444-3969

Nebraska
Mental Health Office
Department of Public Institutions
P.O. Box 94728
Lincoln, NE 68509
402-471-2851

Nevada
Mental Health Office
Mental Hygiene and Mental Retardation
505 E. King Street
Carson City, NV 89710
702-687-5943

New Hampshire
Mental Health Office
Division of Mental Health and Developmental Services
Hazen Drive
Concord, NH 03301
603-271-4681

New Jersey
Mental Health Office
Division of Mental Health and Hospitals
Department of Human Services
Capitol Center, CN-727
Trenton, NJ 08625
609-777-0700

New Mexico
Mental Health Office
Mental Health Bureau
Department of Health
P.O. Box 26110
Santa Fe, NM 87502
505-827-2644

New York
Mental Health Office
Mental Retardation and Developmental Disabilities
44 Holland Avenue
Albany, NY 12229
518-473-1997

North Carolina
Mental Health Office
Mental Health, Retardation and Substance Abuse
Department of Human Resources
325 N. Salisbury Street
Raleigh, NC 27603
919-733-7011

North Dakota
Mental Health Office
Mental Health and Retardation
Department of Human Services
State Capitol, Judicial Wing
600 E. Boulevard
Bismarck, ND 58505
701-224-2766

Ohio
Mental Health Office
Department of Mental Health
30 E. Broad Street, 11th Floor
Columbus, OH 43266
614-466-2337

Oklahoma
Mental Health Office
Department of Mental Health and Substance
Abuse Services
P.O. Box 53277
Oklahoma City, OK 73152
405-271-8644

Oregon
Mental Health Office
Mental Health Division
Department of Human Resources
2575 Bittern Street N.E.
Salem, OR 97310
503-378-2671

Pennsylvania
Mental Health Office
Department of Public Welfare
432 Health and Welfare Building
Harrisburg, PA 17120
717-787-3700

Puerto Rico
Mental Health Office
Mental Health Care
Department of Mental Health
P.O. Box 9342
Santurce, PR 00908
809-781-5660

Rhode Island
Mental Health Office
Retardation Service
Mental Health, Retardation and Hospitals
600 New London Avenue
Cranston, RI 02920
401-464-3234

South Carolina
Mental Health Office
Department of Mental Health
2414 Bull Street
Columbia, SC 29202
803-734-7780

South Dakota
Mental Health Office
Developmental Disabilities
Department of Human Services
Kneip Building
Pierre, SD 57501
605-773-3438

Tennessee
Mental Health Office
Department of Mental Health and Mental Retardation
706 Church Street, Suite 600
Nashville, TN 37243
615-741-3107

Texas
Mental Health Office
Mental Health and Mental Retardation
P.O. Box 12668, Capitol Station
Austin, TX 78711
512-454-3761

Utah
Mental Health Office
Service to the Handicapped
Department of Human Services
120 North 200 West, 4th Floor
Salt Lake City, UT 84103
801-538-4199

Vermont
Mental Health Office
Mental Health and Retardation
Agency of Human Services
103 S. Main Street
Waterbury, VT 05671
802-241-2600

Virgin Islands
Mental Health Office
Department of Health
St. Croix Hospital
St. Croix, VI 00820
809-778-6311

Virginia
Mental Health Office
Mental Health, Retardation and Substance Abuse Services
109 Governor Street
Richmond, VA 23219
804-786-3921

Washington
Mental Health Office
Health and Rehabilitation Services
Social and Health Services Department
OB-2, 4th Floor
Mail Stop OB-44M
Olympia, WA 98504
206-753-3327

West Virginia

Mental Health Office
Health and Human Resources Department
Building 6, Room B-617
State Capitol Complex
Charleston, WV 25305
304-558-2400

Wisconsin

Mental Health Office
Office of Developmental Disabilities
Health and Social Services Department
P.O. Box 7851
Madison, WI 53707
608-266-0805

Wyoming

Mental Health Office
Wyoming Department of Health
Hathaway Building
Cheyenne, WY 82002
307-777-6778

State Occupational and Professional Licensing Offices

These agencies are responsible for licensing and regulating various licensed professionals, including some limited-license health care practitioners (for example, chiropractors, physical therapists, and massage therapists, to name a few). Inquiries and complaints concerning limited-license practitioners should be reported to these offices.

Alaska

Alaska Division of Occupational Licensing
Department of Commerce and Economic Development
State Office Building
333 Willoughby Avenue
Mail to: P.O. Box D-LIC
Juneau, AK 99811
907-465-2534

Arizona

Arizona State Boards Office
Department of Administration
1645 W. Jefferson Street, Room 410
Phoenix, AZ 85007
602-542-3095

California

California Department of Consumer Affairs
1020 N Street, Room 510
Sacramento, CA 95814
916-445-4465

Colorado

Colorado Department of Regulatory Agencies
State Services Building, Room 110
1525 Sherman Street
Denver, CO 80203
303-866-3304

Connecticut

Connecticut Bureau of Licensing and Regulation
Department of Consumer Protection
State Office Building, Room 101
165 Capitol Avenue
Hartford, CT 06106
203-566-7177

Delaware

Delaware Division of Business and
Occupational Regulation
Department of Administrative Services
Margaret M. O'Neill Building
Federal Street
Mail to: P.O. Box 1401
Dover, DE 19903
302-736-4522

District of Columbia

District of Columbia Occupational and Professional Licensing Administration
Department of Consumer and Regulatory Affairs
N. Potomac Building, Room 931
614 H Street N.W.
Mail to: P.O. Box 37200
Washington, DC 20001
202-727-7480

Florida

Florida Department of Professional Regulation
1940 N. Monroe Street
Tallahassee, FL 32399-0750
904-487-2252

Georgia

Georgia Examining Boards Division
Office of Secretary of State
166 Pryor Street S.W.
Atlanta, GA 30303
404-656-3900

Hawaii

Hawaii Department of Commerce and Consumer Affairs
Professional and Vocational Licensing Division
Kamamalu Building
1010 Richards Street
Mail to: P.O. Box 3469
Honolulu, HI 96801
808-548-6520

Idaho

Idaho Bureau of Occupational Licenses
Department of Self-Governing Agencies
2417 Bank Drive, Room 312
Boise, ID 83705
208-334-3233

Illinois

Illinois Department of Registration and Education
320 W. Washington Street
Springfield, IL 62786
217-785-0800

Indiana

Indiana Professional Licensing Agency
State Office Building, Room 1021
100 N. Senate Avenue
Indianapolis, IN 46204-2246
317-232-2980

Iowa

Iowa Professional Licensing and Regulation
Department of Public Health
Lucas State Office Building
1918 S.E. Hulsizer Avenue
Des Moines, IA 50319
515-281-5787

Kentucky

Kentucky Division of Occupations and Professions
Berry Hill Annex
Mail to: P.O. Box 456
Frankfort, KY 40602
501-564-3296

Louisiana

Louisiana Division of Licensing and Certification
Department of Health and Human Resources
1201 Capitol Access Road
Mail to: P.O. Box 3767
Baton Rouge, LA 70802
504-342-6448

Maine

Maine Division of Licensing and Enforcement
Department of Professional and Financial Regulation
Statehouse Station 35
Augusta, ME 04333
207-582-8723

Maryland

Maryland Department of Licensing and Regulation
Stanbalt Building
501 St. Paul Place
Baltimore, MD 21202
410-333-6322

Massachusetts

Massachusetts Board of Allied Health Profession
Division of Registration
Executive Office of Consumer Affairs
Leverett Saltonstall State Office Building, Room 1520
100 Cambridge Street
Boston, MA 02202
617-727-3071

Michigan

Michigan Department of Licensing and Regulation
Ottawa Building N.
611 W. Ottawa Street
Mail to: P.O. Box 30018
Lansing, MI 48909
517-373-1870

Minnesota

Minnesota Department of Commerce
Metro Square Building, Room 500
7th and Robert Streets
St. Paul, MN 55101
612-296-4026

Mississippi

Mississippi Board of Medical Licensure
2688-D Insurance Center Drive
Jackson, MS 39216
601-354-6645

Missouri

Missouri Division of Professional Registration
Department of Economic Development
Barber State Board
3523 North Ten Mile Drive
Mail to: P.O. Box 1335
Jefferson City, MO 65109
314-751-2334

Montana

Montana Business Regulations Division
Department of Commerce
1424 9th Avenue
Helena, MT 59620-0407
406-444-3737

New Jersey

New Jersey State Department of Health
c/o Commissioner's Office, CN-360
Trenton, NJ 08625
609-292-7837

New Mexico

New Mexico Regulation and Licensing Department
Bataan Memorial Building
725 St. Michael's Drive, Room 133
Santa Fe, NM 87503
505-827-7160

New York

New York Division of Professional Licensing Services
State Education Department
Cultural Education Center, Room 3021
Empire State Plaza
Albany, NY 12230
518-474-3830

North Dakota

North Dakota Licensing Department
Office of the Attorney General
600 E. Boulevard, 17th Floor
Bismarck, ND 58505
701-224-2219

Ohio

Ohio Division of Licensing
Department of Commerce
77 S. High Street, 23rd Floor
Columbus, OH 43266-0546
614-466-4130

Pennsylvania

Pennsylvania Bureau of Professional and
Occupational Affairs
Department of State
Transportation and Safety Building, 6th Floor
Commonwealth Avenue and Forster Street
Mail to: P.O. Box 2649
Harrisburg, PA 17105
717-787-8503
800-822-2113

Rhode Island

Rhode Island Division of Professional Regulation
Department of Health
Cannon Building, Room 104
3 Capitol Hill
Providence, RI 02908-5097
401-277-2827

South Dakota

South Dakota Division of Professional and
Occupational Licensing
Department of Commerce and Regulation
State Capitol
910 E. Sioux Avenue
Pierre, SD 57501
605-773-3178

Tennessee

Tennessee Department of Commerce and Insurance
Regulatory Boards
500 James Robertson Parkway
Volunteer Plaza
Nashville, TN 37243-1139
615-741-3449

Utah

Utah Division of Occupational and Professional Licensing
Department of Business Regulation
Heber M. Wells Building
160 East 300 South, 4th Floor
Mail to: P.O. Box 5802
Salt Lake City, UT 84145
801-530-6628

Vermont

Vermont Division of Licensing and Registration
Office of the Secretary of State
Pavilion Office Building
109 State Street
Montpelier, VT 05602
802-828-2363

Virgin Islands

Virgin Islands Division of Licensing
Consumer Services Administration
Subbase, Building 1
Charlotte Amalie
Mail to: P.O. Box 5468
St. Thomas, VI 00801
809-776-7397

Virginia

Virginia Department of Commerce
1601 Rolling Hills Drive, Suite 200
Richmond, VA 23229-5005
804-662-9900

Washington

Washington Professional Programs Management Division
Department of Licensing
1300 Quince Street
Mail to: P.O. Box 9649
Olympia, WA 98504
206-753-3234

Wisconsin

Wisconsin Department of Regulation and Licensing
Washington Square Building, Room 173
1400 E. Washington Avenue
Mail to: P.O. Box 8935
Madison, WI 53708
608-266-8609

State Occupational Safety and Health Offices

These agencies are responsible for inspecting work sites to ensure that workers are protected from hazardous substances and settings. Occupational Safety and Health offices also investigate accidents at work sites to determine how the incident occurred and whether or not any state safety regulations were violated.

Alabama
Occupational Safety and Health
Department of Labor
64 N. Union Street, Room 500
Montgomery, AL 36130
205-242-3460

Alaska
Occupational Safety and Health
Department of Labor
Labor Standards and Safety Division
1111 W. 8th Street
P.O. Box 21149
Juneau, AK 99802-1149
907-465-4855

Arizona
Occupational Safety and Health
Industrial Commission
Safety Division
800 W. Washington
Phoenix, AZ 85007
602-542-5795

Arkansas
Occupational Safety and Health
Department of Labor
10421 W. Markham
Little Rock, AR 72205
501-682-4500

California
Occupational Safety and Health
Department of Industrial Relations
1121 L Street, Number 307
San Francisco, CA 95814
916-324-4163

Colorado
Occupational Safety and Health
Department of Labor and Employment
600 Grant Street, 9th Floor
Denver, CO 80203-3528
303-837-3801

Connecticut
Occupational Safety and Health
Department of Labor
200 Folly Brook Boulevard
Wethersfield, CT 06109-1114
203-566-4550

Delaware
Occupational Safety and Health
Department of Labor
Division of Industrial Affairs
820 N. French Street
Wilmington, DE 19801
302-577-2879

District of Columbia
Occupational Safety and Health
Department of Employment Services
950 Upshur Street N.W.
Washington, DC 20011
202-576-6339

Florida
Occupational Safety and Health
Florida Department of Labor and Employment Security
Division of Safety
Building E, Suite 45
2002 Old St. Augustine
Tallahassee, FL 32399-0663
904-488-3044

Georgia
Occupational Safety and Health
Georgia Department of Labor
Field Services Division
148 International Boulevard
Atlanta, GA 30303
404-656-3014

Hawaii
Occupational Safety and Health
Department of Labor and Industrial Relations
830 Punchbowl Street
Honolulu, HI 96813
808-548-4155

Idaho
Occupational Safety and Health
Department of Labor and Industrial Services
277 N. 6th Street
Boise, ID 83720
208-334-2129

Illinois
Occupational Safety and Health
Department of Labor
One W. Old State Capitol Plaza
Springfield, IL 62701
217-782-6206

Indiana

Occupational Safety and Health
Department of Labor
W479 S. Indiana Government Center
Indianapolis, IN 46204
317-232-2693

Iowa

Occupational Safety and Health
Department of Employment Services
Division of Labor Services
1000 E. Grand Avenue
Des Moines, IA 50319
515-281-3606

Kansas

Occupational Safety and Health
Department of Human Resources
Division of Labor-Management Relations
and Employment Standards
401 Topeka Avenue
Topeka, KS 66603
913-296-4386

Kentucky

Occupational Safety and Health Labor Cabinet
Department of Workplace Standards
1049 U.S. 127 S.
Frankfort, KY 40601
502-564-7360

Louisiana

Occupational Safety and Health
Department of Labor
Office of Labor
P.O. Box 94094
Baton Rouge, LA 70804
504-342-3011

Maine

Occupational Safety and Health
Department of Labor
Labor Standards Bureau
Safety Division
20 Union Street
Augusta, ME 04330
207-289-6460

Maryland

Occupational Safety and Health
Department of Licensing and Regulation
Labor and Industry Division
501 St. Paul Place
Baltimore, MD 21202
410-333-4195

Massachusetts

Occupational Safety and Health
Executive Office of Labor
Labor and Industries Department
Industrial Safety Division
100 Cambridge Street, 11th Floor
Boston, MA 02202
617-727-3460

Michigan

Occupational Health and Safety
Department of Public Health
Environmental and Occupational Health Bureau
3423 N. Logan Street
P.O. Box 30195
Lansing, MI 48909
517-335-9218

Minnesota

Occupational Safety and Health
Department of Labor and Industry
444 Lafayette Road
St. Paul, MN 55101
612-296-2116

Mississippi

Occupational Safety and Health
Department of Health
Bureau of Environmental Health
P.O. Box 1700
Jackson, MS 39215-1700
601-987-3981

Missouri

Occupational Safety and Health
Department of Labor and Industrial Relations
Division of Labor Standards
3315 W. Truman Boulevard
P.O. Box 449
Jefferson, MO 65109
314-751-2461

Montana

Occupational Safety and Health
Department of Health and Environmental Sciences
Environmental Science Division
Occupational Health Bureau
Cogswell Building, Room A113
Helena, MT 59620
406-444-3671

Nebraska

Occupational Safety and Health
Department of Labor
Division of Safety
301 Centennial Mall S, L.L.
P.O. Box 94600
Lincoln, NE 68509-5024
402-471-2239

Nevada
Occupational Safety and Health
Department of Industrial Relations
1370 S. Curry Street
Carson City, NV 89710
702-687-5240

New Hampshire
Occupational Safety and Health
Department of Labor
Inspection Division
19 Pillsbury Street
Concord, NH 03301
603-271-2024

New Jersey
Occupational Safety and Health
Department of Labor
Workplace Standards Division
John Fitch Plaza, CN-110
Trenton, NJ 08625-0110
609-984-3507

New Mexico
Occupational Safety and Health
Department of Health and Environment
Environmental Improvement Division
Harold Runnels Building
1190 St. Francis Drive
Santa Fe, NM 87501
505-827-2877

New York
Occupational Safety and Health
Department of Labor
Campus Labor Department Building
Albany, NY 12240
518-457-3518

North Carolina
Occupational Safety and Health
Department of Labor
Labor Building
4 W. Edenton Street
Raleigh, NC 27601
919-733-4585

North Dakota
Occupational Safety and Health
Department of Health and Consolidated Laboratories
Environmental Health Section
Environmental Engineering Division
Missouri Office Building
1200 Missouri Avenue, Box 5520
Bismarck, ND 58502-5520
701-224-2374

Ohio
Occupational Safety and Health
Industrial Commission
Division of Safety and Hygiene
246 N. High Street
Columbus, OH 43215
614-466-3564

Oklahoma
Occupational Safety and Health
Department of Labor
4001 N. Lincoln Boulevard
Oklahoma City, OK 73105
405-528-1500

Oregon
Occupational Safety and Health
Workers' Compensation Department
480 Church Street S.E.
Salem, OR 97310
503-378-3308

Pennsylvania
Occupational Safety and Health
Department of Labor and Industry
Bureau of Occupational and Industrial Safety
Labor and Industry Building
Harrisburg, PA 17120
717-787-3323
800-426-7362

Puerto Rico
Occupational Safety and Health
Department of Labor and Human Resources
Prudencio Rivera Martínez Building
505 Muñoz Rivera Avenue
Hato Rey, PR 00918
809-754-2171
809-754-2172

Rhode Island
Occupational Safety and Health
Department of Labor
Division of Occupational Safety
220 Elmwood Avenue
Providence, RI 02907
401-457-1829

South Carolina
Occupational Safety and Health
Department of Labor
Landmark Center
3600 Forest Drive
P.O. Box 11329
Columbia, SC 29211-1329
803-734-9644

Tennessee
Occupational Safety and Health
Department of Labor
501 Union Building
Nashville, TN 37243-0655
615-741-2793

Texas
Occupational Safety and Health
Department of Health
Environmental and Consumer Health Protection Division
Environmental Health Bureau
4200 N. Lamar, Suite 200
Austin, TX 78756
512-459-1611

Utah
Occupational Safety and Health
Industrial Commission
160 East 300 South
P.O. Box 510250
Salt Lake City, UT 84151-0910
801-530-6901

Vermont
Occupational Safety and Health
Department of Labor and Industry
State Office Building
120 State Street
Montpelier, VT 05602
802-828-2765

Virgin Islands
Occupational Safety and Health
Department of Labor
Government Complex
Building 2, Room 207
Lagoon Street
Frederiksted
St. Croix, VI 00840
809-772-1315

Virginia
Occupational Safety and Health
Department of Labor and Industry
205 N. 4th Street
P.O. Box 12064
Richmond, VA 23219
804-786-2391

Washington
Occupational Safety and Health
Department of Labor and Industries
Industrial Safety and Health Division
General Administration Building
HC-101
P.O. Box 207
Olympia, WA 98504
206-753-6500

West Virginia
Occupational Safety and Health
Department of Health and Human Resources
Public Health Bureau
Office of Environmental Health
Division of Industrial Hygiene
State Capitol Complex
Building 3, Room 550
Charleston, WV 25305
304-558-3526

Wisconsin
Occupational Safety and Health
Department of Industry, Labor and Human Relations
P.O. Box 7969
Madison, WI 53707
608-266-1816

Wyoming
Occupational Safety and Health
Department of Employment
Herschler Building, 2nd Floor-E
Cheyenne, WY 82002
307-777-7786

State Social Services Offices

These agencies coordinate a variety of community-based social programs designed for children, adults, elderly, and disabled persons. Inquiries concerning information about specific community programs should be directed to these offices.

Alabama
Social Services
Department of Human Resources
James East Folsom Administrative Building
64 N. Union Street
Montgomery, AL 36130-1801
205-242-1160

Alaska
Social Services
Division of Family and Youth Services
Department of Health and Social Services
Alaska Office Building, Room 404
350 Main Street
P.O. Box H-05
Juneau, AK 99811
907-465-3170

Arizona

Social Services
Administration for Children, Youth and Families
Division of Social Services
Department of Economic Security
1717 W. Jefferson Street
Phoenix, AZ 85007
602-542-4791

Arkansas

Social Services
Division of Economic and Medical Services
Department of Human Services
P.O. Box 1437, Slot 316
Little Rock, AR 72203
501-682-8650

California

Social Services
Department of Human Services
744 P Street
Mail Station 17-11
Sacramento, CA 95814
916-445-2077

Colorado

Social Services
State Social Services Building, 8th Floor
1575 Sherman Street
Denver, CO 80203
303-866-5700

Connecticut

Social Services
Department of Human Resources
1049 Asylum Avenue
Hartford, CT 06105
203-566-3318

Delaware

Social Services
Division of Economic Services
Department of Health and Social Services
C T Building
Delaware State Hospital
1901 N. DuPont Highway
P.O. Box 906
New Castle, DE 19720
302-421-6705

District of Columbia

Social Services
Department of Human Services
609 H Street N.E.
Washington, DC 20024
202-727-5930

Florida

Social Services
Children, Youth and Families Health and Rehabilitation
1317 Winewood Boulevard
Building 8, 3rd Floor
Tallahassee, FL 32399
904-488-8762

Georgia

Social Services
Family and Children Services
Department of Human Resources
878 Peachtree Street N.E., Room 624
Atlanta, GA 30309
404-894-6386

Hawaii

Social Services
Department of Human Services
Queen Liliuokalani Building, Room 209
1390 Miller Street
P.O. Box 339
Honolulu, HI 96813
808-548-4997

Idaho

Social Services
Family and Children's Services
Department of Health and Welfare
Towers Building, 10th Floor
450 W. State Street
Boise, ID 83720
208-334-5700

Illinois

Social Services
Department of Children and Family Services
406 E. Monroe Street
Springfield, IL 62701
217-785-2509

Indiana

Social Services
Department of Human Services
IGC-S, E414
302 W. Washington
Indianapolis, IN 46204
317-233-4447

Iowa

Social Services
Department of Human Services
Hoover State Office Building, 5th Floor
1300 E. Walnut Street
Des Moines, IA 50319-0114
515-281-6360

Kansas

Social Services
Department of Social and Rehabilitation Services
Docking State Office Building, 6th Floor
915 Harrison Street
Topeka, KS 66612
913-296-3271

Kentucky

Social Services
Cabinet for Human Resources
Human Resources Building, 6th Floor
275 E. Main Street
Frankfort, KY 40621
502-564-4650

Louisiana

Social Services
Division of Children, Youth and Family Services
Office of Community Services
Department of Social Services
1967 North Street
P.O. Box 3776
Baton Rouge, LA 70821
504-342-0286

Maine

Social Services
Department of Human Services
Human Services Building
221 State Street
Statehouse Station 11
Augusta, ME 04333
207-289-3106

Maryland

Social Services
Department of Human Resources
Saratoga State Center, Room 578
300 W. Preston Street
Baltimore, MD 21201
410-333-0103

Massachusetts

Social Services
Office of Health and Human Services
One Ashburton Place, Room 1109
Boston, MA 02108
617-727-7600

Michigan

Social Services
Commerce Center
300 S. Capitol Avenue
P.O. Box 30037
Lansing, MI 48909
517-373-3500

Minnesota

Social Services
Department of Human Services
658 Cedar Street
St. Paul, MN 55155
612-296-6916

Mississippi

Social Services
Department of Human Services
421 W. Pascagoula Street
Jackson, MS 39203
601-960-4250

Missouri

Social Services
Director's Office
Department of Social Services
Broadway State Office Building
221 W. High Street
P.O. Box 1527
Jefferson City, MO 65102
314-751-4815

Montana

Social Services
Department of Family Services
111 Sanders Street
Helena, MT 59601
406-444-5622

Nebraska

Social Services
Division of Human Services
Department of Social Services
State Office Building
301 Centennial Mall S.
P.O. Box 95026
Lincoln, NE 68509
402-471-3121

Nevada

Social Services
Department of Human Resources
505 E. King Street, Room 600
Carson City, NV 89710
702-687-4400

New Hampshire

Social Services
Division of Human Services
Department of Health and Human Services
Health and Welfare Building
6 Hazen Drive
Concord, NH 03301
603-271-4331
800-852-3345 (in NH)

New Jersey

Social Services
Department of Human Services
Capitol Place One
222 S. Warren Street, CN-700
Trenton, NJ 08625
609-292-3717

New Mexico

Social Services
Human Services Department
725 St. Michael's Drive
P.O. Box 2348
Santa Fe, NM 87504
505-827-8400

New York

Social Services
10 Eyck Building, 16th Floor
40 N. Pearl Street
Albany, NY 12243
518-474-9475

North Carolina

Social Services
Division of Social Services
Department of Human Resources
Albemarle Building, Room 813
325 N. Salisbury Street
Raleigh, NC 27603
919-733-3055

North Dakota

Social Services
Department of Human Services
State Capitol
600 E. Boulevard, Judicial Wing
Bismarck, ND 58505
701-224-2318

Ohio

Social Services
Department of Human Services
State Office Tower
30 E. Broad Street
Columbus, OH 43266
614-466-6282

Oklahoma

Social Services
Family Support Services Division
Department of Human Services
Sequoyah Memorial Office Building
2400 N. Lincoln Boulevard
P.O. Box 25352
Oklahoma City, OK 73125
405-521-2778

Oregon

Social Services
Department of Human Resources
Public Service Building, Room 318
Capitol Mall
Salem, OR 97310
503-378-3034

Pennsylvania

Social Services
Social Programs
Department of Public Welfare
Health and Welfare Building, Room 131
Forster Street and Commonwealth Avenue
P.O. Box 2675
Harrisburg, PA 17105
717-787-3438

Puerto Rico

Social Services
Old Naval Base, Isla Grande
Building 10, 2nd Floor
P.O. Box 11398
Santurce, PR 00910
809-722-7400

Rhode Island

Social Services
Department of Human Services
Aime J. Forand Building
600 New London Avenue
Cranston, RI 02920
401-464-2121

South Carolina

Social Services
North Tower Complex
1535 Confederate Avenue
P.O. Box 1520
Columbia, SC 29202
803-734-5760

South Dakota

Social Services
Richard F. Kneip Building
700 Governor's Drive
Pierre, SD 57501
605-773-3165

Tennessee

Social Services
Division of Child Welfare Services
Human Services Department
111-19 7th Avenue N.
Nashville, TN 37243
615-741-5924

Texas

Social Services
Services to Families and Children
Department of Human Services
P.O. Box 149030
Austin, TX 78714
512-450-3080

Utah

Social Services
Department of Human Services
120 North 200 West, 3rd Floor
Salt Lake City, UT 84103
801-538-3998

Vermont

Social Services
Department of Social and Rehabilitation Services
Osgood Building
103 S. Main Street
Waterbury, VT 05671
802-241-2131

Virgin Islands

Social Services
Department of Human Services
Barbel Plaza S.
St. Thomas, VI 00802
809-774-1166

Virginia

Social Services
Division of Service Programs
Department of Social Services
8007 Discovery Drive
Richmond, VA 23229
804-662-9236

Washington

Social Services
Department of Social and Health Services
Office Building 2, 4th Floor
12th Avenue and Franklin Street
Mail Stop OB-44E
Olympia, WA 98504
206-753-3395

West Virginia

Social Services
Division of Human Services
State Office Building 6, Room B-617
1900 Washington Street E.
Charleston, WV 25305
304-558-7980

Wisconsin

Social Services
Health and Social Services Department
One W. Wilson Street
P.O. Box 7850
Madison, WI 53707
608-266-3681

Wyoming

Social Services
Department of Family Services
Hathaway Building, Room 318
2300 Capitol Avenue
Cheyenne, WY 82002-0710
307-777-6285

State Veterans Affairs Offices

These agencies design and coordinate programs, including education, job training, and health care, for military veterans. All inquiries concerning assistance for veterans should be directed to these offices.

Alabama

Veterans Affairs
770 Washington Street, Suite 530
Montgomery, AL 36130
205-242-5077

Alaska

Veterans Affairs
Dimond Center Tower, Suite 3-450
800 E. Dimond Boulevard
Anchorage, AK 99515
907-249-1241

Arizona

Veterans Affairs
3225 N. Central, Suite 910
Phoenix, AZ 85012
602-255-4713

Arkansas

Veterans Affairs
c/o Veterans Affairs Regional Office
P.O. Box 1280
North Little Rock, AR 72115
501-370-3820

California

Veterans Affairs
1227 O Street
Sacramento, CA 95814
916-445-3111

Colorado
Veterans Affairs
Department of Social Services
1575 Sherman Street, 1st Floor
Denver, CO 80203
303-866-2491

Connecticut
Veterans Affairs
287 West Street
Rocky Hill, CT 06067
203-721-5890

Delaware
Veterans Affairs
Department of State
Townsend Building
Dover, DE 19901
302-739-2792

District of Columbia
Veterans Affairs
Department of Human Services
941 N. Capitol N.E., Room 1211-F
Washington, DC 20002
202-727-0327

Florida
Veterans Affairs
P.O. Box 1437
St. Petersburg, FL 33731
813-898-4443

Georgia
Veterans Affairs
Veterans Memorial Building, Suite 970
Atlanta, GA 30334
404-656-2300

Hawaii
Veterans Affairs
Department of Defense
733 Bishop Street, Suite 1270
Honolulu, HI 96813
808-587-3000

Idaho
Veterans Affairs
Department of Health and Welfare
P.O. Box 7765
Boise, ID 83707
208-334-5000

Illinois
Veterans Affairs
833 S. Spring Street
Springfield, IL 62794
217-785-4114

Indiana
Veterans Affairs
302 W. Washington Street, #3-120
Indianapolis, IN 46204
317-232-3920

Iowa
Veterans Affairs
Department of Public Defense
7700 N.W. Beaver Drive
Johnston, IA 50131
515-242-5333

Kansas
Veterans Affairs
700 S.W. Jackson, Room 701
Topeka, KS 66603
913-296-3976

Kentucky
Veterans Affairs
Boone National Guard Center
Frankfort, KY 40601
502-588-4447

Louisiana
Veterans Affairs
Office of the Governor
P.O. Box 94095
Baton Rouge, LA 70804
504-342-5863

Maine
Veterans Affairs
Department of Defense and Veterans
Statehouse Station 117
Augusta, ME 04333
207-289-4060

Maryland
Veterans Affairs
Federal Building, Room 110
31 Hopkins Plaza
Baltimore, MD 21201
410-333-4429

Massachusetts
Veterans Affairs
100 Cambridge Street, Room 1002
Boston, MA 02202
617-727-3570

Michigan
Veterans Affairs
Department of Management and Budget
P.O. Box 30026
Lansing, MI 48909
517-373-3130

Minnesota
Veterans Affairs
Veterans Building
20 W. 12th Street
St. Paul, MN 55155
612-296-2783

Mississippi
Veterans Affairs
4607 Lindberg Drive
Jackson, MS 39209
601-354-7205

Missouri
Veterans Affairs
Department of Public Safety
P.O. Drawer 147
Jefferson City, MO 65102
314-751-3779

Montana
Veterans Affairs
Department of Military Affairs
1100 N. Last Chance Gulch
Helena, MT 59601
406-444-6926

Nebraska
Veterans Affairs
Nebraska State Office Building, 3rd Floor
P.O. Box 95083
Lincoln, NE 68509
402-471-2458

Nevada
Veterans Affairs
1201 Terminal Way, #108
Reno, NV 89520
702-688-1155

New Hampshire
Veterans Affairs
359 Lincoln Street
Manchester, NH 03103
603-625-8122

New Jersey
Veterans Affairs
Eggert Crossing Road, CN-340
Trenton, NJ 08625
609-292-3888

New Mexico
Veterans Affairs
P.O. Box 2324
Santa Fe, NM 87504
505-827-6300

New York
Veterans Affairs
194 Washington Avenue
Albany, NY 12210
518-474-3725

North Carolina
Veterans Affairs
Department of Administration
325 N. Salisbury Street, #1065
Raleigh, NC 27603
919-733-3851

North Dakota
Veterans Affairs
15 N. Broadway, Suite 613
Fargo, ND 58102
701-239-7165

Ohio
Veterans Affairs
Governor's Office
77 S. High
Columbus, OH 43266
614-644-0898

Oklahoma
Veterans Affairs
2311 N. Central
Oklahoma City, OK 73152
405-521-3684

Oregon
Veterans Affairs
700 Summer Street N.E.
Salem, OR 97310
503-373-2388

Pennsylvania
Veterans Affairs
Department of Military Affairs
Fort Indiantown Gap
Annville, PA 17003
717-274-4500

Puerto Rico
Veterans Affairs
Cobian Plaza, Parada 23
De León Avenue, 1603 Of. UM-7
Santurce, PR 00909
809-725-4400

Rhode Island
Veterans Affairs
Department of Social and Rehabilitative Services
600 New London Avenue
Cranston, RI 02920
401-253-8000

South Carolina
Veterans Affairs
1205 Pendleton Street, Room 227
Columbia, SC 29201
803-734-0200

South Dakota
Veterans Affairs
Military and Veterans Affairs Department
500 E. Capitol Avenue
Pierre, SD 57501
605-773-3269

Tennessee
Veterans Affairs
215 8th Avenue N.
Nashville, TN 37243
615-741-2345

Texas
Veterans Affairs
P.O. Box 12277 Capitol Station
Austin, TX 78711
512-463-5538

Vermont
Veterans Affairs
120 State Street
Montpelier, VT 05620
802-828-3380

Virgin Islands
Veterans Affairs
Department of Labor
22 Hospital
St. Croix, VI 00820
809-773-6663

Virginia
Veterans Affairs
P.O. Box 809
Roanoke, VA 24004
703-982-6383

Washington
Veterans Affairs
505 E. Union, Box 9778
Mail Stop PM-41
Olympia, WA 98504
206-753-4522

West Virginia
Veterans Affairs
1321 Plaza E., #101
Charleston, WV 25301
304-558-3661

Wisconsin
Veterans Affairs
77 N. Dickinson, Room 263
P.O. Box 7843
Madison, WI 53707
608-266-1315

Wyoming
Veterans Affairs
613 Dinwoody Circle
Riverton, WY 82501
307-856-4451

State Vital Statistics Offices

These agencies are responsible for maintaining all pertinent statistics for the state, including birth, marriage, divorce, and death records. Requests for certified copies of certificates should be directed to these offices.

Alabama
Vital Statistics
Alabama Department of Public Health
State Office Building
434 Monroe Street
Montgomery, AL 36130-1701
205-242-5039

Alaska
Vital Statistics
Alaska Department of Health and Social Services
Alaska Office Building, Room 114
P.O. Box H
Juneau, AK 99811-0675
907-465-3392

Arizona
Vital Statistics
Arizona Department of Health Services
1740 W. Adams Street
Phoenix, AZ 85007
602-542-1080

Arkansas
Vital Statistics
Arkansas Department of Health
4815 W. Markham Street
Little Rock, AR 72205
501-661-2120

California

Vital Statistics
California Health and Welfare Agency
Department of Health Services
410 N Street
Sacramento, CA 95814
916-445-1719

Colorado

Vital Statistics
Colorado Department of Health
Office of Health Care Services
Division of Health Policy, Planning and Statistics
4210 E. 11th Avenue
Denver, CO 80220
303-331-4875

Connecticut

Vital Statistics
Connecticut Department of Health Services
150 Washington Street
Hartford, CT 06106
203-566-2334

Delaware

Vital Statistics
Delaware Department of Health and Social Services
Division of Public Health
Jesse Cooper Building
P.O. Box 637
Dover, DE 19903
302-739-4721

District of Columbia

Vital Statistics
District of Columbia Department of Human Services
Division of Research and Statistics
425 I Street N.W., 3rd Floor
Washington, DC 20001
202-757-5319

Florida

Vital Statistics
Florida Department of Health and Rehabilitative Services
1317 Winewood Boulevard
Jacksonville, FL 32299-0700
904-359-6970

Georgia

Vital Statistics
Georgia Department of Human Resources
Division of Public Health
47 Trinity Avenue S.W.
Atlanta, GA 30334-2102
404-656-4750

Hawaii

Vital Statistics
Hawaii Department of Health
Research and Statistics Office
1250 Punchbowl Street
Honolulu, HI 96813
808-548-6501

Idaho

Vital Statistics
Idaho Department of Health and Welfare
Division of Health
450 W. State Street, 1st Floor
Boise, ID 83720
208-334-5976

Illinois

Vital Statistics
Illinois Department of Public Health
Office of Program and Administrative Support
535 W. Jefferson Street
Springfield, IL 62761
217-782-6553

Indiana

Vital Statistics
Indiana State Board of Health
Bureau of Policy Development
1330 W. Michigan Street
P.O. Box 1964
Indianapolis, IN 46206
317-633-8509

Iowa

Vital Statistics
Iowa Department of Public Health
Administration Division
Lucas State Office Building
Des Moines, IA 50319
515-281-4943

Kansas

Vital Statistics
Kansas Department of Health and Environment
Division of Health
Bureau of Community Health
Landon State Office Building
900 S.W. Jackson Street
Topeka, KS 66612
913-296-1414

Kentucky

Vital Statistics
Kentucky Human Resources Cabinet
Department for Health Services
275 E. Main Street
Frankfort, KY 40621
502-564-4212

Louisiana
Vital Statistics
Louisiana Department of Health and Hospitals
Office of Public Health Services
P.O. Box 60630
New Orleans, LA 70160
504-568-5172

Maine
Vital Statistics
Maine Department of Human Services
Bureau of Medical Services
Statehouse Station 11
Augusta, ME 04333
207-289-3184

Maryland
Vital Statistics
Maryland Hall of Records
350 Rowe Boulevard
Annapolis, MD 21401
410-974-3914

Massachusetts
Vital Statistics
Massachusetts Executive Office of Human Services
Department of Public Health
Bureau of Health Statistics, Research and Evaluation
150 Tremont Street, Room B-3
Boston, MA 02111
617-727-0036

Michigan
Vital Statistics
Michigan Department of Public Health
State Registrar and Center for Health Statistics
3423 N. Logan Street
P.O. Box 30195
Lansing, MI 48909
517-335-8676

Minnesota
Vital Statistics
Minnesota Department of Health
Administration Bureau
717 Delaware Street S.E.
Minneapolis, MN 55440
612-623-5121

Mississippi
Vital Statistics
Mississippi Department of Health
Bureau of Information Resources
P.O. Box 1700
Jackson, MS 39215-1700
601-960-7960

Missouri
Vital Statistics
Missouri Department of Health
Health Resources Division
1730 E. Elm Street
P.O. Box 570
Jefferson City, MO 65102
314-751-6383

Montana
Vital Statistics
Montana Department of Health and
Environmental Sciences
Centralized Services Division
Cogswell Building, Room C-118
Helena, MT 59620
406-444-2618

Nebraska
Vital Statistics
Nebraska Department of Health
301 Centennial Mall S., 3rd Floor
P.O. Box 95007
Lincoln, NE 68509-5007
402-471-2871

Nevada
Vital Statistics
Nevada Department of Human Resources
Division of Health
505 E. King Street, Room 201
Carson City, NV 89710
702-687-4480

New Hampshire
Vital Statistics
New Hampshire Department of Health and
Human Services
Division of Public Health Services
6 Hazen Drive
Concord, NH 03301
603-271-4651

New Jersey
Vital Statistics
New Jersey Department of Health
John Fitch Plaza, CN-360
Trenton, NJ 08625
609-292-4087

New Mexico
Vital Statistics
New Mexico Department of Health and Environment
Division of Public Health
Harold Runnels Building
1190 St. Francis Drive
Santa Fe, NM 87501
505-827-2338

New York

Vital Statistics
New York State Department of Health
Corning Tower
Empire State Plaza
Albany, NY 12237
518-474-1094

North Carolina

Vital Statistics
North Carolina Department of Environment, Health,
and Natural Resources
Office of Health Director
Epidemiology Division
Cooper Building
225 N. McDowell Street
Raleigh, NC 27602
919-733-3000

North Dakota

Vital Statistics
North Dakota Department of Health and
Consolidated Laboratories
Administrative Services Section
State Capitol, Judicial Wing, 2nd Floor
Bismarck, ND 58505-0200
701-224-2360

Ohio

Vital Statistics
Ohio Department of Health
Bureau of Supportive Services
246 N. High Street
P.O. Box 118
Columbus, OH 43266-0588
614-466-2533

Oklahoma

Vital Statistics
Oklahoma Department of Health
1000 N.E. 10th Street
P.O. Box 53551
Oklahoma City, OK 73152
405-271-4040

Oregon

Vital Statistics
Oregon Department of Human Resources
Division of Health
1400 5th Avenue S.W.
Portland, OR 97201
503-229-6558

Pennsylvania

Vital Statistics
Pennsylvania Department of Health
State Health Data Center
P.O. Box 1528
New Castle, PA 16103
412-686-3111

Rhode Island

Vital Statistics
Rhode Island Department of Health
3 Capitol Hill
Providence, RI 02908
401-277-2812

South Carolina

Vital Statistics
South Carolina Department of Health and
Environmental Control
J. Marion Sims Building and R. J. Aycock Building
2600 Bull Street
Columbia, SC 29201
803-734 4810

South Dakota

Vital Statistics
South Dakota Department of Health
Policy and Statistics Division
Foss Building
523 E. Capitol
Pierre, SD 57501-3182
605-773-4961

Tennessee

Vital Statistics
Tennessee Department of Health and Environment
Administrative Services Bureau
Health Statistics Division
344 Cordell Hull Building
Nashville, TN 37247-0101
615-741-1763

Texas

Vital Statistics
Texas Department of Health
1100 W. 49th Street
Austin, TX 78756
512-458-7692

Utah

Vital Statistics
Utah Department of Health
Administrative Services Division
P.O. Box 16700
Salt Lake City, UT 84116-0700
801-538-6360

Vermont
Vital Statistics
Vermont Agency of Human Services
Department of Health
Division of Public Health Statistics
60 Main Street
P.O. Box 70
Burlington, VT 05402
802-863-7300

Virginia
Vital Statistics
Virginia Department of Health
James Madison Building
109 Governor Street
Richmond, VA 23219
804-786-3369

Washington
Vital Statistics
Washington Department of Social and Health Services
Mail Stop OB-44
Olympia, WA 98504
206-753-5936

West Virginia
Vital Statistics
West Virginia Department of Health and Human Resources
Public Health Bureau
Office of Epidemiology and Health Promotion
1411 E. Virginia Street
Charleston, WV 25301
304-558-9100

Wisconsin
Vital Statistics
Wisconsin Department of Health and Social Services
Division of Health
One W. Wilson Street
P.O. Box 7850
Madison, WI 53707
608-266-1334

Wyoming
Vital Statistics
Wyoming Department of Health
Division of Health and Medical Services
Hathaway Building
Cheyenne, WY 82002
307-777-7591

State Vocational Rehabilitation Offices

These agencies are responsible for creating and administering education and retraining programs for workers who have been injured and are unable to continue employment in their chosen profession. Information concerning specific career retraining opportunities may be obtained by contacting these offices.

Alabama
Vocational Rehabilitation Agency
Rehabilitation Services
P.O. Box 11586
Montgomery, AL 36111-0586
205-281-8780

Alaska
Vocational Rehabilitation Agency
Division of Vocational Rehabilitation
Box F, Mail Stop 0581
Juneau, AK 99811-0500
907-465-2814

Arizona
Vocational Rehabilitation Agency
Rehabilitation Services Administration
1789 W. Jefferson, North Wing
Phoenix, AZ 85007
602-542-3332

Arkansas
Vocational Rehabilitation Agency
Division of Rehabilitation Services
Department of Human Services
P.O. Box 3781
Little Rock, AR 72203
501-682-6709

California
Vocational Rehabilitation Agency
Department of Rehabilitation
830 K Street Mall
Sacramento, CA 95814
916-445-3971

Colorado
Vocational Rehabilitation Agency
Department of Social and Rehabilitative Services
1575 Sherman Street, 4th Floor
Denver, CO 80203-1714
303-866-2866

Connecticut

Vocational Rehabilitation Agency
Bureau of Client Services
State Department of Education
Division of Rehabilitation Services
10 Griffin Road N.
Windsor, CT 06095
203-298-2000

Delaware

Vocational Rehabilitation Agency
Division of Vocational Rehabilitation
Delaware Elwyn Institutes
321 E. 11th Street, 4th Floor
Wilmington, DE 19801
302-577-2851

District of Columbia

Vocational Rehabilitation Agency
DC Rehabilitation Services Administration
Department of Human Services
605 G Street N.W., Suite 1111
Washington, DC 20001
202-727-3227

Florida

Vocational Rehabilitation Agency
Division of Vocational Rehabilitation
Department of Labor and Employment Security
1709 "A" Mahan Drive
Tallahassee, FL 32399-0696
904-488-6210

Georgia

Vocational Rehabilitation Agency
Division of Rehabilitation Services
Department of Human Resources
878 Peachtree Street N.E., Room 706
Atlanta, GA 30309
404-894-6670

Hawaii

Vocational Rehabilitation Agency
Division of Vocational Rehabilitation and
Services for the Blind
Department of Human Resources
P.O. Box 339
Honolulu, HI 96809
808-586-5355

Idaho

Vocational Rehabilitation Agency
Division of Vocational Rehabilitation
Len B. Jordan Building, Room 150
650 W. State
Boise, ID 83720-3650
208-334-3390

Illinois

Vocational Rehabilitation Agency
Department of Rehabilitation Services
623 E. Adams Street
Springfield, IL 62794
217-785-0218

Indiana

Vocational Rehabilitation Agency
Department of Human Resources
402 W. Washington Street
P.O. Box 7083
Indianapolis, IN 46207-7083
317-232-6500
800-545-7763

Iowa

Vocational Rehabilitation Agency
Department of Education
510 E. 12th Street
Des Moines, IA 50319
515-281-4311

Kansas

Vocational Rehabilitation Agency
Rehabilitation Services
Department of Social and Rehabilitation Services
300 S.W. Oakley
Topeka, KS 66606
913-296-3911

Kentucky

Vocational Rehabilitation Agency
Capital Plaza Tower, 9th Floor
Frankfort, KY 40601
502-564-4566
800-372-7172 (in KY)

Louisiana

Vocational Rehabilitation Agency
Louisiana Rehabilitation Services
Department of Social Services
P.O. Box 94371
Baton Rouge, LA 70804-9071
504-342-2285

Maine

Vocational Rehabilitation Agency
Bureau of Rehabilitation Services
Department of Human Services
35 Anthony Avenue
Augusta, ME 04333-0011
207-626-5300

Maryland

Vocational Rehabilitation Agency
Division of Vocational Rehabilitation
State Department of Education
2301 Argonne Drive
Baltimore, MD 21218
410-554-3276

Massachusetts

Vocational Rehabilitation Agency
Commissioner for the Blind
88 Kingston Street
Boston, MA 02111-2227
617-727-5550
800-392-6450 (in MA)

Michigan

Vocational Rehabilitation Agency
Bureau of Rehabilitation and Disability Determination
Department of Education
P.O. Box 30010
Lansing, MI 48909
517-373-3390

Minnesota

Vocational Rehabilitation Agency
Department of Jobs and Training
Division of Rehabilitation Services
390 N. Robert Street, 5th Floor
St. Paul, MN 55101
612-296-1822

Mississippi

Vocational Rehabilitation Agency
P.O. Box 4872
Jackson, MS 39296
601-354-6411

Missouri

Vocational Rehabilitation Agency
Division of Vocational Rehabilitation
State Department of Education
2401 E. McCarty
Jefferson City, MO 65101
314-751-3251

Montana

Vocational Rehabilitation Agency
Department of Social and Rehabilitation Services
Rehabilitative/Visual Services Division
P.O. Box 4210
Helena, MT 59604
406-444-2590

Nebraska

Vocational Rehabilitation Agency
Division of Rehabilitation Services
State Department of Education
P.O. Box 94987
Lincoln, NE 68509
402-471-3649

Nevada

Vocational Rehabilitation Agency
Department of Human Services
Rehabilitation Division
505 E. King Street, Room 502
Carson City, NV 89710
702-687-4440

New Hampshire

Vocational Rehabilitation Agency
State Department of Education
78 Regional Drive
Concord, NH 03301
603-271-3800

New Jersey

Vocational Rehabilitation Agency
New Jersey Commission for the Blind and
Visually Impaired
153 Halsey Street, 6th Floor
P.O. Box 47017
Newark, NJ 07101
201-648-3333
800-962-1233 (in NJ)

New Mexico

Vocational Rehabilitation Agency
Department of Education
604 W. San Mateo
Santa Fe, NM 87503
505-827-3500
800-235-5387 (in NM)

New York

Vocational Rehabilitation Agency
Office of Vocational and Educational Services
for Individuals with Disabilities
New York State Department of Education
One Commerce Plaza, Room 1606
A.bany, NY 12234
518-474-2714
800-222-JOBS (in NY)

North Carolina

Vocational Rehabilitation Agency
Division of Vocational Rehabilitation
Department of Human Resources
State Office
P.O. Box 26053
Raleigh, NC 27611
919-733-3364

North Dakota

Vocational Rehabilitation Agency
Department of Human Services
600 E. Boulevard
State Capitol Building
Bismarck, ND 58505
701-224-2907
800-472-2622 (in ND)

Ohio

Vocational Rehabilitation Agency
Rehabilitation Services Commission
400 E. Campus View Boulevard
Columbus, OH 43235-4604
614-438-1210
800-282-4536 ext. 1210 (in OH)

Oklahoma

Vocational Rehabilitation Agency
Department of Human Services
Division of Rehabilitation Services
P.O. Box 25352
Oklahoma City, OK 73125
405-424-6647

Oregon

Vocational Rehabilitation Agency
Commission for the Blind
535 S.E. 12th Avenue
Portland, OR 97214
503-238-8380

Pennsylvania

Vocational Rehabilitation Agency
Labor and Industry Building
7th and Forster Streets
Harrisburg, PA 17120
717-787-5244
800-442-6351 (in PA)

Puerto Rico

Vocational Rehabilitation Agency
Department of Social Services
P.O. Box 1118, Building 10
Hato Rey, PR 00919
809-725-1792

Rhode Island

Vocational Rehabilitation Agency
Department of Human Services
Division of Community Services
40 Fountain Street
Providence, RI 02903
401-421-7005

South Carolina

Vocational Rehabilitation Agency
Commission for the Blind
1430 Confederate Avenue
Columbia, SC 29201
803-734-7522
800-922-2222 (in SC)

South Dakota

Vocational Rehabilitation Agency
Division of Rehabilitation Services
Department of Human Services
700 Governor's Drive
Pierre, SD 57501-2291
605-773-3195

Tennessee

Vocational Rehabilitation Agency
Department of Human Services
Citizens Plaza State Office Building, 15th Floor
400 Deaderick Street
Nashville, TN 37248-0060
615-741-2019

Texas

Vocational Rehabilitation Agency
Rehabilitation Commission
4900 N. Lamar
Austin, TX 78751
512-445-8100
800-735-2988
800-628-5115 (in TX)

Utah

Vocational Rehabilitation Agency
Division of Rehabilitation Services
State Office of Education
250 East 500 South
Salt Lake City, UT 84111
801-538-7530

Vermont

Vocational Rehabilitation Agency
103 S. Main Street
Waterbury, VT 05671-2303
802-241-2189

Virgin Islands

Vocational Rehabilitation Agency
Division for Disabilities and Rehabilitation Services
Virgin Islands Department of Human Services
Barbel Plaza S.
St. Thomas, VI 00802
809-774-0930

Virginia
Vocational Rehabilitation Agency
Department of Rehabilitative Services
4901 Fitzhugh Avenue
P.O. Box 11045
Richmond, VA 23230
804-367-0316
800-552-5019 (in VA)

Washington
Vocational Rehabilitation Agency
Department of Social and Health Services
Mail Stop OB 21-C
Olympia, WA 98504
206-753-0293
800-637-5627 (in WA)

West Virginia
Vocational Rehabilitation Agency
Division of Rehabilitation Services
State Board of Rehabilitation
State Capitol
Charleston, WV 25305
304-558-2992
800-642-3021 (in WV)

Wisconsin
Vocational Rehabilitation Agency
Department of Health and Social Services
One W. Wilson, 8th Floor
Madison, WI 53707-7852
608-266-5466
800-362-7433 (in WI)

Wyoming
Vocational Rehabilitation Agency
Department of Employment
One E. Herschler Building
Cheyenne, WY 82002
307-777-7385

Federal Government Health Offices

The following list contains the names of the major health officials currently serving in the United States government. You may from time to time have reason to contact these officials for information or to report a possible problem with the health care delivery system.

U.S. Department of Health and Human Services
Donna E. Shalala, Secretary
200 Independence Avenue S.W.
Washington, DC 20201
202-690-7000

Office of the Inspector General
U.S. Department of Health and Human Services
June Gibbs Brown, Inspector General
200 Independence Avenue S.W.
Washington, DC 20201
202-619-3148

U.S. Public Health Service
Phillip R. Lee, M.D., Assistant Secretary for Health
200 Independence Avenue S.W.
Washington, DC 20201
202-690-7694

U.S. Public Health Service
Office of the Surgeon General
Joycelyn Elders, M.D., Surgeon General
200 Independence Avenue S.W.
Washington, DC 20201
202-690-6467

Health Resources and Services Administration
Robert Harmon, M.D., Administrator
Parklawn Building
5600 Fishers Lane
Rockville, MD 20857
301-443-2216

Centers for Disease Control and Prevention
David Satcher, M.D., Ph.D., Director
1600 Clifton Road N.E.
Atlanta, GA 30333
404-639-3291

National Institutes of Health
Harold Eliot Varmus, M.D., Director
9000 Rockville Pike
Bethesda, MD 20892
301-496-2433

Food and Drug Administration
David Kessler, M.D., Commissioner
5600 Fishers Lane
Rockville, MD 20857
301-443-1544

Health Care Financing Administration
Bruce C. Vladek, Ph.D., Administrator
200 Independence Avenue S.W.
Washington, DC 20201
202-690-6726

Social Security Administration
Shirley S. Chater, Commissioner
6401 Security Boulevard
Baltimore, MD 21235
410-965-3120

Major Congressional Health-Related Subcommittees

The following House and Senate subcommittees are primarily concerned with health policy and health care legislation.

House Subcommittees

Labor, Health and Human Services, Education Subcommittee
2358 Rayburn House Office Building
Independence and S. Capitol Street S.W.
Washington, DC 20515
202-225-3508

Health and Environment Subcommittee
2415 Rayburn House Office Building
Independence and S. Capitol Street S.W.
Washington, DC 20515
202-225-4952

Health Subcommittee
1114 Longworth House Office Building
Independence and New Jersey Avenue S.E.
Washington, DC 20515
202-225-7785

Senate Subcommittees

Labor, Health and Human Services, Education Subcommittee
SD-186, Dirksen Building
First and C Streets N.E.
Washington, DC 20510
202-224-7283

Health for Families and the Uninsured Subcommittee
SD-205, Hart Building
First and C Streets N.E.
Washington, DC 20510
202-224-4515

Aging Subcommittee
SH-615, Hart Building
First and C Streets N.E.
Washington, DC 20510
202-224-3239

Children, Family, Drugs and Alcoholism Subcommittee
Sh-639, Hart Building
First and C Streets, N.E.
Washington, DC 20510
202-224-5630

Senate Special Committee on Aging
SD-G31, Dirksen Building
First and C Streets N.E.
Washington, DC 20510
202-224-5364

Source: 103rd Congress Standard Version, 1st Session, 1993. Capitol Advantage, McLean, VA.

Index